Thieme

Corrective Osteotomies for Rigid Spinal Deformities

Leon Kaplan, MD
Professor of Orthopaedic Surgery
Surgeon-in-Chief and Director of Spine Surgery Unit
Department of Orthopaedic Surgery
Hadassah-Hebrew University Medical Center
Jerusalem, Israel

Lawrence G. Lenke, MD
Professor of Orthopaedic Surgery
Director of Spinal Deformity Surgery
Columbia University Vagelos College of Physicians and Surgeons;
Surgeon-in-Chief, Och Spine Hospital at New York Presbyterian Allen
New York, New York, USA

With special thanks to Dr. Josh Schroeder for his contribution to the book.

543 illustrations

Thieme
Stuttgart • New York • Delhi • Rio de Janeiro

Library of Congress Cataloging-in-Publication Data is available with the publisher.

Important note: Medicine is an ever-changing science undergoing continual development. Research and clinical experience are continually expanding our knowledge, in particular our knowledge of proper treatment and drug therapy. Insofar as this book mentions any dosage or application, readers may rest assured that the authors, editors, and publishers have made every effort to ensure that such references are in accordance with **the state of knowledge at the time of production of the book.**

Nevertheless, this does not involve, imply, or express any guarantee or responsibility on the part of the publishers in respect to any dosage instructions and forms of applications stated in the book. **Every user is requested to examine carefully** the manufacturers' leaflets accompanying each drug and to check, if necessary in consultation with a physician or specialist, whether the dosage schedules mentioned therein or the contraindications stated by the manufacturers differ from the statements made in the present book. Such examination is particularly important with drugs that are either rarely used or have been newly released on the market. Every dosage schedule or every form of application used is entirely at the user's own risk and responsibility. The authors and publishers request every user to report to the publishers any discrepancies or inaccuracies noticed. If errors in this work are found after publication, errata will be posted at www.thieme.com on the product description page.

Some of the product names, patents, and registered designs referred to in this book are in fact registered trademarks or proprietary names even though specific reference to this fact is not always made in the text. Therefore, the appearance of a name without designation as proprietary is not to be construed as a representation by the publisher that it is in the public domain.

Thieme addresses people of all gender identities equally. We encourage our authors to use gender neutral or gender-equal expressions wherever the context allows.

Georg Thieme Verlag KG
Rüdigerstrasse 14, 70469 Stuttgart, Germany
+49 [0]711 8931 421, customerservice@thieme.de

Cover design: © Thieme
Cover image source: © Thieme
Typesetting by DiTech Process Solutions, India

Printed in Germany by Beltz Grafische Betriebe 5 4 3 2 1

DOI: 10.1055/b-006-163752

ISBN: 978-3-13-173081-7

Also available as an e-book:
eISBN (PDF): 978-3-13-173091-6
eISBN (epub): 978-3-13-245439-2

My work is dedicated to my lovely Innula, my wife and best friend.
Thank you, from the bottom of my heart, for your everlasting love, support, and encouragement;
for always standing by my side and having my back (just as a back surgeon needs).
I wouldn't dream of doing this without you.
I would also like to thank my wonderful children and grandchildren.
I am truly a lucky man for having all of you in my life.

Leon Kaplan, MD

I would like to dedicate this textbook to all patients suffering from severe and rigid spinal deformities,
for they are the reason that all of us work so tirelessly to provide the best care possible.
Also, to all the past and current spinal deformity surgeons who have helped contribute to the clinical care, research,
and education of our colleagues. Our patients and our profession have benefitted tremendously from your efforts.

Lawrence G. Lenke, MD

Contents

Foreword xvii

Preface xviii

Introduction xix

Acknowledgments xx

Contributors xxi

1. Congenital Spinal Deformities 1
Ibrahim Obeid, Louis Boissiere, Derek T. Cawley

1.1 Introduction 1

1.2 Deciding on Surgery 1

1.3 Prognosis 3

1.4 Congenital Kyphosis and Kyphoscoliosis 4

1.5 Further Perioperative Considerations 4

1.6 Treatment Options and Principles 6

1.6.1 Observation 6
1.6.2 Epiphysiodesis 6
1.6.3 Hemivertebra Resection 6
1.6.4 Pedicle Subtraction Osteotomy 8
1.6.5 Vertebral Column Resection 9
1.6.6 Vertebral Column Decancellation 11

1.7 Conclusion 11

2. Neuromuscular Spinal Deformities 13
Athanasios I. Tsirikos

2.1 Introduction 13

2.2 Clinical Problems Associated with Spinal Deformity 13

2.3 Etiology and Natural History of Spinal Deformity 13

2.4 Patterns of Spinal Deformity 14

2.5 Specific Types of Spinal Deformity 15

2.5.1 Spina Bifida (Myelomeningocele) 15
2.5.2 Neurofibromatosis 15

2.6 Treatment Principles 16

2.6.1 Nonoperative Treatment 16
2.6.2 Surgical Treatment 16

2.7 Medical Considerations—Preoperative Assessment 17

2.8 Complications during and after Scoliosis Surgery 17

2.9 Deformity Correction Techniques 18

2.9.1 First- and Second-Generation Instrumentation Techniques 18
2.9.2 Third-Generation Instrumentation 18

2.10 Additional Surgical Considerations 19

2.10.1 Intraoperative Management 19
2.10.2 Levels of Fusion 19
2.10.3 Anterior Correction 19
2.10.4 Posterior Vertebral Column Resection 20
2.10.5 Growth Preservation/Modulation Techniques 20

2.11 Quality of Life Assessment/Life Expectancy after Scoliosis Surgery 20

2.12 Conclusion 21

3. Idiopathic Spinal Deformities Treated with Spinal Osteotomies ... 22

Paul J. Park, Eduardo C. Beauchamp, Meghan Cerpa, Lawrence G. Lenke

3.1 Introduction ... 22

3.2 Posterior Column Osteotomy ... 22

3.2.1 Indications in Idiopathic Deformity ... 22
3.2.2 Technique ... 23
3.2.3 Case Illustration ... 23

3.3 Pedicle Subtraction Osteotomy ... 23

3.3.1 Indications in Idiopathic Deformity ... 25
3.3.2 Technique ... 25
3.3.3 Case Illustration ... 26

3.4 Preoperative Considerations and Postoperative Complications ... 26

3.4.1 PCO versus PSO ... 26
3.4.2 Complications ... 27

3.5 Conclusions ... 28

4. The Natural History of Rigid Spinal Deformities ... 33

Jean Dubousset

4.1 Definition and Measurement ... 33

4.2 Natural History, Physiopathology ... 33

4.3 Natural History, Assessment of Flexibility/Rigidity ... 34

4.3.1 Reduction of the Deformity Will Be Checked: Locally and Globally ... 34

4.4 Natural History According to the Growing Spine and Etiologies ... 34

4.5 Natural History According to the Mature Spine and Etiologies ... 34

4.6 Natural History According to the Aging Spine and Etiologies ... 35

4.7 Subsequent Indications for Surgical Treatment ... 35

4.7.1 Treatment and Election of Surgical Approaches ... 35

4.8 Choice of Surgical Techniques and Approaches ... 36

4.8.1 For Localized Rigid Pathology ... 36
4.8.2 For Lesions Extending to Multiple Levels (Scoliotic, Kyphoscoliotic, or Lordoscoliotic Curve) ... 36

4.9 Conclusion ... 38

5. Surgical Management of Children with Congenital Deformities of the Upper Thoracic Spine and Vertebral Malformations ... 39

Sergei Vissarionov

5.1 Introduction ... 39

5.2 Outcomes of Surgical Management ... 43

6. Osteotomies in Children under the Age of 10 Years ... 49

Josh Schroeder, Leon Kaplan

6.1 Background ... 49

6.2 Overall Management of the Rigid Spine Deformity ... 49

6.3 Halo Traction ... 50

6.3.1 Halo Placement Technique ... 50
6.3.2 Complications with Halo Frames ... 50

6.4 Osteotomies for Correction of Rigid Spinal Deformities ... 50

6.4.1 Partial Facet Joint Resection ... 50
6.4.2 Complete Facet Joint Resection (Posterior Elementectomy) ... 50
6.4.3 Three-Column Osteotomies ... 51

6.5 Outcome and Complications ... 56

7. Surgical Treatment of Rigid Spinal Deformities in Patients with Thoracic Insufficiency Syndrome 58
Leon Kaplan, Josh Schroeder

7.1 Thoracic Insufficiency Syndrome 58

7.2 Care 58

7.3 Treatment Options 59

7.3.1 Casting 59
7.3.2 Surgery 59

7.4 Conclusion 60

8. Vertebral Column Resection as a Treatment for Neurologic Deficit in Severe Spinal Deformity 63
Eduardo C. Beauchamp, Paul J. Park, Meghan Cerpa, Lawrence G. Lenke

8.1 Introduction 63

8.2 Preoperative Evaluation 63

8.2.1 History and Physical Examination 63
8.2.2 Imaging 64

8.3 Halo-Gravity Traction 64

8.4 Surgical Technique 65

8.5 Spinal Cord Monitoring 67

8.6 Vertebral Column Resection for Progressive Myelopathy 68

8.7 Case Illustration 69

8.8 Conclusion 70

9. Osteotomies in Syndromic Patients 75
Dino Colo, René M. Castelein

9.1 Introduction 75

9.2 Definition, Classification, and Indication 75

9.3 Rigid Deformities in Syndromic Patients 75

9.4 Choice of Osteotomy: Type and Goal 78

9.5 Preoperative Workup 78

9.5.1 Patient History and Physical Findings 78
9.5.2 Imaging Studies 79

9.6 Surgical Aspects and Technique 80

9.6.1 Positioning and Perioperative Measures 80

9.7 Surgical Technique 80

9.7.1 Smith–Petersen Osteotomy and Ponte Osteotomy 80
9.7.2 Pedicle Subtraction Osteotomy 81
9.7.3 Bone–Disk–Bone Osteotomy 81
9.7.4 Vertebral Column Resection 81

9.8 Postoperative Care 82

9.9 Complications 82

9.10 Outcome 83

9.11 Conclusion 83

10. Rigid Spine Deformities in Early-Onset Scoliosis 84
Pooria Hosseini, Behrooz A. Akbarnia

10.1 Introduction 84

10.2 Clinical and Radiographic Evaluation 84

10.2.1 History and Physical Examination 84
10.2.2 Plain Radiographs 85
10.2.3 EOS Imaging System/Three-Dimensional Modeling Techniques 85
10.2.4 CT Scan 85
10.2.5 MRI 85

10.3 Treatment of Rigid Spine Deformities in EOS 85

10.3.1 Nonoperative Treatments 85
10.3.2 Operative Treatments 86

10.4 Extra Procedures Considered in the Treatment of Rigid Curves 90

10.4.1 Traction 90
10.4.2 Surgical Release of Soft Tissues 91
10.4.3 Temporary Internal Distraction Rod 91
10.4.4 Osteotomies 91

10.5 Discussion 91

11. Secondary Correction of Rigid Spinal Deformity after Failed Instrumentation 93

Meric Enercan, Azmi Hamzaoglu

11.1 Introduction 93

11.2 Preoperative Evaluation 93

11.2.1 History 93
11.2.2 Physical Examination 93
11.2.3 Imaging Studies 94

11.3 Surgical Technique 94

11.3.1 Correction of Scoliosis Deformity 95
11.3.2 Correction of Kyphoscoliosis Deformity 95
11.3.3 Correction of Kyphosis Deformity 96
11.3.4 Correction of Lordosis/Lordoscoliosis Deformity 97
11.3.5 Correction of Severe Rigid Pelvic Obliquity in Neglected Congenital Scoliosis 98
11.3.6 Reconstruction Laminectomy Defect following Posterior Vertebral Column Resection 98

11.4 Complications 99

11.5 Conclusion 100

12. Kyphectomy in Patients with Myelomeningocele 102

Josh Schroeder, Leon Kaplan

12.1 Introduction 102

12.2 Kyphectomy 102

12.3 Surgical Technique 103

12.4 Outcome 105

13. Pitfalls and Difficulties in the Surgical Management of Severe Adolescent Idiopathic Scoliosis 108

Mario Di Silvestre

13.1 Definition of Severe Idiopathic Scoliosis . 108

13.1.1 Preoperative Study 108
13.1.2 Preoperative Halo Traction 109

13.2 Surgical Treatment 110

13.2.1 Introduction 110

13.3 Posterior-Only Procedures 110

13.3.1 Pedicle Screws 111
13.3.2 Posterior Staged Technique 111

13.4 Preferred Operative Technique 111

13.4.1 Magnetically Controlled Growing Rod 113
13.4.2 Intraoperative Monitoring of Spinal Cord Function 114
13.4.3 First Posterior Surgery 114
13.4.4 Second Stage of Posterior Surgery 116

13.5 Conclusion 117

14. Posttraumatic Spine Deformity 120

David B. Bumpass, Lawrence G. Lenke

14.1 Introduction 120

14.2 Epidemiology 120

14.3 Evaluation of Posttraumatic Deformity .. 121

14.3.1 Normal Thoracolumbar Alignment 121
14.3.2 Classification 121
14.3.3 Biomechanics and Pathology 121
14.3.4 Presentation and Physical Exam 122
14.3.5 Radiographic Evaluation 122

14.4 Nonoperative Management 123

14.5 Operative Management 123

14.5.1 Surgical Indications and Planning 123
14.5.2 Anterior Surgical Approaches 126
14.5.3 Combined Anterior–Posterior Surgical Approaches 126
14.5.4 Posterior Surgical Approaches 126
14.5.5 Technical Considerations 127
14.5.6 Complications 128

15. Osteoporotic Rigid Spinal Deformities 130

Marco Brayda-Bruno, Andrea Luca, Gabriele Ristori, Lisa Babbi, Alessio Lovi

15.1 Introduction 130

15.2 Epidemiology and Etiology of Osteoporotic Deformities 130

15.3 Our Philosophy of Treatment in Osteoporotic VCFs and Related Kyphotic Deformities 130

15.4 How to Improve Pedicle Screw Stability 131

15.5 Osteoporotic Spine Deformity Correction 132

15.6 Complications and Conclusions 132

16. Spinal Deformities in Patients with Parkinson's Disease 135

Stéphane Wolff, Peter Upex, Guillaume Riouallon

16.1 Introduction 135

16.2 Surgical Considerations 135

16.3 Surgical Technique 136

16.4 Conclusion 136

17. Surgical Planning for En Bloc Resection of Spinal Tumors: Tailoring the Osteotomy to Tumor Extensions 138

Stefano Boriani, Alessandro Gasbarrini, Riccardo Ghermandi, Shifra Fraifeld, José E. Cohen, Eyal Itshayek

17.1 Introduction 138

17.2 Planning En Bloc Resection 139

17.2.1 Steps for Surgical Planning 139
17.2.2 Essential Surgical Criteria 140
17.2.3 Surgical Tips and Techniques 140
17.2.4 Surgical Approach 140
17.2.5 Osteotomy of the Spine to Finalize the En Bloc Resection 147

17.3 Case Report 147

17.4 Discussion and Conclusions 148

17.4.1 Conflicts of Interest 149
17.4.2 Acknowledgments 149

18. Corrective Osteotomies in the Cervical Spine 151

Venu M. Nemani, Peter B. Derman, Han Jo Kim

18.1 Introduction 151

18.2 Clinical Symptoms and Natural History 151

18.3 Physical Exam 151

18.4 Radiographic Evaluation 152

18.5 Assessment and Preoperative Planning 154

18.5.1 Location of the Deformity 154
18.5.2 Previous Surgery 155
18.5.3 Curve Rigidity and Degree of Deformity 155
18.5.4 Neurologic Status 155

18.6 Osteotomy Types 155

18.6.1 Anterior Osteotomies 155
18.6.2 Posterior Osteotomies 156
18.6.3 Combined Osteotomies 157

18.7 Conclusion 157

19. Junctional Corrective Osteotomies (Cervicothoracic, Thoracolumbar, Lumbosacral)...... 159
Claudio Lamartina, Riccardo Cecchinato

19.1 Introduction 159

19.2 Preoperative Evaluation.................. 159

19.3 Cervicothoracic Kyphotic Deformity and Corrective Osteotomies.................. 160

19.3.1 Patient Preparation 160
19.3.2 Technical Considerations.................... 160

19.4 Thoracolumbar Corrective Osteotomies. 162

19.4.1 Patient Preparation 163
19.4.2 Technical Considerations.................... 164

19.5 Lumbosacral Corrective Osteotomies.... 165

19.5.1 Patient Preparation 166
19.5.2 Technical Considerations.................... 166

20. Corrective Strategies and Management of Rigid Sacropelvic Pathologies 170
Yechiel N. Gellman, Josh Schroeder, Meir Liebergall

20.1 Introduction 170

20.2 Presenting Symptoms 170

20.3 Radiographic Evaluation 171

20.4 Management............................ 171

20.4.1 Reconstruction of the Pelvic Girdle.......... 171
20.4.2 Sacral Osteotomies.......................... 172
20.4.3 Pelvic Osteotomies.......................... 172
20.4.4 Other Salvage Procedures 172
20.4.5 Computer-Assisted Surgery.................. 173

20.5 Summary 174

21. Ankylosing Spinal Disorders 176
Roongrath Chitragran, Rune Hedlund

21.1 Introduction 176

21.2 Ankylosing Spondylitis with Fracture.... 176

21.3 Ankylosing Spondylitis with Kyphotic Deformity............................... 178

21.4 Diffuse Idiopathic Skeletal Hyperostosis with Fracture 180

22. Osteotomies in Revision Surgery 184
Ahmet Alanay, Çağlar Yılgör

22.1 Introduction 184

22.2 General Indications 184

22.3 Osteotomies............................ 185

22.3.1 Grade 1 Osteotomies....................... 185
22.3.2 Grade 2 Osteotomies....................... 185
22.3.3 Grade 3 Osteotomies....................... 185
22.3.4 Grade 4 Osteotomies....................... 186
22.3.5 Grade 5 and 6 Osteotomies................. 186

22.4 Difficulties in Performing Osteotomies in Revision Cases......................... 187

22.5 Conclusions............................ 188

23. Classification and Definition of Rigid Spine Deformity 189
Josh Schroeder, Janina Kueper, Leon Kaplan

23.1 Introduction 189

23.2 Definition.............................. 189

23.2.1 Pediatric Rigid Spinal Deformity 189
23.2.2 Idiopathic Scoliosis 190
23.2.3 Congenital Deformity 190
23.2.4 Neuromuscular and Paralytic Scoliosis....... 190
23.2.5 Scheuermann's Kyphosis.................... 190
23.2.6 Adult Spinal Deformity..................... 190

23.3 Classification ... 191

23.3.1 Pediatric Spinal Deformity Classifications ... 191

23.4 Conclusions ... 192

24. Strategies in the Correction of Rigid Spinal Deformities—Controversies between Anterior and Posterior Approach ... 194

Sebastien Charosky

24.1 Introduction ... 194

24.2 Patient Assessment and Surgical Strategy ... 194

24.2.1 Location of the Deformity ... 194

24.2.2 Shape and Severity of the Deformity ... 195

24.2.3 Flexibility of the Deformity and Balance of the Trunk ... 197

24.3 Conclusion ... 200

25. Anesthesia for Spinal Surgery ... 203

Ruth Shaylor, Benjamin Drenger

25.1 Introduction ... 203

25.2 Spinal Cord ... 203

25.3 Blood Supply ... 203

25.4 Preoperative Assessment ... 203

25.4.1 Preexisting Conditions ... 203

25.4.2 Airway ... 204

25.4.3 Respiratory System ... 204

25.4.4 Cardiovascular System ... 204

25.4.5 Neurologic System ... 204

25.4.6 Trauma ... 204

25.5 Induction and Maintenance ... 205

25.5.1 Neurophysiologic Monitoring ... 205

25.5.2 Bispectral Index (BIS) Monitoring ... 205

25.5.3 Other Monitoring ... 206

25.6 Positioning ... 206

25.7 Blood Conservation Techniques ... 206

25.8 Wake-Up Test ... 207

25.9 Postoperative Considerations and Complications ... 207

25.10 Conclusions ... 208

26. Neuromonitoring in Rigid Spine Deformity Correction ... 209

Akiva Korn, Joseph Danto

26.1 Introduction ... 209

26.2 NIOM Tools ... 209

26.2.1 Somatosensory Evoked Potentials ... 209

26.2.2 Transcranial Electric Motor Evoked Potentials ... 210

26.2.3 Electromyography ... 212

26.2.4 Multimodality Approach ... 212

26.3 Clinical Applications ... 212

26.4 Conclusion ... 212

27. Neurological Complications after Surgery or Trauma to the Rigid Spine ... 214

Avi Ohry, W. S. El Masri, Stephen Eisenstein

27.1 Introduction ... 214

27.2 Spondyloarthropathies ... 214

27.3 Scoliosis ... 215

27.4 Posttraumatic Kyphosis (Hermann Kummell's Disease; 1895) ... 216

27.5 Rehabilitation Medicine Perspective ... 216

28. **Importance of the Sagittal Balance in Correction of Rigid Spine** 218
Pierre Roussouly, Amer Sebaaly

28.1 **Introduction** 218
28.2 **Pelvic Sagittal Parameters: The Plinth of Sagittal Balance** 218
28.3 **Spinal Sagittal Parameters: Are We Speaking the Same Language?** 219
28.4 **Spinal Balance Parameters: Metric versus Angular** 221
28.5 **Spinal Shapes in the Normal Population** . 223
28.6 **Degenerative Spinal Evolution** 224
28.7 **Surgical Strategies in Correcting Rigid Spinal Sagittal Deformity** 226
28.7.1 When the Pelvic Incidence Is Small (<50 degrees) 227
28.7.2 When the Pelvic Incidence Is High (>50 degrees) 228
28.8 **Proximal Junctional Kyphosis: A Complication of Faulty Surgical Strategy** 228
28.9 **Conclusion** 229

29. **Robot-Guided Surgery in Rigid Spinal Deformities** 231
Yair Barzilay, Sajan K. Hegde, Isador H. Lieberman, Pramod K. Sudarshan, Harel Arzi, Samuel S. Bederman

29.1 **Introduction** 231
29.2 **Robotic Guidance in Spine Surgery** 231
29.2.1 Robotic Systems in Clinical Use 231
29.3 **Robotic Surgery in Spinal Deformity** 232
29.4 **Special Considerations** 234
29.4.1 Pelvic Fixation 234
29.4.2 Revision Spinal Surgery—Redrilling Pedicles, Retained Instrumentation 234
29.5 **Case Illustrations** 235
29.5.1 Case 1 235
29.5.2 Case 2 235
29.5.3 Case 3 237
29.5.4 Case 4 237
29.5.5 Case 5 237
29.6 **Robot-Guided Osteotomies for Rigid Deformities** 242
29.7 **Conclusion** 243

30. **Biological Aspects of Spine Fusion—Methods to Enhance Fusion Rates** 244
Venu M. Nemani, Matthew E. Cunningham

30.1 **Introduction** 244
30.2 **Fusion Formation** 244
30.3 **Properties of Bone Grafts** 245
30.4 **Types of Grafts** 245
30.4.1 Autograft 245
30.5 **Osteoinductive Agents** 246
30.5.1 Bone Morphogenetic Proteins 246
30.5.2 Demineralized Bone Matrix 246
30.6 **Osteoconductive Agents** 247
30.6.1 Allograft Bone 247
30.6.2 Synthetic Bone Grafts 247
30.7 **Osteopromotive Agents** 247
30.8 **Systemic Agents** 247
30.8.1 Bisphosphonates 248
30.8.2 Parathyroid Hormone 248
30.9 **Conclusions** 248

31. Role of Anterior Approach in the Correction of Adult Spinal Deformities 251
Sleiman Haddad, Ferran Pellisé

31.1 Introduction 251
31.2 Adult Spinal Deformity 252
31.3 Reconstruction of the Lower Lumbar Spine and Lumbosacral Junction 252
31.3.1 Access to the Lower Lumbar Spine 252
31.3.2 Restoration of Anterior Column Support..... 253
31.3.3 Reconstruction of Lumbosacral Segmental Sagittal Alignment 253
31.4 Thoracolumbar Kyphoscoliosis and Anterior Release 254
31.4.1 Complications of the Anterior Approaches... 255
31.4.2 Comparative Studies: Combined Approaches 256
31.5 Case Studies 256
31.5.1 Case 1.................................... 256
31.5.2 Case 2.................................... 256
31.5.3 Case 3.................................... 256
31.5.4 Case 4.................................... 257
31.5.5 Case 5.................................... 257
31.6 Conclusion 259

32. Osteotomies in Spinal Tuberculosis—Adult Care 261
S. Rajasekaran, Rishi Mugesh Kanna, Ajoy Prasad Shetty

32.1 Introduction 261
32.2 Pathophysiology of Kyphosis in Spinal Tuberculosis.............................. 261
32.2.1 Kyphosis during the Acute Phase of Tuberculosis............................... 261
32.2.2 Healing Patterns in Spinal Tuberculosis...... 262
32.2.3 Kyphosis Progression in the “Healed” Phase 262
32.3 Surgical Treatment of Kyphosis in Spinal Tuberculosis.............................. 262
32.3.1 Principles of Surgery in Active Tuberculosis.. 262
32.3.2 Single-Stage Kyphosis Correction by Anterior Approach and Stabilization......... 263
32.3.3 Single-Stage Transpedicular Approach and Posterior Correction (Posterior Closing Wedge Osteotomy) 263
32.3.4 Single-Stage Kyphosis Correction by Posterior-Only Transforaminal Approach and Interbody Fusion 265
32.3.5 Single-Stage Kyphosis Correction by Posterior Costotransversectomy or Anterolateral Approach and Posterior Stabilization........ 265
32.3.6 Kyphosis Correction by Combined Anterior and Posterior Approach 267
32.4 Surgery for Kyphosis Correction in Healed Tuberculosis...................... 267
32.4.1 Transpedicular Decancellation Osteotomy ... 268
32.4.2 Pedicle Subtraction Osteotomy 268
32.4.3 Single-Stage Kyphosis Correction through Extrapleural Approach 268
32.4.4 Closing Opening Wedge Osteotomy (Vertebral Column Resection)............... 268
32.5 Conclusion 270

33. Osteotomies in Tuberculosis—Pediatric Care 271
Alexander Mushkin

33.1 Introduction 271
33.2 Diagnosis of Spinal Tuberculosis in Children................................. 271
33.3 Principles of Treatment 271
33.3.1 Surgical Treatment of the Consequences of Tuberculosis Spondylitis in Children......... 273

34. Osteotomies for Adult Degenerative Scoliosis 276
Yigal Mirovsky, Yossi Smorgick

34.1 Introduction 276
34.2 Selection of Fusion Levels............... 276

34.3 Spine with Mobile Disks 277

34.3.1 Two Main Surgical Techniques Described in This Category........ 277

34.4 Spine with Decreased Disk Mobility 277

34.4.1 Pedicle Subtraction Osteotomy 277

34.5 Complications 279

34.5.1 Early Complications........ 280

34.5.2 Late Complications........ 280

34.6 Conclusion 281

Index 283

Foreword

Advances in orthopaedics and orthopaedic surgery have a long and impressive history. From the days of primitive man and the times of the Egyptians, the Greeks, the Romans, and throughout the Middle Ages—all have studied medicine and practiced orthopaedic techniques, and applied them in healing. Spine surgery truly progressed in the 19th and 20th centuries, leading to the progression of spinal surgery toward three basic goals: decompression, stabilization, and correction of deformities.

It is a great pleasure and honor for me to write the foreword of this textbook because for almost 40 years, I struggled to put into the minds of my colleagues the importance of 3D alignment and balance in the treatment of spinal deformities, more than pure improvement of the Cobb angle. For this reason, this textbook is focused entirely on the correction of the most difficult spinal deformities, notably the rigid ones, typically utilizing osteotomies of various types to achieve this goal, which require sufficient expertise not only about the strategies for their use, but also about the technical skills required.

No matter the etiology, any spinal deformity can evolve into a rigid deformity not correctible in the usual ways of 3D correction of spinal units, thanks to distraction, compression, and axial rotation maneuvers. In this textbook, readers will be exposed to the indications of various etiologies as well as meticulous descriptions of the technical tips and tricks to achieve proper corrections in 3D in almost any place of the spine. The difference between young children, adolescents, adults, and even elderly patients are well described here with their respective solutions. Moreover, readers will find the proper strategies to prevent complications as well as the means to treat them.

The authors of the 34 chapters of this textbook, great orthopaedists from all over the world, in particular the main authors and initiators of this book, Leon Kaplan and Lawrence G. Lenke, have attempted to bring forth as complete a survey of the rigid spine deformities issue as possible, such as treatment solutions, various patient populations, anesthesia, robot-guided surgical techniques, and neuromonitoring, among others. Consequently, the reader will find precise, reliable answers to solve the problems presented by the status of the patients the physician has to treat.

Here is a typical textbook that any spinal surgeon dealing with rigid spine deformity patients should have in their office.

Jean Dubousset, MD
Orthopaedic Spine Surgeon
Professor of Spinal Pediatric Orthopaedics
Académie Nationale de Médecine
Paris, France

Preface

In our work, *Corrective Osteotomies for Rigid Spinal Deformities*, we would like to present the natural history, surgical strategies, and tactics for managing difficult spinal pathologies. There are approximately 4000 orthopaedic surgeons and a comparable number of neurosurgeons in the United States who perform spine surgery. Yet only 5 to 10% of these surgeons have specific expertise and experience in deformity correction.

Unfortunately, in the modern world, despite the attempts for early detection of spine deformities in the younger and older populations, we come across difficult spine pathologies among all ages and areas, including congenital, neuromuscular, syndrome-associated, infection, or neoplasm-related pathologies.

In this book, we didactically address the different surgical approaches, including anterior, posterior, and combined approaches for correction of rigid deformities. We also address the anesthesiological aspects of spine corrections in different stages of surgery, and the importance of spinal neuromonitoring that is becoming a gold standard, allowing surgeons to make more impressive corrections with greater confidence.

Specific surgical approaches to the various types of rigid spine deformities are presented with the rationale, techniques, and results for each.

In addition, we present new technologies like computer-assisted robotic surgery, evaluation and treatment of tuberculosis in children and adults, biological aspects that speed up spine fusion, complications of cord injuries and rehabilitation approach, and others.

All contributors to this work are recognized experts in the evaluation and treatment of various spinal deformities and pathologies. In this work, they present their own personal experiences through many years of practice in clinical evaluation and surgical treatment in spine disorders.

Scoliotic surgery, especially osteotomies of rigid spinal deformities, is, without doubt, a unified part of general spine surgery and otherwise includes the philosophy of meticulous planning, execution, and management.

This book, as a surgical manual, was created and meant for advanced spine surgeons in the field of spine deformity correction in children, youth, and adults with various spine pathologies.

I am certain that many spine surgeons, and especially the more experienced ones, will highly benefit from the didactic review of our experts.

We hope you enjoy reading our textbook and gain much from reading it.

Leon Kaplan, MD

Introduction

The field of spinal deformity has evolved markedly over the past few decades. With increasing clinical and research efforts worldwide, most patients undergoing spinal deformity reconstructions are obtaining far better correction with less or no reliance on any external immobilization postoperatively along with far fewer intraoperative and postoperative complications, leading to better overall outcomes. Within spinal deformity surgery, further subspecialization includes pediatric deformity, adult deformity, cervical deformity, and application of minimally invasive surgical techniques to many conditions as well. During this time, spinal surgeons taking care of patients with deformity have also recognized that there is a subset of patients who have stiff or "rigid" spinal columns that present a greater challenge than those with flexible deformities, as would be somewhat intuitive. Thus, the rationale for this new novel textbook is to further highlight the inherent challenges and complexities, and provide solutions for safe and optimal treatment of those patients with *rigid spine deformities*. In this compendium of advanced and expertly written chapters, the multiple senior authors, all leading spinal deformity specialists, provide their own insight gained through many decades of surgical care of these types of patients. Important topics covered include the natural history of these rigid deformities, and those associated with common diagnoses such as: congenital, idiopathic, neuromuscular, early-onset, osteoporotic, post-traumatic, Parkinson's related, and ankylosing conditions. Anatomic-based considerations are covered in chapters on rigid deformities, including the cervical spine, the upper thoracic spine, and junctional regions of the cervicothoracic, thoracolumbar, and lumbosacral regions. In addition, other more esoteric, but still essential, topics such as kyphectomies for spina bifida patients, surgery for patients younger than 10 years, those who have preexisting neurologic deficits due to their rigid and angular deformities, and those with tumors of the spinal column are expertly presented as well. Lastly, a common scenario of patients with rigid deformities undergoing revision surgery along with various spinal osteotomies are covered in two separate chapters.

The content of this textbook is complete and detailed, and is recommended for any orthopaedic or neurosurgical spinal surgeon or trainee involved in the care of these specific types of patients. I congratulate Prof. Leon Kaplan on his vision and efforts to create and complete this incredibly educational textbook.

Lawrence G. Lenke, MD

Acknowledgments

There were many people involved in getting this book together and making sure it would see the light of day. But there are two, in particular, without whom you would not be reading these lines...

Shelly Tannenbaum, my editor. Shelly is the backbone of this book. On top of doing the standard editorial work, she has also handled all the coordination with the other book contributors and managed the various book logistics. I would like to thank her for her endless help and professionalism, her immense talent, and the sheer magic powers she has shown driving this book to its completion. She was a pleasure to work with, and has played a key role without which this book would not have been published.

Noa Bineth, my medical student. Noa, at her young age, excelled in every aspect of her life and education. She has offered her talents in support of this book and showed once again how everything she touches turns to gold. She managed the majority of the cooperation between me and the other doctors, and has helped drive the work on this book forward. I would like to thank Noa for her support and help throughout this process.

Ladies, this book would not have happened without you.

Leon Kaplan, MD

Contributors

Behrooz A. Akbarnia, MD
Clinical Professor
Department of Orthopaedic Surgery
University of California, San Diego;
Medical Director Emeritus
San Diego Center for Spinal Disorders
San Diego, California, USA

Ahmet Alanay, MD
Professor of Orthopaedics and Traumatology
Pediatric and Adult Spinal Disorders
Acıbadem University School of Medicine
Department of Orthopaedics and Traumatology
Comprehensive Spine Center at Acıbadem Maslak Hospital, Acıbadem University
Istanbul, Turkey

Harel Arzi, MD
Spine Surgeon
Director of Pediatric Spine Unit
Spine Surgery Unit
Department of Orthopaedic Surgery
Shaare Zedek Medical Center
Jerusalem, Israel

Lisa Babbi, MD
Junior Fellow
Spine Surgery III - Scoliosis Unit
IRCCS Galeazzi Orthopaedic Institute
Milan, Italy

Yair Barzilay, MD
Spine Surgeon
Director of Spine Surgery Unit
Department of Orthopaedic Surgery
Shaare Zedek Medical Center
Jerusalem, Israel

Eduardo C. Beauchamp, MD
Adult and Pediatric Spine Surgeon
Department of Orthopaedic Surgery
Columbia University Medical Center
The Daniel and Jane Och Spine Hospital at New York Presbyterian/The Allen Hospital
New York, New York, USA

Samuel S. Bederman, MD, PhD, FRCSC
Scoliosis and Spine Surgeon
RESTORE Orthopedics and Spine Center
Orange, California, USA

Louis Boissiere, MD
Orthopaedic and Spine Surgeon
Bordeaux University Hospital
Clinique du Dos-Bordeaux Orthopole
Bordeaux, France

Stefano Boriani, MD
Orthopaedic and Spine Surgeon
Professor of Orthopaedic Surgery
Director of Oncologic, Degenerative and Spine Surgery Departments
Rizzoli Institute
Bologna, Italy

Marco Brayda-Bruno, MD
Orthopaedic and Spine Surgeon
Chief Spine Surgery GSpine III – Scoliosis
Director of Spine Care Group
Coordinator, Spinal Research
IRCCS Galeazzi Orthopaedic Institute
Milan, Italy

David B. Bumpass, MD
Vice Chair of Orthopaedic Research
Associate Professor of Orthopaedic Surgery & Neurosurgery
UAMS Department of Orthopaedic Surgery
Arkansas Children's Hospital
Little Rock, Arkansas, USA

René M. Castelein, MD, PhD
Orthopaedic and Spine Surgeon
Professor of Orthopaedic Surgery
Chair, Department of Orthopaedics
University Medical Center Utrecht
Utrecht, The Netherlands

Derek T. Cawley, MMedSc, MCh, FRCS Orth
Consultant Spine Surgeon
Mater Private Hospital
Dublin, Republic of Ireland

Riccardo Cecchinato, MD
Specialist in Orthopaedics, Traumatology, and Vertebral Surgery
Medical Director of the GSpine4 Operational Unit
IRCCS Galeazzi Orthopaedic Institute
Milan, Italy

Meghan Cerpa, MPH
Research Coordinator
Department of Orthopaedic Surgery
Columbia University Medical Center
The Daniel and Jane Och Spine Hospital at New York Presbyterian/The Allen Hospital
New York, New York, USA

Sebastien Charosky, MD
Orthopaedic and Spine Surgeon
Centre Toulousain du Rachis
Clinique La Croix du Sud
Quint-Fonsegrives, France

Roongrath Chitragran, MD
Spine Surgeon
Chief of Spine Surgery Unit
Department of Orthopaedics
Phramongkutklao Hospital and College of Medicine
Bangkok, Thailand

José E. Cohen, MD
Neurosurgeon
Professor of Neurosurgery
Department of Neurosurgery
Hadassah-Hebrew University Medical Center
Jerusalem, Israel

Dino Colo, MD
Otrhopadeic Surgeon
Department of Orthopaedic Surgery
University Medical Center Utrecht
Utrecht, The Netherlands

Matthew E. Cunningham, MD, PhD
Associate Attending Orthopaedic Surgeon
Associate Professor of Orthopaedic Surgery
Weill Cornell Medical College
Hospital for Special Surgery
New York, New York, USA

Joseph Danto, PhD
Director
Surgical Monitoring Services
Beit Shemesh, Israel

Peter B. Derman, MD, MBA
Spine Surgeon
Texas Back Institute
Plano, Texas, USA

Benjamin Drenger, MD
Professor of Anesthesiology
President of Israeli Anesthesiology Society
Department of Anesthesiology and Critical Care Medicine
Hadassah-Hebrew University Medical Center
Jerusalem, Israel

Jean Dubousset, MD
Orthopaedic and Surgeon
Professor of Spinal Pediatric Orthopaedics
Académie Nationale de Médecine
Paris, France

Stephen Eisenstein, MB BCh, PhD, FRCS (Edin)
Emeritus Professor
Consultant Spine Surgeon
Robert Jones & Agnes Hunt Orthopaedic Hospital
Oswestry, Shropshire, United Kingdom

Meric Enercan, MD
Professor of Orthopaedics
Department of Orthopaedics and Traumatology
Faculty of Medicine
Demiroglu Science University
Istanbul, Turkey

Shifra Fraifeld, MBA
Medical Writing and Editing
Jerusalem, Israel

Alessandro Gasbarrini, MD
Orthopaedic and Spine Surgeon
Oncologic and Degenerative Spine Surgery Unit
Rizzoli Institute
Bologna, Italy

Yechiel N. Gellman, MD, MSc
Senior Orthopaedic Surgeon
Foot and Ankle, Sports and Reconstructive Senior Surgeon
Orthopaedic Department Complex
Hadassah-Hebrew University Medical Center
Jerusalem, Israel

Riccardo Ghermandi, MD
Orthopaedic and Spine Surgeon
Oncologic and Degenerative Spine Surgery Unit
Rizzoli Institute
Bologna, Italy

Sleiman Haddad, MD, PhD, FRCS
Orthopaedic and Spine Surgeon
Spinal Surgery Unit
Department of Orthopaedic
Vall d'Hebron University Hospital;
Spine Unit, Quiron Hospital
Barcelona, Spain

Azmi Hamzaoglu, MD
Orthopaedic and Spine Surgeon
Professor of Orthopaedic Surgery
Surgeon-in-Chief and Head of Istanbul Spine Center
Istanbul Florence Nightingale Hospital
Istanbul, Turkey

Rune Hedlund, MD
Orthopaedic and Spine Surgeon
Professor of Orthopaedic Surgery
Sahlgrenska University Hospital
Göteborg, Sweden

Sajan K. Hegde, MD
Orthopaedic and Spine Surgeon
Surgeon-in-Chief and Head of Spine
Apollo Institute of Spine Surgery
Centre for Robotic and Complex Spine Surgeries
Apollo Hospitals
Chennai, India

Pooria Hosseini, MD, MSc
Research Fellow
San Diego Spine Foundation
San Diego, California, USA

Eyal Itshayek, MD
Spine Neurosurgeon
Professor of Neurosurgery
Surgeon-in-Chief and Director of Spine Surgery Unit
Department of Neurosurgery
Rabin Medical Center
Petah Tikva, Israel

Rishi Mugesh Kanna, MS, MRCS, FNB
Associate Consultant Spine Surgeon
Department of Orthopaedics, Traumatology, and Spine Surgery
Ganga Hospital
Coimbatore, India

Leon Kaplan, MD
Professor of Orthopaedic Surgery
Surgeon-in-Chief and Director of Spine Surgery Unit
Department of Orthopaedic Surgery
Hadassah-Hebrew University Medical Center
Jerusalem, Israel

Han Jo Kim, MD
Associate Professor of Orthopaedic Surgery
David B. Levine Endowed Chair
Spine Fellowship Director
Hospital for Special Surgery
New York, New York, USA

Akiva Korn, MMedSc, D-ABNM
Surgical Monitoring Services Ltd
Beit Shemesh, Israel;
Division of Neurosurgery
Tel Aviv University and Medical Center
Tel Aviv, Israel

Janina Kueper, MD
Department of Orthopaedic Surgery
Spine and Scoliosis Service
Hospital for Special Surgery
Weill Cornell Medical College
New York, New York, USA

Claudio Lamartina, MD
Orthopaedic Surgeon
Professor of Orthopaedics
EFM Universities of Milan and Turin;
Chief of Department of Spine Surgery
G4Spine 4, IRCCS Galeazzi Orthopedic Institute
Milan, Italy

Lawrence G. Lenke, MD
Professor of Orthopaedic Surgery
Director of Spinal Deformity Surgery
Columbia University Vagelos College of Physicians and Surgeons;
Surgeon-in-Chief, Och Spine Hospital at New York Presbyterian Allen
New York, New York, USA

Meir Liebergall, MD
Orthopaedic Surgeon
Professor of Orthopaedic Surgery
Surgeon-in-Chief and Director of Orthopaedic Complex
Hadassah-Hebrew University Medical Center
Jerusalem, Israel

Isador H. Lieberman, MD, MBA, FRCSC
Orthopaedic and Spinal Surgeon
President of Texas Back Institute
Plano, Texas, USA

Alessio Lovi, MD
Senior Fellow
Spine Surgery III - Scoliosis Unit
IRCCS Galeazzi Orthopaedic Institute
Milan, Italy

Andrea Luca, MD
Spine Fellow
Spine Surgery III - Scoliosis Unit
IRCCS Galeazzi Orthopaedic Institute
Milan, Italy

W. S. El Masri, FRCS Ed, FRCP
Emeritus Clinical Professor of Spinal Injuries
Keele University;
Consultant Surgeon in Spinal Injuries
Midlands Centre for Spinal Injuries (MCSI)
Robert Jones & Agnes Hunt Orthopaedic Hospital
Oswestry, Shropshire, United Kingdom

Yigal Mirovsky, MD
Orthopaedic Spine Surgeon
Professor of Orthopaedic Surgery
Director of Department of Orthopaedic Surgery and the Spine Unit
Assaf Harofeh (Shamir) Medical Center
Zerifin, affiliated to the Sackler Faculty of Medicine
Tel Aviv University
Tel Aviv, Israel

Alexander Mushkin, MD
Orthopaedic Surgeon
Professor of Orthopaedic Surgery
Surgeon-in-Chief and Doctor of Science
Chief of the Spine Center-Pediatric Surgery and Orthopaedic Clinic
Research Institute of Tuberculosis
Saint Petersburg, Russia

Venu M. Nemani, MD, PhD
Spine Surgeon
Center for Neurosciences and Spine
Virginia Mason Medical Center
Seattle, Washington, USA

Ibrahim Obeid, MD
Orthopaedic and Spine Surgeon
Director of Spine and Scoliosis Surgery
Clinique du Dos-Bordeaux Terrefort
Bordeaux, France

Avi Ohry, MD
Emeritus Professor
Rehabilitation Medicine, Faculty of Medicine
Tel Aviv University
Tel Aviv, Israel

Paul J. Park, MD, MMS
Adult & Pediatric Comprehensive Spine Fellow
Columbia University Irving Medical Center
The Daniel and Jane Och Spine Hospital at New York Presbyterian/The Allen Hospital
New York, New York, USA

Ferran Pellisé, MD, PhD
Orthopaedic Surgeon
Professor of Orthopaedic Surgery
Surgeon-in-Chief of Spinal Surgery Unit
Department of Orthopaedics
Vall d'Hebron University Hospital;
Spine Unit: Quiron Hospital
Barcelona, Spain

S. Rajasekaran, MS, MCh, FRCS, FACS, PhD
Director and Head
Department of Orthopaedics, Traumatology, and Spine Surgery
Ganga Hospital
Coimbatore, India

Guillaume Riouallon, MD
Spine Surgeon
Spine Surgery Unit
Saint Joseph Hospital
Paris, France

Gabriele Ristori, MD
Spine Resident
Spine Surgery III - Scoliosis Unit
IRCCS Galeazzi Orthopaedic Institute
Milan, Italy

Pierre Roussouly, MD
Spine Surgeon
Professor of Orthopaedic Surgery
Surgeon-in-Chief of Spinal Surgery Unit
Chief of Spine Surgery Department
Department of Orthopaedic Surgery
Massues Medicosurgical Clinic
Lyon, France

Josh Schroeder, MD
Senior Spine Surgeon
Senior Lecturer
Director of Spinal Deformities Surgeries
Department of Orthopaedic Complex
Hadassah University Hospital
Jerusalem, Israel

Amer Sebaaly, MD
Spine Surgeon
Department of Orthopaedic Surgery
Clinique médicochirurgicale des Massues
Lyon, France

Ruth Shaylor, BMBS, BMSc, DESA
Division of Anesthesia, Intensive Care, and Pain Management
Tel-Aviv Medical Center
Tel Aviv University
Tel Aviv, Israel

Ajoy Prasad Shetty, MS (Ortho), DNB (Ortho)
Consultant in Spine Surgery
Department of Orthopaedics, Traumatology and Spine Surgery
Ganga Hospital
Coimbatore, India

Mario Di Silvestre, MD
Orthopaedic Surgeon
Professor of Orthopaedic Surgery
Chief of Spine Surgery Department
Santa Corona Hospital
Pietra Ligure (SV), Italy

Yossi Smorgick, MD
Orthopaedic and Spine Surgeon
Department of Orthopaedic Surgery and the Spine Unit
Assaf Harofeh (Shamir) Medical Center
Zerifin, affiliated to the Sackler Faculty of Medicine
Tel Aviv University
Tel Aviv, Israel

Pramod K. Sudarshan, MD, MS Ortho
Fellow in Spine Surgery (ASSI)
Fellow in Spinal Deformity Surgery (IGASS, SICOT)
Consultant Spine Surgeon
Aster MIMS Calicut
Kerala, India

Athanasios I. Tsirikos, MD
Senior Spine Surgeon
Professor of Orthopaedic Surgery
Director of Spinal Neuromuscular Department
Royal University Hospital
Edinburg, Scotland

Peter Upex, MD
Spine Surgeon
Spine Surgery Unit
Saint Joseph Hospital
Paris, France

Sergei Vissarionov, MD, PhD, DSc
Orthopaedic and Spine Surgeon
Professor of Traumatology and Orthopaedic Surgery
Surgeon-in-Chief of Spinal Pediatric Surgery Department
Corresponding Member of the Russian Academy of Sciences
H. Turner National Medical Research Center for Children's Orthopaedics and Trauma Surgery
Saint Petersburg, Russia

Stéphane Wolff, MD
Spine Surgeon
Spine Surgery Unit
Saint Joseph Hospital
Paris, France

Çağlar Yılgör, MD
Spine Surgeon
Comprehensive Spine Center at Acibadem Maslak Hospital
Department of Orthopaedics and Traumatology
Acıbadem University
Istanbul, Turkey

1 Congenital Spinal Deformities

Ibrahim Obeid, Louis Boissiere, Derek T. Cawley

Abstract

Congenital spinal deformities are a fascinating area of the science of the vertebral column. Their diagnoses and management require a deep understanding of the growth patterns, starting from intrauterine vertebral formation and segmentation to causes of pain and disability. Abnormalities of formation and segmentation apply here as much as in any endochondral growth environment. Decisions on the role and timing of surgery are best made as part of a multidisciplinary process. In particular, it is important to recognize how inherently different congenital kyphosis can behave compared to congenital scoliosis in causing neurologic deficit if left untreated. Once the goals of surgery have been identified, it requires careful planning to execute an optimal procedure. The described procedures depend on the deformity, the compensatory curves, and the potential for further deformity. The treatment options include epiphysiodesis to balance an asymmetric physis, and hemivertebral resection or pedicle subtraction osteotomy in unbalanced primary curve progression. In severe and complex deformities, vertebral column resection and vertebral column decancellation are usually the accepted options. However, one must recognize limitations including the patient's physiologic and spinal cord tolerance, availability of surgical and technical skills, and perioperative considerations. Image-guided navigation is a new tool to help implant insertion and in particular to control vertebral resection, which improves correction while decreasing risk. In most cases, we have the privilege of developing a rich relationship with the patients and their relatives over multiple visits.

Keywords: congenital spinal deformities, congenital scoliosis, hemivertebra, butterfly vertebra, congenital concave bar, vertebral column resection, pedicle subtraction osteotomy, convex growth arrest

1.1 Introduction

Congenital spinal deformity is defined as a deviation of the spine from its normal planes associated with one of a broad range of congenital vertebral malformations (CVMs) that form in utero. While the deformity may not be present at birth, the vertebral anomaly is present and may be isolated or part of a syndromic abnormality. Congenital spinal deformity occurs only where growth asymmetry from a CVM occurs. At least 40 syndromes of CVMs have been described, accounting for 61% of cases.[1,2] It is commonly accepted that disruption of somatogenesis at approximately 5 to 8 weeks of gestation is the overriding cause of CVMs from genetic predispositions or teratogenic exposures. Thus the diagnosis of and management decisions for CVMs must be made in the context of a comprehensive analysis of affected individuals—their growth, their expectations, their prognosis and potential pain or disability.

Vertebral growth depends on multiple ossification centers (▶ Fig. 1.1), from uterine life to the end of puberty. During childhood and puberty, vertebral growth depends on growth from the secondary ossification centers. The growth plates of the vertebral body are located at the upper and lower vertebral end plates. Growth can be separated into its coronal and sagittal planes. In the sagittal plane, the anterior and posterior growth patterns should reflect the normal contour of the spine, with physiological lordotic cervical, kyphotic thoracic, and lordotic lumbar curves. The coronal plane reflects symmetric growth between the left and right sides.

Up to 38% of CVMs have been shown to have an intraspinal anomaly, particularly cervical and thoracic, with half displaying clinical evidence of this.[3] The vertebral anomalies* that result in the development of a kyphosis are fully established at birth, developing during a later stage of chondrification than scoliosis, which is thought to develop at an earlier mesenchymal stage.[4] This may explain why the incidence of intraspinal abnormalities is higher in congenital scoliosis than in congenital kyphosis.[5,6] These must be fully investigated with MRI of the whole spine prior to surgery.

Tolerance for blood loss in these patients is often low, and this must be included in the decision-making process prior to the surgery. Identifying how much surgery a patient with CVM can tolerate is guided by comorbidities. The morbidity of increased spinal deformities is largely related to pulmonary effects, including alveolar multiplication and truncal constriction. When compared to a similar idiopathic scoliotic deformity, CVM has a 15% higher loss in vital capacity.

1.2 Deciding on Surgery

Patients with CVM present with radiological abnormalities (usually from chest or abdominal radiographs), cosmetic deformities, pain, or neurological sequelae. The goals of surgery are to stabilize the spine, adjust for growth asymmetry, and correct the deformity so that patient-related outcomes are met.

Eighty percent of spinal deformities are caused by congenital scoliosis, with 15% causing kyphoscoliosis and kyphosis in 5%, depending on the type of vertebral anomaly and its position. A posterior hemivertebra (HV) and/or anterior unsegmented bar will leave a kyphotic deformity. An anterior HV (very uncommon) or posterior bar will leave a lordotic deformity. A lateral-sided HV or a contralateral bar will leave a scoliosis, with its convex apex at the HV or concavity at the site of the bar. Depending on the relative anterior or posterior nature of a lateral-sided HV or bar, the deformity will be either a kypho- or a lordoscoliosis.

Biplanar radiographs have been the foundation for classification and prognostication for CVMs. More recently, three-dimensional systems such as CT have been used to generate a more comprehensive picture of the deformity and to help surgical planning given their ability to demonstrate bony

* Associated spinal cord anomalies include diastematomyelia (most common), intraspinal lipoma (thickened and fatty filum—second most common), tethered cord, Chiari malformation, syringomyelia, dermoid or epidermoid cyst, arachnoid cyst, Dandy–Walker malformation, and a low conus.

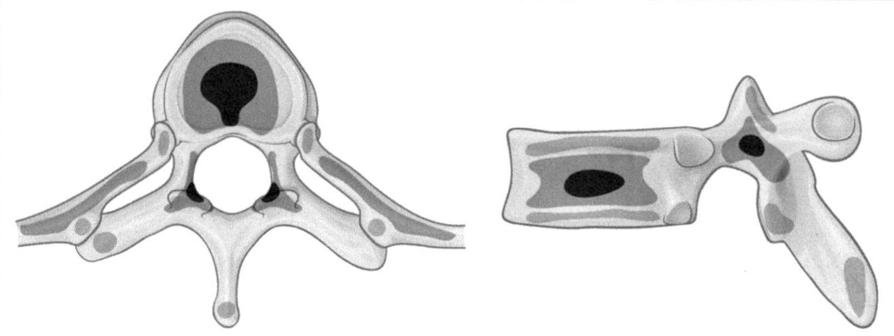

Fig. 1.1 Primary ossification centers (*black*), growth areas from primary ossification centers (*dark gray*) and secondary ossification centers (*light gray*).

architecture for resectional purposes and pedicle morphology to aid pedicle screw insertion.[7]

The most useful and predictive classification system, which outlines failures of formation, failures of segmentation, or combinations of malformations, was designed by Winter et al,[8] then modified by McMaster and Ohtsuka.[9] Thus these descriptions capture the potential for asymmetric growth in any plane, creating abnormal lordosis, kyphosis, or scoliosis. Deformity progression occurs most rapidly during the most rapid periods of growth, from 0 to 5 and 10 to 14 years. Rapid prepubertal progression carries a poor prognosis, and surgical intervention is recommended. In general, defects of segmentation carry a poorer prognosis, with greater potential for deformity than defects of formation.

1. A failure of formation consists of an HV, wedge, and butterfly vertebra, where the abnormality is an aplasia of a part of the vertebra. This allows formation of a unilateral pedicle with a hemilamina, or the presence of either the anterior or posterior elements. Formation of one pedicle usually accompanies an attached rib, leaving an unequal number of ribs. The three types of HV, in order of reducing deformity potential, include a fully segmented HV (most common), a semisegmented HV, and a nonsegmented (or incarcerated) HV.
   - The fully segmented HV has a normal disk above and below, with longitudinal growth occurring on the upper and lower surfaces. As the HV grows, it acts as an enlarging wedge, producing a scoliosis, progressing at approximately 1 to 2 degrees per year. The affected HV will protrude slightly at the apex as it grows. This is more problematic with a posterior HV where the dura and spinal cord may be draped over the kyphosis, potentially culminating in a neurologic deficit. Two adjacent unilateral HVs have four unopposed growth plates, invariably exceeding 50 degrees at maturity. Conversely, opposing HV may cause deformity, depending on the number of levels between them. When close together (one or two interposed vertebrae), they tend to balance each other with small curvatures, whereas when occurring at different regions, they may create unbalanced deformities.
   - A semisegmented HV is fused to an adjacent vertebra, either above or below, and there is only one disk space. The two growth plates are obliterated on the convex side, and, theoretically, there is a balanced spinal growth. However, the slight wedge can maintain a tilt at the apex, which can slowly progress. At maturity, the curve does not usually exceed 40 degrees. Prognosis is usually good except at the lumbosacral junction, where there is an oblique takeoff of the spine from its base at the sacrum and a long compensatory curve at the thoracolumbar junction.
   - An anteroposterior discordance or anteroposterior dissociated HV occurs when the supplementary hemiposterior arch does not correspond to the supplementary hemianterior body. It is best to visualize this on a three-dimensional (3D) CT reconstruction, or in some cases, a 3D printout if one is planning surgery. It is helpful to work out the anterior and posterior relations of the affected pedicle during resection planning (▶ Fig. 1.2).
   - Nonsegmented or incarcerated HVs are fused to the vertebrae above and below, thus set in a niche, scalloped out of the adjacent compensatory vertebrae. There is a low growth potential with low deformity progression, usually less than 20 degrees at maturity.
   - Wedge vertebrae are a result of partial failure of formation on one side of the vertebra (hypoplastic), containing two pedicles, and demonstrate slow longitudinal growth on the wedged side of the vertebra, with low progression of the curve. Depending on the location of the wedge, it may still require surgical deformity correction, especially if there is a compensatory curve.
   - Butterfly HV is a failure of midline fusion that results in two side-by-side HVs (▶ Fig. 1.3). These are often posterior, with a defect of formation of the anterior body, and mainly lead to a kyphotic deformity. They may be asymmetric, thereby producing a kyphoscoliotic deformity.
2. Growth inhibition is due to a failure of segmentation because separate diskovertebral units did not form, and thus a bar extends across adjacent vertebrae, tethering them together. Coexistent rib fusions are often found at the same site. Growth then occurs at the opposite side. Curves progress at approximately 5 degrees per year, frequently resulting in a final deformity of over 50 degrees if left untreated. These mainly occur at the thoracic or thoracolumbar spine. A block vertebra will not usually create a deformity because there is bilateral or circumferential failure of segmentation and uniformly reduced potential for growth across the involved vertebrae, progressing at 0.5 degrees per year.[6]
3. Some (10–20%) are unclassifiable. These often present with multiple curves. Thoracic curves are prevalent but are more common on the left side (unlike adolescent idiopathic scoliosis).[10]

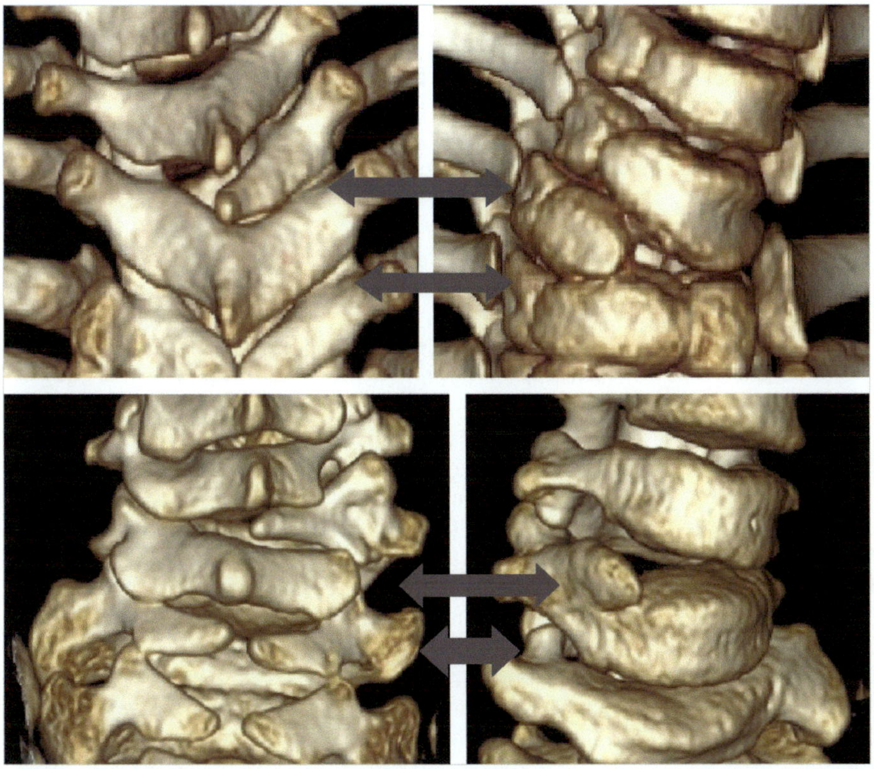

Fig. 1.2 Two cases of anteroposterior discordance as shown on three-dimensional CT reconstructions. The upper case involves the thoracic and the lower involves the lumbar spine.

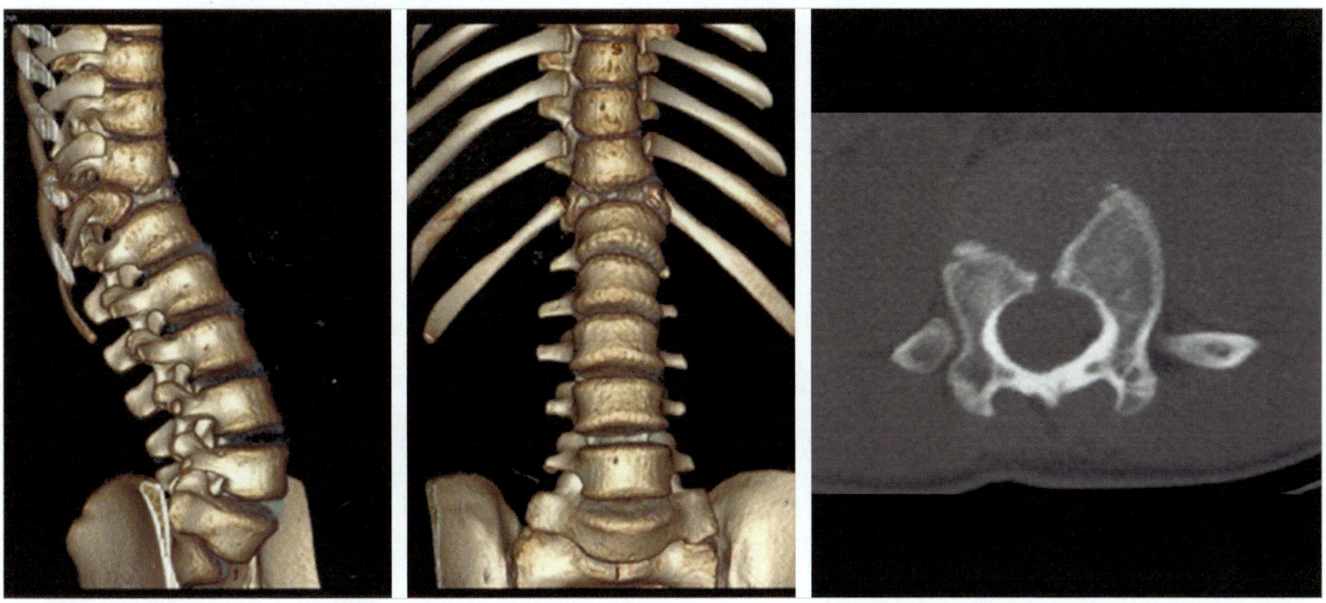

Fig. 1.3 A T 12 butterfly vertebra with central and anterior failure of formation causing thoracolumbar junction kyphosis.

1.3 Prognosis

The prognosis depends on three main factors:

1. The type of vertebral anomaly (growth imbalance magnitude).
2. The site of the anomaly.
3. The age of the patient at the time of diagnosis.

Other prognostic factors include the risk of neurologic complications, mostly with kyphosis and kyphoscoliosis, and associated extraspinal congenital anomalies. The risks of curve progression beyond 40 degrees vary from 37 to 84%.[5,11,12]

Prognosis based on the CVM, from worst to best (approximately), is as follows:

1. Fully segmented HV (two growth plates) with a contralateral bar (10 degrees/year).
2. Double HV with a unilateral bar, especially if fully segmented.
3. Unilateral unsegmented bar.
4. Two consecutive fully segmented HVs.

5. Fully segmented HV.
6. Semisegmented HV.
7. Wedge vertebra (corresponding to a partial failure of formation).
8. Incarcerated HV.[13]

Prognosis based on the site of the anomaly, from worst to best, is as follows:

1. Lumbosacral junction.
2. Thoracolumbar junction.
3. Lower thoracic segment.
4. Lumbar segment.
5. Upper thoracic segment.

The effects of age on deformity progression are not constant. Acceleration of the progression is seen the year before and during puberty during the adolescent growth spurt. Progression of the curve will also depend on the severity of the spinal growth imbalance. Compensatory curves outside the CVM also become stiff with time. This is largely due to the asymmetric load placed on the concavities at the apex and contralateral compensatory curve apices, adhering to the Hueter–Volkmann principle: growth is retarded by increased mechanical compression and accelerated by reduced loading in comparison with normal values.[14]

Severe deformities lead to severe vertebral rotation and distortion of the rib cage. Fused, hypoplastic, or supplementary ribs can result, depending on the level of the CVM. These usually occur within the concavity, but they may occur on both sides of the deformity. While fused ribs may be observed within the concavity, they *accompany* (as opposed to *cause*) the spinal deformity and are therefore not considered when deciding on the curve prognosis. The presence of a rib anomaly increases the likelihood of a renal abnormality.[15]

1.4 Congenital Kyphosis and Kyphoscoliosis

This is an abnormal posterior convex angulation, secondary to a slow anterior column growth, and is often asymmetric, later leading to combined coronal and sagittal deformities. This is observed later in intrauterine growth, mostly at thoracic or thoracolumbar segments. Progressive spinal cord compression causes progressive neurologic deficit.

Multiple HVs have been shown to occur most frequently (44%), followed by anterior segmentation defects (32%) and single HVs (18%).[2] While congenital kyphosis can occur in any part of the spinal column, the apex is often located between T 10 and L 1. The anterior aspect of the spine fails either in formation (65%) or in segmentation (20%) or a combination of both (10%). Inherently different from congenital scoliosis is the potential for congenital kyphosis to cause neurologic deficit if left untreated. This is especially true if the kyphosis is located in the narrow high or midthoracic spine or the lower thoracic spine, where the blood supply is poor.[16] This is the main indication for prophylactic surgery with CVMs. Patients with a preoperative neurologic deficit have a higher potential for intraoperative neurologic complications. HVs, butterfly vertebrae, and wedge vertebrae occur due to the formation failure of the vertebral body.[4]

Winter et al classified these anomalies as failures of formation, segmentation, and combinations thereof, types 1, 2, and 3, respectively.[17]

- Type 1 (anterior failure of formation) can cause rigid annular deformity, with posterolateral quadrant HVs progressing at 2.5 degrees per year until age 10, then increasing to 5 degrees, causing spinal cord compression in 25% of cases.[18] The pathogenesis of these anomalies is thought to occur because of a localized failure of vascularization of the developing cartilaginous centrum. Because the posterior arch develops separately, this is relatively unaffected.
- Type 2 (anterior or anterolateral failure of segmentation) have a smoother kyphosis, often extending over multiple segments. Given the smooth contour and stable configuration conferred by the bar, neurologic deterioration has not been seen in the series by McMaster or Winter et al.[5,18] These are thought to occur because of bone metaplasia changes at the anterior annulus fibrosis and ring apophysis during late chondrification and ossification.[19] The anterior bars progress at ~1 degree per year before 10 years and can be variable after this time. Thicker bars can approximate a block-type anomaly, thus displaying less potential to progress.
- Type 3 mixed anomalies display a sharp angular kyphoscoliosis, usually like kyphosis, and are least common.

1.5 Further Perioperative Considerations

With surgery for deformity correction, it is very important to preserve the periosteal layer beyond the operative site, to avoid spontaneous fusion and allow for normal growth.

If using pedicle screws, allow for availability of sizes smaller than the standard range given the young age of the patient and the morphology of congenitally abnormal anatomy.

Congenital vascular anomalies will usually accompany congenital vertebral anomalies.[20] This is particularly relevant when considering anterior approaches. Noordeen et al concluded that in congenital kyphotic deformities, the blood supply is possibly compromised by three factors:

1. Elongation and compression of the longitudinal arterial trunks, with kinking or stretching of the sulcal arteries.
2. Instability causing microcirculatory perfusion deficits.
3. Congenitally deficient segmental blood supply at the level of the deformity.[21]

Intraoperative scanning with navigation-guided surgery is a helpful conventional technique for inserting pedicle screws in these cases of abnormal anatomy and also for checking bone resection margins. The instrumentation should be compliant with the navigation system. In cervicothoracic kyphosis cases, the head may be positioned on a Mayfield frame that, given the relative anterior positioning of the head on the body, may be much lower on the operating table than the body. This is an important consideration for positioning the reference frame for navigation to allow placement of difficult pedicle screws. A scoliotic hyperlordotic lumbosacral spine may mean that screw placement is deep, and with abnormal anatomy, navigation is helpful here also. Revision surgery is a further justification for navigation surgery (▶ Fig. 1.4, ▶ Fig. 1.5).

Perioperative and intraoperative halo-gravity traction may have a role for patients with severe deformities or those with significant intraspinal pathology.[22]

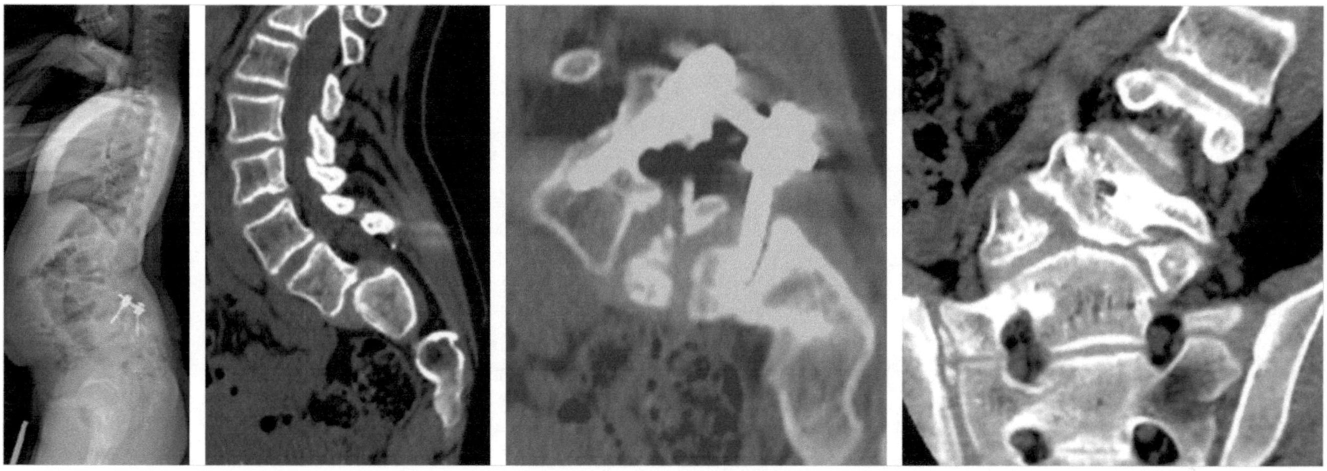

Fig. 1.4 A 13-year-old boy with a lumbosacral junction right hemivertebra. Two insufficient previous resections were performed (late, incomplete correction, implant failure). Progression of the oblique takeoff of the spine is observed with a lumbar compensatory curve that has since become structural. Global coronal malalignment is also present. CT coronal and sagittal images demonstrate lumbosacral oblique takeoff (coronal) and kyphosis (sagittal).

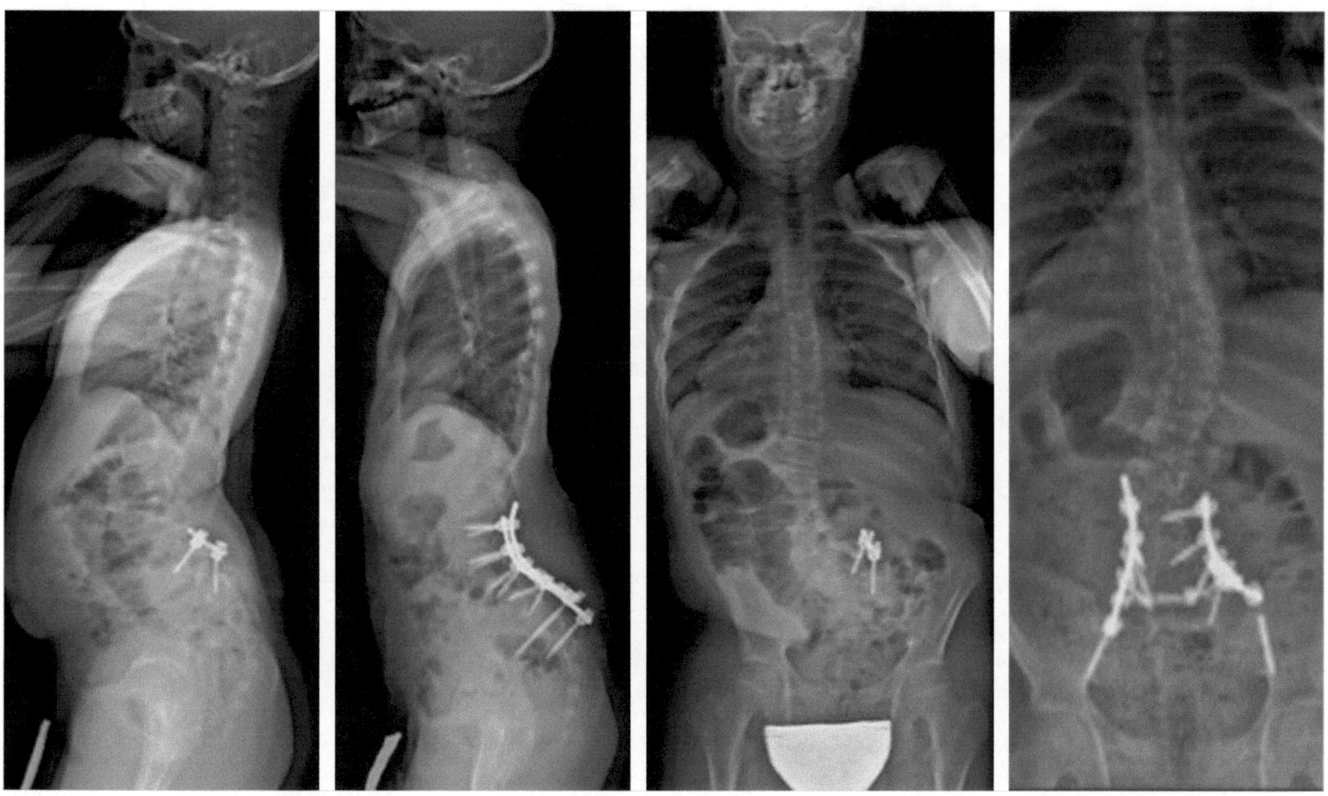

Fig. 1.5 Revision surgery by combined anterior and posterior approach allowed correction of the coronal and sagittal malalignment. At 4-year follow-up the result is maintained despite the right iliac screw fracture (image on the right). Correction of the compensatory curve remains partial because of the old age of the patient at the time of the surgery.

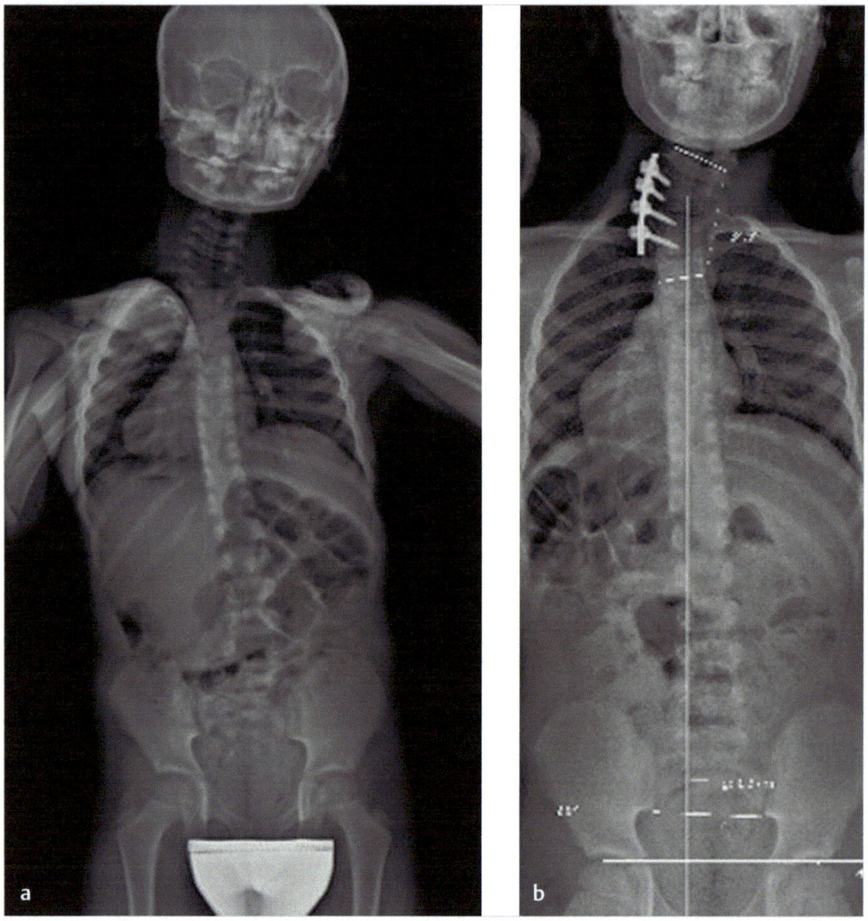

Fig. 1.6 A 7-year-old boy with a congenital unilateral, unsegmented bar at the cervicothoracic junction (a) as a result of a slightly delayed diagnosis. Convex side epiphysiodesis was performed. Four-year follow-up radiographs (b) confirmed that the deformity remained stable.

1.6 Treatment Options and Principles

1.6.1 Observation

Deformity observation is required in isolation or before and after surgical treatment. Clinical evaluation of the child is also important for encompassing characteristics, such as sexual development, cosmetic concerns, pain, and quality of life. Repeated observation alone is appropriate for incarcerated thoracic HVs, complete block vertebrae, or adjacent bilateral HVs. Deformity observation is also very important for monitoring the fusion at the operated level and the behavior of the compensatory curve after surgery.

1.6.2 Epiphysiodesis

The goal of convex epiphysiodesis is to stop the spinal growth at the convex side anteriorly and posteriorly. This can be done with combined anterior and posterior, or posterior alone approaches, depending on the deforming factor. Convex growth arrest by unilateral epiphysiodesis can stop curve progression by canceling growth asymmetry, but cannot correct the deformity (▶ Fig. 1.4). The use of pedicle screws and rigid posterior instrumentation enables posterior and anterior growth arrest by blocking the vertebral body cartilage as it is commonly used in long bone metaphysis by a Blount staple. In older patients, potential for slow correction with growth on the concave aspect is negligible. Epiphysiodesis is best performed before 5 years of age for optimal results or in cases where the anatomy of the location of the pathology is difficult, such as the cervicothoracic junction (▶ Fig. 1.6, ▶ Fig. 1.7).[16] Traditionally, in children who are less than 5 years of age, noninstrumented epiphysiodesis for kyphoscoliosis is appropriate if the kyphotic angle is small—less than 45 degrees according to McMaster and Ohtsuka[9] or 55 degrees according to Winter et al.[18] A combined strategy with growing rods and apical correction and short fusion may be used in complex situations. Short anterior instrumented fusion and posterior convex noninstrumented fusion of HV for congenital scoliosis in very young children has been described. Anterior instrumentation is a safe and effective technique capable of transmitting a high amount of convex compression allowing short-segment fusion.[19]

1.6.3 Hemivertebra Resection

HV resection and three-column osteotomy allow deformity correction and stop spinal growth at the fused segment. Early surgical excision has the advantage of avoiding the structural compensatory curve, particularly for two adjacent HVs or HVs at the thoracolumbar or lumbosacral junctions. Early resection may also be indicated for congenital kyphosis where there is a posterior HV with instability and potential neurologic risk. The aim of the treatment is to achieve a straight spine with respect

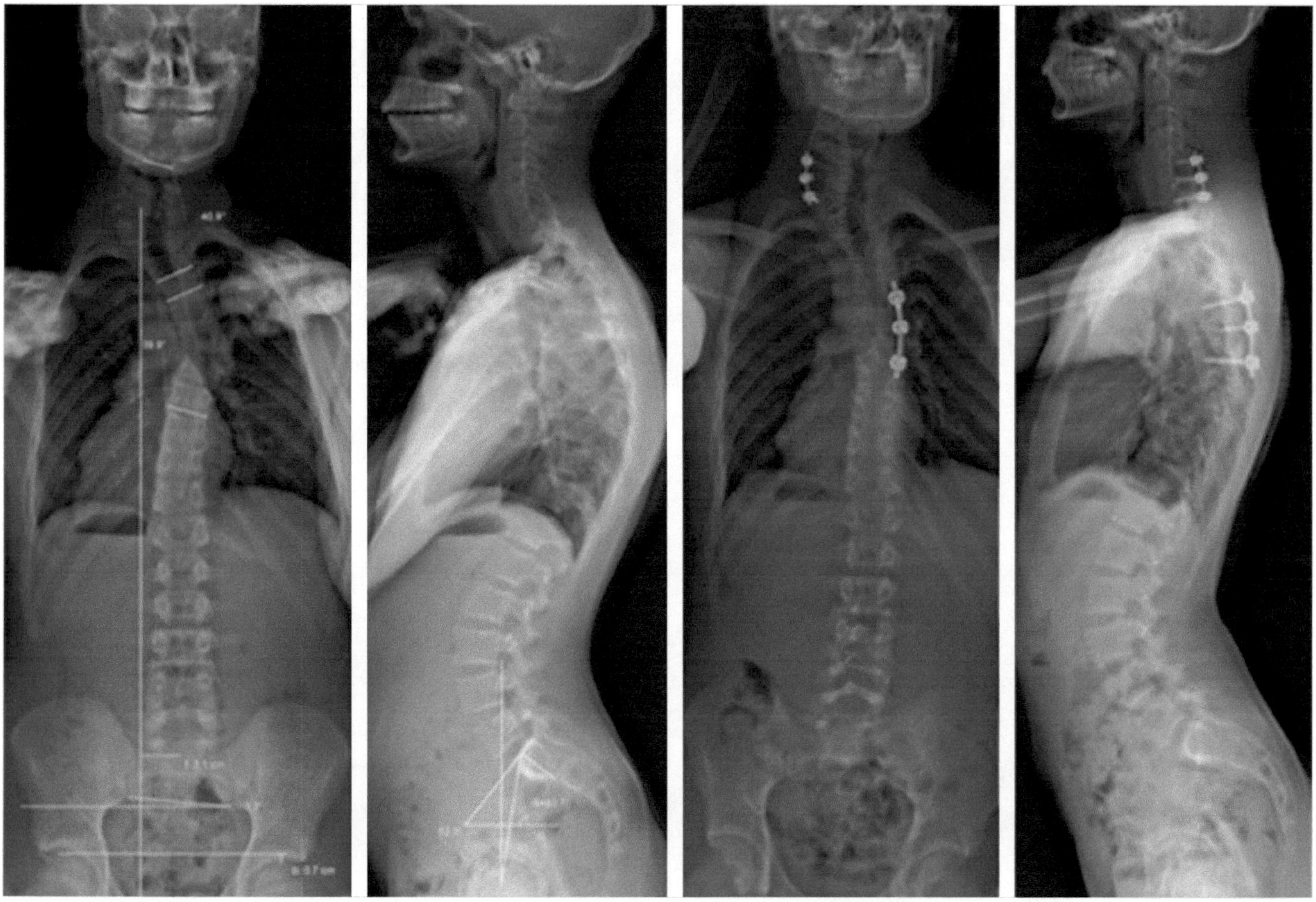

Fig. 1.7 Pre- and postoperative radiographs of a 13-year-old boy with cervicothoracic congenital scoliosis, treated with epiphysiodesis. This is performed with a unilateral posterior approach at the convex side of each curve. Pedicle screws were inserted unilaterally at the level of the hemivertebra and adjacent levels, one above and one below. In the cervicothoracic curve a unilateral growth arrest can be performed using intraoperative navigation for pedicle screw insertion. Fusion with local bone graft is then done posteriorly.

to sagittal contour, and as short a construct as possible. This can be achieved by transpedicular instrumentation, even in very young patients down to 1 year old.[23] Hedequist et al identified the optimal age range as 4 to 6 years.[24]

Thoracic HV resection can be treated by a posterior-only approach with short instrumentation from one level above to one level below using segmental pedicle screws (▶ Fig. 1.8). The surgery is performed under motor-evoked potentials and somatosensory-evoked potentials neuromonitoring. After a standard midline incision, a full-thickness subperiosteal dissection running lateral to the transverse processes exposes the HV with the vertebra above and below it. Care is taken to limit dissection to the concerned levels because spontaneous fusion after exposure only is common in young children. Inferior facetectomies of the HV level and the cephalad level are performed to provide maximum flexibility to the spine. The spinous processes are also resected, and the bone recovered is prepared for use as a graft at the end of the procedure. Pedicle screws are then placed one level above and below the HV. Resection is first performed by removing the proximal part of the same-level rib and the transverse process, followed by the hemilamina. Both foramina, above and below the HV, are opened by removing the superior articular processes. After a careful and complete removal of the rib head, a Cobb elevator is placed outside the lateral portion of the HV and moved anteriorly to the anterolateral quadrant. The pedicle of the HV is then removed with a rongeur, and the nerve roots above and below are identified. The body of the HV is then removed with the use of osteotomes, including the disks above and below, which must include the concave disk material. No retraction of the dural sac is authorized in this region. Venous bleeding in the epidural space should be controlled by bipolar cautery. The convex rod is then placed into the screws. Gradual compression is done to close the resection site, with careful control of the exiting nerve roots and dura. During the closure of the resection site, either convex side pedicle above can fracture in relation to the high strains due to the important reduction needed. Pedicle fracture can be avoided by using a three-rod technique, with opposing supralaminar and infralaminar fixation involving only those vertebrae already used for pedicle screw fixation. Thus a more controlled correction can be achieved through simultaneous compression on pedicles and hooks applied on the posterior arch.[16,25,26]

When checking with fluoroscopy, the inferior end plate of the level above and the superior end plate of the level below should be parallel at the end of the correction maneuver. The posterior elements are then decorticated, and autograft from

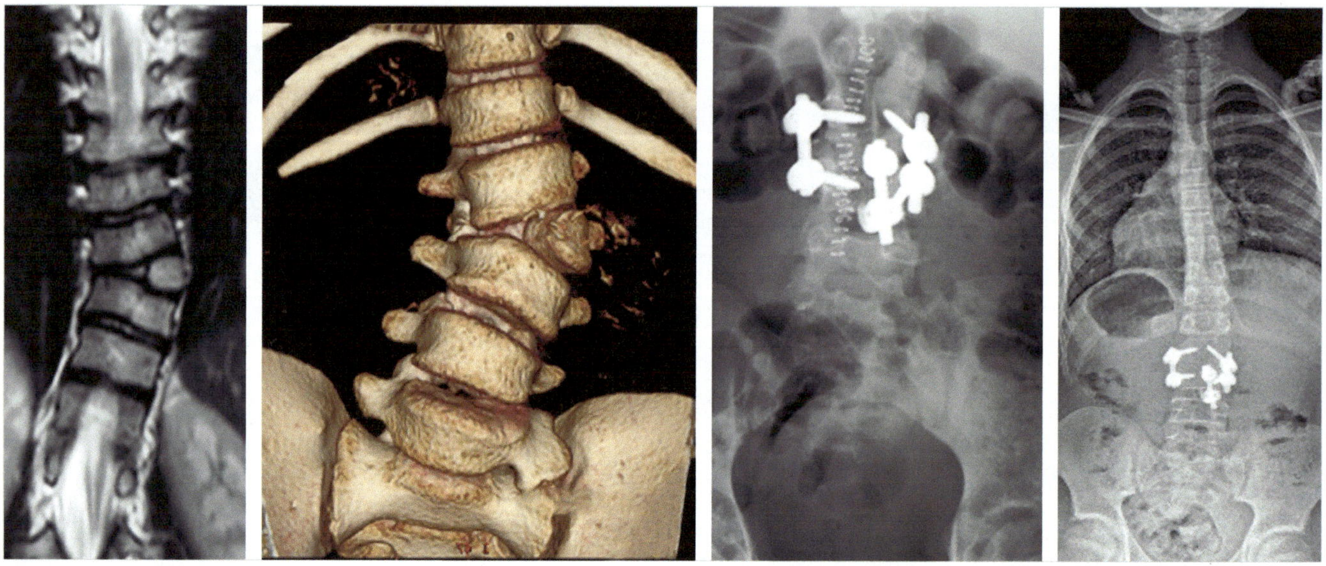

Fig. 1.8 A 7-year-old girl with congenital hemivertebra with scoliosis underwent a posterior complete resection of the bone and of the disk spaces above and below. This allowed a complete and immediate correction of the scoliosis, maintained at 4-year follow-up. This underlines the importance of complete resection and correction of the deformity at a young age before the compensatory curves become structural.

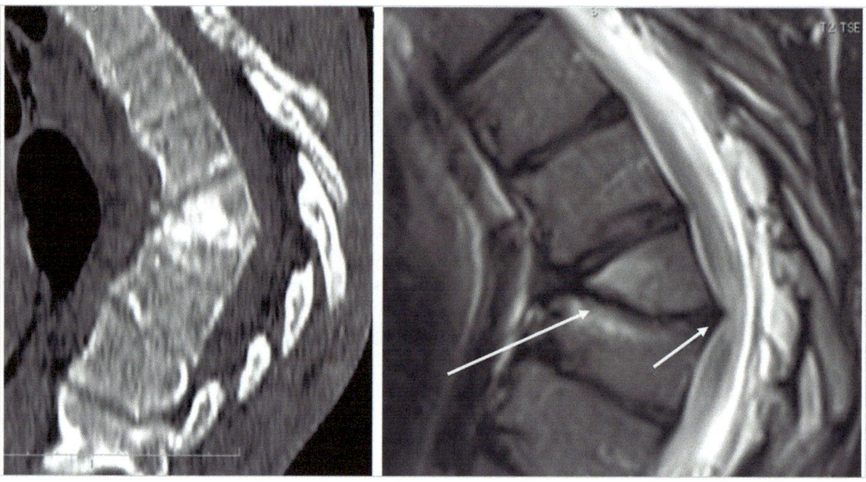

Fig. 1.9 CT and T2-weighted MRI sagittal images demonstrate a posterolateral quadrant hemivertebra causing kyphoscoliotic deformity of the thoracic spine. The increased signal at the anterior column defect (*long arrow*) and within the spinal cord (*short arrow*) indicates spinal instability and cord myelopathy, respectively.

the resected vertebra is applied. Remaining bone defect at the anterior column is filled by autologous bone graft to obtain anterior bony contact and avoid pseudarthrosis. Complete disk and cartilage removal, anterior bony contact either by direct contact or by bone grafting, complete correction of the deformity, and solid fixation are key to a satisfactory long-term result. Compared to convex epiphysiodesis, HV resection allows better correction with shorter fusion. Compared to the double approach, this technique achieves the same result with less morbidity but is technically more demanding.

1.6.4 Pedicle Subtraction Osteotomy

After skeletal maturity, a three-column osteotomy is usually necessary. In the adult setting the choice either includes an osteotomy or a vertebral column resection at the apex (▶ Fig. 1.9, ▶ Fig. 1.10).

In some cases the deformity may be so severe that one pedicle subtraction osteotomy (PSO) would be inadequate to obtain acceptable correction. Adjacent osteotomies can be performed at the same setting. This technique enables bone-on-bone contact between two PSO sites and between the proximal PSO and the level above after the closure, which significantly decreases the pseudarthrosis rate and avoids a complementary anterior approach for grafting. This technique permits use of the vertebral body between the two PSOs as a bony cage, decreasing the risk of spinal cord kinking and increasing fusion rate. The desired correction is slightly kyphotic or neutral, as opposed to lordotic, and thus is not ideal in the lumbar spine. It is preferably indicated in the thoracic and thoracolumbar junction. Furthermore, it is more difficult at the lumbar spine because of the lordotic shape of these segments.

L5 or S1 congenital deformities are difficult to correct. A transdiskal osteotomy utilizes the disk as a further source of correction.[27] A working knowledge of the spinal osteotomy classification by Schwab et al is helpful.[28]

Like any complex surgical procedure, the execution of two-level PSO requires comprehensive *preoperative* (not

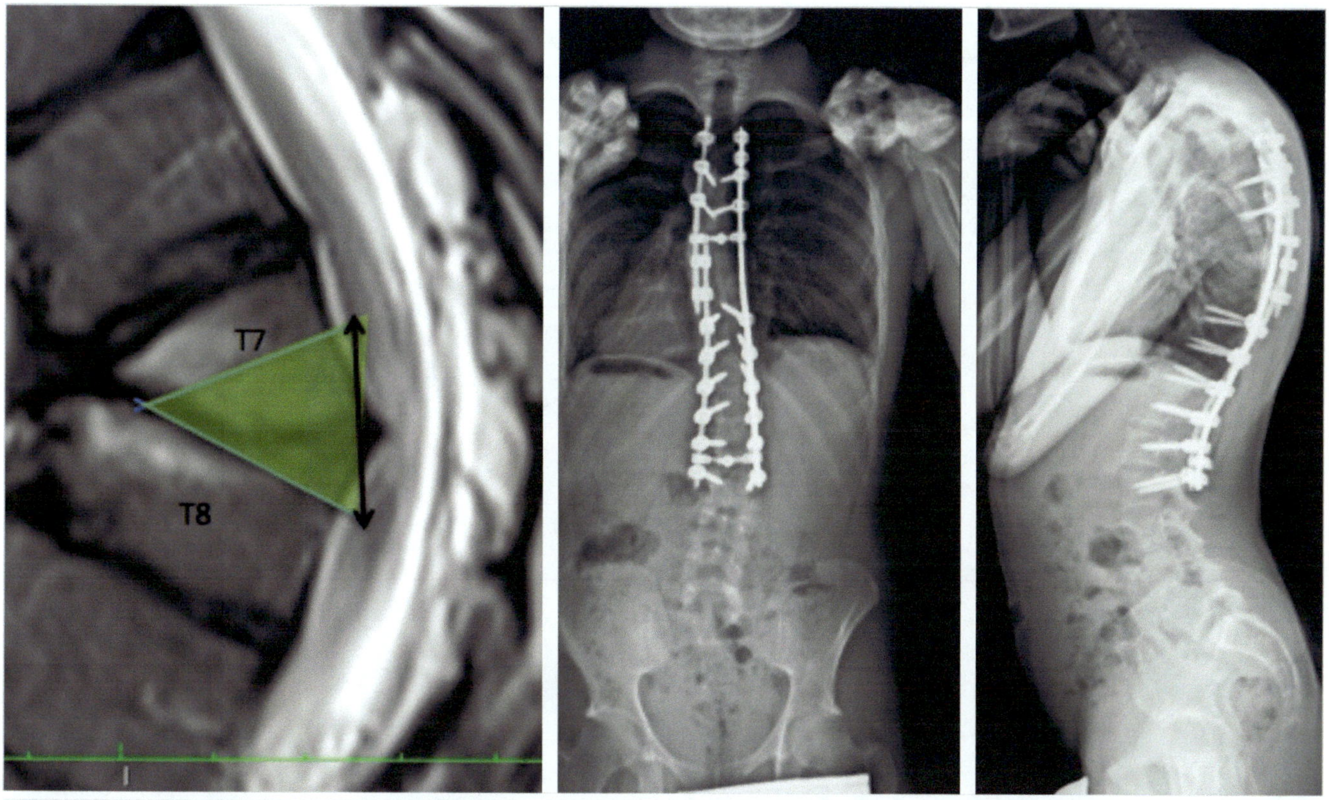

Fig. 1.10 A three-column osteotomy was required to decompress the spinal cord and correct the deformity as projected on the MRI sagittal section. Two-year follow-up radiographs demonstrate a stable correction.

intraoperative) planning, given the usual average bleeding rate for a single PSO (2.4 L).[29] Thus the PSO levels and types should be clearly defined, potentially using a modified PSO including the disk at the proximal level, with PSO for the level below, which allows removal of the disk between the osteotomies, thereby enabling bone-on-bone contact after closure and decreasing the pseudarthrosis rate.[30] One could potentially conserve the distal part of the pedicle of the distal vertebra, keeping intact the posterior arch, without need of opening both distal foramina. This variation helps to decrease the bleeding that may come from the foramina or from the extensive opening of the canal, and extensive exposure of the dura is also avoided. As the disk above is removed, a good correction could still be reached and is not compromised by the partial removal of the pedicle. Usually, with this two-level PSO technique, a correction between 60 and 70 degrees can be achieved. The main advantage compared to vertebral column resection (VCR) is that it does not create the same level of instability, without the need for a temporary rod or for an anterior cage (▶ Fig. 1.11, ▶ Fig. 1.12).[31]

1.6.5 Vertebral Column Resection

VCR may be employed for severe and progressive deformities.

Thoracic posterior VCR carries a higher risk of neurologic injury, particularly with patients over 18 years or in the presence of pulmonary dysfunction and estimated blood loss greater than 50% of the circulating volume.[32] When considering combined anterior and posterior techniques versus posterior alone, it has been suggested that a surgeon at an earlier point on the learning curve would consider combined procedures. Naturally, operative time and surgical blood loss are higher with combined procedures but not necessarily higher in neurovascular complications.[33] A simultaneous anterior and posterior approach through a costotransversectomy is also described as a safe, versatile, and effective approach for accessing congenital kyphosis.[34]

A VCR would be the only corrective technique for a sharp angular deformity or a severe scoliosis (>100 degrees) that would enable a satisfactory result. VCR is a demanding and complex surgery with high neurologic and vascular risks, and it should be performed by experienced spinal deformity surgeons. Ponte-type osteotomies are first performed to provide maximum release and to aid in pedicle screw insertion. The resection vertebra(e) are spared. In the thoracic spine, 5 cm of the proximal rib should be resected to access the lateral wall prior to the laminectomy. A subperiosteal lateral dissection is performed to gain circumferential access. A wide laminectomy is then performed, with the laminae above and below. Pedicles are then removed in a piecemeal fashion, followed by the vertebral body. Prior to removing the anterior body, a temporary, stabilizing rod is placed and attached to at least two or three pedicle screws both above and below the resection area. The cancellous bone is progressively removed from the body and saved for bone graft. In a scoliosis, the temporary rod is usually put on the concave side as the major part of the resection is made at the convex side. One should always remember that the spinal cord is resting on the concave apical pedicle. The concave

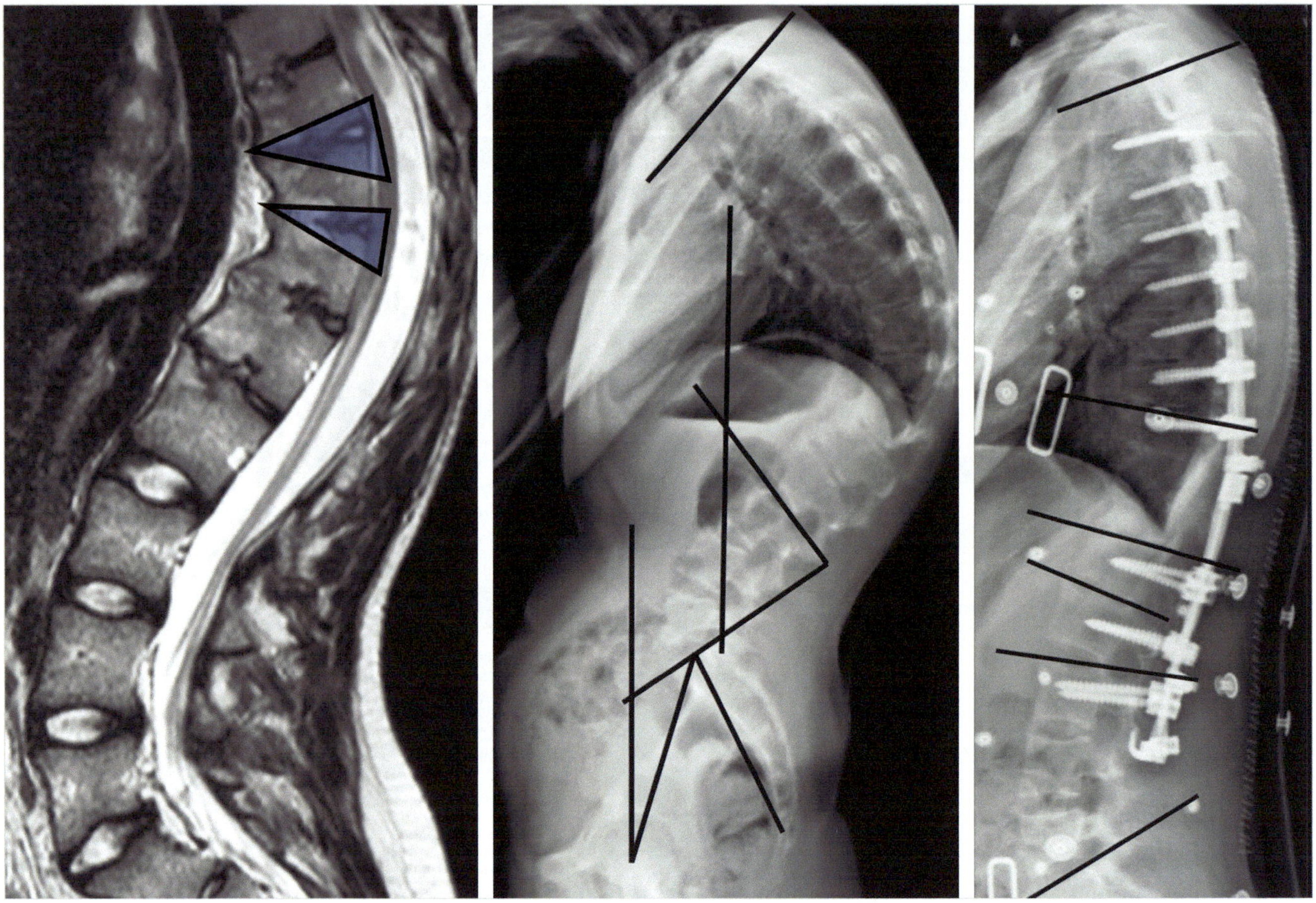

Fig. 1.11 A 16-year-old boy with 70-degree T 10–L 2 kyphosis (*blue arrowheads*) as a result of a two-level anterior unsegmented bar.

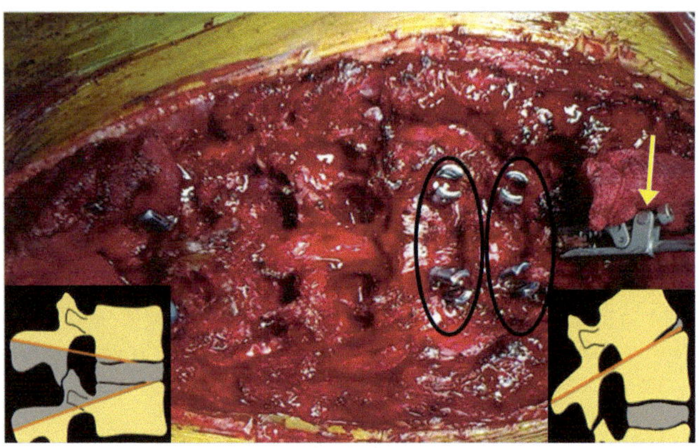

Fig. 1.12 Intraoperative image of the exposed posterior spinal elements with adjacent osteotomies, traversing dura, pedicle screws above and below, and a navigation reference guide placed at the cephalad extremity of the wound. Two adjacent pedicle subtraction osteotomies were performed at T 11 and T 12 for thoracic and thoracolumbar kyphosis. In this case the disks were removed above the vertebrae. At T 12, the distal third of the pedicle was left intact, and the posterior arch was left attached (*arrow*).

pedicle is then removed carefully, with attention to the deep vessels. It is usually enough to thin it with a bur so that it can easily break. The anterior cortex is made as thin as possible but is not completely removed. Diskectomies are performed above and below using curets. The last part of the vertebra to be resected is the posterior vertebral body wall. This part should be completely removed, usually with reverse-angled curets to impale the posterior wall into the ventral defect that had been created. It is imperative that the ventral spinal cord be completely free of any bony prominences to avoid impingement during closure. For reduction, convex compression is performed. This is done by a construct-to-construct closure using side-to-side dominoes at the apex of the resected area after cutting the temporary rod with the assistant holding the two parts of the broken rod. It is imperative to compress slowly because subluxation and/or dural impingement can occur at any time. In case of severe kyphosis, an anterior cage should be placed to prevent overshortening of the deformity and to act as an anterior hinge to provide further kyphosis correction. Once closure is completed, a contralateral rod is implanted after removal of the broken temporary rod. Appropriate compression and distraction forces, in situ contouring, and other correction techniques may be performed with an eye toward any resultant effect on the resected area with respect to subluxation or dural impingement. The spine is then decorticated, and the local graft obtained from the resection procedure is put in place after covering the spinal cord with gel sealant to avoid direct contact with the graft and maintain a continuous posterior graft (▸ Fig. 1.13).[35]

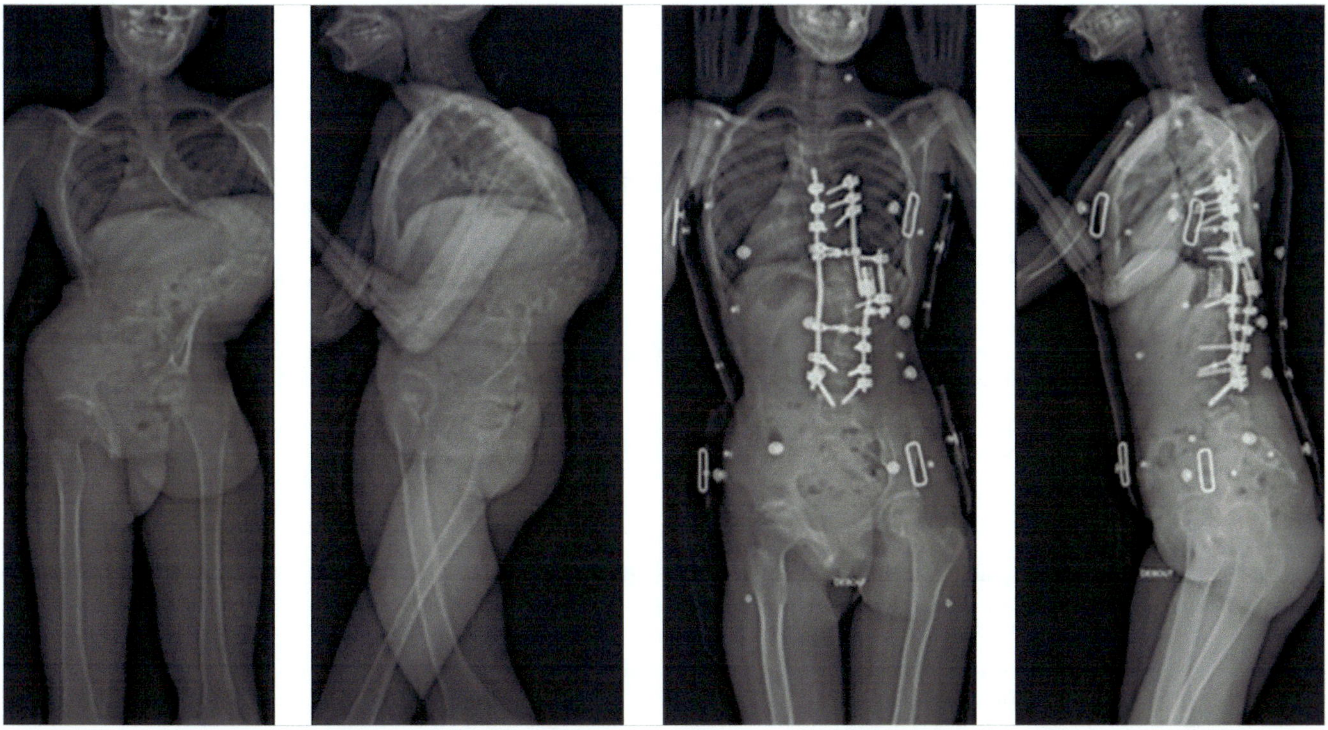

Fig. 1.13 In a 13-year-old girl with neglected kyphoscoliosis, T 11 and T 12 posterior vertebral column resection allows correction in both planes. Vertebral rotation allowed anterior instrumentation by a posterior approach.

1.6.6 Vertebral Column Decancellation

Vertebral column decancellation (VCD) or "eggshell procedure" is a variation of the VCR,[36] but it is less destabilizing, with a lesser amount of resected bone and without the need for an anterior support. With the use of a high-speed bur, it is based on progressive decancellation of the vertebral body. Both pedicles are entered, cancellous bone is removed, the cortex of the anterior and lateral walls is thinned, and the posterior wall is removed, so that the vertebra is rendered sufficiently fragile that it can collapse under pressure during the reduction maneuver. This technique can be applied at multiple adjacent levels, and what remains can serve as natural anterior support structures.

1.7 Conclusion

Congenital scoliosis surgery is indicated for deformity progression, high progression risk, or deformity at an unfavorable anatomical location. Congenital kyphosis and kyphoscoliosis surgeries are also used for neurologic risk progression, mostly for anterior failures of formation. Early treatment is indicated to avoid a compensatory curve becoming structural or to avoid more complex and potentially hazardous anterior and posterior procedures on the spine to correct and stabilize the deformity. Three-dimensional understanding of the diagnosis will allow a greater understanding of how the deformity is likely to progress. Thus picking the most suitable surgical technique is contingent on the patient's tolerance, technical abilities, and surgical goals. All posterior techniques can achieve powerful sustainable corrections, but combined anteroposterior approaches are valid to practice safe surgery.

References

[1] Jones K, Smith DW. Smith's Recognizable Patterns of Human Malformation, 5th ed. Philadelphia, PA: Saunders; 1997

[2] Beals RK, Robbins JR, Rolfe B. Anomalies associated with vertebral malformations. Spine. 1993; 18(10):1329–1332

[3] Basu PS, Elsebaie H, Noordeen MH. Congenital spinal deformity: a comprehensive assessment at presentation. Spine. 2002; 27(20):2255–2259

[4] Tsou PM, Yau A, Hodgson AR. Embryogenesis and prenatal development of congenital vertebral anomalies and their classification. Clin Orthop Relat Res. 1980(152):211–231

[5] McMaster MJ, Singh H. Natural history of congenital kyphosis and kyphoscoliosis. A study of one hundred and twelve patients. J Bone Joint Surg Am. 1999; 81(10):1367–1383

[6] Blake NS, Lynch AS, Dowling FE. Spinal cord abnormalities in congenital scoliosis. Ann Radiol (Paris). 1986; 29(3–4):377–379

[7] Kawakami N, Tsuji T, Imagama S, Lenke LG, Puno RM, Kuklo TR, Spinal Deformity Study Group. Classification of congenital scoliosis and kyphosis: a new approach to the three-dimensional classification for progressive vertebral anomalies requiring operative treatment. Spine. 2009; 34(17):1756–1765

[8] Winter RB, Moe JH, Eilers VE. Congenital scoliosis. A study of 234 patients treated and untreated. J Bone Joint Surg Am. 1968; 59:15–47

[9] McMaster MJ, Ohtsuka K. The natural history of congenital scoliosis. A study of two hundred and fifty-one patients. J Bone Joint Surg Am. 1982; 64 (8):1128–1147

[10] Shahcheraghi GH, Hobbi MH. Patterns and progression in congenital scoliosis. J Pediatr Orthop. 1999; 19(6):766–775

[11] Kuhns JG, Hormell RS. Management of congenital scoliosis; review of one hundred seventy cases. AMA Arch Surg. 1952; 65(2):250–263

[12] Winter RB, Moe JH. Congenital scoliosis a study of 234 patients treated and untreated. Part I: natural history. J Bone Joint Surg. 1968; 50(1):1–15

[13] Arlet V, Odent T, Aebi M. Congenital scoliosis. Eur Spine J. 2003; 12(5):456–463

[14] Mehlman CT, Araghi A, Roy DR. Hyphenated history: the Hueter-Volkmann law. Am J Orthop. 1997; 26(11):798–800
[15] McMaster MJ. Occult intraspinal anomalies and congenital scoliosis. J Bone Joint Surg Am. 1984; 66(4):588–601
[16] Obeid I, Taieb A, Vital JM. Circumferential convex growth arrest by posterior approach for double cervicothoracic curves in congenital scoliosis. Eur Spine J. 2013; 22(9):2126–2129
[17] Winter RB, Moe JH, Wang JF. Congenital kyphosis. Its natural history and treatment as observed in a study of one hundred and thirty patients. J Bone Joint Surg Am. 1973; 55(2):223–256
[18] Winter RB, Moe JH, Lonstein JE. The surgical treatment of congenital kyphosis. A review of 94 patients age 5 years or older, with 2 years or more follow-up in 77 patients. Spine. 1985; 10(3):224–231
[19] Garrido E, Tome-Bermejo F, Tucker SK, Noordeen HN, Morley TR. Short anterior instrumented fusion and posterior convex non-instrumented fusion of hemivertebra for congenital scoliosis in very young children. Eur Spine J. 2008; 17(11):1507–1514
[20] Tanaka T, Uhthoff HK. The pathogenesis of congenital vertebral malformations. A study based on observations made in 11 human embryos and fetuses. Acta Orthop Scand. 1981; 52(4):413–425
[21] Noordeen MH, Garrido E, Tucker SK, Elsebaie HB. The surgical treatment of congenital kyphosis. Spine. 2009; 34(17):1808–1814
[22] Rinella A, Lenke L, Whitaker C, et al. Perioperative halo-gravity traction in the treatment of severe scoliosis and kyphosis. Spine. 2005; 30(4):475–482
[23] Ruf M, Harms J. Posterior hemivertebra resection with transpedicular instrumentation: early correction in children aged 1 to 6 years. Spine. 2003; 28 (18):2132–2138
[24] Hedequist D, Emans J, Proctor M. Three rod technique facilitates hemivertebra wedge excision in young children through a posterior only approach. Spine. 2009; 34(6):E225–E229
[25] Obeid I, Bourghli A, Vital JM. Thoracic hemivertebra resection by posterior approach for congenital scoliosis. Eur Spine J. 2013; 22(3):678–680
[26] Obeid I, Bourghli A, Vital JM. Lumbar hemivertebra resection by posterior approach for congenital scoliosis. Eur Spine J. 2012; 21(12):2721–2723
[27] Alzakri A, Boissière L, Cawley DT, et al. L5 pedicle subtraction osteotomy: indication, surgical technique and specificities. Eur Spine J. 2018; 27(3):644–651
[28] Schwab F, Blondel B, Chay E, et al. The comprehensive anatomical spinal osteotomy classification. Neurosurgery. 2015; 76 Suppl 1:S33–S41, discussion S41
[29] Bridwell KH, Lewis SJ, Lenke LG, Baldus C, Blanke K. Pedicle subtraction osteotomy for the treatment of fixed sagittal imbalance. J Bone Joint Surg Am. 2003; 85-A(3):454–463
[30] Obeid I, Diebo BG, Boissiere L, et al. Single Level Proximal Thoracic Pedicle Subtraction Osteotomy for Fixed Hyperkyphotic Deformity: Surgical Technique and Patient Series. Oper Neurosurg (Hagerstown). 2018; 14(5):515–523
[31] Obeid I, Boissière L, Vital JM, Bourghli A. Osteotomy of the spine for multifocal deformities. Eur Spine J. 2015; 24 Suppl 1:S83–S92
[32] Zhang BB, Zhang T, Tao HR, et al. Neurological complications of thoracic posterior vertebral column resection for severe congenital spinal deformities. Eur Spine J. 2017; 26(7):1871–1877
[33] Demirkiran G, Dede O, Karadeniz E, Olgun D, Ayvaz M, Yazici M. Anterior and posterior vertebral column resection versus posterior-only technique: a comparison of clinical outcomes and complications in congenital kyphoscoliosis. Clin Spine Surg. 2017; 30(7):285–290
[34] Smith JT, Gollogly S, Dunn HK. Simultaneous anterior-posterior approach through a costotransversectomy for the treatment of congenital kyphosis and acquired kyphoscoliotic deformities. J Bone Joint Surg Am. 2005; 87 (10):2281–2289
[35] Obeid I, Bourghli A, Boissière L, Vital JM, Barrey C. Complex osteotomies vertebral column resection and decancellation. Eur J Orthop Surg Traumatol. 2014; 24 Suppl 1:S49–S57
[36] Wang Y, Lenke LG. Vertebral column decancellation for the management of sharp angular spinal deformity. Eur Spine J. 2011; 20(10):1703–1710

2 Neuromuscular Spinal Deformities

Athanasios I. Tsirikos

Abstract

Children and adolescents with neurological or myopathic conditions often develop severe spinal deformities due to muscle weakness, poor neuromuscular control, and spasticity. Scoliosis is the most common type, occasionally associated with increased kyphosis or lordosis and commonly extending to the sacrum and pelvis. The development of spinopelvic imbalance can produce back pain and costopelvic impingement, affecting the patients' ability to function as well as their quality of life while maximizing the need for nursing care. It can also cause significant respiratory complications. Surgical correction is indicated in the presence of a progressive deformity, which produces functional limitations and persistent pain, especially in growing children. This involves a major procedure with considerable risks of intraoperative and postoperative complications directly related to the degree of deformity, the presence of associated comorbidities, and the severity of neurodisability. A thorough medical evaluation is critical in order to establish patient's suitability for major spinal surgery. A well-coordinated multidisciplinary approach will reduce the risks of significant morbidity and mortality, which can occur either during scoliosis surgery primarily related to excessive blood loss in patients with low blood volume or post-surgery mainly due to pulmonary complications, as well as the risk of infection and generalized sepsis in patients who are immunologically compromised. Deformity correction and spinal fusion should only be performed in major centers with adequate medical support by surgeons who have extensive experience in the care of this group of children in order to minimize the risk of complications and produce an optimum outcome.

Keywords: neuromuscular conditions, scoliosis, spinal deformity, surgical treatment, complications, outcome

2.1 Introduction

The development of spinal deformity is a very common orthopaedic problem in patients with impaired neurologic control or inherent muscular dysfunction. This is usually in the form of a scoliosis. Spinal imbalance affecting the sagittal plane, including hyperkyphosis and hyperlordosis, can often occur in association with a scoliosis. Neuromuscular scoliosis is the second most frequent type of deformity (idiopathic scoliosis being the most common) affecting the immature spine. It can produce significant functional limitations in patients with underlying conditions involving the *upper motor neuron*, such as cerebral palsy, Friedreich's ataxia, spinal cord tumor or trauma, as well as the *lower motor neuron*, such as myelodysplasia, spinal muscular atrophy, or poliomyelitis. It is also a very common musculoskeletal manifestation in young patients with *myopathic conditions*, such as Duchenne muscular dystrophy, congenital myopathies, or arthrogryposis multiplex congenita.

2.2 Clinical Problems Associated with Spinal Deformity

The development of a spinal deformity in children and adolescents with a neuromuscular condition can further compromise their limited ability to function. Patients who have preserved ambulatory ability can develop severe back pain and spinal imbalance, which in turn have a significant impact on their postural support and capacity to walk. Wheelchair-bound children may lose their ability to sit comfortably as the developing spinopelvic decompensation has a major effect on their seating balance and postural support. The development of back and rib impingement pain may further affect the patient's function and quality of life. Sitting capability increasingly diminishes with the patient gradually confined to bed, whereas global trunk and pelvic imbalance can result in mechanical back or costopelvic pain as well as cardiac and pulmonary complications. As the deformity progresses and extends to the pelvis, producing a global trunk decompensation, the patient becomes bedridden or is converted to "hand-dependent sitters" (e.g., patients with spina bifida who use their intact upper limb strength to support their body in the sitting position, thereby losing functional ability).[1,2]

The marked global distortion of spinal balance usually affects the thoracic cage, which is also deformed. This results in severe respiratory compromise in patients whose pulmonary function is already affected by the underlying neuromuscular disease. Rapid loss of pulmonary function occurs mainly in patients with myopathic conditions (e.g., Duchenne muscular dystrophy–spinal muscular atrophy) during accelerated stages of skeletal growth around puberty, and this is aggravated by the acute progression of spinal deformity. Chest function is further exacerbated by the patient's immobility and lying in a flat position to avoid mechanical pain produced by the deformity. Preexisting gastrointestinal problems, including gastroesophageal reflux, swallowing disorders, and gastric dysmotility, are also often exacerbated as the scoliosis progresses. The patient's ability to eat can be diminished in the presence of upper gastrointestinal dysmotility and severe reflux as the spinal deformity progresses. Seizure activity may be aggravated due to associated uncontrolled pain as a consequence of the deformity and poor body posture. Asymmetrical loading in the area of the buttocks due to marked pelvic obliquity can cause pressure sores, especially in patients with skin insensitivity (e.g., in spina bifida). The need for parental and nursing care is subsequently maximized.

2.3 Etiology and Natural History of Spinal Deformity

The spinal deformity in growing children with neurologic or muscular conditions develops as the result of poor muscular control along the trunk and pelvis; inherent weakness of the dorsal and abdominal muscles, which do not provide postural support to the spine; and the presence of spasticity (spastic cerebral palsy). The development of scoliosis is less common in patients with isolated dystonia or ataxia. The spinal curve affecting the coronal or both the coronal and the sagittal planes results from the effect of gravity on the vertebral column, which is inadequately supported due to generalized weakness of the trunk muscles during a period of rapid skeletal growth. The onset of scoliosis depends on the evolution, extent, and severity of the condition, all of which determine the level of involvement of the skeletal muscles. Spinal deformity is directly related to the degree of underlying neuromuscular involvement as well as the patient's ambulatory function.[3] Ambulatory children are less likely to develop severe deformities. In contrast, patients who are confined to their wheelchair, regardless of the underlying neurologic or muscular diagnosis, usually develop early-onset scoliosis, which is highly aggressive during growth, especially around puberty and often beyond skeletal maturity, and extends to include the lumbosacral junction and pelvis. In this group of nonambulatory children the spinal deformity is most likely to produce maximum functional and medical complications, responds poorly to conservative treatment, and often requires early surgical management.

In regard to the growth-related development of scoliosis in these groups of patients, a flexible postural curve commonly starts in early childhood, and this retains flexibility demonstrated by near complete correction of the curve in the supine position or when vertical traction is applied. At this stage of skeletal growth, no treatment is needed other than close patient monitoring and provision of postural support when sitting. As the child grows and approaches later childhood a structural component is applied to the deformity. Over time this structural component becomes more rigid and fixed, especially as the patient approaches puberty and the adolescent growth spurt. Apart from progression of the curve on the frontal and lateral planes, which maximally occurs during the accelerated pubertal skeletal growth, the rotatory component of the deformity is also aggravated, leading to severe thoracic distortion and subsequent respiratory complications. Scoliosis of around 40 to 50 degrees at skeletal maturity tends to deteriorate at a slower rate even into adult life due to the presence of the underlying incompetent neuromuscular control.

2.4 Patterns of Spinal Deformity

The typical scoliosis seen in most patients with neuromuscular conditions involves a collapsing, long, sweeping, C-shaped curve often associated with marked pelvic obliquity, with the elevated side corresponding to the concavity of the scoliosis. The trunk collapses on the concave side of the curve, and the deformity stops only when the lower concave ribs are sitting against the elevated hemipelvis. The rib impingement creates a mechanical block that slows, and eventually arrests, further scoliosis deterioration. As the trunk lists toward the concavity of the deformity and the convex shoulder is elevated, trunk balance is further compromised and spinal and thoracic decompensation is exacerbated.

Distal extension of the coronal curve across the lumbosacral junction to include the sacrum and pelvis can give rise to obliquity of the pelvis. Alternatively, obliquity of the pelvis can be caused by hip imbalance, with asymmetrical contractures of the hip adductors, abductors, and flexors often leading to a "windswept/windblown" posture.[4] A combination of both causative factors is very common. If a collapsing scoliosis with severe pelvic tilt occurs in conjunction with a symptomatic hip subluxation or dislocation it is usually preferable to prioritize correction of the spinopelvic deformity to produce a level pelvis, which will make relocation of the hips technically easier and more likely to produce a sustainable effect.

Sagittal spinal deformity can arise mostly in association with a scoliosis.[5] Increased thoracic or thoracolumbar kyphosis is the most frequent type of sagittal deformity. Such a deformity can aggravate preexisting respiratory compromise because it limits the longitudinal thoracic space available for the lungs. An increasing collapsing kyphosis produces positive global sagittal balance of the spine, especially in children with poor neck and head control who lose their ability to look forward and interact with the environment. A long kyphoscoliosis with the apex in the thoracolumbar spine is very common in patients with quadriplegia; in patients with generalized low muscle tone; and in patients with spasticity or fixed contractures of the hamstrings producing a posterior pelvic tilt, decreased lumbar lordosis, and a compensatory thoracolumbar kyphosis. Children who have undergone extensive laminectomies for dorsal rhizotomies may also develop an isolated thoracolumbar kyphosis.

Lumbar hyperlordosis is less common and can develop either in isolation or in conjunction with a scoliosis. This lordosis may be totally asymptomatic for a number of years, during which time it produces few problems until it becomes acutely painful, usually around the period of rapid adolescent growth. At this stage, the progressive deformity produces a marked negative global sagittal balance of the spine with compensatory cervical kyphosis, which may significantly affect sitting balance and produces severe mechanical back pain. Adaptations to the patient's wheelchair cannot effectively address seating intolerance and increasing pain due to increased lordosis; thus, surgical correction is often required as the only means to alleviate pain and restore function.

Increased lumbar lordosis can develop in children with flexion contractures of the hips and marked anterior pelvic tilt as seen in ambulatory diplegia, as well as some forms of congenital myopathy (e. g., facioscapulohumeral muscular dystrophy). Patients with severe extensor posturing may also develop total spinal lordosis. Ambulatory patients with lumbar hyperlordosis are at greater risk of developing isthmic spondylolysis and spondylolisthesis, which can contribute to their frequent complaint of low back pain. Lumbar hyperlordosis or lordoscoliosis is the most difficult type of spinal deformity to correct surgically and has been associated with the highest rate of technical complications related to pelvic fixation, especially when the unit rod technique is used.[6]

Adolescent patients with a lesser degree of neurologic involvement, such as hemiplegic cerebral palsy, Friedreich's ataxia, neurofibromatosis (nondystrophic), arthrogryposis, or syndromic conditions (e. g., Prader–Willi syndrome) can develop a scoliosis that resembles in pattern idiopathic curves in that it does not involve the sacrum and pelvis and, therefore, requires a shorter fusion during correction. However, the scoliosis in these groups of patients will still progress much more rapidly, show little or no response to bracing, reach extreme levels if left untreated, and become rigid quite early when compared to adolescent idiopathic curvatures.[7,8,9] Surgical treatment is almost always required in order to restore spinal balance and prevent clinical symptoms.

2.5 Specific Types of Spinal Deformity

2.5.1 Spina Bifida (Myelomeningocele)

As described previously, children with myelomeningocele can develop a collapsing scoliosis producing global trunk imbalance. They may also have associated congenital vertebral anomalies (apart from the posterior element defects), including failures of formation or segmentation (e. g., an isolated hemivertebra or a unilateral unsegmented bar with or without a contralateral hemivertebra), which can in turn produce a congenital spinal deformity with a superimposed collapsing component due to the inherent muscle weakness. Intraspinal abnormalities (e. g., Arnold–Chiari malformation or tethered cord) are not uncommon in this group of patients and can play a further causative factor in the development of the spinal deformity. These intraspinal anomalies may also require neurosurgical treatment prior to scoliosis correction. Associated hydrocephalus and optimal function of ventriculoperitoneal shunts have to be taken into account when spinal surgery is planned. The scoliosis is frequently combined with a long, collapsing kyphosis, which affects spinal balance and impairs respiratory function.

A unique type of deformity seen in patients with a high-level myelomeningocele is a severe, progressive lumbar kyphosis, which affects seating balance and function. It can also jeopardize skin cover due to the development of pressure areas across the apex of the kyphosis that corresponds to the primary neural closure. These patients often present to the spinal clinic with long-standing infected pressure sores across the lumbar spine that result in multiorganism bacteremia and a chronic spondylodiskitis. The treatment of a symptomatic lumbar kyphosis involves a kyphectomy with resection of the apical first to third vertebral bodies and adjacent intervertebral disks through a posterior approach to the spine followed by spinal instrumentation and arthrodesis (▶ Fig. 2.1). Distal fixation of the rods can be achieved either directly within the sacrum or in front of the sacral ala. The technique of placement of sacral (S 2) alar-iliac screws for distal stabilization of the lumbosacral junction is very useful in patients with poor soft tissue cover as it significantly reduces the profile of the instrumentation and provides solid sacropelvic fixation.[10] The aim of the surgery is to remove the lumbar gibbus and produce a flat lumbar spine that will allow skin integrity. Skin and soft tissue cover on top of the instrumentation may be challenging as the initial neural sac closure leads to extensive scarring and poor vascular supply. Mobilizing local musculocutaneous flaps or secondary closure over a vacuum pump in the presence of a preexisting, active infection are valuable techniques that can achieve adequate skin healing. A long course of antibiotics is frequently required to treat a chronic or prevent a postoperative infection.

2.5.2 Neurofibromatosis

Neurofibromatosis type 1 (NF-1) is the most common autosomal-dominant inherited condition often associated with the development of spinal deformity. Scoliotic curves can be *nondystrophic,* which resemble idiopathic scoliosis yet have an earlier presentation and more rapid progression, or *dystrophic* which are more severe, short-segmented, sharply angulated, often associated with kyphosis and dystrophic features, such as penciling of the ribs, anterior/posterior/lateral vertebral scalloping, vertebral wedging, spindling of the transverse processes, thinning of the pedicles, widening of the canal, and enlargement of the foramina.

Treatment of the deformity should be based on a meticulous clinical assessment and evaluation of the spine with plain radiography and MRI to rule out dysplastic changes that will deter-

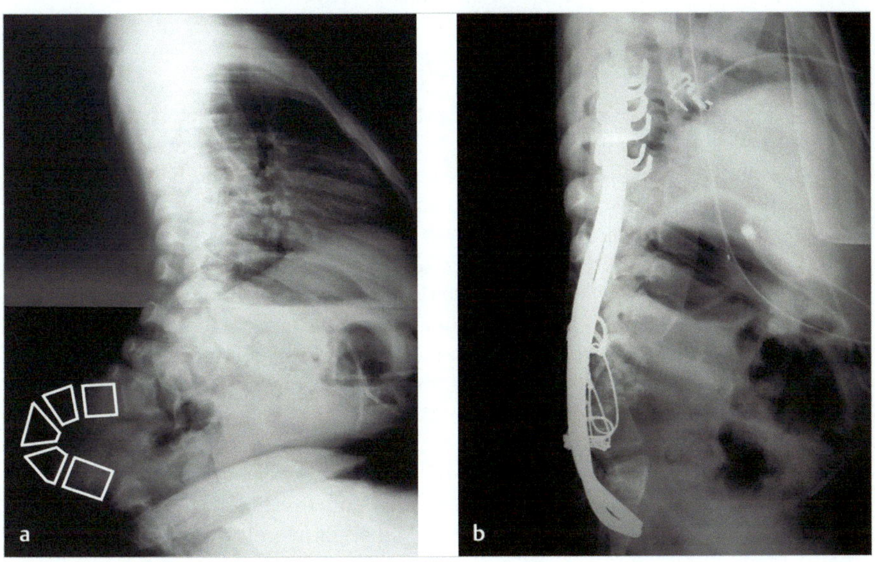

Fig. 2.1 **(a)** Preoperative lateral radiograph of the spine on a patient with myelomeningocele shows a very severe lumbar kyphosis producing pressure sores. **(b)** The patient underwent a three-level kyphectomy across the apex of the deformity followed by posterior instrumented arthrodesis to the sacrum with a good outcome.

mine prognosis and surgical planning. Patients with NF-1 may present with preexisting neurologic deficits. An MRI scan of the whole spine is necessary to demonstrate intraspinal or paraspinal lesions, such as neurofibromas, dural ectasia, and rib protrusion into the canal (additional imaging with CT would be useful), which could cause an increased neurologic risk or excessive blood loss during scoliosis surgery. Nondystrophic curvatures can be treated with decision-making criteria similar to those applied in patients with idiopathic scoliosis. Close observation is necessary due to the possibility of modulation with further growth, as well as the increased risk of pseudarthrosis after spinal fusion. The relentless aggressive nature of dystrophic curves necessitates early operative treatment. Bracing of dystrophic curves does not stop progression. Combined anterior/posterior spinal arthrodesis including the entire structural component of the deformity is often indicated, particularly in the presence of a severe kyphoscoliosis.[11] Abundant autologous bone and segmental posterior instrumentation fixation can reduce the risk of pseudarthrosis and recurrence of the deformity.

2.6 Treatment Principles

The decision-making for scoliosis treatment in patients with complex neuromuscular disorders and associated medical comorbidities has to be tailored to the individual conditions and needs of each patient. It has to take into account the stage of skeletal development and the amount of remaining growth, which will directly affect the risk and rate of scoliosis progression. The presence of associated medical problems, mainly related to cardiorespiratory function, will determine the life span, as well as the patient's fitness to undergo major scoliosis surgery. The natural history of the underlying neuromuscular condition will also dictate patient suitability for surgery, as well as the age when this can be most beneficial. As an example, in patients with Duchenne muscular dystrophy and Friedreich's ataxia who develop gradually progressive cardiomyopathy and respiratory decline, scoliosis correction is usually indicated at a younger age in order to prevent pulmonary compromise due to the development of the scoliosis and in anticipation of their shorter life expectancy.

2.6.1 Nonoperative Treatment

Observation and monitoring are appropriate in young children with mild, flexible curves that do not cause functional limitations. An initial review every 9 to 12 months is usually indicated, with serial radiographs if needed, and this can often be performed as part of a joint neurodisability clinic in conjunction with neurologists and pediatric orthopaedic surgeons to avoid numerous trips to the hospital for families.

Seating adaptations for wheelchair-bound patients are essential, with the aim to maintain a balanced posture and allow interaction with the environment. Wheelchair modifications include offset lateral supports for the chest, shoulder harnesses in an X configuration, a waist strap, head and feet supports, as well as the ability of the chair to recline to provide spinal stretch and patient rest in the course of the day and passively correct kyphotic deformities, particularly in patients with poor head and neck control. A soft neck collar may improve head support and allow better forward vision. A molded seat can provide maximum trunk support for older patients who reach skeletal maturity with terminally fixed curves for which surgical correction is not planned. This would be contraindicated in growing children with progressive deformities in whom the shape of their spine is constantly changing.

Bracing can be used in young children with small, flexible curves to improve postural stability in an attempt to slow scoliosis deterioration and delay surgical correction while maximizing skeletal growth. Bracing is of limited benefit in the natural history of neuromuscular scoliosis; even in ambulatory patients, most curves are going to progress with growth due to deficient underlying muscle control.[8,9,12] It is, therefore, important for patients and their families to recognize that brace treatment is mainly a temporizing measure with the aim to improve postural balance of the trunk, maintain growth of the spine, and allow for surgical correction to be performed as late in skeletal development as possible.

The conventional custom-molded Boston-type thoracolumbosacral orthosis commonly used in patients with idiopathic scoliosis is manufactured of a rigid plastic material with apical paddings and a three-point fixation. These require tight fitting and are not indicated in patients with neuromuscular scoliosis because they can restrict chest expansion, cause skin irritation, and aggravate gastroesophageal reflux and other feeding/swallowing disorders. Compliance with a standard thoracolumbosacral orthosis in this group of patients can be very challenging. In addition, bracing can be detrimental in children with myopathic conditions and significant respiratory compromise because it can produce rib cage molding during critical stages of growth and adversely affect chest development. It can also have a negative impact on gastrointestinal function in patients with reflux and feeding tubes. Whenever bracing is selected, a soft Plastazote whole-body contact or a bivalved brace can be used because these are better tolerated by children with impaired neurologic function as an alternative to the modular seating adjustments whenever these patients are not using their wheelchair. Since the postural support provided by the orthosis is used for the benefit of sitting, there is no indication to wear the brace when the child is lying or during nighttime.

2.6.2 Surgical Treatment

Scoliosis correction with the use of instrumentation followed by spinal arthrodesis is the only effective treatment in young patients with severe spinal deformities that produce back or costopelvic pain, major functional limitations, and respiratory complications, as well as challenge the ability to provide adequate nursing care. Scoliosis surgery can produce a balanced spine with level shoulders and pelvis, relieve pain, and restore patients' functional ability within the limitations of the underlying neurological condition. It can also straighten the thoracic spine and stabilize the chest, thereby preventing respiratory compromise that would result from rib cage distortion as a consequence of the severe spinal imbalance. Spinal surgery is, however, associated with increased morbidity and a high rate of perioperative complications that are directly related to the degree of deformity and inherent neurologic involvement, which in turn dictates the severity of associated medical comorbidities.

Patients with extreme and fixed deformities are usually most severely affected by the underlying neurodisability. In these patients, scoliosis surgery is associated with the highest risk of life-threatening complications because children in this group often have the most severe related medical problems (children who are severely mentally retarded, cannot feed orally, cannot speak or communicate, cannot sit independently). In the presence of such rigid curvatures the ability to correct the deformity is often limited, even with a combined anterior–posterior spinal approach. In this group, the risks of surgery probably outweigh any anticipated benefits, and these patients should be considered poor candidates for scoliosis correction.

2.7 Medical Considerations—Preoperative Assessment

The risks and benefits of scoliosis correction have to be carefully weighed in the context of the existing medical condition and associated comorbidities. It is often very difficult to decide the most appropriate treatment strategy, especially in patients who have severe mental impairment, profound neurologic disabilities, and no communication. A detailed discussion of the pros and cons of surgery must be conducted with the patients and their families before any decision is reached given the narrow margin of error in these medically fragile patients. A detailed preoperative medical assessment of surgical candidates is critical, with involvement of allied disciplines, to determine the patient's suitability for scoliosis correction and to provide a comprehensive estimation of the risk-to-benefit ratio.

In our practice, all patients undergo a thorough respiratory, cardiac, and anesthetic review, including sleep studies, an electrocardiogram, and a cardiac ultrasound. Nutritional evaluation is conducted by the gastroenterology and dietician teams to address gastroesophageal reflux, swallowing/feeding disorders, or gastric dysmotility and to increase nutritional intake before surgery. It is paramount to optimize the patient's preoperative nutritional state and have a clear plan on how postoperative feedings will be delivered as soon after surgery as possible as this may require placement of a gastrostomy/jejunostomy or planning for a nasogastric/nasojejunal tube or even total parenteral nutrition (TPN) through a central venous access. Neurologists are needed to manage patients with seizure activity and address issues related to the presence of ventriculoperitoneal shunts, intrathecal baclofen pumps, and vagal nerve stimulators; a ketogenic diet for refractory epilepsy; and severe dystonia or behavioral problems. A metabolic assessment may be required in patients with poor bone quality and a history of fractures due to disuse osteopenia or medication-induced osteomalacia (e.g., antiepileptic medication) who may benefit from bisphosphonate treatment preoperatively. The results of all tests are discussed at a joined multidisciplinary meeting before a final decision is made. The input of these other specialties is equally essential after surgery and as the patient recovers from a very major procedure. Preoperative bowel preparation is indicated in children with chronic constipation to allow early establishment of feedings in the postoperative period and prevent overflow diarrhea, which can contaminate the spinal wound and jeopardize skin healing. A preoperative review by the intensivists is occasionally helpful for very complex patients in whom a higher risk of medical complications is anticipated; these patients may require a prolonged intensive care unit stay.

2.8 Complications during and after Scoliosis Surgery

The rate of intra- and postoperative complications is directly related to the degree of neurologic impairment, as well as the presence of severe medical comorbidities. The neurologic risk of scoliosis correction is more significant in patients who have ambulatory function and those who have good bladder/bowel control. Attention is needed for accurate placement of the instrumentation to avoid injury to the spinal cord and nerve roots, as well as during correction maneuvers that can produce a neural deficit. Intraoperative spinal cord monitoring is recommended in patients with good motor/sensory function and bladder/bowel continence.

Excessive blood loss can be expected during scoliosis correction in this group of handicapped children, who often have inherent or acquired disorders of coagulation. Even if the patient's clotting times are within normal limits this can be life threatening. Red blood cells, fresh frozen plasma, and clotting factors should be readily available during surgery and in the postoperative period. The use of cell saver, controlled hypotensive anesthesia, muscle relaxation, antifibrinolytic agents (e.g., tranexamic or aminocaproic acid), as well as meticulous hemostasis during careful tissue dissection can reduce the risk of intraoperative bleeding.

Scoliosis surgery in patients with significant underlying pulmonary compromise results in further reduction in their respiratory reserves in the immediate postoperative period and during initial recovery, with the maximum drop at 5 to 7 days postsurgery, during which time the patients will often benefit from noninvasive ventilation (NIV). A trial of NIV is often helpful preoperatively to familiarize the patient with the technique and assess compliance issues. Keeping the patient electively intubated/ventilated in the immediate postoperative period with gradual weaning to NIV is usually beneficial, especially to optimize medical management for children with severe respiratory compromise who are medically unstable and have undergone extensive surgery with considerable blood loss. Placement of a preoperative tracheostomy may be indicated in children with complex upper airway anomalies. Aggressive pulmonary toilet as well as early patient mobilization will reduce the risk of atelectasis and chest infection.

Gastric dysmotility and persistent gastroesophageal reflux often result in insufficient nutritional intake as well as aspiration pneumonias and must be treated before surgery. Placement of a gastrostomy/jejunostomy or a Nissen fundoplication may improve the symptoms. We recommend reestablishment of normal nutrition in patients who are on a ketogenic diet to treat refractory epilepsy long before scoliosis surgery because this can significantly increase the risk of a wound infection. Resuming optimum feedings in the postoperative period may be challenging and often requires placement of a nasojejunal or nasogastric feeding tube. Enteral feedings are always preferable and better tolerated compared to gastric feedings. TPN can provide an alternative in the immediate postoperative period if there is persistent paralytic ileus and nutritional malabsorption.

Poor nutrition predisposes to delayed wound healing and increases the risk of infection in a group of patients who are immunologically compromised due to the inherent neurodisability. Gallbladder disease and subclinical pancreatitis possibly related to an ischemic reperfusion syndrome are also relatively common complications after scoliosis surgery. There is controversy around enteral feeding in the face of increased amylase and lipase blood levels and a subclinical pancreatitis, and this would be an additional indication to consider TPN.

Significant correction of severe spinal deformities (especially hyperlordosis) can result in the development of superior mesenteric artery syndrome due to compression of the third portion of the duodenum between the aorta and the superior mesenteric artery. This will usually require gastric decompression through a nasogastric tube, feedings through a nasojejunal tube, and nil by mouth; it is expected to resolve within 2 weeks from instigation of treatment.

The presence of mental impairment, behavioral disorders, and learning difficulties can make the cooperation of these patients particularly challenging, and a close cooperation between the parents/caregivers and the clinical teams is critical to secure effective postoperative physiotherapy, wound management, mobilization, and establishment of feedings. The dose delivered through intrathecal baclofen pumps in quadriplegic patients usually has to be elevated in the postoperative period to accommodate increased seizure activity related to surgical pain.

In a recent review of 110 consecutive patients who underwent surgical treatment for neuromuscular scoliosis, we recorded a 22% rate of complications, with deep wound infection (8%), gastrointestinal complications (4.5%), and hepatotoxicity (3.6%) being the most common.[13] The complication rate was higher in Duchenne muscular dystrophy patients (total: 38.5%; deep wound infection: 19%, all hepatotoxicity events) compared to other neuromuscular conditions (total: 16.7%; deep wound infection: 5%).

2.9 Deformity Correction Techniques

2.9.1 First- and Second-Generation Instrumentation Techniques

Harrington instrumentation was initially used in the treatment of neuromuscular scoliosis, but the incidence of pseudarthrosis and curve deterioration remained high. Luque[14] introduced the concept of segmental spinal stabilization, applying translational corrective forces using sublaminar wires and two unconnected soft rods. The rods could move independently and failed to provide stability, resulting in high rates of nonunion, crank-shafting, and deformity recurrence. The Galveston technique of intrailiac rod placement allowed for secure pelvic fixation to correct associated pelvic obliquity and was incorporated in the unit rod, which used a single stiff, precontoured rod. This achieved excellent deformity correction with low rates of complications and reoperations.[6,15,16,17] Based on these results extrapolated from studies primarily including children with quadriplegic cerebral palsy, the unit rod has been considered the gold standard of care in patients with neuromuscular deformity, mainly in North America. A valid alternative to the unit rod, which in our experience has produced comparable results, applies two rigid rods with bilateral segmental, sublaminar wire fixation, cross-connected in the upper thoracic and lower lumbar spine and secured to the pelvis through bilateral iliac bolts.

2.9.2 Third-Generation Instrumentation

The use of all pedicle screw or hybrid (proximal hook/distal screw) constructs has been popularized in the treatment of idiopathic scoliosis and has been introduced more recently in the correction of neuromuscular scoliosis.[18,19,20] These constructs follow the Luque principle of segmental fixation, allowing for gradual deformity correction along multiple levels combined with iliac bolts for lumbopelvic or sacroiliac plates for sacropelvic stabilization. In previous series of patients with cerebral palsy, hybrid instrumentation has produced lesser spinopelvic deformity correction when compared to the unit rod, with a similar rate and type of complications.[6,19,20] In contrast, all-pedicle-screw constructs have achieved better initial deformity correction with clinically insignificant loss at follow-up, as well as lesser rates and severity of complications and fewer reoperations compared to the unit rod technique.[5] In addition, if repeat surgery is required it is technically easier and neurologically safer to revise pedicle screws or hooks compared to sublaminar wires. The greater degree of deformity correction and lesser rate of complications and reoperations due to nonunion, prominent instrumentation, or failed pelvic fixation using a pedicle screw compared to the unit rod technique have to be balanced against the increased implant cost. Segmental sublaminar wires can be combined with a pedicle screw construct across levels where stability of the construct rather than correction of the deformity is required, and this can reduce the overall instrumentation cost by limiting the total number of screws used without compromising surgical outcomes.

Revision of the instrumentation in thin patients with inadequate soft tissue cover over the heads of the iliac screws and the lateral connectors to the distal end of the rods due to prominence of the implants is not uncommon. The technique of placement of sacral (S 2) alar-iliac screws reduces the profile of the instrumentation across the lumbosacral junction and allows direct connection to the caudal end of the spinal rods (with or without additional S 1 screws), which precludes the need for lateral cross-links. This is mechanically an attractive alternative to iliac bolts in patients who are markedly underweight, and may help reduce the risk of reoperation due to the need for prominent implant removal causing localized pain and skin breakdown.

Neuromuscular lordoscoliosis or hyperlordosis produces a very rigid and highly symptomatic deformity that is usually associated with fixed anterolateral or anterior pelvic tilt and is among the most challenging patterns of deformity to correct. Previous series have suggested the need for combined anterior and posterior surgery to allow for correction. We recently reported 13 patients with quadriplegic cerebral palsy and severe lordoscoliosis (12 patients)/hyperlordosis (1 patient) producing refractory pain that did not respond to conservative measures. The patients were treated through an isolated posterior spinal arthrodesis.[21] Sagittal imbalance was the major component of the deformity that correlated with perioperative morbidity. All patients achieved good coronal and sagittal balance of the spine and pelvis, which was maintained at follow-up and was associated with excellent reported feedback from the patients and their parents.

2.10 Additional Surgical Considerations

2.10.1 Intraoperative Management

Our patients receive prophylactic intravenous antibiotics (cefuroxime) during surgery and for 24 hours postoperatively. Arterial and central venous lines are placed for administration and close monitoring of fluids. A nasogastric tube is used to decompress the stomach and a Foley catheter to monitor urine output. We use spinal cord monitoring intraoperatively in ambulatory patients, recording somatosensory and motor evoked potentials. We also monitor continent patients with myopathic conditions using somatosensory recording. Locally harvested autologous bone is placed mainly across the lumbosacral junction, where the risk of nonunion is highest, and this is supplemented by fresh frozen allograft bone impregnated with antibiotics (cefuroxime–gentamicin) to achieve a solid bony fusion across the instrumented levels. We perform extensive facetectomies and posterior closing wedge osteotomies in the presence of rigid deformities. We recently started using vancomycin powder, which is placed across the surgical wound before deep tissue closure to further reduce the risk of deep infection. A superficial wound drain is used on top of the lumbosacral fascia and is maintained for 3 to 4 days after surgery.

2.10.2 Levels of Fusion

Instrumented arthrodesis in patients with typical long collapsing thoracolumbar scoliosis and associated significant pelvic deformity extends from the proximal thoracic spine (T2/T3 in order to prevent the development of junctional kyphosis) down to the sacrum, with pelvic fixation of the rods. Previous reports have confirmed that long fusions from T1/T2 to include the lumbosacral junction and extend to the pelvis with the use of the unit rod in children with cerebral palsy do not compromise their walking ability as long as an adequate global sagittal balance has been achieved. Children who have minimal or no pelvic obliquity do not require fusion to the sacrum; in these patients the instrumentation extends caudally to the lower lumbar spine and preserves distal lumbar/lumbosacral mobility, which is beneficial for maintaining functional skills. The treatment of patients with curves that resemble adolescent idiopathic scoliosis follows the same principles with shorter fusions down to the midlumbar spine and a comparatively uneventful postoperative recovery as these patients have a much better general medical condition.

2.10.3 Anterior Correction

A combined anterior and posterior spinal arthrodesis is rarely indicated in patients with neuromuscular scoliosis as this significantly increases the risk of major morbidity and mortality, especially in patients with myopathic conditions or very severe neurodisability. When selected for severe and rigid curves it is probably safer to be performed staged under two anesthetics 5 to 7 days apart in order to give time for medical stabilization of the patient, particularly in the presence of significant medical comorbidities.[22] A thoracotomy or thoracoabdominal approach considerably increases the rate of pulmonary complications, and this may be contraindicated in the presence of severe inherent respiratory compromise due to the underlying condition. Anterior instrumentation is often impossible due to osteopenia or technically difficult due to the acute angle and severity of the scoliosis, which provides limited access; however, it provides a major mechanical advantage if it can produce a nearly straight apical segment across the deformity, which increases stability of the spine and can achieve a circumferential fusion (▶ Fig. 2.2).[5]

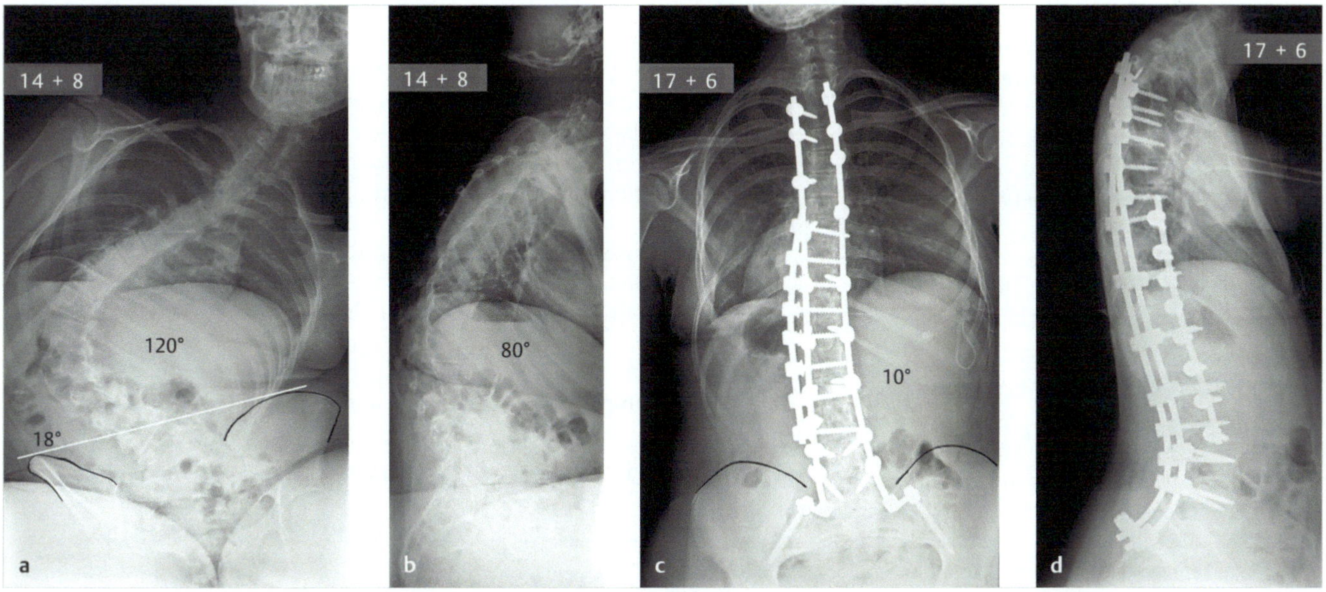

Fig. 2.2 **(a)** Posteroanterior and **(b)** lateral radiographs of the spine on a patient with quadriplegic cerebral palsy, good general medical condition, and normal intellect show a very severe kyphoscoliosis with associated pelvic obliquity. The patient underwent a two-stage combined anterior and posterior spinal arthrodesis using circumferential instrumentation extending to the sacrum/pelvis with the use of iliac screws. **(c)** Excellent deformity correction on the coronal and **(d)** sagittal plains was achieved and maintained at follow-up.

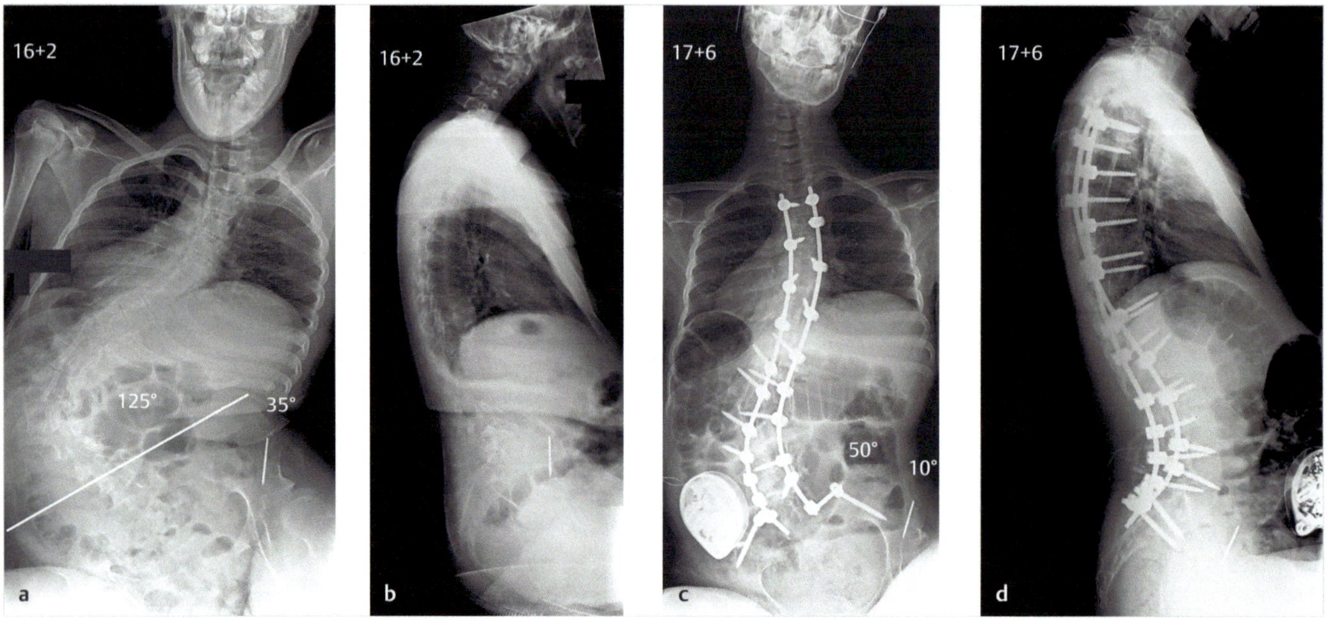

Fig. 2.3 **(a)** Posteroanterior and **(b)** lateral radiographs of the spine on a patient with quadriplegic cerebral palsy and associated co-morbidities including respiratory compromise that precluded an anterior spinal procedure, and good intellect show a very severe kyphoscoliosis with associated pelvic obliquity. The patient underwent a posterior spinal arthrodesis with apical vertebrectomy using segmental pedicle screw/rod instrumentation extending to the sacrum with pelvic fixation through iliac screws. **(c, d)** Excellent correction of the deformity was achieved and maintained at follow-up.

2.10.4 Posterior Vertebral Column Resection

A posterior apical vertebrectomy is the alternative to a combined anterior and posterior instrumented fusion for very severe and rigid deformities (▶ Fig. 2.3). This has the advantage of preventing the need for the anterior procedure, but in severely affected neuromuscular patients it results in excessive blood loss that occurs over an acute period of time and can be life threatening. The presence of two experienced surgical teams would allow performing a simultaneous vertebral resection bilaterally and speed up the procedure. The vertebrectomy allows satisfactory coronal and sagittal correction of a sharply angulated, short-segmented deformity. However, it has a lesser ability to mobilize the spine globally and allow for correction of a severe, fixed pelvic obliquity. In the presence of a fixed deformity that spans longer segments of the spine and is combined with severe pelvic obliquity, it is our experience that combined anterior and posterior arthrodesis with the use of circumferential instrumentation has a better ability to correct the global spinopelvic deformity.

2.10.5 Growth Preservation/ Modulation Techniques

Growth-sparing techniques in the form of growing rods and the vertical expandable prosthetic titanium rib have been tried in very young children with rapidly progressive neuromuscular scoliosis with the aim to better control the curvature and delay the definitive fusion for a later stage of growth, mainly in order to preserve chest and lung development. In our opinion, there is a limited role for these techniques in children who have severe associated comorbidities as part of the underlying neurologic impairment. In these patients, the cumulative risks of repetitive anesthetics and complicated surgery (repeat hospital stays, rod breakage, hook/screw loosening, skin-healing problems or infections, psychological effects of multiple surgeries) should be weighed over the shortcomings of an earlier definitive spinal fusion, which is usually preferable. The advent of magnetic expandable rods, which are lengthened with an external actuator under fluoroscopic or ultrasound control, limits the number of repeat surgeries and provides a more valid therapeutic option in young children, enabling postponement of the final fusion for an older age.

Growth modulation has been a successful technique in the correction of limb deformities. It gradually becomes a compelling concept in scoliosis treatment as more devices (spinal staples, screw–plate or screw–cord constructs) are developed, but the data currently available are limited to document safety and performance as they are mainly preclinical and focus on animal models. Harnessing growth in order to prevent deformity progression or even correct an existing curvature may be feasible through manipulation of the vertebral growth plates by applying convex compressive forces (convex epiphysiodesis), which can produce a balancing effect while preserving residual concave spinal growth. Such techniques would be appealing in the treatment of young children with nonidiopathic scoliosis in order to avoid ineffective brace wear and major fusion surgery.

2.11 Quality of Life Assessment/ Life Expectancy after Scoliosis Surgery

Introduction of modern respiratory management with sophisticated NIV techniques, as well as close cardiac monitoring and early treatment, has resulted in marked improvement in life expectancy for several groups of primarily myopathic patients who can now survive into their third decade and often beyond. Newly introduced genetic treatments promise to alter the dismal natural history of genetic conditions such as Duchenne muscular dystrophy, increase patient functionality, and prolong survivorship. Treatment of spinal deformity is, therefore, becoming a necessity with the aim to optimize function within the limitations of the underlying condition, prevent respiratory decline due to the development of spinal deformity, and improve quality of life.

A predicted 70% survival at 11.2 years has been reported following scoliosis surgery among children and adolescents with quadriplegic cerebral palsy.[23] The best predictor of a poor outcome and short survival rates after spinal correction was the number of days the patients spent postoperatively in the intensive care unit, which reflects their general medical condition, primarily related to respiratory compromise.

Quality of life assessment data exist mainly for patients with quadriplegia. These date demonstrate across previous studies a strong positive impact of scoliosis surgery on the patients' quality of life as perceived by their parents and caretakers.[7] Limitations of all previous retrospective series are the fact that they assess functional improvements following surgery using nonvalidated questionnaires, which are the only ones available in the literature. These reports also present outcomes based primarily on the parents' and caregivers' perception of the benefits of scoliosis surgery, as many of the patients with neuromuscular conditions have severe learning and communication disabilities that prevent their participation in these surveys.

2.12 Conclusion

The development of a spinal deformity is a very common and possibly the most severe musculoskeletal condition affecting children with severe neurodisability or myopathic disorders. This can be in the form of scoliosis, often associated with increased kyphosis or lordosis and pelvic tilt. Surgical correction is indicated in the presence of a progressive deformity that produces functional limitations and severe symptoms, especially in growing children. This involves a major procedure with considerable risks of intraoperative and postoperative complications directly related to the severity of the deformity, as well as the presence of associated comorbidities and the degree of neurologic impairment. A thorough medical assessment is critical to establish the patient's suitability for such major surgery. A well-coordinated multidisciplinary approach will reduce the risks of major morbidity and mortality, which can occur either during scoliosis surgery (primarily related to excessive blood loss) or in the postoperative period (mainly due to pulmonary complications), as well as the risk of infection and generalized sepsis in patients with inherently poor immunological response. Prolonged postoperative recovery can be expected, and patients and their parents should be informed of the anticipated benefits and possible risks, with the decision for each patient being individualized. Deformity correction and spinal fusion should be performed only in major spinal centers with adequate medical support by well-trained surgeons who are familiar with the surgical techniques in order to minimize the risk of complications and produce an optimum outcome. The selection of operative technique and type of instrumentation depends on the experience of individual surgeons and aims to achieve adequate deformity correction while decreasing complication rates.

References

[1] Kalen V, Conklin MM, Sherman FC. Untreated scoliosis in severe cerebral palsy. J Pediatr Orthop. 1992; 12(3):337–340

[2] Comstock CP, Leach J, Wenger DR. Scoliosis in total-body-involvement cerebral palsy. Analysis of surgical treatment and patient and caregiver satisfaction. Spine. 1998; 23(12):1412–1424, discussion 1424–1425

[3] Madigan RR, Wallace SL. Scoliosis in the institutionalized cerebral palsy population. Spine. 1981; 6(6):583–590

[4] Letts M, Shapiro L, Mulder K, Klassen O. The windblown hip syndrome in total body cerebral palsy. J Pediatr Orthop. 1984; 4(1):55–62

[5] Tsirikos AI, Mains E. Surgical correction of spinal deformity in patients with cerebral palsy using pedicle screw instrumentation. J Spinal Disord Tech. 2012; 25(7):401–408

[6] Tsirikos AI, Lipton G, Chang WN, Dabney KW, Miller F. Surgical correction of scoliosis in pediatric patients with cerebral palsy using the unit rod instrumentation. Spine. 2008; 33(10):1133–1140

[7] Lonstein JE, Akbarnia A. Operative treatment of spinal deformities in patients with cerebral palsy or mental retardation. An analysis of one hundred and seven cases. J Bone Joint Surg Am. 1983; 65(1):43–55

[8] Labelle H, Tohmé S, Duhaime M, Allard P. Natural history of scoliosis in Friedreich's ataxia. J Bone Joint Surg Am. 1986; 68(4):564–572

[9] Tsirikos AI, Smith G. Scoliosis in patients with Friedreich's ataxia. J Bone Joint Surg Br. 2012; 94(5):684–689

[10] Chang TL, Sponseller PD, Kebaish KM, Fishman EK. Low profile pelvic fixation: anatomic parameters for sacral alar-iliac fixation versus traditional iliac fixation. Spine. 2009; 34(5):436–440

[11] Tsirikos AI, Saifuddin A, Noordeen MH. Spinal deformity in neurofibromatosis type-1: diagnosis and treatment. Eur Spine J. 2005; 14(5):427–439

[12] Miller A, Temple T, Miller F. Impact of orthoses on the rate of scoliosis progression in children with cerebral palsy. J Pediatr Orthop. 1996; 16(3):332–335

[13] Duckworth AD, Mitchell MJ, Tsirikos AI. Incidence and risk factors for postoperative complications in patients with Duchenne muscular dystrophy: a comparison with other neuromuscular conditions. Bone Joint J. 2014; 96-B (7):943–949

[14] Luque ER. Segmental spinal instrumentation for correction of scoliosis. Clin Orthop Relat Res. 1982(163):192–198

[15] Allen BL, Jr, Ferguson RL. L-rod instrumentation for scoliosis in cerebral palsy. J Pediatr Orthop. 1982; 2(1):87–96

[16] Gau YL, Lonstein JE, Winter RB, Koop S, Denis F. Luque-Galveston procedure for correction and stabilization of neuromuscular scoliosis and pelvic obliquity: a review of 68 patients. J Spinal Disord. 1991; 4(4):399–410

[17] Bell DF, Moseley CF, Koreska J. Unit rod segmental spinal instrumentation in the management of patients with progressive neuromuscular spinal deformity. Spine. 1989; 14(12):1301–1307

[18] Modi HN, Hong JY, Mehta SS, et al. Surgical correction and fusion using posterior-only pedicle screw construct for neuropathic scoliosis in patients with cerebral palsy: a three-year follow-up study. Spine. 2009; 34(11):1167–1175

[19] Teli M, Elsebaie H, Biant L, Noordeen H. Neuromuscular scoliosis treated by segmental third-generation instrumented spinal fusion. J Spinal Disord Tech. 2005; 18(5):430–438

[20] Teli MG, Cinnella P, Vincitorio F, Lovi A, Grava G, Brayda-Bruno M. Spinal fusion with Cotrel-Dubousset instrumentation for neuropathic scoliosis in patients with cerebral palsy. Spine. 2006; 31(14):E441–E447

[21] Karampalis C, Tsirikos AI. The surgical treatment of lordoscoliosis and hyperlordosis in patients with quadriplegic cerebral palsy. Bone Joint J. 2014; 96-B (6):800–806

[22] Tsirikos AI, Chang W-N, Dabney KW, Miller F. Comparison of one-stage versus two-stage anteroposterior spinal fusion in pediatric patients with cerebral palsy and neuromuscular scoliosis. Spine. 2003; 28(12):1300–1305

[23] Tsirikos AI, Chang WN, Dabney KW, Miller F, Glutting J. Life expectancy in pediatric patients with cerebral palsy and neuromuscular scoliosis who underwent spinal fusion. Dev Med Child Neurol. 2003; 45(10):677–682

[24] Tsirikos AI, Chang WN, Dabney KW, Miller F. Comparison of parents' and caregivers' satisfaction after spinal fusion in children with cerebral palsy. J Pediatr Orthop. 2004; 24(1):54–58

3 Idiopathic Spinal Deformities Treated with Spinal Osteotomies

Paul J. Park, Eduardo C. Beauchamp, Meghan Cerpa, Lawrence G. Lenke

Abstract

Various osteotomy techniques, combined with pedicle screw fixation, have greatly increased the amount of correction that can be obtained in all three planes in spinal deformity patients. The posterior column osteotomy, which involves releasing the posterior elements of spine, can be applied for a more gradual correction over multiple levels, and is most effective in patients with a flexible anterior column. In patients with stiffer, more angular deformities, the pedicle subtraction osteotomy (PSO) may be employed, addressing all three columns, and allowing for greater angular correction at a single level. Understanding these techniques, and when to use them, can greatly improve alignment in both the pediatric and adult spinal deformity patients.

Keywords: posterior column osteotomy, pedicle subtraction osteotomy, spinal deformity, scoliosis, kyphosis, revision spinal surgery

3.1 Introduction

With the advent of segmental, all-pedicle-screw constructs, increasingly complex scoliosis deformities have been corrected using varying forms of spinal osteotomies. Pedicle screws allow for three-column fixation and correction in three planes: coronal deformity, sagittal plane deformity, and axial rotation.[1,2] By preserving distal motion segments in some spinal deformities, decreased stress distal to the construct prevents further degeneration.[3,4,5] This level of control and strength in constructs, in combination with various osteotomy techniques, has been shown to be a powerful tool in adolescent idiopathic scoliosis (AIS) deformity correction. With the incorporation of partial facetectomies in scoliosis surgery, initially described by Hibbs and Moe as early as 1924,[6,7] the use of more advanced osteotomies has progressed rapidly in the past several decades and has been applied to increasingly complex deformities.

3.2 Posterior Column Osteotomy

First described by Smith-Petersen and colleagues in 1945, the use of corrective osteotomies in the posterior elements was seen in patients with ankylosing spondylitis (AS).[8] In the years following, several other authors performed posterior osteotomies in patients with ankylosing spondylitis (AS).[9,10,11] In these early years, surgeons were able to achieve sagittal corrections from 25 to 55 degrees.[12,13,14,15] In 1946, La Chapelle reported using a two-stage posterior wedge osteotomy, in which a second operation through an anterior approach was used to release the ossified anterior longitudinal ligament.[16] Another variation described by Adams in 1952 used a lateral approach to perform this osteotomy.[17] As spinal fusions became more common, the Smith-Petersen technique was expanded to patients who had had previous spinal fusions.[18] Meiss described a two-stage operation allowing for biplanar correction in patients with severe kyphoscoliosis.[18] Eventually, instrumented fixation was combined with these early osteotomy techniques to aid in osteotomy closure and postoperative stability; both McMaster and Bradford et al then described a combination with Harrington rods in the 1980s.[19,20] Ponte et al eventually adapted the technique to patients who had had no previous fusion in the setting of severe kyphotic deformity, such as Scheuermann kyphosis, involving a posterior release with complete facetectomies to allow for shortening of the posterior column and subsequent restoration of lordosis.[21,22,23] By the early 1990 s, lumbar pedicle screw fixation was gaining popularity and was also being combined with posterior osteotomies.[24,25] The use of pedicle screw fixation following spinal osteotomies was then described in the AIS patient in the late 1990 s by Shufflebarger.[26,27] Often called Smith-Petersen osteotomies in patients with previous spinal fusion (i.e., AS), the same technique in an unfused spine is referred to as a Ponte osteotomy; hereafter these techniques will be interchangeably referred to as a posterior column osteotomy (PCO).

3.2.1 Indications in Idiopathic Deformity

In patients with idiopathic scoliosis, for each 1 mm resected in a PCO a corresponding sagittal correction of approximately 1 degree is seen.[28,29] This amount of correction is possible when there is significant healthy disk anteriorly and 5 mm in height without osteophyte bridging.[30] As such, a collapsed disk or prior previous arthrodesis may significantly limit the amount of correction attainable.[31] Whereas in AS the anterior release can be achieved by osteoclasis, either indirectly by positioning or by a two-stage procedure with an anterior approach, in the idiopathic patient the amount of correction hinges on the "give" or health of the disk anteriorly. This can be combined with PCOs at multiple levels to achieve greater segmental deformity correction. Aside from benefits in the sagittal plane, the PCO provides increased flexibility to allow for coronal correction and derotation as well. A cadaveric biomechanical study assessing range of motion with three sequential PCOs showed increases of up to 69% in flexion, 56% in extension, and 65% in axial rotation.[32] The PCO is particularly applicable to AIS in that it allows for lordosis to be increased in the lumbar spine, whereas a thoracic PCO allows for increase of kyphosis by distraction. In AS, the closing wedge osteotomy allows for increased lordosis; on the other hand, the complete and extensive posterior release of the PCO gives correction to the hypokyphotic thoracic curves often seen in patients with AIS.

A study by Shah et al reviewed 87 AIS patients with Lenke type 1–4 curves undergoing PCOs for curve correction and found a significant improvement in Cobb angle, as well as apical vertebral translation over 2 years.[33] Of note, they also found significant increases in T5–T12 kyphosis.[33] A recent multicenter retrospective study by Samdani et al looked at 191 patients with Lenke 1A and 1B curve types who underwent PCOs (average 4.3 levels per patient). Curve correction was similar between the osteotomy and control groups; however, there was a significantly higher level of lordosis and stiffness and better Cobb angle correction at 2 years postoperatively in the osteotomy group, along with a corresponding increase in T5–T12 kyphosis and rib hump prominence, illustrating the power of the three-dimensional plane correction of the PCO.[34] Demura et al reviewed 26 patients with Lenke type 1 or 2 curves and found significant correction in the coronal, sagittal (thoracic kyphosis), and axial rotational plane as seen by rib hump prominence as well.[35] The authors describe a multifactorial approach to support the PCO by increasing the strength of the construct using differential rod overcontouring combined with uniplanar screws and stiff steel rods.[35]

3.2.2 Technique

The patient is positioned prone on the operating table with the abdomen free and all bony prominences well padded. Neurophysiologic monitoring baseline data are obtained prior to starting the case. Selection of osteotomy levels is based on the apex and flexibility of the deformity. In idiopathic deformity, PCOs are more commonly performed in the thoracic spine. Standard subperiosteal dissection is performed to expose the spine with electrocautery, out to the transverse processes at each level. Careful hemostasis is maintained throughout every step of the osteotomy. Facetectomies are performed to remove the inferior articular process, exposing the superior articular process of the distal vertebra ventrally. Soft tissues and interspinous ligaments between the levels of the osteotomy are removed. The spinous process of the vertebra just cephalad to the osteotomy site is removed to expose the underlying ligamentum flavum. The midportion of the ligamentum flavum is carefully removed with a Leksell rongeur to gain access to the epidural space. Once the epidural space is visualized, a Woodson elevator can be carefully introduced into the epidural space to separate the dura from the ligamentum or bony structures. This maneuver is extremely helpful in revision cases where the dura may be adhered to adjacent structures. A Kerrison rongeur is then used to remove the ligamentum flavum and superior articular process from medial to lateral, toward the intervertebral foramen. The Woodson elevator is used to palpate the superior and medial aspect of the pedicle as well as the intervertebral foramen to avoid inadvertent extension of the osteotomy into the pedicle. The bone in the concavity of the deformity may become thicker and sclerotic, making its resection with a Kerrison rongeur difficult. In these cases, a high-speed bur may be used to thin down or remove the sclerotic bone while carefully protecting the dura with a Woodson elevator. Epidural hemostasis is maintained with the use of bipolar cautery, hemostatic matrix, and cottonoids. The osteotomy proceeds laterally and cranially, assuming a chevron-like configuration. Throughout the osteotomy, care should be taken to keep the wedge resection symmetrical unless coronal plane correction is desired. In cases with significant rotation, the osteotomy should be greater on the convex side in order to avoid decompensation in the coronal plane with osteotomy closure. The same procedure is performed in each predetermined osteotomy level. The osteotomies are undercut to prevent subsequent compression during the closure. Pedicle screw fixation is obtained using the freehand technique. Rods are placed and corrective maneuvers are performed. In cases of severe kyphosis where multiple PCOs are required, we consider placing a contralateral temporary rod as to avoid distraction and stretching of the cord once the osteotomies are completed. It is imperative to inspect the dura during and after closure to avoid inadvertent impingement. With multiple PCOs a gradual harmonious correction in both sagittal and coronal planes can be achieved.

3.2.3 Case Illustration

The patient is a 62-year-old woman with a history of adult idiopathic scoliosis with thoracic and lumbar degeneration. The patient presented with increasing back pain, exacerbated by sitting and standing. On physical examination she stood with a noticeable right thoracolumbar trunk shift and had a normal neurologic exam. Upright posteroanterior and lateral radiographs demonstrated a 70-degree thoracolumbar scoliosis curve, a 46-degree fractional lumbosacral curve, and subluxation of L3 and L4. The sagittal plane showed a 56-degree thoracic kyphosis and 30 degrees of lumbar lordosis. There was moderate correction of the deformity seen in the supine position on comparison between standing and supine films (▶ Fig. 3.1). Bone density examination revealed osteopenia. A posterior spinal instrumented fusion from T2 to S1 with an L5–S1 transforaminal interbody fusion was performed. Multiple apical PCOs were performed to achieve harmonious correction in both the coronal and the sagittal plane without the need for a three-column osteotomy (▶ Fig. 3.2). Bilateral S2 alar-iliac screws and a right-sided formal iliac screw were used to obtain sacral pelvic fixation and maintain correction. Restoration of both coronal and sagittal alignment was achieved with complete resolution of her symptoms and evidence of stable alignment and fixation at 10 months postoperatively (▶ Fig. 3.3).

3.3 Pedicle Subtraction Osteotomy

For severe deformity, more powerful osteotomy techniques have been described. The pedicle subtraction osteotomy (PSO) begins with a PCO, then progresses to the removal of the entire posterior elements and ligaments and a portion of the superior vertebral body anteriorly for greater flexibility and three-column deformity correction. As described previously, the limiting factor of the PCO ends up being the anterior column—the PSO attempts to address this and eliminate the need for a higher-risk anterior approach.[33,36] The additional benefit of the PSO is that it allows for significant coronal correction as well. Earlier iterations of the PSO, described as an eggshell procedure for the way the vertebral body is hollowed out,[35] included a controlled fracture of the anterior cortex. In 1985 Thomasen first described the PSO as a circumferential wedge excision to provide additional lordosis.[37] Similarly to the development of PCOs, a PSO was initially developed for fixed sagittal deformity in AS patients.[37] This excision creates a large foramen for two

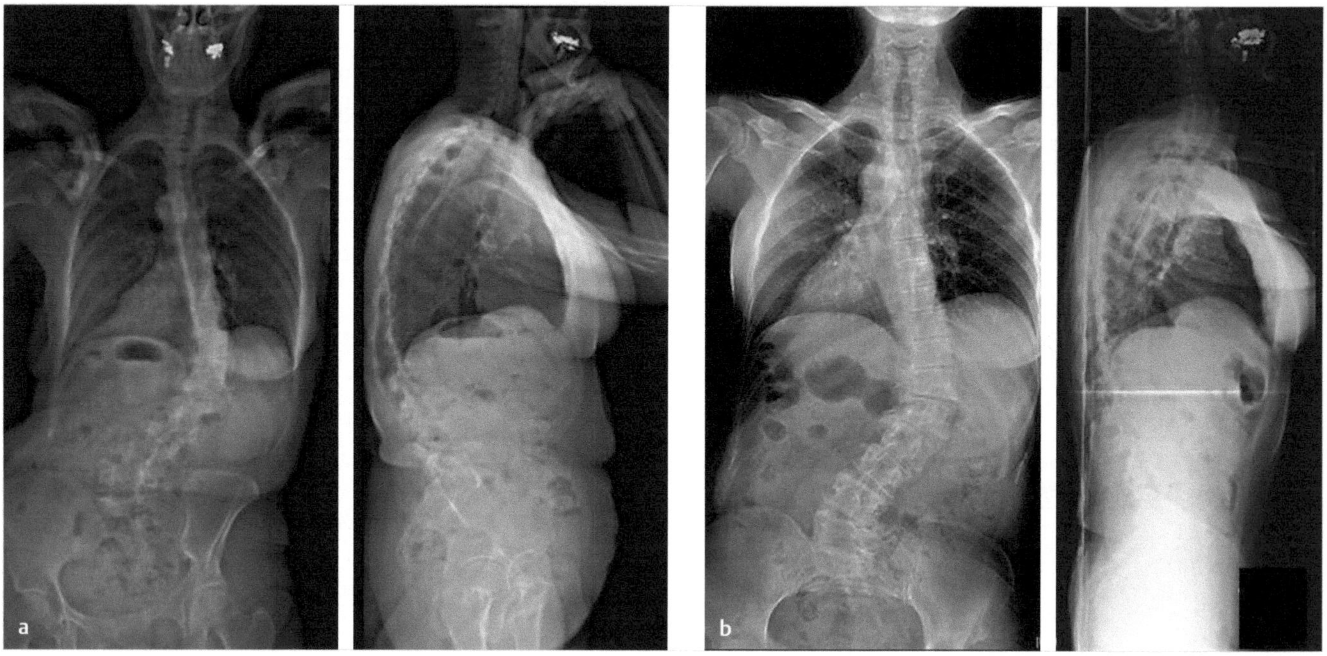

Fig. 3.1 **(a)** Standing and **(b)** supine preoperative full-spine radiographs. There is adequate correction of the deformity in the sagittal plane with the patient lying supine, whereas the coronal plane deformity remains fairly rigid **(b)**.

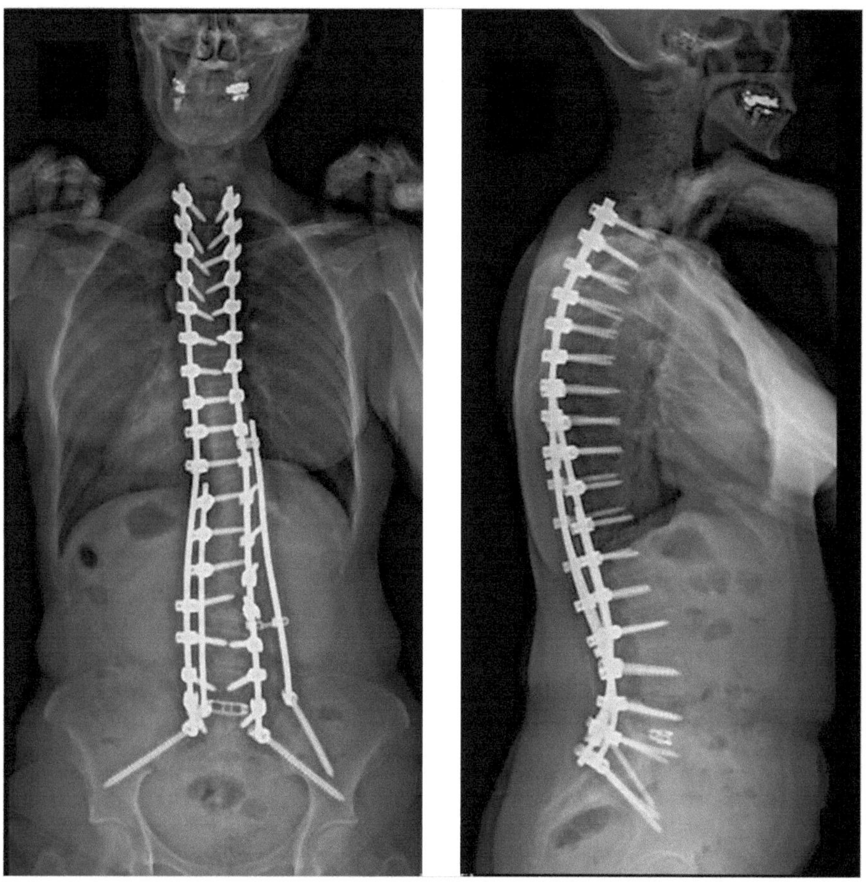

Fig. 3.2 One year postoperative radiographs after a T 2–sacrum posterior instrumented spinal fusion with multiple posterior column osteotomies (PCOs) due to adult idiopathic scoliosis. Even with a rigid coronal and sagittal deformity, a significant amount of correction in both planes is obtained with multilevel sequential PCOs.

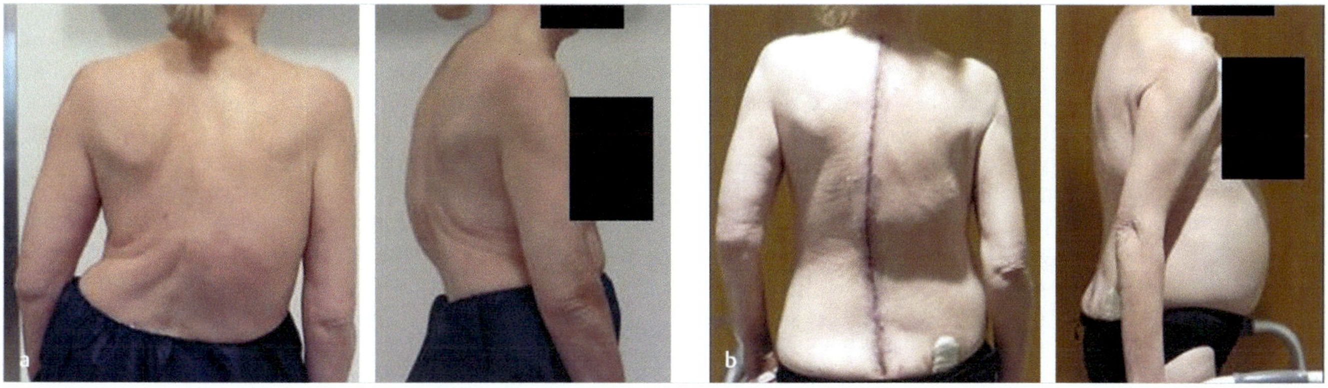

Fig. 3.3 (a) Preoperative and (b) postoperative clinical images.

levels of exiting nerve roots, to prevent neural compression and also to increase cancellous bone contact and fusion.[38,39] By including the cephalad disk an "extended PSO" can be performed to allow for even greater deformity correction and to procure an anterior arthrodesis of the cephalad motion segment of a PSO (i. e., L 3–L 4 disk for an L 4 PSO).

3.3.1 Indications in Idiopathic Deformity

The PSO's main goal is to relieve hypolordotic or frank kyphotic deformities in the thoracolumbar and lumbar spine. These hypolordotic deformities are commonly seen as a result of Harrington distraction and instrumentation, thoracolumbar fractures, or a previous laminectomy that caused rigid lumbar kyphosis. A PSO allows for significantly more posterior closure than a single PCO. A one-level PSO has been shown to allow for almost 30 to 40 degrees of lumbar lordosis production, specifically in patients with severe fixed sagittal plane deformities and a positive sagittal imbalance of greater than 12 cm.[29,40,41,42,43,44,45,46] The PSO is ideally performed at a level caudad to the conus medullaris to prevent neurologic complications.[47] Understanding the appropriate role for multiple PCOs versus a single PSO has been an ongoing question that is answered mainly by anterior flexibility in the setting of AS, revision AIS fusions, and adults with previous fusions or flatback deformities from previous Harrington rods.[29,48]

3.3.2 Technique

The patient is positioned prone on a Jackson table with the hips extended to allow for lumbar lordosis. Neurophysiologic monitoring baseline data are obtained prior to starting the case. Adequate exposure is obtained by the standard subperiosteal technique. Pedicle screws are placed spanning two to three levels above and below the PSO site for proper control following the osteotomy. PSOs have traditionally been performed at L 2 or L 3; hence, fixation often spans from T 10 to the pelvis. However, many surgeons are now doing these at L 4 or L 5, where more lordosis normally resides. In addition, the more distal osteotomy provides a greater degree of global sagittal rebalancing.

Inferior facetectomies are performed at the level of the PSO and the level above. Pedicle preparatory holes at the level of the osteotomy are placed to aid in orientation. The PSO begins similarly to the PCO, except for the addition of a central laminectomy. The central laminectomy is extended from the inferior aspect of the pedicle above to the superior aspect of the pedicle below, completely visualizing the thecal sac. This permits adequate visualization of the dura during eventual closure of the osteotomy. The laminectomy is subsequently widened laterally to expose the exiting nerve roots. The ascending articular process of and cranial portion of the pedicle are removed using a Leksell rongeur. A Kerrison rongeur is then used to remove the bone along the inferior margin of the pedicle cephalad to the PSO, removing all ligamentum flavum and thereby allowing visualization of the superiorly exiting nerve root. This is often kept in a tuft of perineural fat to keep the nerve root from entering the field of the PSO.

The lateral exposure of the vertebral body begins with the dissociation of the transverse process with the lateral pedicle using a high-speed drill. A Penfield elevator is then used to dissect a subperiosteal plane along the lateral vertebral wall. Segmental vessels should be dissected away laterally; the soft tissue and any residual bleeding are addressed with bipolar electrocautery, hemostatic matrix, packing, and bone wax. The dissection is brought anteriorly along the vertebral body until the body is ventral, while only partially exposing the intervertebral disks above and below the PSO level. Malleable retractors may then be placed anterior to the vertebral body to expose the lateral vertebral body, without placing excess tension on the exiting nerve roots—one must be conscious of how long the retractors are in place. Sponges are inserted laterally in this newly created space to maintain the area once the retractors are removed. Often, for L 4 and L 5 PSOs, we will not expose the lateral body but will instead decancellate the entire body through the pedicles while also thinning out the lateral vertebral walls from the inside out.

Attention is then turned back to the pedicles previously exposed. A curet is placed in the established pedicle hole into the cancellous bone of the vertebral body. This bone is subsequently removed, and the pedicle is then resected to lie flush with the posterior vertebral body. The pedicle resection is then expanded to confirm that the exiting nerve root at the PSO level is free. A temporary unilateral rod is then placed to prevent premature closure posteriorly during decancellation of the contralateral side. The lateral retractors are replaced, and the sponge packing is then removed. A nerve root retractor is then used to pull the thecal sac medially as an osteotome is used to cut a wedge-shaped osteotomy in the lateral vertebral wall. The shape of these osteotomies will vary, depending on the desired sagittal and coronal correction. The remainder of the vertebral body cancellous bone can then be removed, using curets, up to the anterior vertebral cortex and posterior body wall. A high-speed drill is then used to remove the anterior vertebral body cortex to the lateral aspect of the anterior longitudinal ligament. The rod is switched to the ipsilateral side, and the contralateral rod is removed. The posterior vertebral body wall is then addressed. The thecal sac is carefully circumferentially freed and separated from the posterior longitudinal ligament and the epidural venous complex with a Woodson elevator. A curved, reverse-angle curet, Kerrison rongeur, or specialized posterior wall impactor is then used to remove the posterior vertebral wall.

Finally, osteotomy closure is performed. With bilateral temporary rods in place, the set screws are released. There are several ways to perform the closure either alone or in conjunction with other methods: manual reduction, using a lordotically contoured rod to cantilever across the PSO, hyperextending the chest and lower extremities, or gentle compression between screws. To relieve focal stress across one bone–screw interface, temporary rods may be placed above and below the PSO and compressed to each other using a domino connector. Once the closure is complete, the thecal sac and nerve roots are carefully examined with the Woodson and Penfield elevators. If sufficient posterior decompression and a wide laminectomy were performed initially, this should allow for dural redundancy and prevent possible impingement during this step. Any additional bone needs to be removed in order to allow space for the neural elements.

3.3.3 Case Illustration

The patient is a 54-year-old woman with a history of previous L4–L5 decompression with posterolateral and interbody fusion 11 years prior. She is now presenting with progressive back and leg pain. The patient's chief complaint was slow deterioration of her posture over the last 5 years with an inability to remain standing or walk for prolonged periods of time (▶ Fig. 3.4). She had tried multiple nonsurgical interventions, including physical therapy, thoracolumbar orthoses, and epidural injections, among others, none of which provided relief of her symptoms. Upright posteroanterior and lateral radiographs (▶ Fig. 3.5) as well three-dimensional CT reconstruction (▶ Fig. 3.6) show a fixed coronal and sagittal deformity. There is a global thoracolumbar kyphosis of 49 degrees with a positive sagittal balance of 20 cm. In the coronal plane there is a 24-degree thoracic, a 32-degree lumbar scoliosis, and a coronal imbalance of 9 cm. Due to the fixed kyphotic deformity and fused lower lumbar segment, the decision was made to perform an extended PSO at L4. This allowed for significant correction of her lumbar lordosis through a three-column osteotomy. PCOs were performed at the remaining flexible lumbar segments (▶ Fig. 3.7) and a posterior instrumented spinal fusion from T4 to the sacrum with iliac instrumentation was performed. Excellent restoration of both coronal and sagittal alignment was achieved with complete resolution of her symptoms and evidence of stable alignment and fixation at 1 year postoperatively (▶ Fig. 3.8).

3.4 Preoperative Considerations and Postoperative Complications

The increased flexibility and curve correction afforded by osteotomies are powerful tools; however, careful consideration must be given to determine the appropriate treatment for each patient. The potential for increased blood loss, increased operating time, proximity of dissection to the nerve roots and spinal cord, along with increased importance of construct fixation and stability are all factors one must consider with corrective osteotomies. It is critical to have an experienced neuromonitoring team throughout these cases because neuromonitoring changes are increased in patients undergoing osteotomy,[49] as well as an anesthesia team to maintain specific mean arterial pressure (MAP) goals throughout different portions of the case.[50] The anesthesia team needs to be well versed in the medications used so that the neuromonitoring results will not be masked or produce false readings, as the level of sedation and paralysis may affect these measures.

3.4.1 PCO versus PSO

The decision to perform PCOs versus PSOs depends on several factors. As global sagittal imbalances become more severe and stiffer there is a natural progression in technique from a less extensive (PCO) to a more extensive osteotomy (PSO). As such, flexibility is a major deciding factor that needs to be assessed with imaging and a physical exam. On average, a PCO allows for 10 degrees of curve correction per level, whereas a PSO allows for approximately 30 degrees per level. A recent study by Cho et al found three PCOs had similar sagittal correction to one PSO, though this was in a retrospective study in which the preoperative sagittal imbalance was significantly greater in the PSO group.[29] The study also found similar operative times for the two surgeries, however the blood loss was substantially greater in the PSO group. Therefore, additional considerations include understanding the patient's reserve and what type of intraoperative blood loss the patient could tolerate safely.[29]

Osteotomies work in two different ways; patients with AIS or adult thoracic idiopathic scoliosis often have hypokyphotic sagittal curves, in which a posterior release is more useful rather than a closing wedge to elongate the posterior column. PCOs tend to work better for smoother, rounded scoliotic or kyphotic curves. When considering an osteotomy in the lumbar or tho-

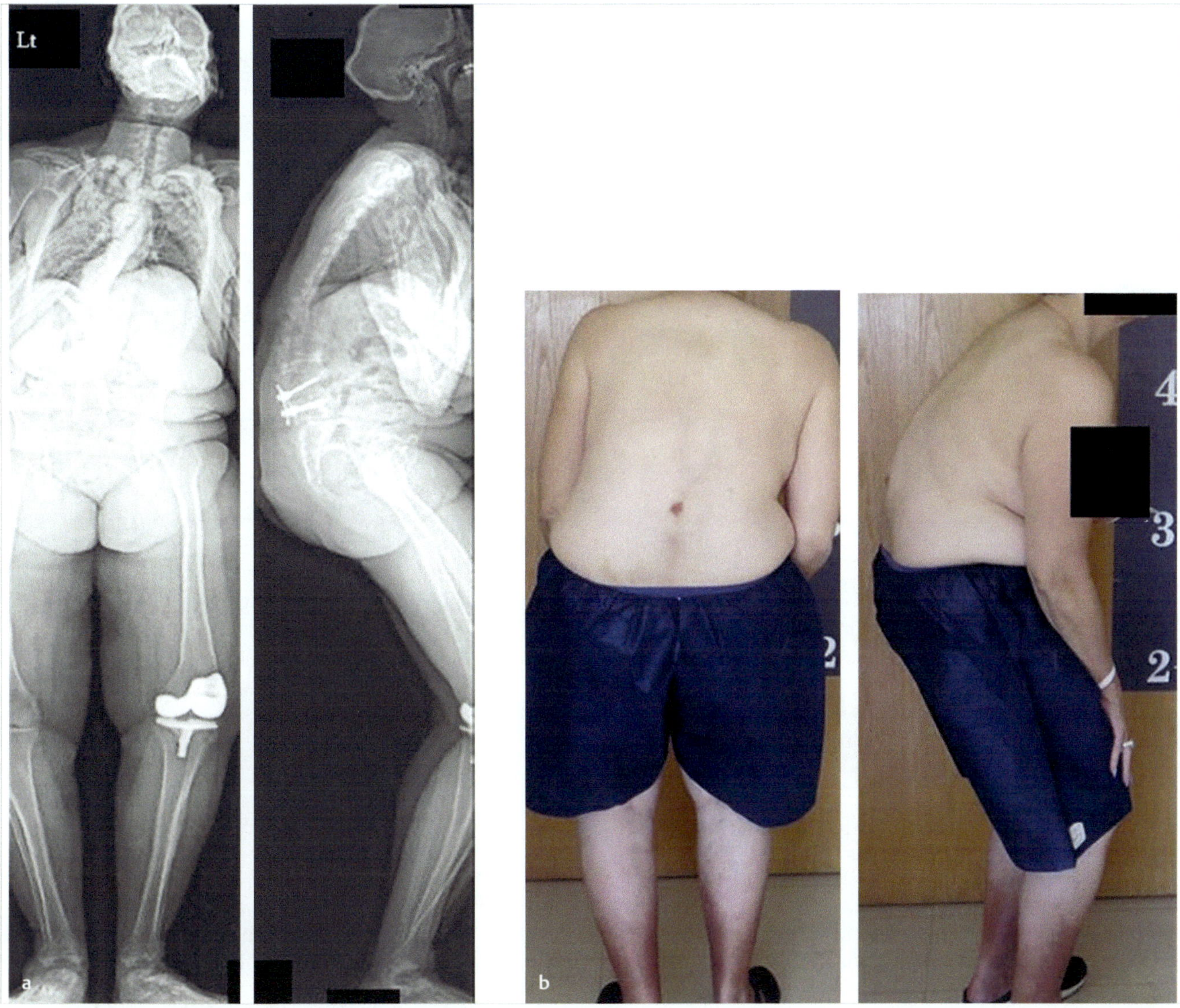

Fig. 3.4 **(a)** Preoperative radiographs and **(b)** clinical images demonstrating a fixed coronal and sagittal imbalance. The patient is trying to compensate for her sagittal imbalance by retroverting her pelvis and flexing her knees.

racic spine, one must also consider the location of the thecal sac. In the thoracic spine, PSOs become more difficult because they necessitate rib resection to provide anterior exposure of the lateral aspects of the vertebral bodies; this is also important so as not to retract the thecal sac too aggressively. One must also consider the higher risk and more severe complications of working around the spinal cord in the thoracic spine versus the cauda equina more caudally. In AIS and adult idiopathic scoliotic patients, there is often a larger and stiffer coronal plane deformity that also requires correction; using an uneven PSO wedge osteotomy can allow for major coronal plane corrections, which may alternatively be more applicable, depending on the curve. PSOs also require fixation both proximally and distally to control the spine once the osteotomy has been corrected. If the PSO level required is lower in the lumbar spine it may be difficult to achieve adequate fixation distally unless one obtains multiple sacral/iliac fixation points.

3.4.2 Complications

As with any procedure, infection and bleeding are major complications that can be associated with these surgeries, especially in relation to the extent of the osteotomies. With the extensive bony and ligamentous dissection required to perform PSOs, dural tears and the potential for nerve injury become even more relevant, stressing the importance of proper neuromonitoring. With PSOs in particular, the amount of bone being resected gives rise to subluxation of the spine as a possible complication, potentially resulting in neurologic deficit that is not often seen in PCOs. The closure of the PSO may also result in dural buckling. These complications appear to happen with more regularity at L4–L5 rather than at L2–L3.[29] Finally, with increased bone removal and instability, implant failure and loss of correction are always considerations given the increased amount of correction and the forces the instrumentation will be

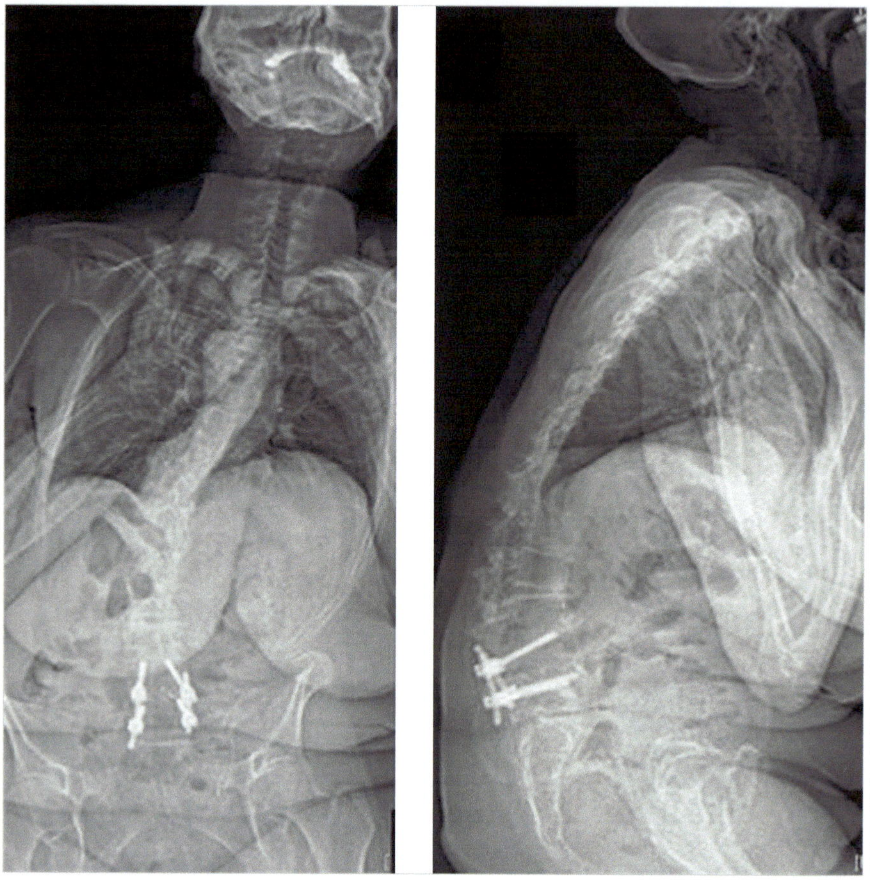

Fig. 3.5 Preoperative posteroanterior and lateral radiographs showing a fixed coronal and sagittal imbalance with a posterolateral and interbody fusion at L4–L5.

working against. Because of the inherent instability with PSOs, it has become commonplace to use multiple rods (typically three to five) spanning the PSO site. Although this hasn't completely eliminated implant failure or pseudarthrosis across PSO sites in the lumbar spine, the occurrence is markedly lessened.[43] With increased mobility of the spine there is a real risk of stretch or compression of the spinal cord and cauda equina; thus it is important to increase the central canal as well as exiting neuroforamina.[17,22,41]

Coronal decompensation is a complex concept that also needs to be addressed for PCOs and PSOs in the setting of idiopathic scoliosis.[46,51] Scoliosis is a complex, three-dimensional deformity where the apex of the coronal curve often correlates with axial rotation, in which the vertebral body rotates toward the convexity and the posterior spine is rotated to the concavity. When performing a PCO or PSO, one is ultimately either shortening the posterior elements to increase lordosis or lengthening the posterior elements to increase kyphosis. As a result, in the coronal plane there is preferential lengthening due to rotation as well (if the osteotomy is performed symmetrically). Berven et al found an average coronal imbalance correction of 1.8 cm (2.9 cm average coronal imbalance preoperatively).[52] In theory, with the larger resection of bone involved in a PSO, one would expect a preexisting coronal decompensation to be more pronounced. Options for addressing this would include an asymmetrical wedge osteotomy in which more bone is resected on the convex side, or, preferably, to perform the osteotomies at neutral vertebra.

The benefit in idiopathic deformity is that patients are often otherwise healthy, and their neural axis can tolerate the large amount of manipulation that occurs with osteotomies. However, the ultimate goal of any deformity correction is still fusion, optimized with (near) bone-on-bone contact. To ensure that this occurs, in multilevel PCO and PSO surgery in adults we attempt to span the osteotomy site with an autologous strut of local bone (from a different area of fusion in a revision or congenital setting); we may even use allograft ribs or tibia for this same purpose.

3.5 Conclusions

As fixation techniques and technology have advanced over the past several decades, the utility of osteotomies to address highly complex spinal deformities has increased. Initially, these methods developed out of necessity while addressing the fixed sagittal deformities seen in patients with AS. The ability to restore lumbar lordosis played a critical role in helping these patients achieve sagittal realignment, improved posture, and forward gaze. Over time, however, the techniques have been applied to the thoracic spine as well, allowing for improvement in hypokyphotic curves seen frequently in AIS and adult idiopathic scoliosis. As such, the PCO and PSO, and varying combinations of the two techniques, have become versatile and useful tools when treating idiopathic scoliosis and other related spinal deformities, allowing for increased flexibility and correction in all three planes.

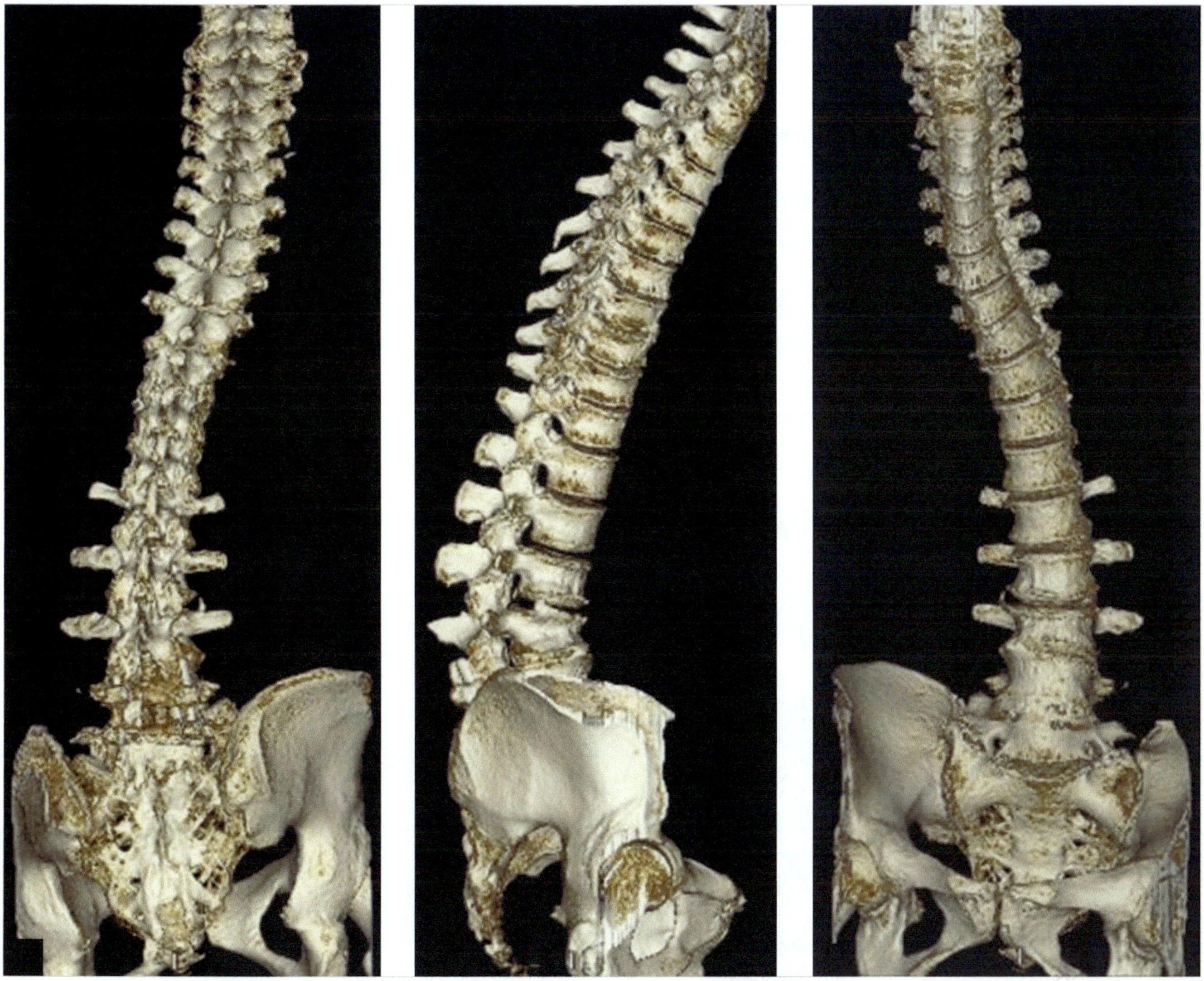

Fig. 3.6 Three-dimensional CT reconstructions reveal a completely fused and rigid L 4–L 5 segment and minimal passive correction of the sagittal and coronal deformity while lying supine.

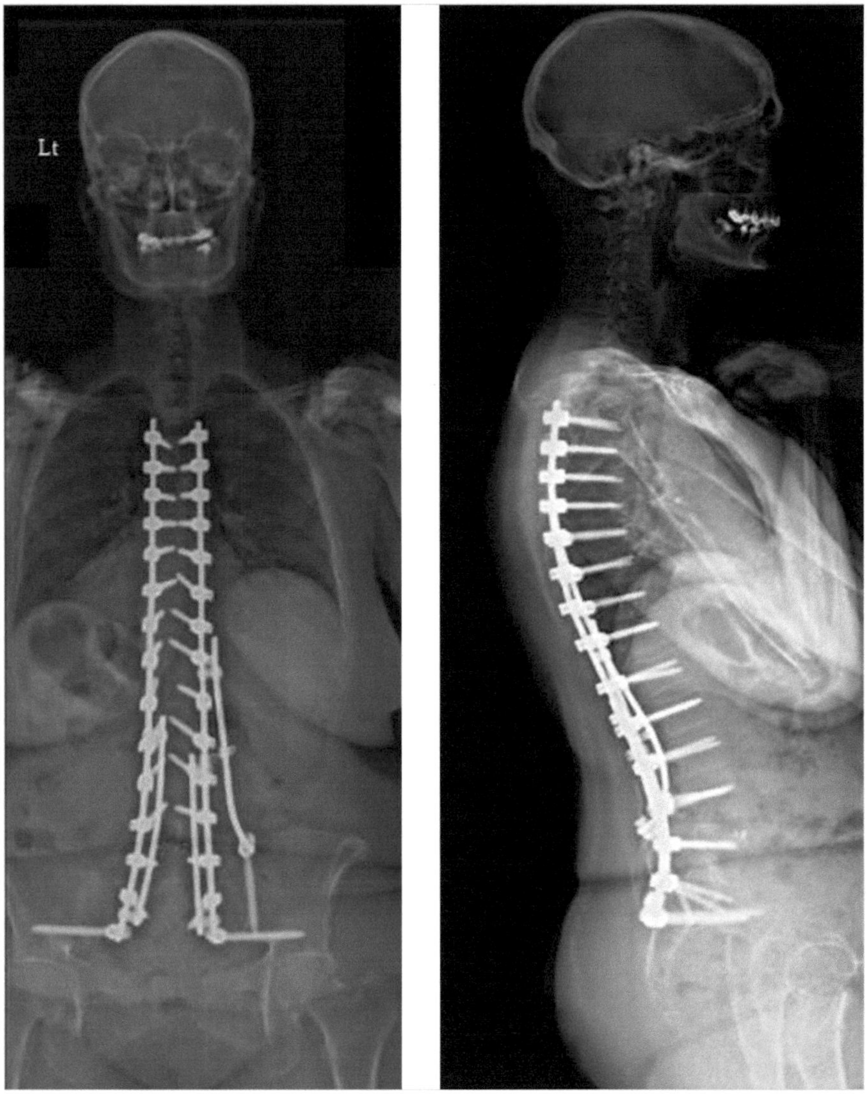

Fig. 3.7 One-year postoperative radiographs after a T4 to sacrum posterior instrumented spinal fusion with and extended L4 pedicle subtraction osteotomy and multiple posterior column osteotomies. Four rods were placed spanning the osteotomy site and a "Kick-stand" pelvic instrumentation was used to correct the rigid pelvic obliquity.

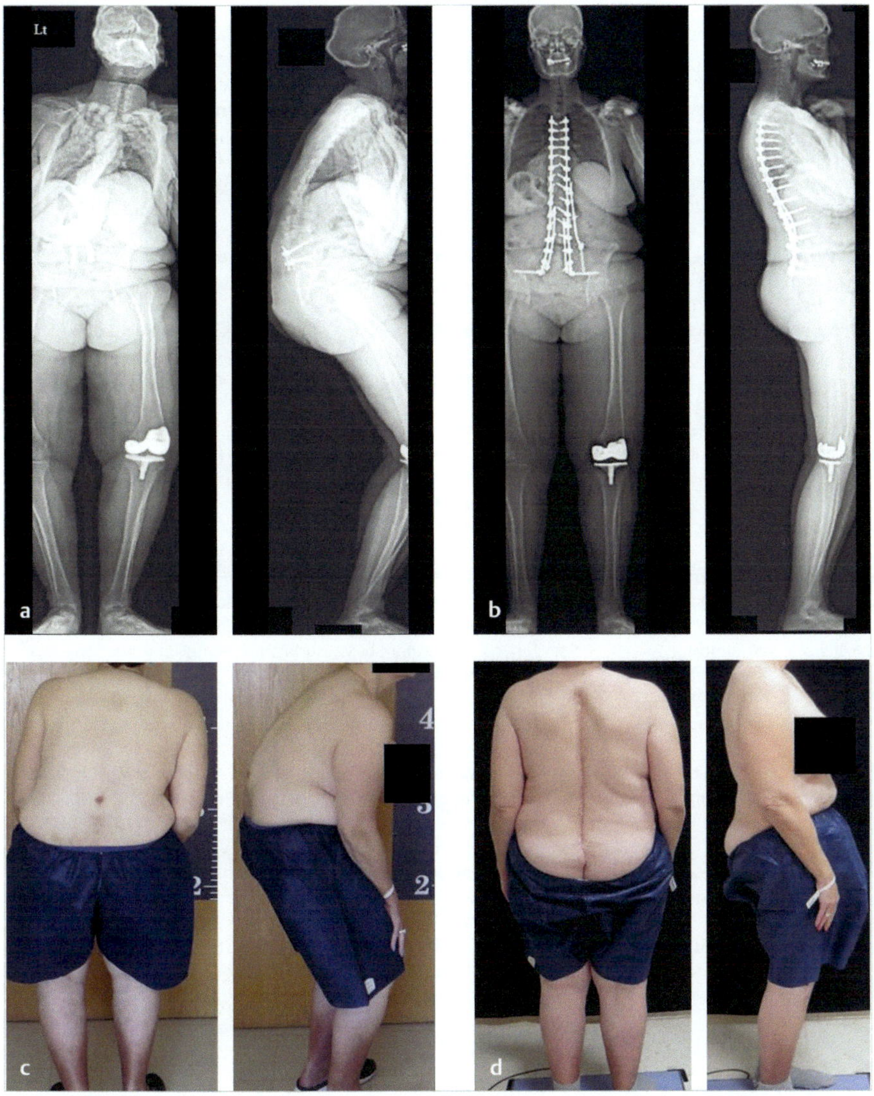

Fig. 3.8 **(a)** Preoperative and **(b)** 1 year postoperative full-body radiographs. Notice the lordosis obtained on the previously fused L4–L5 segment **(b)**. **(c)** Preoperative and **(d)** 1 year postoperative clinical images showing excellent restoration of her sagittal and coronal balance.

References

[1] Kuklo TR, Potter BK, Polly DW, Jr, Lenke LG. Monaxial versus multiaxial thoracic pedicle screws in the correction of adolescent idiopathic scoliosis. Spine. 2005; 30(18):2113–2120

[2] Lee SM, Suk SI, Chung ER. Direct vertebral rotation: a new technique of three-dimensional deformity correction with segmental pedicle screw fixation in adolescent idiopathic scoliosis. Spine. 2004; 29(3):343–349

[3] Suk SI, Lee CK, Kim WJ, Chung YJ, Park YB. Segmental pedicle screw fixation in the treatment of thoracic idiopathic scoliosis. Spine. 1995; 20(12):1399–1405

[4] Liljenqvist U, Lepsien U, Hackenberg L, Niemeyer T, Halm H. Comparative analysis of pedicle screw and hook instrumentation in posterior correction and fusion of idiopathic thoracic scoliosis. Eur Spine J. 2002; 11(4):336–343

[5] Kim YJ, Lenke LG, Kim J, et al. Comparative analysis of pedicle screw versus hybrid instrumentation in posterior spinal fusion of adolescent idiopathic scoliosis. Spine. 2006; 31(3):291–298

[6] Hibbs RA. A report of fifty-nine cases of scoliosis treated by the fusion operation. J Bone Joint Surg Am. 1924; 6:3–34

[7] Moe JH. A critical analysis of methods of fusion for scoliosis; an evaluation in two hundred and sixty-six patients. J Bone Joint Surg Am. 1958; 40-A (3):529–554, passim

[8] Smith-Petersen MN, Larson CB, Aufranc OE. Osteotomy of the spine for correction of flexion deformity in rheumatoid arthritis. J Bone Joint Surg Am. 1945; 27:1–11

[9] Herbert JJ. Vertebral osteotomy; technique, indications and results. J Bone Joint Surg Am. 1948; 30A(3):680–689

[10] McMaster PE. Osteotomy of the spine for correction of fixed flexion deformity. AMA Arch Surg. 1958; 76(4):603–610

[11] Sotelo-Ortiz F. Results of osteotomy of the spine according to the type of curvature. Surg Gynecol Obstet. 1958; 107(1):47–54

[12] Alexander WA. Lumbar spinal osteotomy. J Bone Joint Surg Br. 1959; 41-B (2):270–278

[13] Goel MK. Vertebral osteotomy for correction of fixed flexion deformity of the spine. J Bone Joint Surg Am. 1968; 50(2):287–294

[14] Emnéus H. Wedge osteotomy of spine in ankylosing spondylitis. Acta Orthop Scand. 1968; 39(3):321–326

[15] Camargo FP, Cordeiro EN, Napoli MMM. Corrective osteotomy of the spine in ankylosing spondylitis. Experience with 66 cases. Clin Orthop Relat Res. 1986 (208):157–167

[16] La Chapelle EH. Osteotomy of the lumbar spine for correction of kyphosis in a case of ankylosing spondylarthritis. J Bone Joint Surg Am. 1946; 28(4):851–858

[17] Adams JC. Technique, dangers and safeguards in osteotomy of the spine. J Bone Joint Surg Br. 1952; 34-B(2):226–232

[18] Meiss WC. Spinal osteotomy following fusion for paralytic scoliosis. J Bone Joint Surg Am. 1955; 37-A(1):73–77

[19] McMaster MJ. A technique for lumbar spinal osteotomy in ankylosing spondylitis. J Bone Joint Surg Br. 1985; 67(2):204–210

[20] Bradford DS, Schumacher WL, Lonstein JE, Winter RB. Ankylosing spondylitis: experience in surgical management of 21 patients. Spine. 1987; 12(3):238–243

[21] Ponte A, Vero B, Siccardi GL. Surgical treatment of Scheuermann's hyperkyphosis. In: Winter RB, ed. Kyphosis (Progress in Spinal Pathology). Bologna, Italy: Aulo Gaggi; 1984:75–80

[22] Ponte A. Posterior column shortening for Scheuermann's kyphosis: an innovative one-stage technique. In: Haher T, Merola A, eds. Surgical Techniques for the Spine. 1st ed. New York: Thieme; 2003:107–113

[23] Geck MJ, Macagno A, Ponte A, Shufflebarger HL. The Ponte procedure: posterior only treatment of Scheuermann's kyphosis using segmental posterior shortening and pedicle screw instrumentation. J Spinal Disord Tech. 2007; 20 (8):586–593

[24] Hehne HJ, Zielke K, Böhm H. Polysegmental lumbar osteotomies and transpedicled fixation for correction of long-curved kyphotic deformities in ankylosing spondylitis. Report on 177 cases. Clin Orthop Relat Res. 1990(258):49–55

[25] van Royen BJ, de Kleuver M, Slot GH. Polysegmental lumbar posterior wedge osteotomies for correction of kyphosis in ankylosing spondylitis. Eur Spine J. 1998; 7(2):104–110

[26] Shufflebarger HL, Clark CE. Effect of wide posterior release on correction in adolescent idiopathic scoliosis. J Pediatr Orthop B. 1998; 7(2):117–123

[27] Shufflebarger HL, Geck MJ, Clark CE. The posterior approach for lumbar and thoracolumbar adolescent idiopathic scoliosis: posterior shortening and pedicle screws. Spine. 2004; 29(3):269–276, discussion 276

[28] Gill JB, Levin A, Burd T, Longley M. Corrective osteotomies in spine surgery. J Bone Joint Surg Am. 2008; 90(11):2509–2520

[29] Cho KJ, Bridwell KH, Lenke LG, Berra A, Baldus C. Comparison of Smith-Petersen versus pedicle subtraction osteotomy for the correction of fixed sagittal imbalance. Spine. 2005; 30(18):2030–2037, discussion 2038

[30] Bridwell KH. Osteotomies for fixed deformities in the thoracic and lumbar spine. In: Bridwell KH, Dewald RL, eds. The Textbook of Spinal Surgery. 2nd ed. Philadelphia, PA: Lippincott-Raven, 1997:821–835

[31] Macagno AE, O'Brien MF. Thoracic and thoracolumbar kyphosis in adults. Spine. 2006; 31(19) Suppl:S161–S170

[32] Sangiorgio SN, Borkowski SL, Bowen RE, Scaduto AA, Frost NL, Ebramzadeh E. Quantification of Increase in Three-dimensional Spine Flexibility Following Sequential Ponte Osteotomies in a Cadaveric Model. Spine Deform. 2013; 1 (3):171–178

[33] Shah SA, Dhawale AA, Oda JE, et al. Ponte Osteotomies With Pedicle Screw Instrumentation in the Treatment of Adolescent Idiopathic Scoliosis. Spine Deform. 2013; 1(3):196–204

[34] Samdani AF, Bennett JT, Singla AR, et al. Do Ponte Osteotomies Enhance Correction in Adolescent Idiopathic Scoliosis? An Analysis of 191 Lenke 1A and 1B Curves. Spine Deform. 2015; 3(5):483–488

[35] Demura S, Yaszay B, Carreau JH, et al. Maintenance of Thoracic Kyphosis in the 3D Correction of Thoracic Adolescent Idiopathic Scoliosis Using Direct Vertebral Derotation. Spine Deform. 2013; 1(1):46–50

[36] Shamji MF, Isaacs RE. Anterior-only approaches to scoliosis. Neurosurgery. 2008; 63(3) Suppl:139–148

[37] Thomasen E. Vertebral osteotomy for correction of kyphosis in ankylosing spondylitis. Clin Orthop Relat Res. 1985(194):142–152

[38] Michele AA, Krueger FJ. Surgical approach to the vertebral body. J Bone Joint Surg Am. 1949; 31A(4):873–878

[39] Tsuzuki N, Kostuik JP. Laminoplasty of the thoracic and lumbar spine. In: Frymoyer JW, ed. The Adult Spine: Principles and Practice. Philadelphia, PA: Lippincott-Raven; 1997:2089–2109

[40] Boachie-Adjei O, Ferguson JA, Pigeon RG, Peskin MR. Transpedicular lumbar wedge resection osteotomy for fixed sagittal imbalance: surgical technique and early results. Spine. 2006; 31(4):485–492

[41] Bridwell KH, Lewis SJ, Edwards C, et al. Complications and outcomes of pedicle subtraction osteotomies for fixed sagittal imbalance. Spine. 2003; 28 (18):2093–2101

[42] Kim KT, Suk KS, Cho YJ, Hong GP, Park BJ. Clinical outcome results of pedicle subtraction osteotomy in ankylosing spondylitis with kyphotic deformity. Spine. 2002; 27(6):612–618

[43] Kim YJ, Bridwell KH, Lenke LG, Cheh G, Baldus C. Results of lumbar pedicle subtraction osteotomies for fixed sagittal imbalance: a minimum 5-year follow-up study. Spine. 2007; 32(20):2189–2197

[44] Murrey DB, Brigham CD, Kiebzak GM, Finger F, Chewning SJ. Transpedicular decompression and pedicle subtraction osteotomy (eggshell procedure): a retrospective review of 59 patients. Spine. 2002; 27(21):2338–2345

[45] Bridwell KH. Decision making regarding Smith-Petersen vs. pedicle subtraction osteotomy vs. vertebral column resection for spinal deformity. Spine. 2006; 31(19) Suppl:S171–S178

[46] Chen IH, Chien JT, Yu TC. Transpedicular wedge osteotomy for correction of thoracolumbar kyphosis in ankylosing spondylitis: experience with 78 patients. Spine. 2001; 26(16):E354–E360

[47] Wang MY, Berven SH. Lumbar pedicle subtraction osteotomy. Neurosurgery. 2007; 60(2) Suppl 1:ONS140–ONS146, discussion ONS146

[48] O'Shaughnessy BA, Ondra SL. Measuring, preserving, and restoring sagittal spinal balance. Neurosurg Clin N Am. 2007; 18(2):347–356

[49] Feng B, Qiu G, Shen J, et al. Impact of multimodal intraoperative monitoring during surgery for spine deformity and potential risk factors for neurological monitoring changes. J Spinal Disord Tech. 2012; 25(4):E108–E114

[50] Buckwalter JA, Yaszay B, Ilgenfritz RM, Bastrom TP, Newton PO, Harms Study Group. Analysis of Intraoperative Neuromonitoring Events During Spinal Corrective Surgery for Idiopathic Scoliosis. Spine Deform. 2013; 1(6):434–438

[51] Lagrone MO, Bradford DS, Moe JH, Lonstein JE, Winter RB, Ogilvie JW. Treatment of symptomatic flatback after spinal fusion. J Bone Joint Surg Am. 1988; 70(4):569–580

[52] Berven SH, Deviren V, Smith JA, Emami A, Hu SS, Bradford DS. Management of fixed sagittal plane deformity: results of the transpedicular wedge resection osteotomy. Spine. 2001; 26(18):2036–2043

Further Reading

D'Aliberti G, Talamonti G, Villa F, et al. Anterior approach to thoracic and lumbar spine lesions: results in 145 consecutive cases. J Neurosurg Spine. 2008; 9 (5):466–482

Heinig CF. Eggshell procedure. In: Luque ER, ed. Segmental Spinal Instrumentation. Thorofare, NJ: Slack; 1984:221–230

4 The Natural History of Rigid Spinal Deformities

Jean Dubousset

Abstract

The natural history of the rigid spine depends on its physiopathology where, at whatever age, the structural deformity is localized to few spinal units (three to five), originating from various etiologies (congenital, trauma, infections, and idiopathic, including degeneration over time). Its spontaneous evolution can lead to rigidity. Frequently this rigidity is secondary to a previous surgical treatment performed at an early age with an incomplete correction, leading to the "crankshaft phenomenon." The consequences are not only increasing deformities with respiratory disorders, but also radicular pain or spinal cord compression associated with more or less instability. Assessment of rigidity/ flexibility can be done by bending or performing the Billot test, which is less reliable than the information given by longitudinal traction, either with distraction, or correction in a Stagnara cast or halo brace either in a sitting or lying position. This is often used in practice to prepare for surgical correction. The duration of this preoperative external preparation is monitored by respiratory function improvement. When a plateau is reached for the improvement, surgery may be performed. Surgical treatment depends on the age and localization of the deformity, each having its personalized strategy. Some require anterior, posterior, or combined approaches, including the various types of osteotomies, as well as the associated instrumentation for the particular type of surgery. The final goal of the surgical procedure is to achieve the best balance and stability as possible.

Keywords: spine, rigidity/flexibility, crankshaft phenomenon, balance, cardiorespiratory function, spinal osteotomies

4.1 Definition and Measurement

The rigidity or flexibility of any spinal structure, with or without deformity, can be defined as the amount of change in the structure's shape in any of the three dimensions as a result of *external passive forces* (e.g., longitudinal traction, fulcrum, suspension, or bending forces or the Billot test) *or active forces* (e.g., flexion/extension/axial rotation) in one direction or the other, without any direct surgical or instrumental involvement or approach to that structure.

It is measured by the difference in value of this shape between the initial status (e.g., postural standing or lying) and the secondary status (after the structure's submission to the passive or active movements). The measurements are taken with the same basic references in terms of the levels as well as the two- or three-dimensional (2D or 3D) plane of the measurement (sagittal, frontal, axial). It may also be measured by the percentage of variation between the two statuses: arriving at the same numbers in both statuses indicates complete (100%) rigidity. This provides a good evaluation of the biomechanics of the entire or the localized pathological portion of the spinal structure as well as the 3D anatomical localization of the rigidity: the anterior body and disk; the posterior pedicle, facet, and lamina; or both, and their adjacent soft tissues.

4.2 Natural History, Physiopathology

The natural history must be understood in terms of age (growing, mature, or aging spine) and its effects on the vital functions (cardiopulmonary or metabolic) and on neuro-orthopaedic disabilities in relation to static and dynamic disorders of alignment and balance. Thus, working with these patients requires multidisciplinary involvement for both diagnosis and treatment. It is necessary to monitor the deformity's effect on pulmonary function, bone maturation, and nervous structures (spinal cord or roots) with MRI scans. Instability can be seen on stress films, and potential (hidden) instability, although not demonstrated on stress films, may be revealed by a small trauma or may evolve spontaneously. Finally, the influence of stiffness or instability on the patient's static and dynamic balance must be followed.

The natural history will depend on the anatomopathology of the most frequent etiologies. We have identified four major groups:

1. **Structural deformities localized on a few spinal units (less than three or four)** that may or may not cause a significant change in spinal balance, such as congenital malformations located between the craniocervical and lumbosacral junctions, as well as remnants of infectious, inflammatory, posttraumatic, or dystrophic localized diseases that may have occurred at any age.
2. **Structural deformities involving a significant part of the spine**, such as an idiopathic or degenerative dystrophic, congenital, or neuromuscular scoliosis, kyphosis (e.g., Scheuermann kyphosis), or kyphoscoliosis *where the flexibility is less than 15 to 20%.*
3. **Structural deformities involving the entire spine**, such as inflammatory diseases (e.g., ankylosing spondylitis, rheumatoid arthritis) or muscular diseases (e.g., rigid spine syndrome or other muscular dystrophies). Structural deformity of the entire spine is also observed in some rare congenital disorders, malformations, dysplasias, or dystrophies affecting the entire skeleton.
4. **Structural deformities referred to as iatrogenic because they have already been operated on.** Iatrogenic structural deformities can arise from an insufficient previous correction on an established deformity in an adult patient (e.g., residual posttraumatic kyphosis) or an insufficient first correction performed during childhood for a localized infectious lesion, spondylodiskitis, or Pott's disease. They may also result from an idiopathic or degenerative scoliosis for which a previous surgical treatment with fusion created a rigid deformity from an initially flexible deformity. More often they result from a progressive deformity acquired during the end of growth after an improper surgical treatment during childhood, such as the deformity secondary to a "crankshaft phenomenon" for an infantile or juvenile deformity. For all iatrogenic structural deformities it is necessary to check the deformity's effects on the functional impairment of the cardiopulmonary

apparatus, the neurologic status of the spinal canal shape and contents, and the static as well as dynamic balance of the body.

4.3 Natural History, Assessment of Flexibility/Rigidity

It is necessary to evaluate the levels of flexibility and rigidity, as well as the ways to assess them.

4.3.1 Reduction of the Deformity Will Be Checked: Locally and Globally

Reduction in the alignment (by external maneuver) may vary from no reduction to complete reduction, and will dictate the treatment strategy.

- **Supine traction** is a good method but must be used with great care given the danger of elongation when the spinal cord is lying (more or less attached and fixed by the bilateral roots extending) on the acute apex of a rigid deformity. The traction, as it stretches the mobile segments above and below, will elongate the spinal cord and increase the compression at its apex, creating the potential for local ischemia and subsequent secondary necrosis. The contrary is true when the apex is not rigid but mobile; the traction reduces the stress on the spinal cord.
- **Suspension** provides the same kinds of information on flexibility but is less reliable because of the permanent action of the surrounding protecting muscles. But suspension does provide some information that may better predict the final global alignment.
- The **Billot test, fulcrum, and active or passive bending** are also useful in some cases.
- **Halo traction on the skull combined with, but independent from, the Donaldson–Stagnara distraction cast** provides better results than continuous halo–wheelchair traction (given the viscoelasticity of the spinal structures and alternative relaxation of the soft tissues provided by the chin support of the cast between two successive cast elongations). We have used this technique to obtain complete recovery from paralysis of the lower limbs, including sphincter paralysis secondary to spinal cord compression/elongation as seen in the so-called twisted rotary-dislocation siphon of the spine. This technique helps the surgeon by preventing excessive manipulation of the spinal cord structures during surgical fusion/stabilization. It may be useful in cases where an aggressive, direct surgical procedure on the rigid curve is contraindicated. This technique gives clinical and radiological information useful to perform computer simulation in order to plan surgery, choose the proper level(s) for osteotomies, and predict the global postoperative alignment.

4.4 Natural History According to the Growing Spine and Etiologies

- **For localized lesions:** Many localized rigid lesions are not progressive, and no intervention is required throughout the patient's lifetime. Examples include congenital lesions, spontaneous fusions at one or two levels secondary to spondylodiskitis, and posttraumatic mild kyphosis. But for others, according to the anatomopathology, the natural history is well known, as in some congenital hemivertebrae with or without kyphosis, some asymmetrical defects of segmentation (e. g., an unsegmented posterolateral bar), the three apical vertebrae of a dystrophic spine in type 1 neurofibromatosis, or some cases of childhood tuberculosis that affect multiple consecutive levels and lead to kyphotic deformities that are often severe and can pose a neurologic risk of spinal cord compression. In such cases we can predict the evolution of the deformity, anticipate its progression, and make an immediate treatment decision. In other cases, X-ray screenings at regular intervals will demonstrate whether the lesion is stable or progressive.
- **For more extensive rigid pathology of the spine:** The prognosis may be poor for idiopathic, congenital, or syndromic diseases involving both the spine and the thorax, sometimes with multiple unilateral or bilateral rib fusions, with or without associated muscle disease. This is why surgical expansion of the thoracic skeleton (spine and rib cage) must be done as early as possible. Nevertheless, in many such syndromes (e. g., Jeune syndrome or asphyxiating thoracic dystrophy) the major involvement of the soft tissues, muscles, ligaments, and connective tissues justifies the earliest possible positive pressure respiratory support sustained throughout the growth period. This can help prevent the need for surgical expansion of the thoracic cage in some patients. But in neuromuscular disorders as seen in the rigid spine syndrome, or in some congenital myopathies or dystrophies, the problem, rather than involving spinal cord risk, involves respiratory impairment and its developmental, cardiac, and vital consequences. This is also the case for infantile idiopathic scoliosis. We know that for the malignant type of Min Mehta scoliosis, the apex of the curve is sometimes extremely rigid, and even repeated casting doesn't completely reduce the apex. In these cases, it is tempting to address the deformity surgically during childhood. But this requires caution because early asymmetrical fusion gives rise to numerous complications involving nonfusion distraction devices and the crankshaft phenomenon. An early fusion in the thoracic area can also have disastrous consequences for pulmonary function. Thus nonoperative treatment is advised until patients reach sufficient maturation to tolerate fusion, the definitive correction. It is also advisable to develop a minimally invasive technique for bipolar elongation without fusion, which enabled our first patients to reach the end of the growth stage without the need for fusion, achieving instead a spontaneous stabilizing stiffness or rigidity. The same approach can be used to treat a stiff Scheuermann kyphosis successfully, with repeated casting and bracing during childhood resulting in very few cases requiring surgery by the end of growth.

4.5 Natural History According to the Mature Spine and Etiologies

Rigid deformities may arise from lesions acquired during adulthood, as posttraumatic kyphosis or from postinfectious or inflammatory diseases, but more generally from diseases developed during childhood where the involved part and not the affected part became progressively less reducible and subsequently stiff and rigid. The natural history led to deformity with more or less pain (sometimes radicular pain secondary to root compression in the foramen on the concave side) or elongation on the convex side with more or fewer osteophyte lesions. But often the pain is located purely paravertebral as a nonspecific low back pain. Direct cord compression signs must be checked, especially in localized postinfectious, posttraumatic, or dystrophic lesions, where a true kyphosis of the canal exists. These cord compression signs are exceptional in the so-called idiopathic kyphoscoliosis. This progressive stiffness is typical in idiopathic scoliosis, in the thoracic or thoracolumbar area, where, inside the curve, the soft tissues retract and the facet joints degenerate with arthritis and lose their motion abilities, as well as inside and outside the intervertebral disk structures. There is often significant impairment of pulmonary function. This evolution may occur at the levels of the compensatory curves where a progressive stiffness leads to imbalance and decompensation, but in some patients the reducibility remains intact for a long time. The speed of such change is variable among patients. In some patients, the deformity increases regularly at the rate of 0.5 to 1.5 degrees a year, but in others the deformity can increase suddenly by as much as 10 degrees in 6 months (this is particularly evident for some women around menopause. Thus each case must be checked for passive reduction both locally and globally for the entire spine to decide whether only local treatment of the rigidity is suitable, depending on the possibilities for compensation residing in the regions above and below. This is very clear for Scheuermann kyphosis, where in cases of surgical treatment the posterior instrumentation must be extended far below the pathological segment to achieve a balanced spine.

4.6 Natural History According to the Aging Spine and Etiologies

Of course the same pathoanatomy amplifies with age; stiffness and rigidity increase, and sometimes instability appears because of the degeneration of the soft connective tissue of the disks and ligaments and weakening of the muscles. The radicular signs are more frequently observed in a global "back pain" feeling, with a progressive loss of height, global kyphosis, and decline of the active function speed of walking. In some rare cases cord compression signs may be observed, especially for lesions in the cervical area of the aging spine. At any location in the spine, passive or active reducibility testing of the spine deformity demonstrates almost no or minimal change; thus a sufficient correction of the malalignment creating the imbalance cannot be achieved. This determines the necessity to address the rigid zone more directly.

Finally, today a growing number of problems in the aging spine are worsened by previous spinal surgeries, sometimes as simple as disk herniation removal; sometimes one- or two-level fusion; and sometimes more complicated, as in a previous scoliosis that was treated with front and back fusion and secondarily decompensated. For such cases it will be evident that the first response for any kind of treatment is to consider and calculate the surgery's risk–benefit ratio with regard to the vital issues of life versus function.

Thus the impact of the surgical techniques using more or less sophisticated osteotomies of the spine can be of primary importance in the planning and realization of the corrective surgery.

4.7 Subsequent Indications for Surgical Treatment

Some "rigid spines" can be kept intact for the patient's entire life.

- **Localized lesions** if they are stable (whatever the etiology), not progressive, not stenotic for the canal, well included and aligned in a harmonious and well-balanced spine. Examples include congenital, posttraumatic, or postinfectious short kyphoscoliotic fusion masses. But we must monitor degeneration of the adjacent-segment levels with long-term follow-up (cervical spine++).
- **Extended lesions**, when, despite a noticeable rigid deformity (scoliosis, kyphosis, or lordosis, whatever the etiology), the quality of life, including vital functions, cosmetic issues, balance, and level of pain, is acceptable, the risk for progression is low with regard to life expectancy, and the risk of neurologic compromise is exceptional (e.g., in some kyphoscoliosis postpoliomyelitis), or in many cases of Scheuermann kyphosis or even some cases of "rigid spine syndrome" where spine surgery is often unable to bring real improvement to the patient's quality of life.

For all other conditions, when a rigid spine, whatever the age, whatever the localization, leads to either *an immediate or a future danger* to the life or the function of the patient, *surgical treatment is indicated*, with proper measurement of the risk-benefit ratio of the surgical strategies for such treatment.

4.7.1 Treatment and Election of Surgical Approaches

The preoperative evaluation will first consider the following (adapted to the age of the patient): the reasons for consultation, deformity, pain, walking or sitting problems, neurology, imbalance, and cosmetic issues. Second, the physical exam will assess the vital functions, especially cardiorespiratory functions (with their proper corresponding laboratory exams). A complete neurologic exam is performed, followed by a 3D study of alignment, balance, and clinical measurement of real functionality with the chronometer, testing on three maneuvers (from a sitting position to walking 3 m front and back, climbing and descending three stairs, sitting on the floor and getting up, which is probably the most discriminating and is especially important in aging people to evaluate pre- and postoperative functional results. Finally, the possibility of compensation in the joints of the lower limbs is measured (hip joint+++). Third is the imaging examination, which includes X-rays (global and local); anteroposterior/sagittal EOS imaging with 3D reconstruction; and CT, MRI, bone age, and bone density scans, all of which provide a good idea of the anatomy as well as the localization of the rigidity and the possible pitfalls. Sometimes a 3D computer simulation may be helpful for deciding which levels to address for the correction.

4.8 Choice of Surgical Techniques and Approaches

The surgical technique and approach are chosen based on several variables, broadly including whether the pathology is localized or extends to multiple levels. The patient's age is also a key factor.

4.8.1 For Localized Rigid Pathology

For the predicted or controlled progressive cases in which the local lesion is treated surgically, the treatment of choice in children leaves the growth potential of the unaffected regions intact. This is achieved with or without a postoperative cast and brace treatment to treat an incomplete reduction or associated pathology, even if later on the fusion and instrumentation must be extended when growth ends. The approach and technique discussed for each case depend on the anatomy, the location of the rigidity, and the quality of the lesion and always employ effective spinal cord monitoring.

When the rigidity is posterior or posterolateral, most often the correction can be performed with a unique posterior approach that is more or less extended laterally to reach the anterior column if necessary. An example would be a congenital hemivertebra excision and fusion one level above and below with compression instrumentation by hooks or pedicle screws and rods and autogenous bone graft. For a congenital posterior or posterolateral defect of segmentation with a pedicle bar, one could use a posterolateral subtraction osteotomy, with removal or not of the pedicle and postinstrumentation to realign perfectly. Whatever the etiology, the control of the dural sac must be excellent under direct vision, as well as the proper front and back resection of the bone or disk with a postsubtraction osteotomy or a pedicle subtraction osteotomy, and their subsequent approximation during the reduction maneuver. This surgery can be safely performed even in cases of instability, thanks to the strong bilateral fixation and the immediate stability provided by the pedicle screw and rod frames (sometimes alternatively used unilaterally, when one is working in the front on one side), which are ultimately strongly aligned in the ideal position to recover the best 3D alignment possible. The extent of the instrumentation will depend on the global 3D alignment of the body and the dynamic possibilities of adaptation in the chain of balance.

When the rigidity is clearly anterior, an anterior congenital bar or an acquired acute anterior fusion is used for a predominant acute kyphosis (whatever the etiology). For special localizations, such as the cervical spine (with or without neurologic signs), a clear decompression of the dura and the spinal cord is necessary and requires the anterior or anterolateral approach first for decompression, with a simultaneous posterior approach postinstrumentation. This allows direct control of the spinal cord under vision during the reduction maneuver of the kyphosis. In children, the length of the posterior instrumentation and fusion depends on the amount of reduction of the deformity. If reduction is completely achieved the fusion is short (only the levels involved). In the case of a residual kyphosis, if complete reduction is not achieved, the postinstrumentation and fusion must be extended one or more levels above and below so that the epiphysiodesis effect contributes to the progressive reduction of the residual kyphosis, thanks to the residual growth potential. This group of patients includes some cases of dystrophic spines as neurofibromatosis 1 with acute rotatory dislocation where short front and back fusions with separate approaches are often necessary to regulate or prevent the evolution of the deformity. Of course, in young children a postoperative cast immobilization is useful for a few months, followed (or not) by a brace, depending on the associated neuromuscular or dystrophic pathologies and any local or global alteration of the posture. This is opposite to the case in adults, where the strong fixation doesn't necessitate any external support.

Special mention is required for the craniocervical junction, where correction may include a combination of anterior surgery through the mouth, and a posterior approach to fuse and stabilize, with or without instrumentation of the junction. Doing this inside a preoperative halo cast with a perfectly organized strategy provides a great deal of comfort for the patient, the anesthesiology team, and the surgeon.

4.8.2 For Lesions Extending to Multiple Levels (Scoliotic, Kyphoscoliotic, or Lordoscoliotic Curve)

For lesions that extend to multiple levels, the surgical technique and approach vary according to factors associated with the patient's age, which are discussed here for lesions in young children, older children and adults, and older adults.

Young Children

The typical example in the young child is the malignant infantile scoliotic curve resistant to repeated cast and brace treatment. We know that the apex of the curve has a severe torsion on the three apical vertebrae, especially in the horizontal plane, and it is the goal of the Shilla technique to surgically address these three apical vertebrae with a posterior approach, pedicle screw direct derotation with interbody and postfusion. This part of the procedure is often successful, but the portion of the Shilla technique that involves instrumentation without fusion of the unaffected parts of the spine above and below the apex is too extensive in this author's opinion. For these patients we prefer to use nonoperative treatment with repeated casting followed by bracing and active and continued respiratory management, until a proper age is reached to perform the final instrumentation and fusion. In this method, the apical area is perhaps not absolutely corrected but is included in a well balanced (of course not "straight") but harmonious fusion mass. We have the same thinking regarding some other techniques, such as dual distraction rods (magnetic or not) used for such deformities, with some exceptions for neuromuscular or dystrophic collapsing with or without a rigid spine, where these posterior devices can be used (with a minimally invasive approach to prevent spontaneous fusions) to assist the bracing treatment until the final fusion can be performed safely at a reasonable age. We regard the minimally invasive bipolar fusionless technique as the best way to address this problem. It starts with casting in children up to 6 years old, followed by the bipolar minimally invasive technique with upper fixation at the upper end of the curve on two consecutive vertebrae using two pediculosupralaminar hook claws on each side, and two pedicular screws at the lower end of the curve on each side, with a proper bend of the two intramuscular rod-fitted parallels in between and linked with a "click domino," allowing mechanical, continuous elongation without any anesthesia or surgical action. No cast and no brace are required, and spontaneous stiffness and stabilization of the spine are obtained by the end of growth without fusion. It should be noted that the same application is used for neuromuscular curves with pelvic obliquity, the only difference being in the bilateral pelvic fixation, thanks to two iliosacral screws.

For Older Children, Adolescents, and Adults with "Abandoned" Curves

For patients with curves where the rigidity (less than a 20-degree difference in the Cobb angle after traction, bending, etc.) lies as in the front as in the back of the spinal structures (the typical example is the rigid Scheuermann kyphosis), in the past the surgical treatment began with an anterior release disk excision and fusion, followed by posterior compressive instrumentation and fusion. Today the treatment is purely posterior thanks to multiple Ponte osteotomies and compression instrumentation, with results as good as those with the earlier procedure with no loss of pulmonary function, which is sometimes permanent after a chest opening (minimally invasive or not). For rigid scoliosis curves in the past the treatment was preoperative continuous halo traction (with or without a distraction cast continued until the improvement of pulmonary function plateaued), then a posterior surgery was performed with a complete extensive facet excision (and root release in cases of radiculopathy) and post-only instrumentation and fusion with a hybrid or pedicle-screws-only montage. This was the method of choice because a simultaneous anterior release (open or video assisted through the tube) has not been proven to be beneficial for pulmonary function. The length of the instrumentation and fusion follows the rules of spinal surgery for deformities according to balance and stability. The cosmetic aspect was only moderately improved, but pain, pulmonary function, and balance were greatly improved.

Techniques currently in use include postsubtraction osteotomy, pedicle subtraction osteotomy, and, in some cases, vertebral column resection (for experimental teams only) and provide better cosmetic results, but they can generate more complications. In rare cases, when pyramidal signs are observed in relation with the rigid zone and are still present after preoperative traction, decompression is required. But in some cases, mainly at the lumbar and thoracolumbar localization, the deformity's origin is purely disk degeneration, with secondary bone deformity, rotatory dislocation, and apparent global rigidity. In fact when corrected level by level with a precise release and a strong posterior bilateral pedicle fixation only, it appears that the correction can be properly performed without any bone osteotomy.

For cases needing revision after a prior surgery (e.g., short posterior or anterior and posterior fusion for disk disease or degenerative spine), in general the rigid portion is included with more or less pedicle subtraction osteotomy, in an extension of the instrumentation both above and below (sometimes down to the sacrum). It should be noted that the most challenging revision surgery is the one secondary to a significant crankshaft phenomenon with imbalance. The choice lies between keeping the deformity and extending the fusion above and below or, more often, using a simultaneous anterior and posterior approach to perform anterior release on the disk space and multiple posterior osteotomies and posterior hybrid or pedicle screw instrumentation. Some cases of vertebral column resection have been reported. But the results are never perfect, regardless of the technique used, demonstrating once again that prevention is the best approach in spinal surgery.

The most evident rigid spine deformity in the adult arises from kyphosis secondary to ankylosing spondylitis, with deformity in only one plane and often very severe, requiring corrective posterior osteotomies. At the cervicothoracic junction for a predominant upper deformity, halo fixation allows manipulation of the head during the reduction. At the lumbar region, for the most frequent lower deformity remaining after hip surgery, the level and number of osteotomies and the correct amount of lordosis were at one time obtained using scissors as the X-ray phantom. Computer simulations have replaced this method. They are either multiples, from a Smith–Petersen type, with a harmonious correction, or unique, with an acute correction that is less harmonious and perhaps more dangerous than the multiples for the aorta.

For the Aging Spine

The speed and the nature of deterioration of anatomy and function with aging vary greatly from one person to the next; thus the functional tests already described are important for measuring these factors. Even if the chronological age is not a critical criterion, when the patient is over 70 years old, there are four key principles to consider:

1. **Use surgery sparingly.** There is a higher risk for general complications (vascular, pulmonary, cognitive) following general anesthesia. Surgery should be decided on only after conservative procedures have been exhausted (including local infiltrations for radiculopathies, bracing and physiotherapy for alignment and balance). Only in the face of a severe disability should surgery be considered. Thus measuring the functional score at regular intervals in aging patients provides guidance for choosing the optimal surgical date, when the score is clearly declining and before the patient reaches the age where the complication rate becomes too high.
2. **Avoid the anterior approach if possible.** It is preferable to avoid an anterior approach, despite the fact that in some cases of degenerative spine a minimally invasive anterior disk excision done on a few levels with anterior-only realignment and interbody fusion with cages can solve the problems of pain and imbalance, with a minimal complication rate.
3. **Use the shortest posterior approach possible.** Use a minimally invasive technique to restore alignment and balance to prevent a junctional kyphosis, especially above the instrumented spine. This can be achieved by choosing the levels for instrumentation by obtaining a precise assessment of the

amount of possible passive, but mainly active, compensation above and below the proposed instrumented zone.

4. **Avoid as much as possible long instrumentations/fusions down to the sacrum.** Often the alignment obtained looks good on the X-rays, but the resulting level of function is not optimal because the rigidity has been extended to a previously mobile segment of the spine, especially when the reserve in extension at the hip joint level was missing.

4.9 Conclusion

There are four main messages for the treatment of such rigid spinal deformities, whatever the patient's age:

1. Identify clearly the reasons for treatment.
2. Identify the pathoanatomy of the deformity locally and globally for balance, and function of the patient currently, and predict these factors for the future.
3. Decide the indications and process of treatment with the help of a multidisciplinary team, considering all aspects of the consequences of the disease for the patient and the patient's family.
4. Choose the technique and strategy with regard to the expertise of the surgical team and the preoperative, perioperative, and postoperative environmental conditions.

5 Surgical Management of Children with Congenital Deformities of the Upper Thoracic Spine and Vertebral Malformations

Sergei Vissarionov

Abstract

Congenital deformities of the thoracic spine in pediatric patients remain a serious issue for spinal surgeons. Unique characteristics of the thoracic region, such as narrow spinal canals, which predispose patients with severe deformities to neurologic deterioration, and proximity to both cervical and lumbar regions with greater mobility, pose a challenge for treatment.

Early surgical treatment is essential, allowing achievement of good cosmetic and functional results. The ideology of surgical treatment of congenital deformity of the upper thoracic spine caused by lateral and posterolateral vertebrae is based on three main principles: extirpation of the abnormal vertebra, radical correction of the deformity using metal construct, and autologous bone grafting (360-degree fusion). Due to smaller size of vertebral pedicles in children and abnormal anatomy, it is sometimes very hard to get appropriate fixation points. It is critical to shorten the length of instrumentation as much as possible, and not to disturb remaining growth of the thoracic spine.

One of the most common anomalies is hemivertebrae. When located in the upper thoracic region, a single dorsal approach can be utilized to achieve correction and fusion. Mid-thoracic and thoracolumbar hemivertebrae usually require a combined approach, which allows good exposure, total resection, and mobilization of the segment.

Further, we describe indications for treatment, surgical technique, and long-term results in patients treated at our institution. Both scoliotic and kyphotic curves were reduced significantly. Solid bone fusion in all patients allowed the performance of implant removal at 1.5 to 2 years without altering spine stability and preserving spinal growth.

Keywords: congenital scoliosis, children, spine, surgery, malformations, thorax, hemivertebrae

5.1 Introduction

The most common congenital anomalies of the thoracic spine that cause spinal deformity are those associated with vertebral malformation. The course of congenital spinal deformity depends on the location of the anomaly, the initial degree of curvature, and the rate of its progression as the child grows.

Early diagnosis and timely, adequate surgical management can correct the deformity, form the natural frontal and sagittal profiles of the functional spinal unit that was operated on, and ensure further normal growth of the spine. Correction of congenital spinal deformity in pediatric patients is used to prevent severe and rigid scoliosis and neurologic disorders from occurring as the patient ages.[1,2,3]

The upper thoracic spine is a unique spinal segment from both the anatomical and the biomechanical points of view. First, the locations of thoracic vertebrae and spinal cord segments are mismatched at this level. The upper thoracic spinal cord segments are located two vertebrae higher than their corresponding vertebrae of the same number; the lower thoracic cord segments are located three vertebrae below their corresponding vertebrae. The spinal canal is very narrow at the thoracic region: it is only 10 to 11 mm at the level of the upper thoracic vertebrae, whereas the anteroposterior diameter of the thoracic spinal cord is 6 mm and that of the dural sac is 9 mm. It should be mentioned that the thoracic spine is a transient area between the upper-lying natural cervical lordosis and the lower-lying thoracic kyphosis. The greatest range of motion in the thoracic spine is possible only in its upper and lower functional spinal units. In the most mobile segment, T 11–T 12, the highest extension angle is 4.8 degrees, whereas the highest flexion angle is 5 degrees. Segment mobility is much lower at the T 1–T 4 level and negligible at the medium thoracic level. The total range of motion during lateral flexion in the entire thoracic spine is less than 30 degrees.

Few studies have been devoted to developmental anomalies in children with vertebral malformations in the thoracic spine, and in the upper thoracic spine (T 1–T 4) in particular. Different researchers reported different rates of deformity progression in the thoracic spine. According to some, the rate of deformity progression in the upper and lower thoracic spine is 1.8 and 2.8 degrees per year, respectively.[4] Despite the lack of consistency in opinions about the course of congenital thoracic spine deformities, this malformation often causes the development of secondary spinal curvatures, shoulder girdle imbalance, functional disorders in the cervical spine, and severe cosmetic defects, even if the initial degree of deformity was small.

The few studies focused on outcomes of surgical treatment of congenital spinal deformity caused by vertebral malformation include both thoracic and lumbar anomalies.[5] Most publications deal with extirpation of a thoracolumbar or lumbar vertebra through the combined (anterolateral and dorsal) approach.[5,6,7,8,9,10,11] A comparative analysis of surgical management of congenital scoliosis through the combined and dorsal approaches was carried out in some studies.[12]

We monitored 28 patients from 1 year 4 months to 3 years (mean age, 2 years 7 months) with congenital anomalies of the upper thoracic spine. A single spinal anomaly was observed in all cases: either a lateral hemivertebra (in 11 patients) or a posterior hemivertebra (in 17 patients). Gender distribution showed that girls (16 cases) had this anomaly more frequently than boys (12 cases) (▶ Table 5.1).

The hemivertebrae were located on the right side in 16 cases and on the left side in 12 cases. The abnormal hemivertebrae were located mostly at the T 3 level and caused development of a scoliotic or kyphoscoliotic deformity in the upper thoracic spine.

Table 5.1 Age distribution of patients with congenital vertebral malformations in the upper thoracic spine

	Age 0–2 years	Age 2–3 years	Total
Boys	4	8	12 (43 %)
Girls	5	11	16 (57 %)
Total	9	19	28 (100 %)

Table 5.2 Localization of posterolateral and lateral hemivertebrae in the upper thoracic spine

	Right-sided anomaly	Left-sided anomaly	Total*
Normal T 2 vertebra	3	3	10 (36 %)
Extra T 2 vertebra	2	2	
Normal T 3 vertebra	3	2	13 (46 %)
Extra T 3 vertebra	5	3	
Normal T 4 vertebra	2	1	5 (18 %)
Extra T 4 vertebra	2	-	
Total	17 (61 %)	11 (39 %)	28 (100 %)

*Each number in the Total column refers to the sum of Right-sided and Left-sided columns.

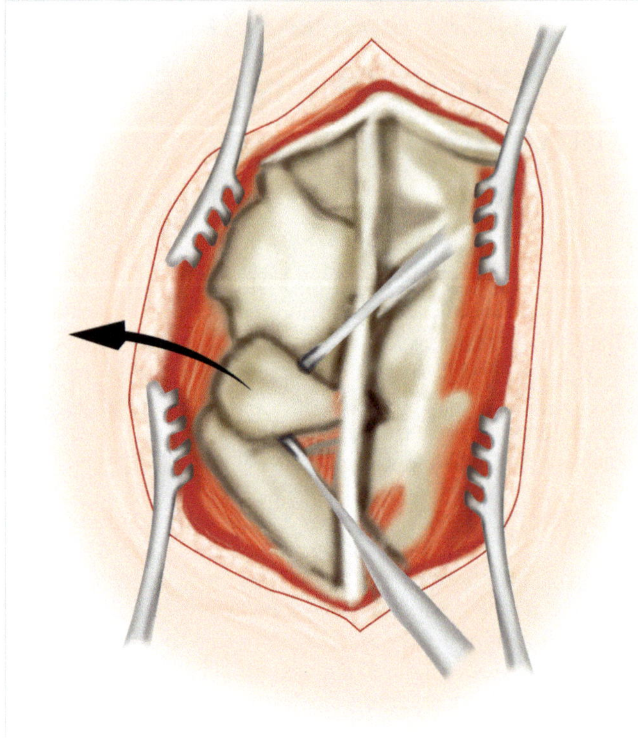

Fig. 5.1 The posterior vertebral column after the hemivertebral hemiarch was extirpated.

▶ Table 5.2 lists the data on localization of abnormal hemivertebrae. The spinal deformity curve was right sided in 61% of patients and left sided in 39% of patients. Prior to surgical management, all patients had compensatory curves balancing the main congenital curvature: 9 patients had a cranial and a caudal counter curve; 17 patients had a counter curve in the caudal spine portion with respect to the abnormal vertebra; 2 patients had a counter curve only in the cranial spine portion with respect to the abnormal vertebra.

All patients underwent clinical, biomechanical, and X-ray examination (X-ray films of the spine in two planes) and CT scans before and after surgery. The preoperative CT scan assessed the anatomical and anthropometric and spatial relations between the bone structure of the abnormal vertebra and the adjacent functional spinal units, and evaluated the rate of bone block formation after the surgery. Furthermore, all children underwent preoperative MRI scanning to rule out malformation of the medullary canal and the spinal cord.

The indications for surgery included a Cobb angle greater than 25 degrees in patients with lateral hemivertebrae and a Cobb angle greater than 20 degrees in children with kyphoscoliosis caused by posterolateral hemivertebrae.

Surgery was performed using a dorsal-only approach in all patients. With the patient lying prone, a longitudinal skin incision was made along the line of the spinous processes running through the apex of the deformity. The posterior supporting structures of the abnormal vertebra and the adjacent intact bone structures of neighboring vertebrae on both sides with respect to the line of spinous processes were skeletonized. The approach to the posterior supporting elements of the adjacent vertebrae was performed within two to three functional spinal units above and below the hemivertebra.

Following the approach, the transverse rib junction at the abnormal vertebra was resected. The transverse process and the hemivertebral arch (up to its base) were sequentially extirpated (▶ Fig. 5.1). This was followed by subperiosteal resection of a 7- to 10-cm portion of the rib running to the hemivertebral body, then partial rib resection to provide more convenient access to the abnormal vertebral body as well as material for bone grafting.

The posterior portion of the hemivertebral body with the adjacent intervertebral disks was exposed after bony structures of the posterior vertebral column had been removed (▶ Fig. 5.2).

The hemivertebral body was extirpated by medially displacing the dural sac, protecting the lower-lying spinal nerve root with spatulas, and extrapleurally covering the lower-lying vessels. The body of an abnormal vertebra was removed using bone scrapers, a conchotome, and Luer and Kerrison forceps. The spongy portion of the abnormal vertebra was completely removed through the base of the hemivertebral arch using the bone scrapers. The procedure was started in the lateral portion of the hemivertebra, and the entire spongy bone tissue was gradually removed. The cortical layers of the abnormal vertebra were then removed in the same order: from the lateral cortical plate to the anterior and medial portions. The cortical plate, which lay adjacent to the dural sac and was the anterior wall of the spinal canal, was eventually removed. The upper- and lower-lying disks adjacent to the hemivertebra were completely resected, together with the end plates, to reach the opposite side with respect to the abnormal vertebra (▶ Fig. 5.3). After radical resection of the hemivertebral body with the adjacent disks and its posterior bony structures, partial resection of the

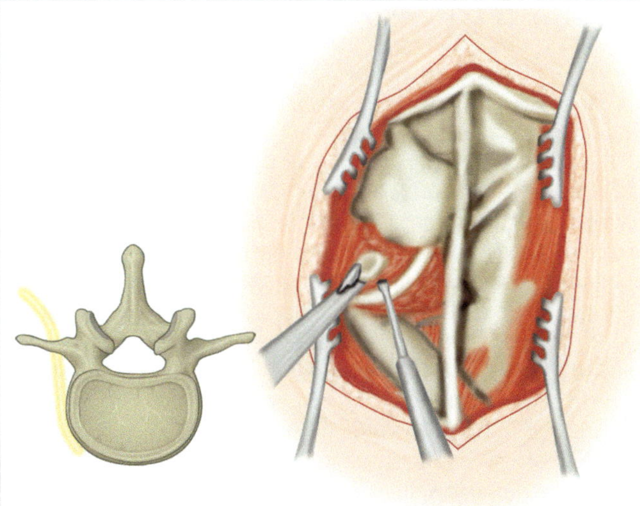

Fig. 5.2 Posterior portion of the hemivertebral body after the posterior bony structures were extirpated.

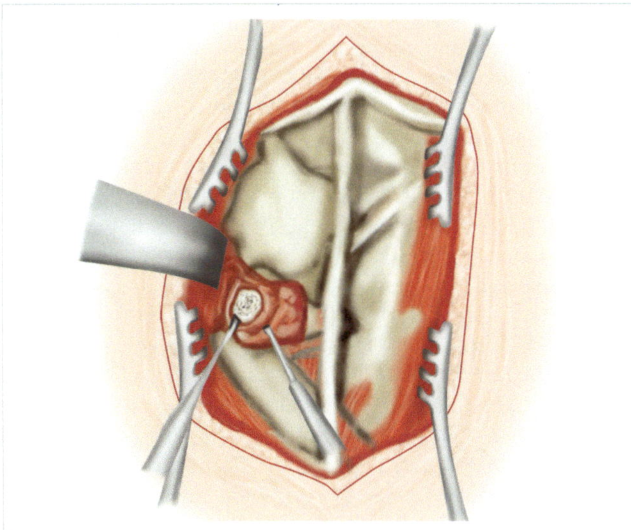

Fig. 5.3 Extirpation of the hemivertebral body.

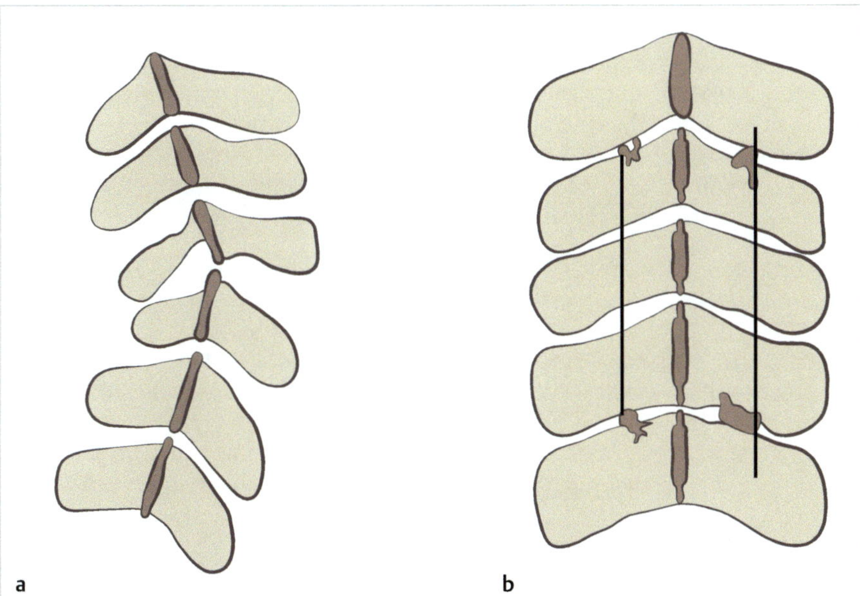

Fig. 5.4 (a) Deviation of the upper and lower spine portions with respect to the abnormal vertebra. (b) Spine region after partial wedge resection of the neighboring arches, longitudinal osteotomy of the upper and lower vertebral arches, and installation of the multiple screw fixation system (dorsal view).

lower portion of the arch of the upper-lying body and the upper portion of the arch of the lower-lying vertebra (by one-third width) was additionally performed on the side opposite to the extirpated hemivertebra through the dorsal approach. A triangular-shaped defect with its base facing the line of spinous processes was eventually formed.

Osteotomy of the lower-lying arch by two-thirds of its height along the spinous process was additionally performed in patients with the caudal spine diverging from the natural frontal spinal axis starting from the level of the abnormal vertebra. If the cranial spine diverged starting from the level of the abnormal vertebra, osteotomy of the upper-lying arch by two-thirds of its height along the spinous process was additionally performed. When both the cranial and caudal portions of the spine diverged from the natural frontal axis, osteotomy of the upper- and lower-lying arches by two-thirds of the height along the spinous process was performed (▸ Fig. 5.4a, b).

To achieve radical correction of the congenital deformity, fixation constructs were installed after additional mobilization of the posterior supporting complex, which included partial resection and osteotomy of the adjacent vertebral arches.

The hooks were placed into the arches of intact vertebrae adjacent to the osteotomy zone. Titanium alloy constructs with a rod diameter of 3.5 mm (Medtronic Sofamor Danek) were used in all patients to achieve posterior stabilization of the thoracolumbosacral spine. One hook was installed into each arch. The fixation constructs on the side of the abnormal vertebra were placed in such a way that compression was performed after they were connected using a rod. A graft (the rib fragment) was installed between the bodies of the vertebrae adjacent to the abnormal one on the concave side of the deformity prior to performing compression. After the manipulation, the graft was wedged between the intact bodies. Laminar hooks were installed contralaterally to the abnormal vertebra behind the arches of the adjacent vertebrae that had been subjected to partial resection and connected with a rod; then distraction was performed. After performing the multidirectional correcting manipulations along the rods, the construct was stabilized with internal fixation nuts. The final stage of the surgery consisted of forming posterior local fusion with autologous bone grafting along the construct. Postoperatively all patients wore a semirigid Schanz collar and a posture corrector during the entire period of spine fixation with a metal construct (1.5–2 years on average).

All patients preoperatively had a spinal deformity of the upper thoracic spine, which disrupted the biomechanics of the spine (displaced the center of gravity). The clinical changes in children showed total agreement with the radiographic presentation. No neurologic deficit was observed in any patient. None of the children had any pathologies affecting the spinal cord and spinal canal. No cases of congenital myogenic torticollis were observed among the patients.

Eleven patients with lateral hemivertebrae had no kyphotic deformity; the preoperative Cobb angle was 26 to 52 degrees (mean Cobb angle, 36.5 degrees). In 17 patients with posterolateral hemivertebrae, the preoperative Cobb angle was 22 to 46 degrees (mean Cobb angle, 38.2 degrees); the kyphosis angle was 16 to 28 degrees (mean angle, 22.4 degrees).

The symmetry of the shoulder girdle, angles of the scapulae, and waist triangles was observed after the surgical intervention in 82% of patients; the remaining 18% of patients had an insignificant asymmetry of the shoulder girdles and angles of the scapulae.

Instrumented correction of the congenital spinal deformity caused by lateral hemivertebrae resulted in a postoperative Cobb angle of 0 to 6 degrees. The degree of correction was 86 to 100% (▶ Fig. 5.5).

The residual postoperative Cobb angle after extirpation of posterolateral hemivertebrae was 0 to 4 degrees (mean Cobb angle, 2.5 degrees); the local kyphosis angle was 6 to 14 degrees (mean angle, 8.2 degrees). The degree of correction was 62 to 80% (▶ Table 5.3).

The surgery lasted for 90 to 200 minutes (mean duration, 140 min); the blood loss was 150–300 mL (mean volume, 225 mL). Cell salvage was used during surgical intervention in all patients. No infectious, neurologic, or vascular complications were observed postoperatively.

The metal construct was removed 1.5 to 2 years after the surgery, when the bone block in the intervention zone had been formed. After the spinal implant had been removed, children wore a soft Schanz collar for 3 to 4 months. The need for the collar was gradually eliminated through the use of exercise therapy, spine and collar zone massage, and restorative treatment. The patients were followed up after the construct was removed for 60 to 108 months (mean follow-up period, 84 months). No loss of correction was observed after removing the implant; no spinal deformities developed.

The ideology of surgical treatment of congenital deformity of the upper thoracic spine caused by lateral and posterolateral vertebrae is based on three main principles: extirpation of the abnormal vertebra, radical correction of the deformity using a metal construct, and autologous bone grafting (360-degree fusion). However, performing this range of surgical interventions through the classical combined approach (anterolateral and dorsal approaches) in patients with malformation of the upper thoracic spine has a number of limitations. Access to the anterolateral surface of the upper thoracic spine through the anterolateral approach is complicated, and there is a significant risk of intraoperative trauma and blood loss. Furthermore, access to the anterior vertebral column at this level is impeded by the proximity and thus potential injury of mediastinal organs.

The use of the dorsal approach for extirpating an upper thoracic hemivertebra allows one to perform surgical management of the congenital spine deformity by allowing access to all the elements of the abnormal structure while avoiding contact with the internal organs, which is inevitable when the ventral approach is used.

Resection of bones and soft tissues that cause the formation and progression of a congenital anomaly promotes radical cor-

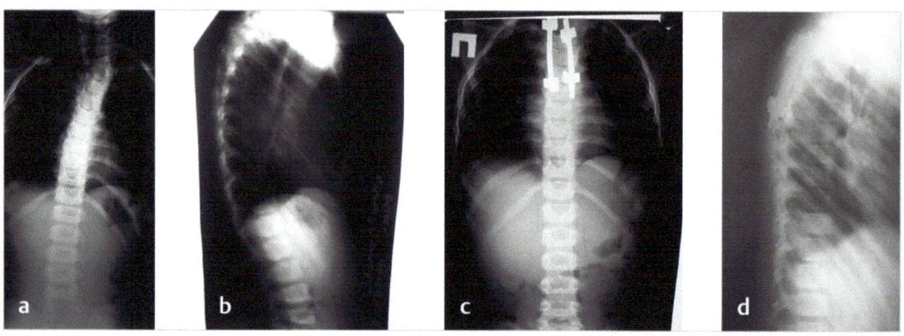

Fig. 5.5 X-ray films of a 3-year-old patient with congenital kyphoscoliosis caused by T3 posterolateral hemivertebra. **(a, b)** Before surgery. **(c, d)** Two years after surgery.

Table 5.3 Outcomes of correction of the congenital deformity in the upper thoracic spine

Groups	Mean preoperative Cobb angle (scoliosis/kyphosis)	Mean residual postoperative Cobb angle (scoliosis/kyphosis)	Mean degree of deformity correction, % (scoliosis/kyphosis)
Lateral hemivertebra	36.5° (24–52°)	4° (0–6°)	93 % (86–100 %)
Posterolateral hemivertebra	38.2° (22–46°)/ 22.4° (16–28°)	2.5° (0–4°)/ 8.2° (6–14°)	93.5 % (87–100 %)/ 55.4 % (50–61 %)

rection of the deformity and prevents its progression during the child's growth and development.

5.2 Outcomes of Surgical Management

Vertebral body malformation is the most common reason for congenital thoracic spine deformity in children.[13] According to Bosch et al, this type of spinal deformity in patients with this localization of the defect is characterized by rapid progression of the deformity (mean rate, ≥ 2.8 degrees/y).[4] Taking this fact into account, secondary counter curves in the portions of the spine that are located cranially and caudally with respect to the abnormal vertebra can be formed in children of early and preschool age.

Some authors believe that surgical management of this pathology aims at extirpation of the abnormal vertebral body, radical correction of the deformity, and stabilization of the minimal number of spinal functional units involved in the curvature.[1,14]

A number of surgeons believe that this outcome can be achieved only through the dorsal approach. After the hemiarch of the abnormal vertebra and its base have been resected, the hemivertebral body is isolated on the medial and lateral sides up to the anterior cortical end plate with the adjacent upper- and lower-lying disks. After diskectomy of the disks adjacent to the hemivertebra and achieving mobility of the body of the abnormal vertebra, the latter is extirpated. The remaining portion of the disk is removed on the concave side of the deformity followed by apophysectomy of the cranial and caudal end plates of the bodies of the adjacent intact vertebrae. Deformity correction is performed using a construct with multiple fixation points; the procedure is accompanied by contraction along the convex deformity side and distraction along the concave deformity side.[15] When using the dorsal approach for radical correction of congenital deformity caused by vertebral malformation, a surgeon contacts the spinal dura mater, which is associated with a high risk of neurologic disorders. For this very reason, there have been no reports that radical correction of the deformity has been achieved with the dorsal approach.

To eliminate congenital deformity in the thoracic spine, Garrido and Tome-Bermejo and colleagues have used ventral instrumented fixation. However, given the long-term treatment outcomes in patients with congenital deformity in the thoracic spine they have added the use of dorsal instrumented fixation.[16]

Many authors consider spinal functional units in the thoracic spine to be the region with the most severe course of congenital deformities in patients with vertebral malformations (posterolateral and lateral hemivertebrae).[14,15,17,18,19,20,21,22] Because thoracic kyphosis borders lumbar lordosis, the segmental stability and sagittal profile of the thoracolumbar spine region are characterized by certain biomechanical features that must taken into account for pediatric patients to ensure correct formation of natural frontal and sagittal spinal curves at early stages of development. It is extremely important that proper spinal curves are formed in preschool-age children to provide the conditions for normal growth and development of the spine and ensure normal load distribution over all spinal functional units.

Some authors believe that it is unreasonable to focus on the thoracolumbar junction because the progression rate of the congenital spinal deformity does not differ significantly from the progression rate of deformity in the thoracic and lumbar spine.[23] Meanwhile, other surgeons have reported that the greatest number of vertebral malformations localize in the thoracolumbar junction.[24,25] However, no clear explanation has been provided for this fact.

First, it is worth mentioning that the thoracolumbar spine region is a junction between the rigid thoracic and the mobile lumbar sections of the spine. A number of authors believe that this feature of the thoracolumbar region causes the formation of compensatory curves in the adjacent spine sections with respect to the main congenital curve.[1,14] Furthermore, a hemivertebra located on the convex side of the curve in this spine section during a child's growth and development exerts mechanical pressure on the lateral surface of the adjacent vertebral bodies on the opposite side. In turn, this pressure causes rapid progression of the deformity in the spine sections adjacent to the abnormal vertebra. The pathological mechanism of these biomechanics may play a key role in the formation of compensatory curves in the adjacent segments. It is extremely important to evaluate the sagittal spine profile in patients with congenital deformities in the thoracolumbar and lumbar spine because there is a high risk of severe kyphosis in these cases. Severe kyphosis does not develop when the deformities localize in the lumbosacral region of the spine.[14]

In this series, 39 patients aged 1 year 4 months to 3 years (mean age, 2 years 3 months) with congenital deformity in the thoracic spine caused by vertebral malformation were operated on. The sex distribution of the patients shows that 24 girls and 15 boys had congenital deformities (▸ Table 5.4). All children had an isolated spine abnormality.

The spine deformity was caused by a lateral hemivertebra in 3 patients, whereas the remaining 36 patients had a posterolateral hemivertebra. Lateral hemivertebrae were located at the T 6, T 8, and T 9 levels (1 case each). All the lateral hemivertebrae were non-extra. The posterolateral hemivertebrae were located as follows: five hemivertebrae (3 extra and 2 non-extra), at the T 5 level; four hemivertebrae (3 extra and 1 non-extra), at the T 6 level; six abnormal vertebrae (4 extra and 2 non-extra), at the T 7 level; six abnormal vertebrae (4 extra and 2 non-extra), at the T 8 level; seven hemivertebrae (5 extra and 2 non-extra), at the T 9 level; and eight hemivertebrae (5 extra and 3 non-extra), at the T 10 level. There was a right-sided hemivertebra in 19 patients, whereas 20 patients had a left-sided vertebra (▸ Table 5.5).

The congenital deformity curved to the right side in 49% of cases and to the left side in 51% of cases. All patients preoperatively had counter curves compensating for the congenital primary curve: 19 patients had cranial and caudal curvature with respect to the abnormal vertebra; 14 patients had a curvature only in the caudal portion of the spine; 6 patients had a counter curve only in the cranial portion of the spine.

Surgical management in 37 patients with congenital scoliosis caused by isolated lateral and posterolateral hemivertebrae in the thoracolumbar junction was analyzed separately. Patients'

Table 5.4 Age distribution of patients with congenital vertebral malformations in the thoracolumbar junction

Age	0–2 years	2–3 years	Total
Boys	5	10	15 (38 %)
Girls	13	11	24 (62 %)
Total	18 (46 %)	21 (54 %)	39(100 %)

Table 5.5 Distribution of posterolateral hemivertebrae with respect to their localization and position

Localization	Dextra	Sinistra	Total
T 5	3	2	5
T 6	1(1)	3	5
T 7	3	3	6
T 8	3	3(1)	7
T 9	4	3(1)	8
T 10	4	4	8
Total	18(1)	18(2)	39

Note: The number of lateral hemivertebrae is shown in parentheses.

age varied from 10 months to 3 years. The distribution by sex was 11 boys and 26 girls (▶ Table 5.6).

Vertebral malformations in the thoracolumbar junction (T 11–L 2) and caused formation of either a local scoliotic or kyphoscoliotic spinal deformity. ▶ Table 5.7 lists the data on localization of abnormal vertebrae.

The deformity curve was right sided in 54% of cases and left sided in 46% of cases. Counter curves compensating for the primary congenital curve were preoperatively observed in all patients: 17 patients had a cranial and caudal curvature; 19 patients had a curvature only in the caudal portion with respect to the abnormal vertebra; one child had a counter curve only in the thoracic spine.

All the pediatric patients preoperatively had a local thoracic spinal deformity clinically manifesting as shoulder girdle asymmetry and scapular height discrepancy. Patients with posterolateral hemivertebrae had increased thoracic kyphosis. No neurologic deficit was observed in any patient.

One-stage surgery was used to manage the deformities in the thoracic and thoracolumbar spine in pediatric patients as described following here.

The patient was lying on the side contralateral to the abnormal vertebra. The anterolateral approach to the apex of the deformity was used. An extrapleural thoracotomic approach was used to reach the thoracic hemivertebrae and those at the T 11 level. Thoracophrenolumbotomy and resection of the diaphragmatic crus from its insertion site to the internal surface of the thoracic cage was performed in patients with an abnormal vertebra at the T 12 or L 1 level. The extraperitoneal lumbotomic approach was used if the abnormality was at the L 2 level. The segmental vessels at the level of the abnormal vertebra were ligated and transected. The anterior longitudinal ligament above the abnormal vertebral body and the neighboring intervertebral disks with the end plates of the adjacent vertebrae was detached. The bodies of the lateral and posterolateral

Table 5.6 Age distribution of patients with congenital vertebral malformations in the thoracolumbar junction

Age	0–2 years	2–3 years	Total
Boys	4	7	11 (29.7 %)
Girls	14	12	26 (70.3 %)
Total	18 (49 %)	19 (51 %)	37 (100 %)

Table 5.7 Localization of the posterolateral and lateral hemivertebrae in the thoracolumbar junction

	Right-sided anomaly	Left-sided anomaly	Total
Non-extra T 11 vertebra	3	4	10 (27 %)
Extra T 11 vertebra	3	–	
Non-extra T 12 vertebra	1	–	3 (8.1 %)
Extra T 12 vertebra	1	1	
Non-extra L 1 vertebra	3	2	13 (35.2 %)
Extra L 1 vertebra	5	3	
Non-extra L 2 vertebra	2	6	11 (29.7 %)
Extra L 2 vertebra	2	1	
Total	20 (54 %)	17 (46 %)	37 (100 %)

hemivertebrae with the adjacent disks were extirpated; the posterior portion of the hemivertebral body adjacent to the spinal canal was resected.

The child was then placed in a prone position. An incision with its center passing through the apex of the deformity was made along the spinous processes of the vertebral bodies. The hemivertebral hemiarch and the remnants of its base were resected. Partial resection of the lower portion of the arch of the upper-lying vertebra and the upper portion of the arch of the lower-lying vertebra contralateral to the extirpated hemivertebra was then performed through the dorsal approach from the line of the spinous processes laterally to the arch edge. The partial resection was performed for one-third of the width of the lower portion of the upper-lying normal arch and for one-third of the width of the upper portion of the lower-lying normal arch. A triangular-shaped defect with its base facing the spinous processes was eventually formed. The partial wedge resection of the posterior vertebral column on the side contralateral to the abnormal vertebra provided additional mobility of the functional spinal unit when deformity correction was performed. Furthermore, longitudinal osteotomy of the neighboring normal vertebral arch (or two arches) that diverged from the correct vertical spinal axis, starting with the level of the abnormal vertebra and depending on the existing counter curves, was performed ipsilateral to the resected hemivertebra.

Osteotomy was performed strictly along the line of the spinous process for two-thirds of the height of a normal vertebral arch. If the cranially located spine portion diverged from the normal sagittal vertical axis starting from the level of the abnormal process (for patients with a thoracic compensatory curve), osteotomy was performed along the line of the spinous process of the upper-lying arch for two-thirds of its height. If the caudally located spine portion diverged from the normal sagittal vertical axis (in patients with a lumbar compensatory curve), osteotomy was performed along the spinous process of the lower-lying arch for two-thirds of its height. If both the cranially and caudally located spine portions (in patients with thoracic and lumbar compensatory curves) diverged from the normal sagittal vertical axis, osteotomy was performed along the line of the spinous processes for two-thirds of the height and along the upper- and lower-lying arches of the normal vertebrae. The additional selective osteotomy of the neighboring intact arches of the adjacent vertebrae made it possible to use the personalized approach to correction of the congenital spinal deformity. In addition, this procedure provided additional mobility to the posterior vertebral complex at the level of functional spinal units involved in the primary curve of the congenital deformity.

Metal constructs (hooks and/or screws) were installed after two neighboring arches contralateral to the abnormal hemivertebra had been resected for one-third of their width and after the intact arch or the neighboring arches (for two-thirds of their width) ipsilateral to the abnormal hemivertebra had been osteotomized along the line of the spinous processes. The hooks were placed on the arch of the nonosteotomized intact vertebral body that was directly adjacent to the zone where the abnormal hemivertebral hemiarch had been resected and to the arch located one segment above the osteotomized one. A hook (either infra- or supralaminar) was placed on each arch. The hooks were connected with a rod, and the supporting elements along it were compressed. On the opposite side, laminar hooks were placed on the arches of the vertebral bodies adjacent to the partially resected ones. Laminar constructs were placed on vertebral bodies in such a way that distraction could be performed after they were connected with a rod. In patients whose pedicular anatomy made it possible to place transpedicular instrumentation, correction of congenital spinal deformity was performed using transpedicular metal constructs. The constructs were placed in the bodies of the intact vertebrae whose arches had not been additionally osteotomized. After the deformity correction through the dorsal approach using a metal construct, autologous bone grafts were placed along the spinal implant, and the local fusion was formed.

The patient was returned to the lateral position. After the deformity correction, anterior fusion was performed using an autologous bone graft between the bodies of the upper- and lower-lying intact vertebrae with respect to the extirpated abnormal vertebra. Postoperative drainage was used. The wound was tightly sutured in a stepwise manner.

The temporary instrumentation was removed 1.5 to 2 years after surgical management. A bone block securing the spinal position attained during deformity correction had been formed at the intervention site by that time.

A metal construct with laminar fixation only was used in the thoracic spine (▶ Fig. 5.6). The following instrumentation was used, depending on the type of construct inserted in the thoracolumbar junction: transpedicular screws, 12 (32.4%) patients; hooks, 8 (21.6%) patients; and hook–screw combinations, 17 (46%) patients (▶ Fig. 5.7).

The outcomes of surgical management in patients were evaluated before and after treatment according to the following criteria:

- Correction of scoliotic and kyphotic deformity (Cobb angle).
- Presence or absence of bone or bone fibrous fusion.
- Progression of spinal deformity in the segments adjacent to the abnormal vertebra during child growth.

The outcomes of surgical treatment were evaluated both immediately after the intervention and during the long-term period. The duration of follow-up after the metal constructs had been removed was 60 to 120 months (mean duration, 94 months).

In three patients with congenital deformity in the thoracic spine caused by lateral hemivertebrae, the preoperative Cobb angle ranged from 34 to 59 degrees (mean Cobb angle, 46.8 degrees). In 36 patients with posterolateral hemivertebrae, the preoperative Cobb angle ranged from 26 to 57 degrees (mean Cobb angle, 40.8 degrees); the angle of local pathological

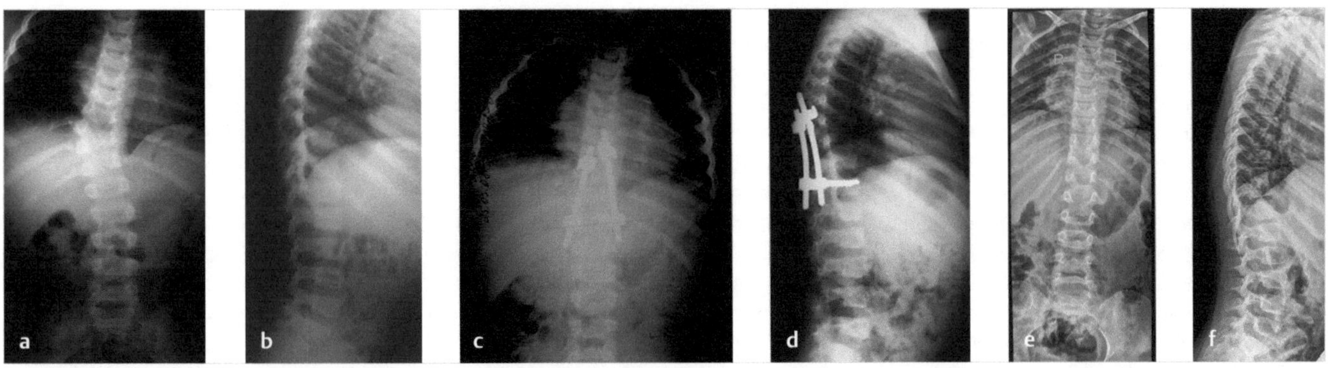

Fig. 5.6 A 16-month-old boy with congenital kyphoscoliosis caused by right-sided T10 posterolateral hemivertebra. X-ray taken before surgery in **(a)** AP and **(b)** lateral views showing local curves. X-rays taken 18 months after extirpation of the hemivertebrae, spinal instrumentation and fusion at T9-T11 level in **(c)** AP and **(d)** lateral views. **(e)** AP and **(f)** lateral views taken after 3 years post removal of implants showing preservation of correction and solid fusion at the level of surgery.

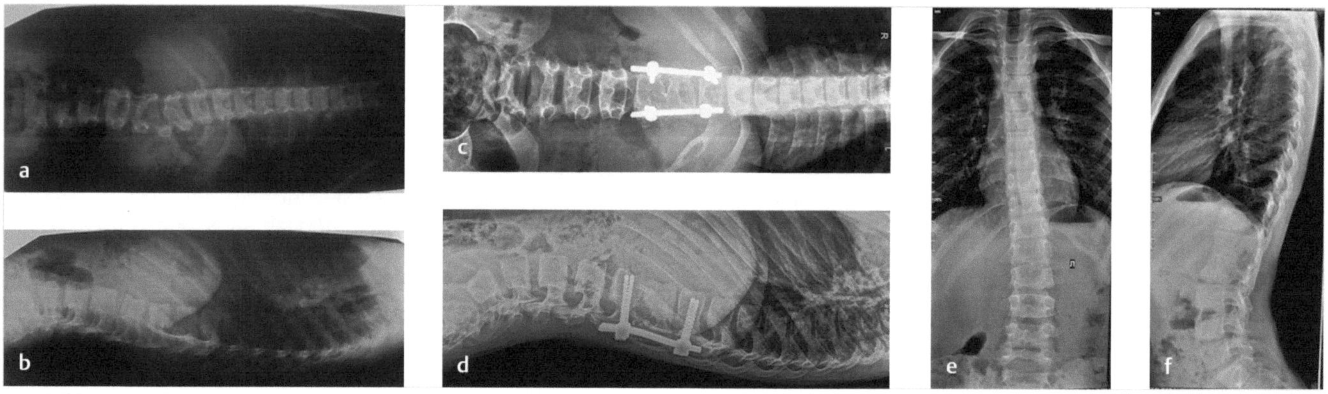

Fig. 5.7 A 2-year-old girl with congenital kyphoscoliosis caused by left-sided L2 posterolateral hemivertebra. **(a)** AP and **(b)** lateral views taken before surgery show prominent local scoliotic deformity and flattening of lumbar lordosis. After extirpation using combined approach complete correction both in **(c)** frontal and **(d)** sagittal planes was achieved. Note that short instrumentation was placed at the T12-L3 levels. 4 years after removal of the implants: **(e)** AP and **(f)** lateral views show solid bone fusion between upper and lower vertebrae, correction is maintained. Surgery helped to prevent inevitable progression of the deformity in this particular child.

kyphosis varied from 18 to 41 degrees (mean angle, 29.6 degrees).

The Cobb angle after instrumented correction of spinal deformity caused by lateral hemivertebrae became 6 to 14 degrees (degree of correction was 82.3–94.7%). After posterolateral hemivertebrae had been extirpated, the residual postoperative Cobb angle varied from 0 to 8 degrees (mean Cobb angle, 4.2 degrees); the degree of correction ranged from 92 to 100%; the angle of local pathological kyphosis at the level of abnormal vertebra was 0 to 9 degrees (mean angle, 4.5 degrees). Stable fixation was achieved in all the patients with congenital thoracic deformity for the entire period of bone fusion formation; 360-degree fusion was observed after the metal constructs had been removed.

The preoperative Cobb angle of the local scoliotic curve in the thoracolumbar junction varied from 18 to 52 degrees (mean Cobb angle, 32.7 degrees ± 5.9 degrees); the Cobb angle of kyphotic deformity varied from 4 to 49 degrees (mean Cobb angle, 22.0 degrees ± 9.4 degrees).

After extirpation of the abnormal hemivertebra, anterior fusion using autologous bone graft, posterior correction, and fixation with a metal construct, the amount of scoliotic deformity correction was 85%; the amount of kyphotic deformity correction was 78.6%. Stable fixation of spinal functional units was achieved in 35 patients during the period when they had a metal construct inserted; the 360-degree bone fusion was formed in the intervention area. Destabilization of a construct caused by household injuries was observed in two children in this group; reoperation was required to stabilize the spinal implant. However, the formation of the anterior and posterior bone fusion during the surgery was not affected.

The compensatory curves (both the cranial and caudal curves) in patients with congenital deformity in the thoracic spine and the thoracolumbar junction were eliminated after the primary curve had been corrected. Long-term follow-up showed no progression of abnormal spine curvature in patients with radically corrected congenital deformity. It is reasonable to use the combined approach to perform surgical intervention in patients with vertebral malformations in the thoracic spine and thoracolumbar junction. As opposed to the isolated dorsal approach, this procedure provided minimal contact with and injury to the spinal cord, and unlike the isolated anterolateral approach it promoted the formation of 360-degree fusion. Extirpation of the abnormal vertebral body with the upper- and lower-lying disks and full correction of the existing deformity are the prerequisites for correction of this type of spine curvature disorder. Selective wedge resection and osteotomy of the neighboring intact vertebral bodies additionally stabilized the posterior supporting complex of the functional spinal unit at the level of the abnormal vertebra to achieve full deformity correction using a construct with multiple fixation points.

The extension of fixation in the thoracic spine and thoracolumbar junction should be selected individually with allowance for the features of compensatory curves in the area of the abnormal vertebra and the range of additional osteotomy of the adjacent arches. The 360-degree spinal fusion formed during temporary fixation is a prerequisite of reliable and stable long-term outcome of surgical management.

Assessment of the long-term outcomes of surgical management of patients younger than 3 years with congenital deformity of the thoracic spine caused by vertebral malformation showed that the postoperative Cobb angle of scoliotic deformity was 0 to 9 degrees (mean Cobb angle, 4.5 degrees ± 3.4 degrees), whereas the Cobb angle of kyphotic deformity varied from 0 to 14 degrees (mean Cobb angle, 4.6 degrees ± 4.3 degrees) (▶ Table 5.8).

Assessment of the long-term outcomes of surgical management of patients younger than 3 years with congenital deformity in the thoracolumbar junction caused by vertebral malformation showed that the postoperative Cobb angle of scoliotic deformity was 0 to 22 degrees (mean Cobb angle, 4.6 degrees ± 4.2 degrees), the Cobb angle of kyphotic deformity varied from − 15 to 23 degrees (mean Cobb angle, 6.5 degrees ± 6.1 degrees) (▶ Table 5.9).

Table 5.8 Outcomes of surgical management of pediatric patients with posterolateral and lateral hemivertebrae in the thoracic spine before surgery, immediately after, and during long-term follow-up

Indicators	Before surgery	Immediately after surgery	Long-term follow-up	Statistical significance
Number of cases (n)	39	39	39	39
Cobb angle of kyphotic deformity, °	18–41	0–9	0–9	*P*<0.001 (Student's *t*-test)
	29.6 ± 8.4	4.5 ± 3.8	4.5 ± 3.4	
Cobb angle of scoliotic deformity, °	26–59	0–14	0–14	*P*<0.001 (Student's *t*-test)
	42.7 ± 5.8	4.9 ± 3.7	4.6 ± 4.3	
Bone block fusion	Fusion in 39 (100 %) patients			

Note: The selected threshold values and the mean ± standard deviation are listed in the table. Patient groups were compared using the Student's t-test for dependent samples.

Table 5.9 Outcomes of surgical management of pediatric patients with posterolateral and lateral hemivertebrae in the thoracolumbar junction before surgery, immediately after, and during long-term follow-up

Indicators	Before surgery	Immediately after surgery	Long-term follow-up	Statistical significance
Number of cases (n)	37	37	37	37
Cobb angle of kyphotic deformity, °	4–49 22.0 ± 9.4	−15–20 4.7 ± 4.8	−15–23 6.5 ± 6.1	*P*<0.001 (Student's *t*-test)
Cobb angle of kyphotic deformity correction, °		17.3	15.5	
Cobb angle of scoliotic deformity, °	18–52 32.7 ± 5.9	0–24 4.9 ± 4.9	4.6 ± 4.2	*P*<0.001(Student's *t*-test)
Cobb angle of scoliotic deformity correction, °		27.8 0–22	28.1	
Bone block fusion	Fusion in 37 (100 %) patients			

Note: The selected threshold values and the mean ± standard deviation are listed in the table. Patient groups were compared using the Student's t-test for dependent samples.

References

[1] Vissarionov SV. Surgical treatment of segmental instability of the thoracic and lumbar spine in children [in Russian]. Doctoral dissertation. Siberian University, Novosibirsk, Russia 2008

[2] Mikhailovskii MV, Fomichev NG. Surgery of Spinal Deformities [in Russian]. Redactio Publishers, Novosibirsk, Russia; 2002

[3] Ul'rikh EV. Spinal Anomalies in Children [in Russian]. Sotis Publishers, St. Petersburg; 1995

[4] Bosch B, Heimkes B, Stotz S. Course and prognosis of congenital scoliosis [in German]. Z Orthop Ihre Grenzgeb. 1994; 132(5):363–370

[5] Ruf M, Harms J. Hemivertebra resection by a posterior approach: innovative operative technique and first results. Spine. 2002; 27(10):1116–1123

[6] Bollini G, Docquier PL, Viehweger E, Launay F, Jouve JL. Lumbar hemivertebra resection. J Bone Joint Surg Am. 2006; 88(5):1043–1052

[7] Bradford DS, Boachie-Adjei O. One-stage anterior and posterior hemivertebral resection and arthrodesis for congenital scoliosis. J Bone Joint Surg Am. 1990; 72(4):536–540

[8] Chen YT, Wang ST, Liu CL, Chen TH. Treatment of congenital scoliosis with single-level hemivertebrae. Arch Orthop Trauma Surg. 2009; 129(4):431–438

[9] King JD, Lowery GL. Results of lumbar hemivertebral excision for congenital scoliosis. Spine. 1991; 16(7):778–782

[10] Leatherman KD, Dickson RA. Two-stage corrective surgery for congenital deformities of the spine. J Bone Joint Surg Br. 1979; 61-B(3):324–328

[11] Slabaugh PB, Winter RB, Lonstein JE, Moe JH. Lumbosacral hemivertebrae. A review of twenty-four patients, with excision in eight. Spine. 1980; 5(3):234–244

[12] Jalanko T, Rintala R, Puisto V, Helenius I. Hemivertebra resection for congenital scoliosis in young children: comparison of clinical, radiographic, and health-related quality of life outcomes between the anteroposterior and posterolateral approaches. Spine. 2011; 36(1):41–49

[13] Mikhailovskii MV, Fomichev NG. Surgery of Spinal Deformities [in Russian]. Redactio Publishers, Novosibirsk, Russia; 2011

[14] Bollini G, Docquier P-L, Viehweger E, Launay F, Jouve J-L. Thoracolumbar hemivertebrae resection by double approach in a single procedure: long-term follow-up. Spine. 2006; 31(15):1745–1757

[15] McMaster MJ, Ohtsuka K. The natural history of congenital scoliosis. A study of two hundred and fifty-one patients. J Bone Joint Surg Am. 1982; 64 (8):1128–1147

[16] Garrido E, Tome-Bermejo F, Tucker SK, Noordeen HN, Morley TR. Short anterior instrumented fusion and posterior convex non-instrumented fusion of hemivertebra for congenital scoliosis in very young children. Eur Spine J. 2008; 17(11):1507–1514

[17] Campos MA, Fernandes P, Dolan LA, Weinstein SL. Infantile thoracolumbar kyphosis secondary to lumbar hypoplasia. J Bone Joint Surg Am. 2008; 90 (8):1726–1729

[18] Cheung KM, Zhang JG, Lu DS, K Luk KD, Y Leong JC. Ten-year follow-up study of lower thoracic hemivertebrae treated by convex fusion and concave distraction. Spine. 2002; 27(7):748–753

[19] MacEwen GD, Winter RB, Hardy JH. Evaluation of kidney anomalies in congenital scoliosis. J Bone Joint Surg Am. 1972; 54(7):1451–1454

[20] McMaster MJ, McMaster ME. Prognosis for congenital scoliosis due to a unilateral failure of vertebral segmentation. J Bone Joint Surg Am. 2013; 95 (11):972–979

[21] Nasca RJ, Stilling FH, III, Stell HH. Progression of congenital scoliosis due to hemivertebrae and hemivertebrae with bars. J Bone Joint Surg Am. 1975; 57 (4):456–466

[22] Winter RB, Moe JJ, Eilers VE. Congenital scoliosis a study of 234 patients treated and untreated. J Bone Joint Surg Am. 1968; 50-A:1–47

[23] Uzumcugil A, Cil A, Yazici M, et al. Convex growth arrest in the treatment of congenital spinal deformities, revisited. J Pediatr Orthop. 2004; 24(6):658–666

[24] Ivashchenko DA. Congenital spine curvatures caused by pathological changes in vertebral bones. Ortopediya I Travmatologiya. 1936(1):68–79

[25] McMaster MJ, Singh H. Natural history of congenital kyphosis and kyphoscoliosis. A study of one hundred and twelve patients. J Bone Joint Surg Am. 1999; 81(10):1367–1383

Suggesed Readings

Holte DC, Winter RB, Lonstein JE, Denis F. Excision of hemivertebrae and wedge resection in the treatment of congenital scoliosis. J Bone Joint Surg Am. 1995; 77 (2):159–171

Ledonio CG, Polly DW, Jr, Vitale MG, Wang Q, Richards BS. Pediatric Pedicle Screws: Comparative Effectiveness and Safety: a systematic literature review from the Scoliosis Research Society and the Pediatric Orthopaedic Society of North America task force. J Bone Joint Surg Am. 2011; 93(13):1227–1234

McMaster MJ. Occult intraspinal anomalies and congenital scoliosis. J Bone Joint Surg Am. 1984; 66(4):588–601

Murrey DB, Brigham CD, Kiebzak GM, Finger F, Chewning SJ. Transpedicular decompression and pedicle subtraction osteotomy (eggshell procedure): a retrospective review of 59 patients. Spine. 2002; 27(21):2338–2345

Suk SI, Kim W-J, Lee S-M, Kim J-H, Chung E-R. Thoracic pedicle screw fixation in spinal deformities: are they really safe? Spine. 2001; 26(18):2049–2057

6 Osteotomies in Children under the Age of 10 Years

Josh Schroeder, Leon Kaplan

Abstract

Pediatric spinal deformities can be rigid and require different grades of soft tissue and bony releases in order to realign the spine. In simple cases, a partial facetectomy is enough; however, in more complex cases, single or multiple vertebrae might need to be removed. In this chapter, we will describe the different kinds of osteotomies in use when realigning the spine.

Keywords: rigid spinal deformity, osteotomy, pedicle subtraction osteotomy, vertebrectomy

6.1 Background

The prevalence of patients with juvenile idiopathic scoliosis has remained relatively constant, ranging from 8 to 16% of all idiopathic scoliosis cases in the literature.[1] It is more common in girls than in boys (at rates of 1:1.6:15.4). Juvenile scoliosis develops before a child is 10 years old and progresses slowly during the period of steady spinal growth. However, after the age of 10 years, progression is rapid during the period of accelerated spinal growth, despite the use of a brace, leading in most cases to the need for spinal athrodesis in order to prevent additional progression.[2]

Poor prognosis (progression of the deformity) in juvenile idiopathic scoliosis includes a serial increase in the rib–vertebrae angle difference at the apex of the primary curve, a thoracic kyphosis of less than 20 degrees, and a left-sided curve in a boy.[3,4] The thoracic spinal deformities are associated with a progression leading to the need for surgical management.

As the spine deformity progresses, the chest wall distortion increases and a restrictive respiratory disease develops.[5] The decrease in respiratory vital capacity in children with juvenile idiopathic scoliosis is greater than the decrease in vital capacity in children with similar Cobb angles who develop scoliosis in adolescence.[6] Children with infantile scoliosis demonstrate asymmetry in right and left lung fields in chest radiographs as the spinal deformity worsens. In severe deformities, a thoracic insufficiency syndrome, defined as the inability of the thorax to support normal respiration or lung growth in a skeletally immature patient, can develop.[7]

Idiopathic scoliosis in patients under 10 years of age has been shown to carry a higher prevalence of concordant intraspinal anomalies when compared to the adolescent age group. These anomalies include Arnold–Chiari malformation (most commonly type II), syringomyelia, tethered cord, and other dysraphic disorders of the cord, including intraspinal neoplasms.[8] These anomalies have been reported in approximately 20% of patients with juvenile idiopathic scoliosis.[9] Neglected early-onset scoliosis can lead to cor pulmonale and early death.[10]

Casting and bracing constitute the initial stage of management of these curves; however, the success rate of such treatment is modest because the curve is not likely to be controlled throughout growth with such measures.

When surgery is considered, nonfusion devices are the first line of care because they allow the vertebrae in the deformity area and the chest cavity to continue to grow.[10] However, unilateral growing rods and Luque trolley systems are predictably disappointing in controlling noncongenital early-onset spinal deformities and in preserving growth. Bilateral growing rods provide a more solid mode of initial fixation.[3] However, the risk of placement and pullout of pedicle screws in patients with small anatomy, repetitive surgery, the rigidity of fixation, and a complication rate of 20% per surgery, promoted the search for alternative methods of fixation.[11]

The Shilla system is based on a single intervention with periapical pedicle screw fixation, local fusion, as well as pedicle screw anchoring at both ends of the curve. Those screw heads provide slide-through of the rods with further growth.[12] In both systems, the reported correction rate is 50 to 60% of the initial deformity.[11,12] However, the studies on this technique are still premature and are gathered from case series at best.

The Vertical Expandable Prosthetic Titanium Rib device (VEPTR; DePuy Synthese) has been tried as a fusion-sparing alternative in patients with juvenile deformities.[13] VEPTR was primarily designed for children with thoracic insufficiency syndrome related to spinal and thoracic abnormalities (and is described in Chapter 7).

In a study by Hasler et al, with 23 children with an average age of 5.4 to 7.6 years at first surgery,[14] the initial average Cobb angle was 68 degrees, with a mix of cases of juvenile, syndromatic, and neuromuscular deformities with a different amount of rigidity. VEPTR indirectly corrected 30% of the initial spinal deformity.

The need for repeated surgeries in the nonfusion devices with a high rate of complications, including soft tissue, bone, and rib fractures; dislodgment of implants; metal implant breakage; and infections, reduces the implication of these systems in all pediatric deformities.

6.2 Overall Management of the Rigid Spine Deformity

A rigid spinal deformity in a child requires an assessment of the underlying pathology that is driving the deformity and whether it is unifocal or multifocal. Is it driven from a congenital spinal deformity or a systemic disease that created a spinal deformity as part of a syndrome? What are the functional demands of the child—is he a walker or will he need a balanced spine for wheelchair sitting? These considerations will guide the surgeon in the process of planning the surgical correction of the deformity. The overall goal of the treatment is to provide a balanced spine on both the coronal and the sagittal planes, allow balanced sitting in nonambulatory patients, prevent skin-related problems caused by asymmetrical compression of the deformity (i.e., pressure sores), facilitate daily activities for the patient and caretakers, improve external appearance, and improve self-image.

An osteotomy should be considered in any situation where release of soft tissue and instrumentation alone are unlikely to adequately correct deformity and restore balance. Osteotomies should be considered in fixed deformities that do not bend down to below 70 degrees on bending or traction films.[14] As a rule of thumb, the greater degree of osteotomies involves a larger risk of complications, such as permanent neurologic damage, increased bleeding, infection, and iatrogenic instability.[15] A detailed preoperative plan should be fabricated, and a discussion with families of the risks and benefits of osteotomies should be considered a mandatory first step in these procedures.

6.3 Halo Traction

Halo traction, which was developed for the unstable cervical spine (resulting from fracture-dislocations and unstable fractures of the vertebrae) can be used for presurgical correction and evaluation of severe scoliosis requiring fusion, or spinal osteotomy and refusion.[16] The halo also allows other forms of skeletal traction to be used.[17] It has been shown to reduce the curve by 30 to 50%[18] and can assist in simplifying the correction of the deformity. The traction can be used as a halo-pelvic or halo-femoral traction, or as a halo-gravity construct allowing mobility of the child while traction is applied (i. e., halo-chair or halo-walker traction allowing mobility and movement during the traction).

6.3.1 Halo Placement Technique

The halo traction apparatus is placed under local or general anesthesia (depending on the child's age). The number of skull pins varies with patient age, with younger patients having more pins placed (up to 6–8 pins) to prevent secondary loosening of the halo apparatus.[19,20] The traction is started at 2 to 4 kg (5–10 lb). The weights are connected to a transferable frame that can be placed on a wheelchair or walker when the patient sits up or walks. The traction is increased as tolerated by the patient until the patient is barely touching the wheelchair seat, or up to 33% of body weight.[21] In bed, the traction is maintained. The patient's neurologic status is monitored in the inpatient unit and on follow-up. Patients may be discharged home in traction after parents are trained and comfortable with the management of halo traction. Routine skull pin care is performed. Decisions as to the length and timing of traction depend on the magnitude of the deformity, the response to traction, and the patient's overall systemic, respiratory, nutritional, and social conditions, as determined by the surgeon in charge of the patient's care.

Long-term traction is used to maximize pulmonary function and nutritional status.[16] At times, the traction can be applied after an anterior release procedure to increase the curve flexibility and achieve a partial correction of the curve, and to allow a better understanding of the skeletal pathology (as the curve uncoils) before the surgical decision is made.

6.3.2 Complications with Halo Frames

Complications related to traction depend on the type of traction, the age of the patient, the duration of treatment, and the amount of traction applied. Skull pin complications include loosening and migration (causing at times unsightly scars), superficial and deep pin tract infections that may lead to skull osteomyelitis, spontaneous ankylosis of the cervical spine, avascular necrosis of the proximal part of the dens, loss of cervical lordosis, and long-term loss of cervical movement. Several neurologic complications are related to halo traction, the most common being preoperative paraplegia, cranial nerve (CN 6) palsies, and supraorbital neuralgia.

6.4 Osteotomies for Correction of Rigid Spinal Deformities

Posterior-based spinal release and osteotomies were first described by Hibbs in the 1920 s. In 1931, Hibbs and Ferguson described a partial facetectomy and inferior joint resection with curettage of the joint cartilage.[22] In the 1940s, Howarth expanded the technique to include resection of the spinous process and the intraspinous ligaments to improve mobility of the spine and the use of local bone graft for fusion.[23] Later on, in 1969 Smith-Petersen et al, modified this technique for lumbar flexion deformity in ankylosis spondylitis,[25,24] allowing a primary correction of the sagittal profile, but this osteotomy may be useful for a coronal plane correction as well.

Three-column osteotomies, were initially described by Michele and Krueger[26] in the late 1940s and were the basis for modern pedicle subtraction osteotomy (PSO). PSO was also known as the eggshell procedure for posterior treatment of vertebral osteomyelitis; later on the technique was modified to become a closing-wedge osteotomy. These approaches were developed to create a posterior-based technique to mobilize and correct a rigid spinal deformity in the sagittal plane.

Schwab et al[27] have also described a classification system spinal osteotomies for corrective sagittal malalignments. Their progressive grading system includes six steps of resection, corresponding to different anatomical bone resections, which reflect increasing degrees of potential destabilization of the spine. This classification system applies only to the sagittal plane.

This chapter presents a grading system of osteotomies for rigid spine deformities that includes correction of coronal, sagittal, and multiplanar deformities.

6.4.1 Partial Facet Joint Resection

Partial facet osteotomies, as described by Hibbs,[28] involve resection of the inferior facet and joint capsule at a given spinal level. This technique has limited power over spinal deformity correction.

Technique

After soft tissue release and removal of the facet capsule, the inferior facet is removed with an osteotome or bur drill, exposing the underlying cartilage. The cartilage is scraped from the joint using a curet or a bur to expose the underlying joint and to provide grounds for facet joint fusion.

6.4.2 Complete Facet Joint Resection (Posterior Elementectomy)

As described by Geck et al[29], this osteotomy removes all of the posterior base confounders from one side of the spine to the other. Such a release requires total removal of the facet joints, the ligamentum flavum, parts of the lamina, and the spinous processes at the resected level. This osteotomy requires preexisting anterior column mobility and is suitable for long deformities, such as hyperkyphosis cases with developmental deformities involving multiple vertebrae (e. g., Scheuermann's kyphosis and osteoporosis).

Technique

This technique was described by Smith-Petersen and refined by Diab et al.[30]

The spine is exposed and screw tracts are developed for subsequent pedicle screw placement. The screw tracts remain empty during the osteotomy procedure; the empty tracts help guide the osteotomy, but screws themselves may block the procedure. The spinous process of the vertebra cephalad to the osteotomy site is resected to allow full exposure of the interspace and to allow closing of the osteotomy. Using Kerrison rongeurs, part or all of the lamina (depending on the amount of correction needed), the ligamentum flavum, and the superior and inferior articular processes are removed bilaterally. The osteotomy is carried laterally to the intervertebral notch. The resection creates a chevron-shaped area, with the point oriented distally. In cases in which an element of coronal plane correction is desired as well, one side of the osteotomy is widened more than the other side, creating an asymmetrical gap allowing closure of the defect. If the osteotomy is performed at a level with significant rotational deformity, the osteotomy should be opened to a greater degree on the side of the convexity in an effort to decrease the rotational aspect of the deformity.[30] Closure of the defect may occur passively as a result of lordosis induced by the surgical frame, or prebent rods can be added to the previously placed bone anchors, and a combination of cantilever correction and compression should achieve the necessary reduction.

6.4.3 Three-Column Osteotomies

Three-column osteotomies involve a partial wedge resection of the posterior vertebral body and the posterior elements with the pedicles.[27] A portion of the vertebral body and the disks above and below the level of the osteotomy remain intact. The following sections describe six subtypes of osteotomies aimed at providing surgeons with the proper techniques to deal with complex deformities.

Type I—Pure Hyperkyphotic Deformity

For pure kyphotic deformity (in the sagittal plane) with a positive sagittal balance, a balanced pedicle subtraction osteotomy is needed, as described by Thomasen.[25] In this osteotomy, as in complete facetectomy, a wide resection of the posterior elements is needed, which involves removing the complete lamina with resection of the facet joints above and below the resected vertebrae. This allows safe neural mobility so that at the end of the procedure both exiting nerve roots will be in the same foramina. This osteotomy allows correction of nearly 30 degrees in the sagittal plane and is suitable for short, sharp, kyphotic deformities (as in cases of posttraumatic kyphosis, ankylosis spondylitis, or congenital kyphosis) (▶ Fig. 6.1).

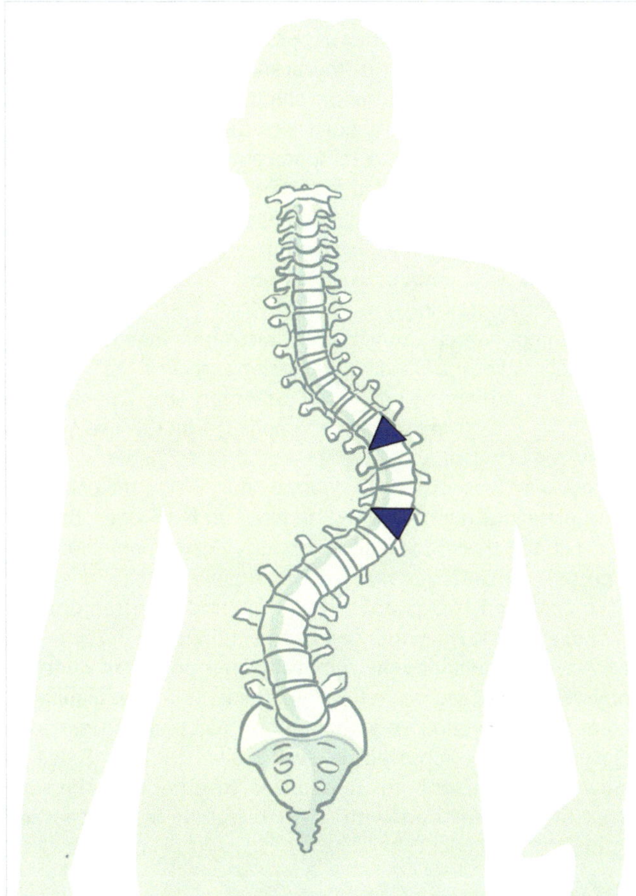

Fig. 6.1 For coronal plane deformities or scoliosis, this is a wedge-type corrective osteotomy that is convexity-based. It may be single or multiple, and can be used to perform an osteotomy of the fusion mass.

Technique

The spine is exposed and the level or levels to be osteotomized are identified. Pedicle screws are placed above and below the osteotomy. A Kerrison rongeur and bur drills are used to perform laminectomies and complete bilateral facetectomies at the osteotomy level. An extensive posterior decompression of the dura above and below the osteotomy is needed to prevent invagination of the dura with osteotomy closure, which can result in kinking of the neural elements inside the dural sac and associated neurologic deficit.[15]

A tract is developed through the pedicle to the vertebral body (as if to place a pedicle screw). The pedicles are decancellated with a bur drill or osteotome and then detached from the transverse processes, and the lateral vertebral walls are exposed by dissecting the psoas muscle away from the lateral aspect of the vertebral body with a sponge stick or periosteal elevator. This separation is maintained by leaving a sponge or malleable retractor in the potential space until closure of the osteotomy. The nerve roots above and below the pedicle are identified. At times in the thoracic spine, the roots are sacrificed to allow a larger working space and better mobility of the cord to prevent a traction injury when the reduction is completed. A wedge of bone is resected from the vertebral body through the pedicles while the dura and nerve roots are protected.

Working underneath the posterior vertebral cortex, the surgeon thins the cortex as much as possible with a curet. After decancellation and thinning of the posterior wall, the portion of the vertebral body underlying the anterior spinal canal is removed by collapsing this bone into the decancellated cavity with a downfacing curet. A temporary rod is placed across the osteotomy site. The fractured posterior cortex is then removed.

The final step in completing the bony resection of the osteotomy is to remove or break the lateral vertebral body walls. The cord at this time should be visualized from all sides (360-degree decompression) to ensure that there is no bony impingement, which can cause a catastrophic event when the osteotomy is being closed. The anterior aspect of the vertebral body acts as a hinge by which the osteotomy site is closed. Closure of the osteotomy can be accomplished by the use of temporary rods to cantilever the spine and/or by hyperextending the chest and legs with the operating table. When the construct is complete and the osteotomy is closed on both sides, the spinal canal, the thecal sac, and the exiting nerve roots should be inspected to ensure that there are no impinged sites.

The extended PSO is defined as in a grade 4 osteotomy by Schwab et al.[27] It is a wider wedge resection through the vertebral body and includes the removal of the posterior vertebral body, removal of the posterior elements with pedicles, and sufficient body resection such that an end plate and at least one adjacent disk are removed. In such cases, the disk above or below is removed, or both are removed, together with the bony PSO. This is associated with a rib resection in the thoracic region.

Type II—Hyperlordotic Deformity

In cases with a pure sagittal deformity in which the sagittal balance is negative, there is a lordotic deformity in the low thoracic or lumbar spine. This can lead to a posterior pelvic tilt (with a horizontal sacrum), leading to a crouched-gate walking pattern and severe back pain and disability. This type of deformity is relatively rare and can be corrected in a combined anterior and posterior approach, or as described here in a posterior-only osteotomy. In such cases, the osteotomy will be ventrally based with anterior spine shortening and straightening and elongating and straightening of the posterior arch. The correction will close the anterior column of the spine and will not greatly distract the posterior elements. This correction is technically demanding (▸ Fig. 6.2).

Technique

The first steps are similar to those for kyphotic deformity correction up to the point in which the osteotomy is made. The osteotomy in the vertebral body is planned in a triangular fashion, aiming at the anterior cortex of the vertebra. The bone is resected from the vertebral body through the pedicles while protecting the dura and nerve roots.

Working underneath the posterior vertebral cortex, the surgeon thins the anterior cortex as much as possible with a curet. After decancellation and thinning of the anterior vertebral wall, the spongy bone of the vertebra is removed. In addition, a portion of the posterior aspect of the vertebra underlying the anterior border of the spinal canal is removed. At this time the cord should be visualized to make certain that it is decompressed from all aspects (i. e., 360 degrees).

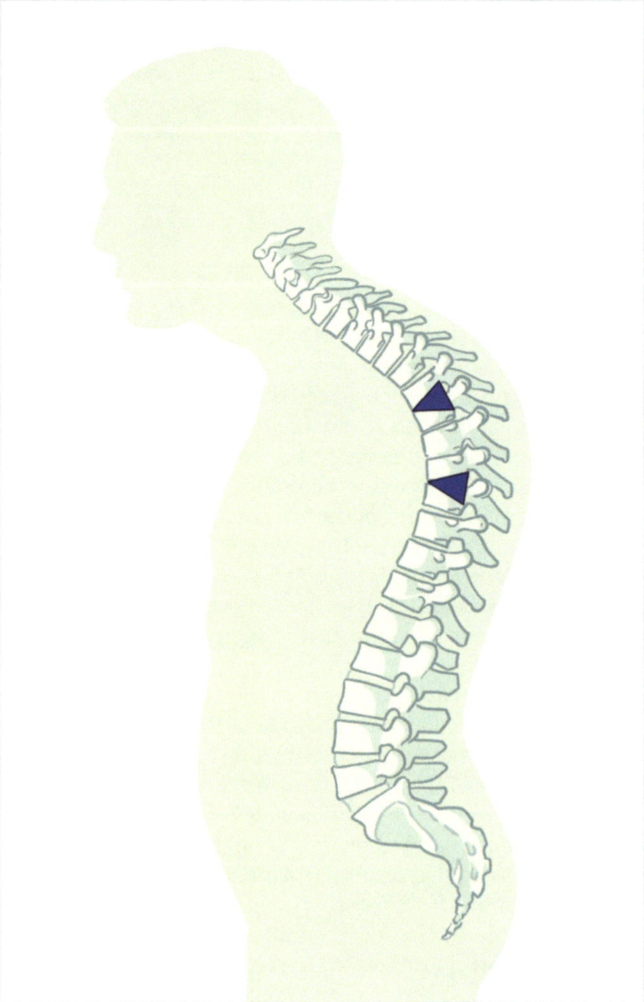

Fig. 6.2 For kyphosis, this dorsally based corrective osteotomy allows posterior arch shortening.

The final step in completing the bony resection of the osteotomy is to remove the lateral vertebral body walls. The dorsal aspect of the vertebral body acts as a hinge by which the osteotomy site is closed. Closure of the osteotomy can be accomplished by the use of temporary rods to cantilever the spine. When the construct is complete and the osteotomy is closed on both sides, the spinal canal, thecal sac, and nerve roots can be inspected to ensure they are not distracted too much when the arch is closed in order to realign the spine. Neuromonitoring of the nerve roots with electromyography is critical for a safe correction during the entire procedure.

Type III—Pure Coronal Plane Deformity

These patients have a deformity in the coronal plane with a normal sagittal plane. This deformity is caused mainly by a congenital anomaly, driving most of the deformity to wedge in the coronal plane, such as a congenital hemivertebra.

The convex-based osteotomy is an asymmetric PSO to remove the extra bone and balance the spine (▸ Fig. 6.3).

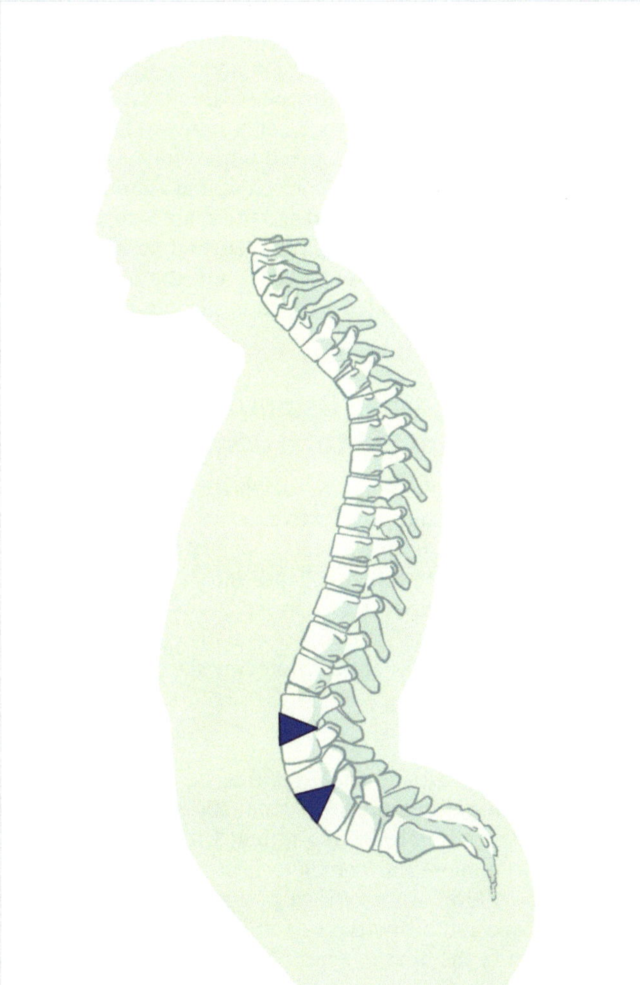

Fig. 6.3 For hyperlordosis, this corrective osteotomy is ventrally-based, allowing anterior spine shortening and posterior arch straightening.

Technique

The first steps are similar to those for a symmetrical PSO, up to the point in which the osteotomy is made. The osteotomy of the vertebral body is planned in a triangular fashion, removing an increased bony portion on the convex side of the deformity. The bone is resected from the vertebral body through the convex pedicle while protecting the dura and nerve roots. In the majority of cases there is a posterior synostosis, mandating a wide excision of the posterior elements to allow adequate mobility of the spinal segment to correct the deformity.

Working underneath the posterior vertebral cortex, the surgeon thins the dorsal cortex as much as possible with a curet until the deformed vertebra is completely removed. The rod is placed and the compression step is performed on the convexity of the spine, to close the gap, reaching bony contact and a coronally balanced spine. When the construct is complete and the osteotomy is closed, the spinal canal and the thecal sac and nerve roots should be inspected to ensure they are not impinged upon.

Type IV—Multiplanar Kyphoscoliotic Deformity

In these cases there is both a sagittal and a coronal plane deformity at the same spinal segment (▶ Fig. 6.4). In such cases the correction can be done in a combined anterior and posterior fashion, in which the corpectomy is performed from the convex side, resecting the bone causing the coronal deformity. Using a posterior approach, a PSO is performed correcting the sagittal deformity. This has been the classical approach; however, there is much morbidity in such extensive approaches. To avoid the morbidity and the complicated approaches, a posterior-only approach has been developed. For such correction a two-plane osteotomy is needed, which requires complex planning and may employ a computer-assisted navigation system.

When approaching this deformity one must remember that the cord always takes the shortest course possible; therefore, it

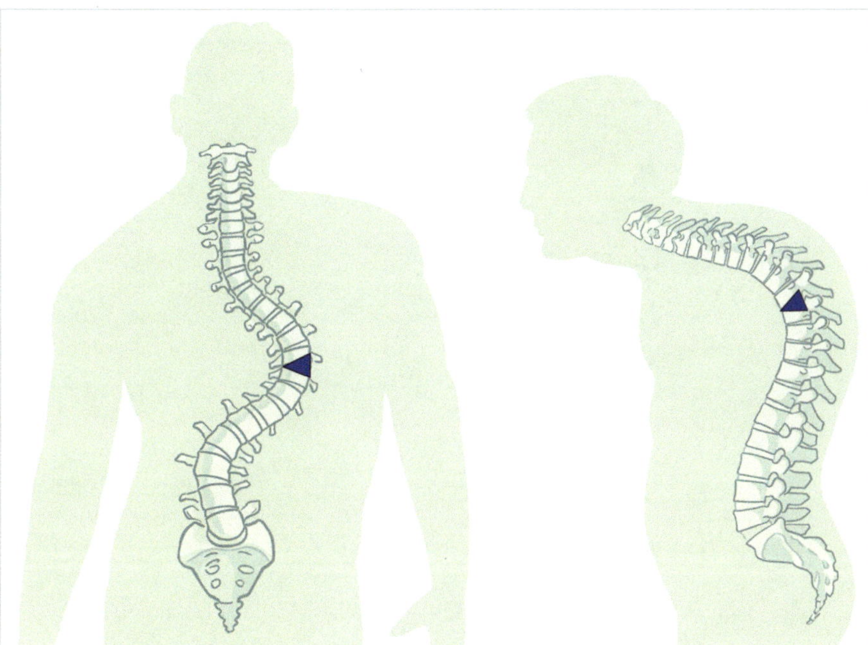

Fig. 6.4 This is a complex wedge corrective osteotomy for complex plane deformities, kyphoscoliosis, or kyphosing scoliosis: Front (corpectomy) + back (wedge osteotomy), or back (corpectomy + 2 plane osteotomies).

lies adjacent to the concavity side and on the kyphotic corner of the deformity. This side should be where bone is first removed, in order to allow cord mobility and prevent impingement of the cord and neurologic damage when the correction is performed. This type of osteotomy is very similar to a vertebral column resection (VCR) or an apical vertebral resection.

Technique—Posterior Only

The first steps are similar to those for a PSO up to the point in which the osteotomy is made. The posterior elements are removed with a triangular-shaped osteotomy, with the wide base directed toward the convexity of the deformity. As stated earlier, the first part of the vertebrectomy needs to be done at the concavity of the deformity removing the pedicle and the kyphotic corner of the deformed spinal segment in order to make sure that there is no impingent of the cord. The osteotomy is continued in the vertebral body in a wide, biplanar fashion, working toward the convexity and dorsally, removing an increased bony portion on the convex side of the deformity. The bone is resected from the vertebral body through the pedicles while protecting the dura and nerve roots. The wedge needs to be planned according to the magnitude of the kyphoscoliosis; removal of one vertebra can possibly correct the deformity by 30 to 40 degrees, and each disk adds 5 to 15 degrees to the correction. The proximal ends of the adjacent ribs from both sides should be removed as well to allow proper mobility.

Working underneath the posterior vertebral cortex, the surgeon thins the cortex as much as possible with a curet. The posterior cortex of the vertebra is removed, decompressing the cord in all directions (i. e., 360 degrees) for circumferential decompression. Nerve roots at the apex of the osteotomy should be ligated and cut (one or two on the concavity and convexity side, as needed), allowing cord mobility and preventing tethering or traction injury of the cord at the time of reduction. The rods are placed, and the compression and reduction steps are performed with a four-rod technique—two rods on each side of the deformity being brought together, progressively and slowly closing the gap. The rods are linked with domino connectors. Secondary in situ progressive correction and compression are performed until the gap is closed and the spine is corrected and balanced. When the construct is complete and the osteotomy is closed on both sides, the spinal canal and the dural sac and nerve roots can be inspected to ensure they are not impinged upon.

Type V—The Eggshell Osteotomy (the Decancellated or Subtotal Corpectomy)

In eggshell osteotomy the entire vertebra is decancellated with preservation of the end plates and external cortex. This allows correction of a focal asymmetrical deformity of the vertebra (of any shape) and a controlled collapse into a flat vertebra.[31,32] The osteotomy is designed to correct a short, sharp, sagittal plane deformity in one step. It allows sufficient bone-on-bone contact and good healing of the osteotomy site (▶ Fig. 6.5).

Technique

The spine is exposed and the level(s) to be osteotomized are identified. Pedicle screws are placed above and below the osteotomy. A Kerrison rongeur and bur drills are used to perform laminectomies, and complete bilateral facetectomies at the osteotomy level. An extensive posterior decompression of the dura above and below the osteotomy is needed to prevent impingement of the dura when the osteotomy is closed, which

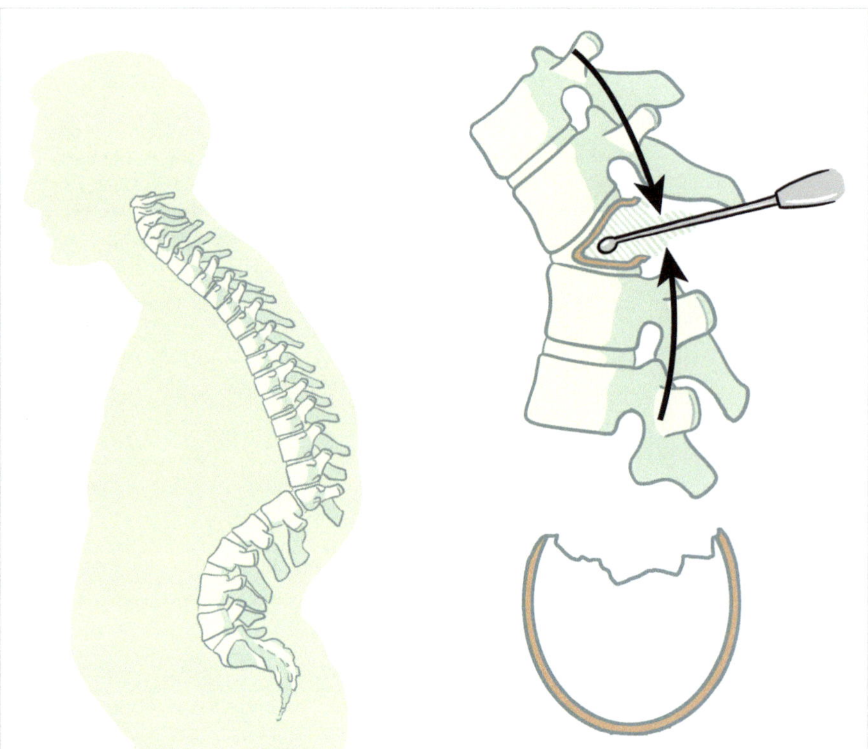

Fig. 6.5 In case of a localized deformity such as a wedge vertebra that causes a sagittal or coronal plane deformity, this eggshell procedure empties the vertebrae allowing localized shortening of the deformity.

can result in kinking of the neural elements and the associated neurologic deficits.

A tract is developed through the pedicle to the vertebral body (as if to place a pedicle screw). The posterior decancellation osteotomy is started on the side of the most accurately detailed anatomy. This pedicle is identified circumferentially and removed with its transverse process while visual protection of the nerve is maintained.

The pedicle opposite the proposed osteotomy is identified, and a similar exposure is performed. After pedicle removal, the vertebral body and the inferior floor of the canal are exposed. The dura is elevated off the posterior wall of the vertebral body. The decancellation of the body is performed through both pedicle remnants. Curets and osteotomes are used to remove the cancellous bone of the body. A temporary rod is placed across the osteotomy site. The floor of the canal is then pushed into the space with reverse curets and removed. After completion of the osteotomy, gentle pressure is applied to the posterior spine or with extension of the hips to close the osteotomy site ("crack phenomenon correction"). Finally, the two rods are placed with appropriate alignment and connected to the screws. The dural sac and nerve roots are visualized to prevent entrapment when the correction is made.

Type VI—Vertebral Column Resection or Apical Vertebral Resection

VCR is a resection of one or more vertebral segments, including the posterior elements (spinous process and laminae), pedicles, vertebral body, and disks, both cephalad and caudad to the resected vertebral body.[33] This allows the greatest correction of the spinal deformity, but it is time consuming and involves a higher risk of local and systemic complications, including nonunion.

The VCR differs significantly from other types of osteotomies in that, because of the complete vertebral segment removal, bone-on-bone contact is not always completely achieved with the closure maneuver. At times it is necessary to reconstruct the anterior spinal column using an interbody device (e.g., an expandable cage, a metal cage, or an allograft or autograft) after a VCR (▶ Fig. 6.6).

A VCR can be performed using combined anterior and posterior approaches or a posterior-only approach. A specific subtype of VCR is used in children with myelomeningocele (MMC) in which a large gibbus is present; this subtype—a kyphectomy—is described extensively in Chapter 12.

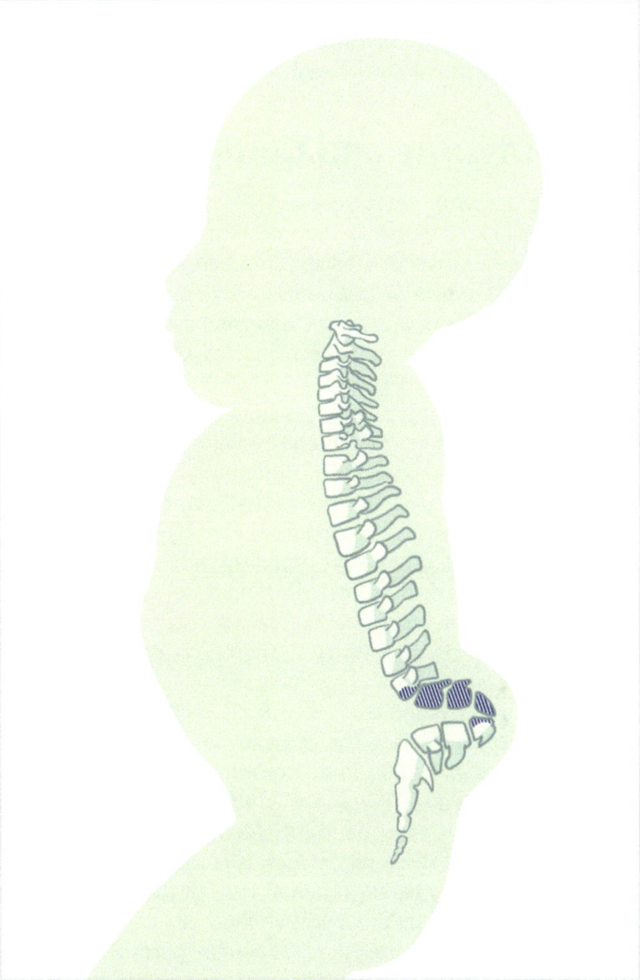

Fig. 6.6 In case of fixed kyphosis, such as MMC, or a kyphectomy, a VCR of several of the vertebrae is performed, allowing full mobility of the spine.

Technique—Posterior Only

Like the PSO the resection begins after placement of the pedicular screws above and below the osteotomy site. This is followed with removal of the posterior elements, including the spinous processes, laminae, facet joints, and transverse processes at the level(s) to be resected. All exiting nerve roots need to be exposed. In the thoracic spine, costotransversectomies facilitate removal of the vertebral body.

Careful subperiosteal dissection is performed on the side of the spine opposite the temporary stabilizing rod, following the lateral wall of the vertebral body until the anterior aspect is easily palpable. The pedicle and lateral aspect of the vertebral body are then removed using an osteotome or a high-speed bur drill. A temporary rod is placed to prevent translation of the cord during the procedure. Resection of the vertebral body and intervening disks is then accomplished in a stepwise fashion, extending toward the medial side and crossing over to the contralateral side. A thin shell of medial bone is left behind to protect the dural sac and is removed as one of the last steps in the procedure. A second temporary rod, contoured to fit the shape of the deformity, is secured into position on the side that has now undergone subperiosteal dissection and partial vertebral body removal. The first temporary rod is then removed to facilitate complete removal of any residual bone or disk. After placement of the rod, the vertebrae is shelled out, and the dorsal part of the vertebrae is removed in order to free the anterior part of the spinal cord.

The deformity is initially gradually corrected by repeated compression and shortening of the vertebral column using the temporary rods. After the resected gap is shortened and compressed, the temporary rods are exchanged, one by one, with precontoured definitive rods. Additional correction of kyphoscoliosis can be achieved through in situ rod bending with segmental correction as needed by compression, distraction or translation.

The techniques described (PSO, VCR, and apical vertical resection) can sometimes be combined with transverse (Ponte) osteotomies to achieve optimal correction.

6.5 Outcome and Complications

The classic approach for a severe deformity consists of combined anterior and posterior approaches; however, extensive posterior-based corrective osteotomies are gaining popularity.[34,35] Because posterior procedures are performed in a single stage, they involve less surgical time and fewer infections.[36] However, reports state that the blood loss is similar in both approaches.[32]

These complex reconstructions have a high rate of complications that can affect 60% of patients. A wide array of complications have been described in osteotomy cases, including sepsis, cerebrovascular accident, malignant hyperthermia, optic deficit, myocardial infarction, severe hypotension, deep venous thrombosis, pulmonary embolism, pneumonia, cardiac arrest, pulmonary embolism, cord and nerve root injury, instrumentation or junctional failure, vascular injury, wound dehiscence, and visceral injury.[37] There is a small mortality rate in these cases.

In the morbidity and mortality Scoliosis Research Society report[38] of pediatric cases, the complication rate was 10.9% in congenital cases and 17.9% in neuromuscular cases. Aggressive osteotomies, including PSOs and VCRs, are associated with higher rates of new-onset neurologic deficits. Thus, when considering the use of these techniques, it is important to recognize the significantly higher inherent risks of these approaches and provide appropriate preoperative counseling.

We think that these procedures should be performed only at high-volume centers with deformity-experienced surgical teams, experienced neurophysiologists, and proper intensive care units in order to provide patients the safest and best care possible.

Despite the high rate of complications, overall the patients are satisfied with the correction achieved with these extensive osteotomies.

References

[1] Lenke LG, Betz RR, Harms J, et al. Adolescent idiopathic scoliosis: a new classification to determine extent of spinal arthrodesis. J Bone Joint Surg Am. 2001; 83(8):1169–1181

[2] Figueiredo UM, James JI. Juvenile idiopathic scoliosis. J Bone Joint Surg Br. 1981; 63-B(1):61–66

[3] Akbarnia BA. Management themes in early onset scoliosis. J Bone Joint Surg Am. 2007; 89 Suppl 1:42–54

[4] Mehta MH. The rib-vertebra angle in the early diagnosis between resolving and progressive infantile scoliosis. J Bone Joint Surg Br. 1972; 54(2):230–243

[5] Davies G, Reid L. Effect of scoliosis on growth of alveoli and pulmonary arteries and on right ventricle. Arch Dis Child. 1971; 46(249):623–632

[6] Gillingham BL, Fan RA, Akbarnia BA. Early onset idiopathic scoliosis. J Am Acad Orthop Surg. 2006; 14(2):101–112

[7] Campbell RM, Jr, Smith MD, Mayes TC, et al. The characteristics of thoracic insufficiency syndrome associated with fused ribs and congenital scoliosis. J Bone Joint Surg Am. 2003; 85(3):399–408

[8] Lewonowski K, King JD, Nelson MD. Routine use of magnetic resonance imaging in idiopathic scoliosis patients less than eleven years of age. Spine. 1992; 17(6) Suppl:S109–S116

[9] Nakahara D, Yonezawa I, Kobanawa K, et al. Magnetic resonance imaging evaluation of patients with idiopathic scoliosis: a prospective study of four hundred seventy-two outpatients. Spine. 2011; 36(7):E482–E485

[10] Pehrsson K, Larsson S, Oden A, Nachemson A. Long-term follow-up of patients with untreated scoliosis. A study of mortality, causes of death, and symptoms. Spine. 1992; 17(9):1091–1096

[11] Bess S, Akbarnia BA, Thompson GH, et al. Complications of growing-rod treatment for early-onset scoliosis: analysis of one hundred and forty patients. J Bone Joint Surg Am. 2010; 92(15):2533–2543

[12] McCarthy RE, Luhmann S, Lenke L, McCullough FL. The Shilla growth guidance technique for early-onset spinal deformities at 2-year follow-up: a preliminary report. J Pediatr Orthop. 2014; 34(1):1–7

[13] Reinker K, Simmons JW, Patil V, Stinson Z. Can VEPTR(®) control progression of early-onset kyphoscoliosis? A cohort study of VEPTR(®) patients with severe kyphoscoliosis. Clin Orthop Relat Res. 2011; 469(5):1342–1348

[14] Hasler CC, Mehrkens A, Hefti F. Efficacy and safety of VEPTR instrumentation for progressive spine deformities in young children without rib fusions. Eur Spine J. 2010; 19(3):400–408

[15] Bridwell KH, Lewis SJ, Edwards C, et al. Complications and outcomes of pedicle subtraction osteotomies for fixed sagittal imbalance. Spine. 2003; 28 (18):2093–2101

[16] Sink EL, Karol LA, Sanders J, Birch JG, Johnston CE, Herring JA. Efficacy of perioperative halo-gravity traction in the treatment of severe scoliosis in children. J Pediatr Orthop. 2001; 21(4):519–524

[17] Mehlman CT, Al-Sayyad MJ, Crawford AH. Effectiveness of spinal release and halo-femoral traction in the management of severe spinal deformity. J Pediatr Orthop. 2004; 24(6):667–673

[18] Watanabe K, Lenke LG, Bridwell KH, Kim YJ, Hensley M, Koester L. Efficacy of perioperative halo-gravity traction for treatment of severe scoliosis (≥ 100°). J Orthop Sci. 2010; 15(6):720–730

[19] Garabekyan T, Hosseinzadeh P, Iwinski HJ, et al. The results of preoperative halo-gravity traction in children with severe spinal deformity. J Pediatr Orthop B. 2014; 23(1):1–5

[20] Rinella A, Lenke L, Whitaker C, et al. Perioperative halo-gravity traction in the treatment of severe scoliosis and kyphosis. Spine. 2005; 30(4):475–482

[21] Takeshita K, Lenke LG, Bridwell KH, Kim YJ, Sides B, Hensley M. Analysis of patients with nonambulatory neuromuscular scoliosis surgically treated to the pelvis with intraoperative halo-femoral traction. Spine. 2006; 31 (20):2381–2385

[22] Hibbs RA, Ferguson AB. Scoliosis treated by the fusion operation an end-result study of three hundred and sixty cases. J Bone Joint Surg Am. 1931; 13 (1):91–104

[23] James JI. Scoliosis in children. Br J Radiol. 1954; 27(321):511–523

[24] Smith-Petersen MN, Larson CB, Aufranc OE. Osteotomy of the spine for correction of flexion deformity in rheumatoid arthritis. Clin Orthop Relat Res. 1969; 66:6–9

[25] Thomasen E. Vertebral osteotomy for correction of kyphosis in ankylosing spondylitis. Clin Orthop Relat Res. 1985(194):142–152

[26] Michele AA, Krueger FJ. Surgical approach to the vertebral body. J Bone Joint Surg Am. 1949; 31A(4):873–878

[27] Schwab F, Blondel B, Chay E, et al. The comprehensive anatomical spinal osteotomy classification. Neurosurgery. 2014; 74(1):112–120, discussion 120

[28] Hibbs RA. An operation for progressive spinal deformities: a preliminary report of three cases from the service of the orthopaedic hospital. 1911. Clin Orthop Relat Res. 2007; 460(460):17–20

[29] Geck MJ, Macagno A, Ponte A, Shufflebarger HL. The Ponte procedure: posterior only treatment of Scheuermann's kyphosis using segmental posterior shortening and pedicle screw instrumentation. J Spinal Disord Tech. 2007; 20(8):586–593

[30] Diab MG, Franzone JM, Vitale MG. The role of posterior spinal osteotomies in pediatric spinal deformity surgery: indications and operative technique. J Pediatr Orthop. 2011; 31(1) Suppl:S88–S98

[31] Murrey DB, Brigham CD, Kiebzak GM, Finger F, Chewning SJ. Transpedicular decompression and pedicle subtraction osteotomy (eggshell procedure): a retrospective review of 59 patients. Spine. 2002; 27(21):2338–2345

[32] Suk SI, Kim JH, Lee SM, Chung ER, Lee JH. Anterior-posterior surgery versus posterior closing wedge osteotomy in posttraumatic kyphosis with neurologic compromised osteoporotic fracture. Spine. 2003; 28(18):2170–2175

[33] Bradford DS, Tribus CB. Vertebral column resection for the treatment of rigid coronal decompensation. Spine. 1997; 22(14):1590–1599

[34] Suk SI, Chung ER, Kim JH, Kim SS, Lee JS, Choi WK. Posterior vertebral column resection for severe rigid scoliosis. Spine. 2005; 30(14):1682–1687

[35] Bridwell KH, Lewis SJ, Lenke LG, Baldus C, Blanke K. Pedicle subtraction osteotomy for the treatment of fixed sagittal imbalance. J Bone Joint Surg Am. 2003; 85(3):454–463

[36] Dobbs MB, Lenke LG, Kim YJ, Luhmann SJ, Bridwell KH. Anterior/posterior spinal instrumentation versus posterior instrumentation alone for the treatment of adolescent idiopathic scoliotic curves more than 90 degrees. Spine. 2006; 31(20):2386–2391

[37] Lenke LG, Newton PO, Sucato DJ, et al. Complications after 147 consecutive vertebral column resections for severe pediatric spinal deformity: a multicenter analysis. Spine. 2013; 38(2):119–132

[38] Reames DL, Smith JS, Fu KM, et al. Scoliosis Research Society Morbidity and Mortality Committee. Complications in the surgical treatment of 19,360 cases of pediatric scoliosis: a review of the Scoliosis Research Society Morbidity and Mortality database. Spine. 2011; 36(18):1484–1491

7 Surgical Treatment of Rigid Spinal Deformities in Patients with Thoracic Insufficiency Syndrome

Leon Kaplan, Josh Schroeder

Abstract

Thoracic insufficiency syndrome (TIS) is defined as the inability of the thorax to support breathing due to a spinal deformity. TIS is generally diagnosed in children with one or more than one complex systemic conditions. The children are often malnourished and quite fragile. TIS is caused by a spinal deformity that leads in turn to severe deformity of both the lungs, resulting in combined restrictive and constrictive lung disease. The contribution possible from nonsurgical care in these patients is supportive at best, leading to chronic ventilation, recurrent infections, and deterioration in the child's well-being. Spine fusion is not a good option, as it stops bone growth and may leave the patient with small and dysplastic lungs. Often the pedicles and laminas of the children are weak and osteoporotic, and devices attached to them during surgery are frequently dislodged. Device fixation to the ribs allows broader attachment with a stronger context. The use of recurrent elongation constructs allows intermittent elongation of the chest as the child grows, facilitating lung expansion and indirect correction of the spine.

Keywords: exotic scoliosis, thoracic insufficiency syndrome (TIS), thoracic expansion procedure, VEPTR

7.1 Thoracic Insufficiency Syndrome

Thoracic insufficiency syndrome (TIS) is defined as the inability of the thorax to support normal respiration and lung growth.[1] TIS can be caused by severe malformations and coalitions of the spine and the rib cage and leads to respiratory failure due to a restrictive lung disease. The three-dimensional deformity in congenital scoliosis includes the spine, ribs, and sternum, and leads to decreased width and depth of the rib cage, which in turn leads to decreased lung volume.[2] In addition, the chest wall deformity leads to restricted rib motion with unilateral loss of the secondary breathing mechanism. The windswept thorax leads to decreased lung volume on both sides of the thorax, on the concavity and the convexity of the deformity, due to the extreme deformity in the chest wall. The combination of these deformities leads to breathing insufficiency.[3]

The causes of TIS are varied and can include unilateral failure of thoracic segmentation (e.g., congenitally fused ribs with a unilateral unsegmented vertebral bar), failure of formation (e.g., hemivertebrae with absent ribs), early-onset scoliosis, fusion of ribs after chest or chest wall procedures, or multiple fractures in the spine (e.g., as seen in patients with osteogenesis imperfecta).[4,5] Because lung growth occurs mostly after birth it is limited by the anatomical boundaries of the thorax; thus any spine or rib cage malformation that reduces the thoracic volume early in life may adversely affect the size and development of the lungs.[6,7] Patients with considerable congenital thoracic spine deformities have a lower vital capacity on pulmonary function testing than do patients with an equivalent degree of idiopathic scoliosis, which may be due to the restrictive lung disease.[7]

7.2 Care

Treatment of TIS is challenging; patients experience a combination of extreme spinal deformities as well as decreased metabolic and pulmonary function. In addition, many of these children have bone, renal, or cardiac function anomalies that must be evaluated prior to surgery.

Patients with TIS should be evaluated by a multidisciplinary team that includes a pediatrician, pediatric anesthesiologist, pulmonologist, dietitian, social worker, physical therapist, and spine surgeon to assess their ability to withstand the surgery and the extended recovery period. The team should also assess the patients' caregivers because care of these patients requires an integral approach.

The main objectives of surgical treatment in this group of patients are to improve lung function and to prevent secondary complications, such as recurrent pneumonia, and not to correct the spinal deformity.

When considering the intervention, the following important points should be discussed with the patients, their parents, and any caregivers:

1. **The severely collapsing chest cavity deformity:** Respiratory failure is one of the leading factors causing death in TIS patients. The extreme deformity of the chest cavity leads to respiratory complications (i.e., recurrent or chronic pneumonia or apnea). These lead to the need for supplemental oxygen, and the use of accessory muscles and arm support to maintain the body in a balanced sitting posture and to enable adequate breathing. Building the chest's muscular envelope prior to surgery is an important step in the preparation for surgery.
2. **The ability to perform corrective spinal surgery:** Surgery may be detrimental to the patient, due to the severity of the deformity, nutritional deficiencies, poor lung function, and extremely poor bone quality. The surgical procedure takes a toll on patients with TIS. Inserting bulky implants in cachectic children, who may be too thin for surgery, leads to hardware prominence lacking proper soft tissue coverage. In addition, fusion at a young age is problematic.
3. **Flexibility of the deformity on bending, traction, or "hanging" radiographs:** Most of the deformities that lead to TIS are rigid; however, if improvement is seen on these dynamic films the deformity is more easily corrected. In ambulatory patients, bending or traction images can be helpful in

planning the surgical procedure and calculating the amount of expected curve correction. However, in nonambulatory (i. e., seated) children, hanging or traction radiographs should be obtained by holding the child at the axillae and allowing gravity to correct the spinal deformity to the extent possible. Alternatively, two people can pull at the patient from the axillae and the legs, with the patient being in the prone position. These radiographs should be taken in the presence of a physician or nurse practioner.

4. **Significant risk of mortality without intervention:** TIS is not an inert condition and cannot be followed without intervention for long because lung capacity decreases over time, causing the need for permanent oxygen support, then intubation, and eventually mechanical ventilation. Thoracic scoliosis of more than 60 degrees or collapsing hemithorax has severe adverse effects on pulmonary function. In severe cases of TIS with poor pulmonary function, the surgical correction of TIS should be considered a lifesaving procedure.

7.3 Treatment Options

7.3.1 Casting

Cast correction can be part of the management of mild or moderate cases of early-onset scoliosis. Its use was quite common before the development of effective spinal instrumentation. Studies have shown that casting is effective in cases of infantile scoliosis but not for neuromuscular or congenital scoliosis. Casting is most effective in young patients, starting care before the age of 2, and in those with curves of 50 degrees or less.[8] Casting requires careful placement because it can create pressure sores, significant rib or mandibular deformities, and can constrict the chest leading to secondary breathing impairment.

There are no studies focused on TIS and casting; however, if the child is diagnosed at an early stage, casting may slow the progression of a TIS deformity that is not due to a congenital malformation of the spine.

7.3.2 Surgery

Fusion

Fusion spine surgery in young children with TIS has had mixed results. Fusion may prevent the progression of the spinal deformity; however, it has been shown to decrease the chest's ability to grow, causing a decrease in forced vital capacity compared with that of healthy individuals and preventing alveolar regeneration. In addition, there was a negative correlation between length of fusion and FVC in these patients.[2,4] Spinal fusion and deformity correction in patients with TIS are associated with a high failure rate. The weak bone results in weak instrumentation and higher rates of hardware dislodgment. In cases of osteogenesis imperfecta,[9] for example, pedicle fractures have been documented, which often occur as soon as the deformity is corrected by the hardware, leading to secondary loss of correction.

In light of these issues, growth-friendly implants are used to control thoracic spinal deformity in TIS patients and minimize the adverse impact on growth and development of the spine and thorax.

Nonfusion Devices—Thoracospinal Elongation

Distraction-based implants correct and maintain spinal deformity via spinal column distraction. These implants can be attached to the ribs, spine, or pelvis, depending on patient age, characteristics of the curve, the child's level of physical function, and available bone stock. The upper fixation points can be on the spine or the adjacent ribs. Fixation on the spine allows direct correction of the deformity; however, a large percentage of these cases undergo spontaneous fusion. Fixation to the ribs is generally more appropriate in younger children, in whom we try to avoid or delay spinal fusion, spinal fixation is limited by an immature spine, and implants may lead to complications. The downside of fixation to the ribs is that correction of the deformity can be achieved only indirectly.

The two common implants used for nondistraction-based devices are growing rods[10] and the Vertical Expandable Prosthetic Titanium Rib (VEPTR; DePuy Synthes).[4] The growing rod is based on screws placed in the lumbar area of the deformity (usually the lower two vertebrae of the deformity) and fixation in the upper thoracic area of the deformity (pedicle screws, hooks, or rib graspers), with the elongation fixation between the fused areas. The child undergoes elongations every 4 to 6 months according to spinal growth. The accepted indications for growing rods include significant remaining axial growth, progressive deformity, a curve greater than 50 degrees, and a flexible or semirigid spinal deformity.[11] These rods may not be applicable in cases of rigid spine deformity.[11] The growing rod concept can be modified as in the Shilla technique,[12] where a short fusion around the apex of the deformity is performed with guided growth above and below in the spine. This is achieved with mismatched rods and screws, allowing the spine to grow in a controlled fusion in the coronal plane. Modern growing rods allow magnetic elongation of the rods, thus preventing the need for repeat surgery.[13]

The VEPTR concept is the gold standard fixation for patients with TIS. As introduced by Campbell et al,[4] the VEPTR was originally indicated for patients with rib fusions, but indications for the VEPTR have widened to surpass those for use of the growing rod. VEPTR features include circumferential rib anchors and a telescopic lengthening mechanism that allows expansion in the kyphotic segment of the thoracic spine, as opposed to axial connectors, which generally need to be placed at the thoracolumbar junction. Several studies[2,3,6] have demonstrated the VEPTR's efficacy in controlling curve magnitude and promoting spine growth. The VEPTR does not correct the deformity, but it allows an indirect correction of nearly 30% of the deformity, which is maintained over several years. Thoracic spine growth is maintained as well. The complications of the VEPTR are similar to those of traditional growing rods, including wound problems, infections, and rib fractures, creeping fusion, and iliac crest migration.

Because the VEPTR is a costly system with a relatively high profile, it is not always suitable for cases of extreme muscle wasting or cases in which the facility or patient cannot afford the VEPTR system. Other constructs that attach the spine to the ribs (or the pelvis to the ribs) have been developed (▶ Fig. 7.1) based on the use of pedicle screws in the lumbar spine and attaching them to hooks surrounding the ribs with double rods that are linked with domino connectors, which will allow secondary lengthening of the system.[5]

In a case series published by the authors,[5] patients with TIS and osteogenesis imperfecta were treated with a VEPTR-like construct, attaching a proximal construct to the five ribs to allowing force dispersion, and a distal construct to the pedicles in the lumbar spine or pelvis (▶ Fig. 7.2, ▶ Fig. 7.3). Despite poor bone quality, patient lung function and metabolism improved, thereby increasing their body mass index and reducing metabolic imbalances often associated with TIS.

Limited data exist regarding the effect of distraction instrumentation on lung function, in part because of the difficulty in measuring pulmonary function in young children. However, from the few case series that have been published on patients treated with these systems, forced vital capacity increases significantly, and the dependency on oxygen support decreases.

7.4 Conclusion

Thoracic insufficiency syndrome remains a challenging problem. The major problem with these children is progressive pulmonary insufficiency, which mandates a timely intervention. A multidisciplinary team should be part of the care pathway for these children. When they are referred for surgery, the VEPTR system is the gold standard of care; however, data from larger series are needed to provide definitive answers for TIS treatment and long-term management of the associated problems.

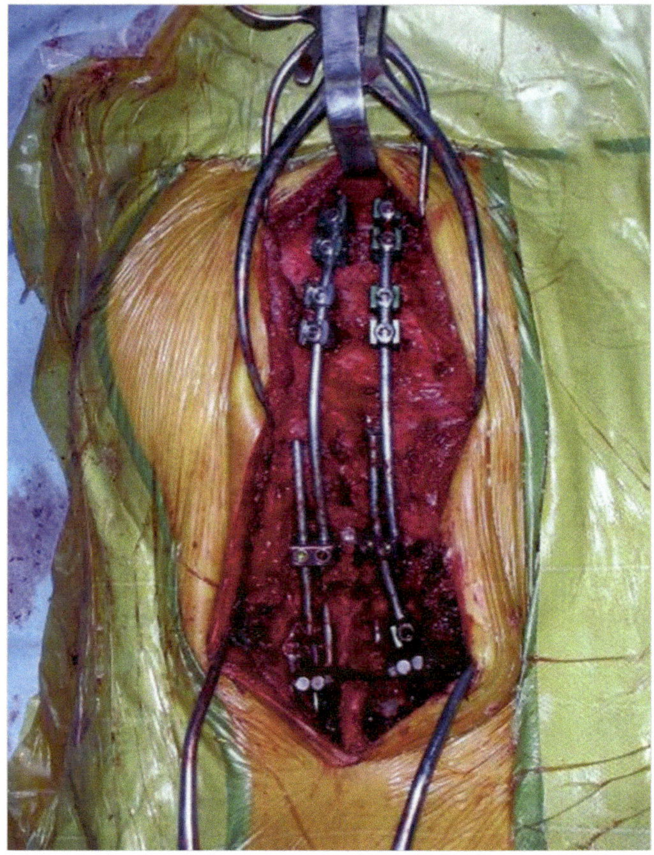

Fig. 7.1 The construct in an exposed spine. There are four rods connected to the screws, and hooks are placed with redundancy allowing future elongation.

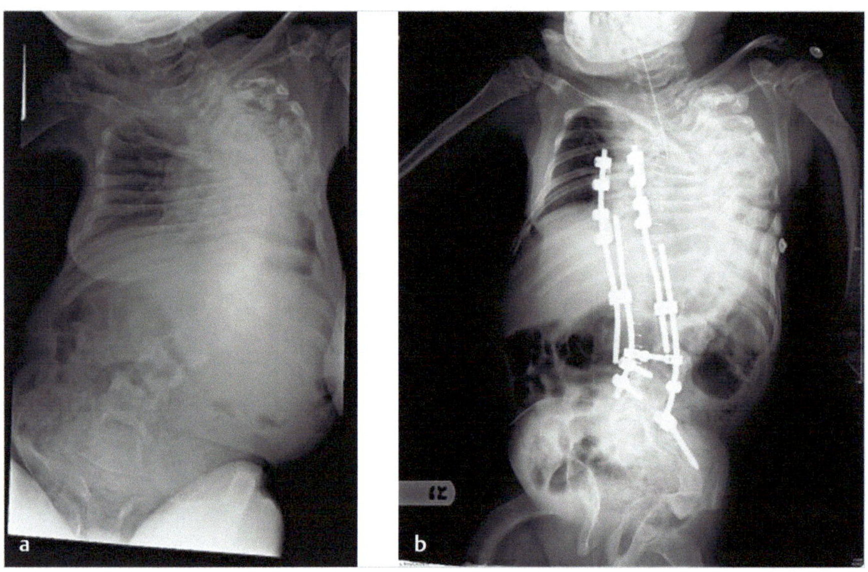

Fig. 7.2 Anteroposterior views of the spine. Image of a child **(a)** before and **(b)** after placement of the construct.

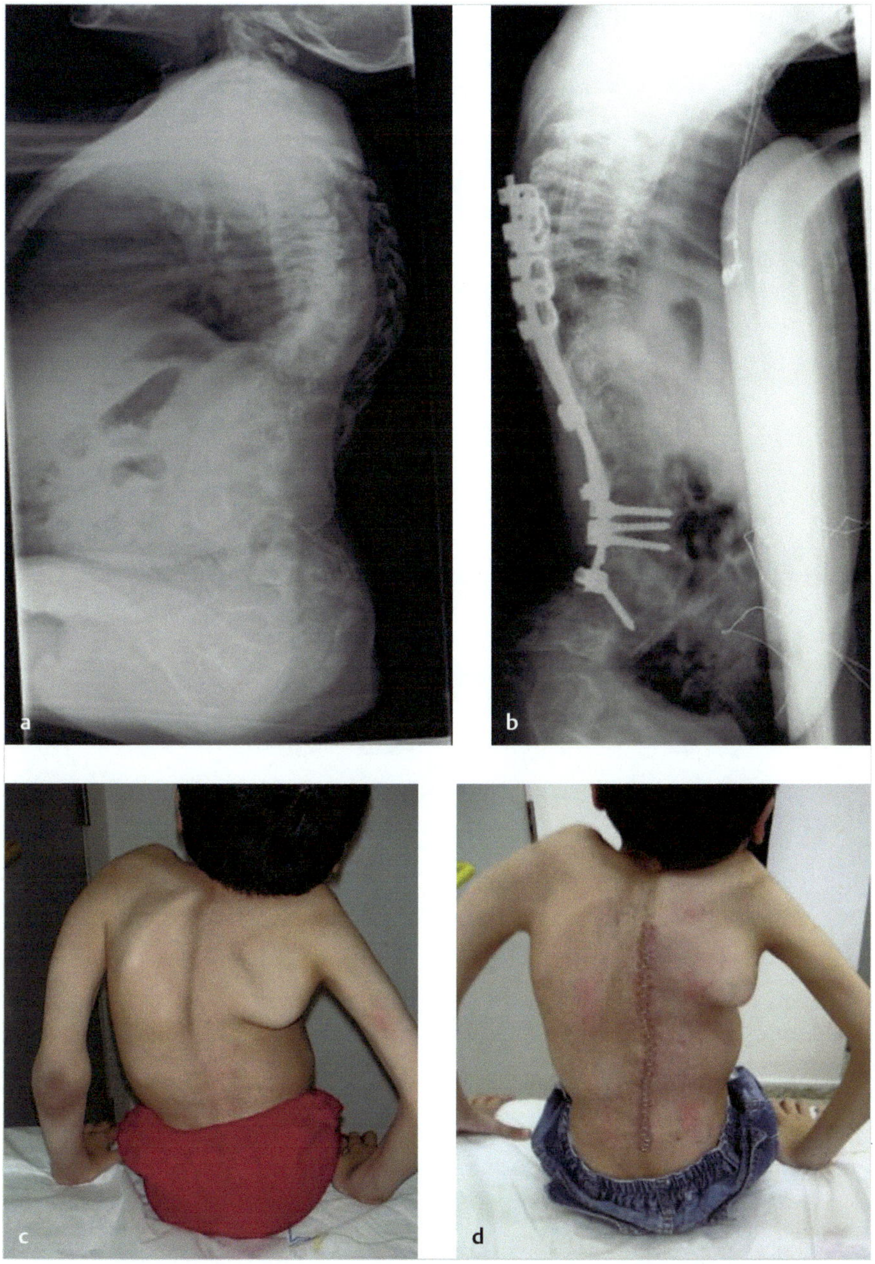

Fig. 7.3 (a, b) Lateral view of a child before and after the construct was placed. **(c, d)** Clinical improvement in the spine of the child before and after surgery.

References

[1] Campbell RM, Jr, Smith MD, Mayes TC, et al. The characteristics of thoracic insufficiency syndrome associated with fused ribs and congenital scoliosis. J Bone Joint Surg Am. 2003; 85(3):399–408

[2] Campbell RM, Jr, Adcox BM, Smith MD, et al. The effect of mid-thoracic VEPTR opening wedge thoracostomy on cervical tilt associated with congenital thoracic scoliosis in patients with thoracic insufficiency syndrome. Spine. 2007; 32(20):2171–2177

[3] Ramírez N, Cornier AS, Campbell RM, Jr, Carlo S, Arroyo S, Romeu J. Natural history of thoracic insufficiency syndrome: a spondylothoracic dysplasia perspective. J Bone Joint Surg Am. 2007; 89(12):2663–2675

[4] Campbell RM, Jr, Smith MD, Hell-Vocke AK. Expansion thoracoplasty: the surgical technique of opening-wedge thoracostomy. Surgical technique. J Bone Joint Surg Am. 2004; 86-A Suppl 1:51–64

[5] Kaplan L, Barzilay Y, Hashroni A, Itshayek E, Schroeder JE. Thoracic elongation in type III osteogenesis imperfecta patients with thoracic insufficiency syndrome. Spine. 2013; 38(2):E94–E100

[6] Emans JB, Caubet JF, Ordonez CL, Lee EY, Ciarlo M. The treatment of spine and chest wall deformities with fused ribs by expansion thoracostomy and insertion of vertical expandable prosthetic titanium rib: growth of thoracic spine and improvement of lung volumes. Spine. 2005; 30(17) Suppl:S58–S68

[7] Redding G, Song K, Inscore S, Effmann E, Campbell R. Lung function asymmetry in children with congenital and infantile scoliosis. Spine J. 2008; 8(4):639–644

[8] Smith JR, Samdani AF, Pahys J, et al. The role of bracing, casting, and vertical expandable prosthetic titanium rib for the treatment of infantile idiopathic scoliosis: a single-institution experience with 31 consecutive patients. Clinical article. J Neurosurg Spine. 2009; 11(1):3–8

[9] Widmann RF, Bitan FD, Laplaza FJ, Burke SW, DiMaio MF, Schneider R. Spinal deformity, pulmonary compromise, and quality of life in osteogenesis imperfecta. Spine. 1999; 24(16):1673–1678

[10] Mehdian H, Stokes OM. Growing rod construct for the treatment of early-onset scoliosis. Eur Spine J. 2015; 24 Suppl 5:647–651

[11] Yazici M, Emans J. Fusionless instrumentation systems for congenital scoliosis: expandable spinal rods and vertical expandable prosthetic titanium rib in the management of congenital spine deformities in the growing child. Spine. 2009; 34(17):1800–1807

[12] McCarthy RE, Luhmann S, Lenke L, McCullough FL. The Shilla growth guidance technique for early-onset spinal deformities at 2-year follow-up: a preliminary report. J Pediatr Orthop. 2014; 34(1):1–7

[13] Rolton D, Richards J, Nnadi C. Magnetic controlled growth rods versus conventional growing rod systems in the treatment of early onset scoliosis: a cost comparison. Eur Spine J. 2015; 24(7):1457–1461

8 Vertebral Column Resection as a Treatment for Neurologic Deficit in Severe Spinal Deformity

Eduardo C. Beauchamp, Paul J. Park, Meghan Cerpa, Lawrence G. Lenke

Abstract

Vertebral column resection as treatment for neurologic deficit and myelopathy in severe spinal deformity is extremely challenging. A multidisciplinary approach and careful preoperative planning are needed for the care of these complicated patients. Posterior vertebral column resection (PVCR) is an effective treatment option for deformity correction and spinal cord decompression. Preoperative imaging studies are necessary to determine the extent of spinal cord compression and the complex anatomy typically associated with severe spinal deformity. Computed tomography with a three-dimensional printed model is a useful tool for preoperative surgical planning. A period of preoperative halo gravity traction may contribute to partial deformity correction, as well as improve respiratory function and provide time to enhance the patient's nutritional status. Circumferential spinal cord decompression may be achieved successfully through a posterior only approach in patients with preexisting neurologic deficits or myelopathy. Often these patients are at a higher risk of postoperative neurologic complications after a PVCR, due to their underlying spinal cord fragility, and the unavailability of obtaining intraoperative spinal cord data in many of them.

Keywords: Vertebral column resection, VCR, Myelopathy, spinal deformity, pediatric spinal deformity, osteotomy, scoliosis, kyphosis, spinal cord monitoring

8.1 Introduction

Since the initial vertebrectomy description in 1922 by MacLennan,[1] vertebral column resection (VCR) has become the most powerful corrective technique in the treatment of severe adult and pediatric spinal deformity. In 1969, Leatherman recognized that in order to minimize neurologic injury while correcting a rigid spine deformity the spinal column must be shortened. He developed a two-stage corrective closing-wedge osteotomy for congenital spine deformities with an average correction of 47%.[2,3] Circumferential VCR as we know it today was first described by Bradford in 1987.[4,5] Boachie-Adjei and Bradford further expanded Bradford's original series by reporting on 16 patients treated with a two-stage circumferential VCR achieving an average scoliosis correction of 43%.[6]

Surgical treatment for severe spinal deformity has historically been performed through a combined anterior and posterior approach. Nevertheless, it has been demonstrated that anterior approaches disrupting the thoracic cage may adversely affect postoperative pulmonary function.[7,8,9,10] Several studies have documented improvements in pulmonary function tests as early as 3 months and maintained up to 20 years following a posterior spinal arthrodesis for idiopathic scoliosis.[11,12,13] Suk et al were the first to report on a single-stage, posterior vertebral column resection (PVCR) for both severe rigid scoliosis[14,15] and fixed lumbosacral deformity.[16] Lenke et al subsequently reported on 35 pediatric[17] and 47 adult and pediatric[18] patients treated with a PVCR and found they had no permanent neurologic sequelae. Over the past two decades, a posterior approach for VCR has become increasingly common for the correction of severe adult and pediatric spine deformity.[14,15,16,17,18,19]

With the advent of three-column fixation provided by pedicle screws, the vast majority of spinal deformity can now be safely addressed through a posterior approach. This avoids the morbidity associated with a circumferential approach, decreases operative time and estimated blood loss, and achieves equivalent deformity correction.[17,18,19,20,21] The dilemma arises when a PVCR is needed on an already myelopathic or neurologically compromised patient since manipulating an already diseased spinal cord is a risk factor for permanent neurologic injury.[14,15,20,22,23]

8.2 Preoperative Evaluation

A thorough preoperative evaluation in patients with severe spinal deformity is crucial, particularly in those with preoperative neurologic deficit. A complete evaluation should include a detailed physical examination and history, followed by careful examination of their imaging studies.

8.2.1 History and Physical Examination

Clinical evaluation should begin with a comprehensive medical history and physical examination. Due to the overall complexity of medical conditions encountered in patients with severe spinal deformity, countless subspecialty consultations are typically required prior to surgery. For example, these may include neurologic, genetic, endocrine, cardiac, pulmonary, psychiatric, and hematologic evaluations. Careful attention is given to the nutritional and pulmonary status of the patient since significant respiratory compromise, secondary to the spine and chest wall deformity, is notorious in this population. Preoperative spirometry exercises and pulmonary function tests are recommended. Any restrictive lung disease should be documented and pulmonary consultation pursued. Bumpass et al showed that pediatric patients who underwent PVCR for severe spinal deformity had a small but statistically significant improvement in their pulmonary function tests 2 years after surgery.[24] Although this was not true for the adult population in their study, they attributed this difference to the ability for further lung capacity and chest wall development after surgery in the pediatric population, which is no longer present in the adult population.

A thorough physical examination should include height, weight, skin evaluation, nutritional assessment, gait assessment, extremity and spine range of motion, and sensory and motor function evaluation. Hyperreflexia, sustained ankle clonus, positive Babinski sign, gait instability, and any other long-tract sign should be assessed and documented. Inspection of the global coronal and sagittal balance is imperative. Many patients with significant coronal and sagittal deformity may also suffer from rib on pelvis deformity, which can be a source of pain and discomfort. Having the patient lie in the prone position on the examination table is helpful to evaluate flexibility and have a preliminary sense of how the deformity will look on the operating table. Having the patient lie in a prone position several times a day prior to surgery may help the patient's body and spinal cord acclimate to the position required for a prolonged period during the surgery.

8.2.2 Imaging

Initial imaging for patients with severe spinal deformity should include standing full spine coronal and sagittal radiographs (▶ Fig. 8.1). Supine radiographs are used to assess the flexibility of the deformity and full-body radiographs to assess the global spine alignment. It is essential to review previous imaging studies to gain a broad perspective on the natural history of the deformity and to document progression. This is particularly important in the pediatric population during periods of rapid growth, since preexisting myelopathy may be at risk of progression with worsening of the deformity. Given the complexity and three-dimensional (3D) nature of these deformities, two-dimensional radiographs are insufficient to fully demonstrate the deformity in these patients. A full-spine CT scan with 3D reconstructions is essential for delineating the extent of the deformity, as well as evaluating structural anomalies, such as laminar defects, hemivertebrae, absent pedicles, and other indications that could affect the surgical plan (▶ Fig. 8.2). A full-sized 3D printed model of the spinal column can be extremely helpful in the personalized treatment of complex spinal deformity. Such a model serves as a preoperative planning tool, assisting in observation of the pathoanatomy, selection of internal fixation and osteotomy levels, and determining the extent of the PVCR. The model may also serve as a tangible intraoperative guide for anatomy identification, instrumentation, and deformity correction (▶ Fig. 8.3).

Imaging of the neuroaxis is most commonly achieved with MRI. A full-spine MRI including the craniocervical junction is essential for the evaluation of patients prior to a PVCR. Pathologies of the neural axis, such as tethered cord, syrinx, or Chiari malformations, may be associated with a severe spine deformity. Such findings may warrant a preemptive neurosurgical consultation. Spinal cord compression caused by the spinal deformity can be visualized on the MRI. On T1- and T2-weighted images, signal intensity changes ("cord signal changes") within the spinal cord are associated with histopathologic changes,[25] and further surgical manipulation in these areas during a PVCR should be avoided if possible, although cord signal changes are often present at the location of maximal angular deformity. MRIs are valuable in patients with severe spinal deformity to preoperatively assess spinal cord health and improve surgical planning.

8.3 Halo-Gravity Traction

In adult and pediatric patients with severe spinal deformity, a period of perioperative halo-gravity traction (HGT) may

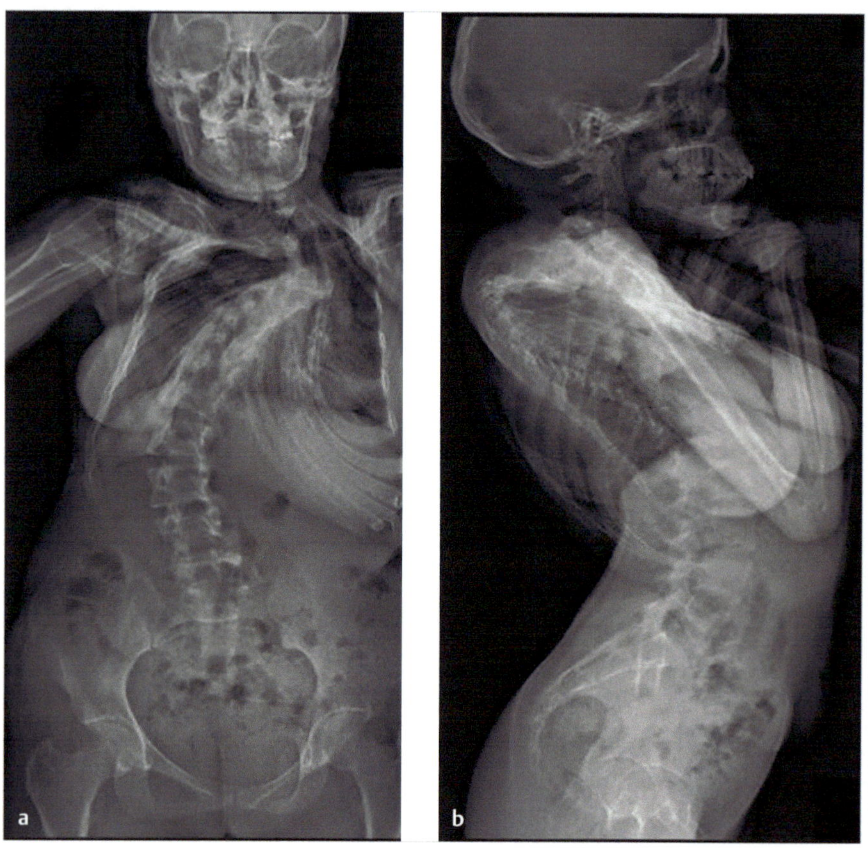

Fig. 8.1 **(a)** Posteroanterior and **(b)** lateral radiograph of a 20-year-old patient with neurofibromatosis and severe progressive kyphoscoliosis.

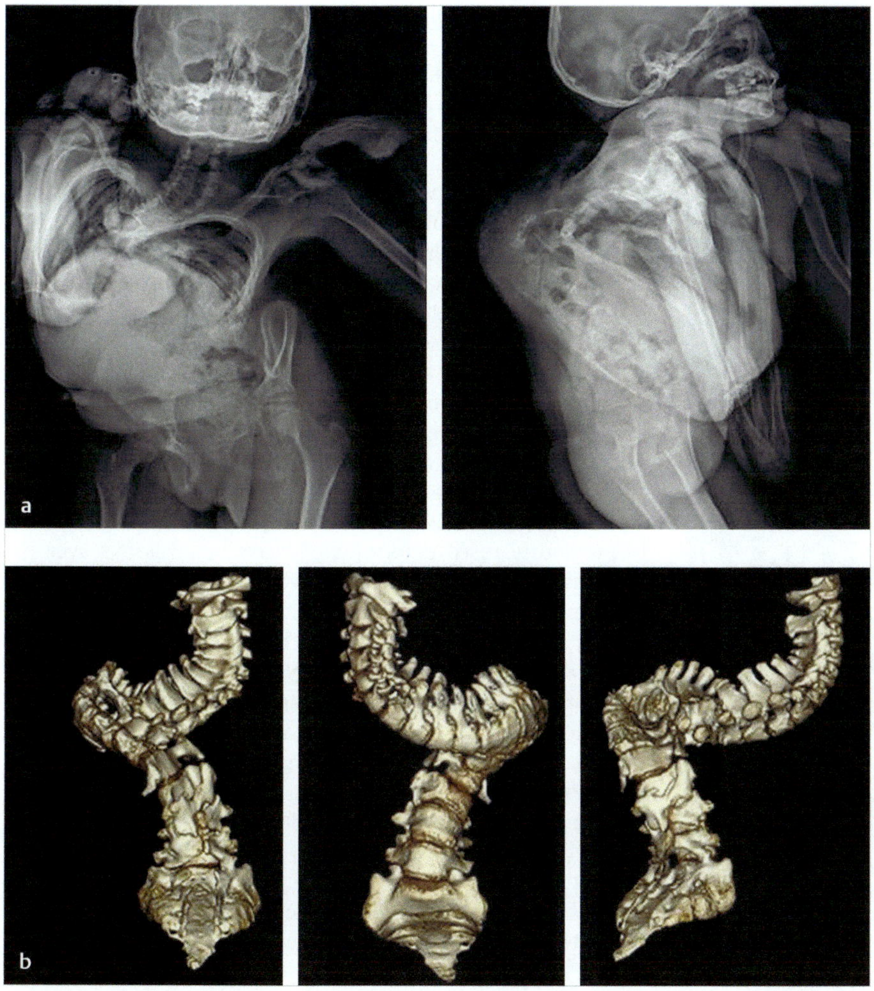

Fig. 8.2 (a) Posteroanterior and lateral radiographs and **(b)** three-dimensional CT reconstructions of a 10-year-old patient with a history of tethered cord and diastematomyelia repaired at 3 years of age. The radiographs show severe kyphoscoliosis, but the three-dimensional CT reconstructions demonstrate segmentation anomalies and laminar defect not appreciated in the radiographs.

be beneficial in ameliorating the magnitude of the deformity (▶ Fig. 8.4). This period of traction can render the patient a more suitable candidate for surgery because HGT can aid in improving respiratory mechanisms and nutritional status.[26,27,28,29,30,31] A recent systematic review and meta-analysis on the use of HGT for severe spinal deformity reported 24.1% and 19.3% correction on coronal and sagittal planes, respectively, attributable only to the preoperative HGT period.[28] Koller et al[26] reported an improvement from 42% predicted to 49.5% predicted forced vital capacity (FVC%) after 19 days of HGT in patients with severe spinal deformity. In a subgroup of patients with an initial FVC < 40% the increase in FVC% during the HGT period was 9%. Length of traction is generally between 2 and 12 weeks depending on the overall preoperative medical condition of the patient.

The traction goal fluctuates between 33 and 50% total body weight, as tolerated by the patient. In our experience, smaller patients may tolerate even greater percentages of total body weight traction, to the point where their buttocks can remain slightly suspended while sitting in a traction wheelchair. Weekly radiographs of the full spine should be ordered to monitor correction of the deformity and unintended cervical lamina and facet over distraction. Daily ambulation using a walking frame is encouraged to avoid deconditioning. Our current protocol is to add 2 lb of traction in the morning and 1 lb in the afternoon with neurologic exams during every 8-hour shift as each additional weight is added. Neurologic exams include evaluation of cranial motor nerves, upper and lower extremity strength, and sensation and reflex assessment. Any deterioration of the baseline neurologic exam should be addressed emergently by reducing the traction weight as there have been reports of cranial nerve palsies and other neurologic symptoms,[29,31,32,33] including one case of paraplegia,[34] due to halo gravity traction. The most common complications are back pain and pin-related issues. These include pin-site infection and loosening, which are typically treated with oral antibiotics and debridement or pin exchange, respectively. Other reported complications are trapezial soreness, dizziness, nausea, and nystagmus, which typically resolve with reduction of traction weight.

8.4 Surgical Technique

Although technically demanding, this posterior only approach has become the gold standard technique for VCR. It requires a proficient surgical team keen on management of severe spinal deformities. Due to the extent of the procedure, adequate patient positioning is crucial. Patients are placed in a Gardner–Wells tong or have already received preoperative HGT, to help relieve pressure on the orbits and facial structures. In both cases

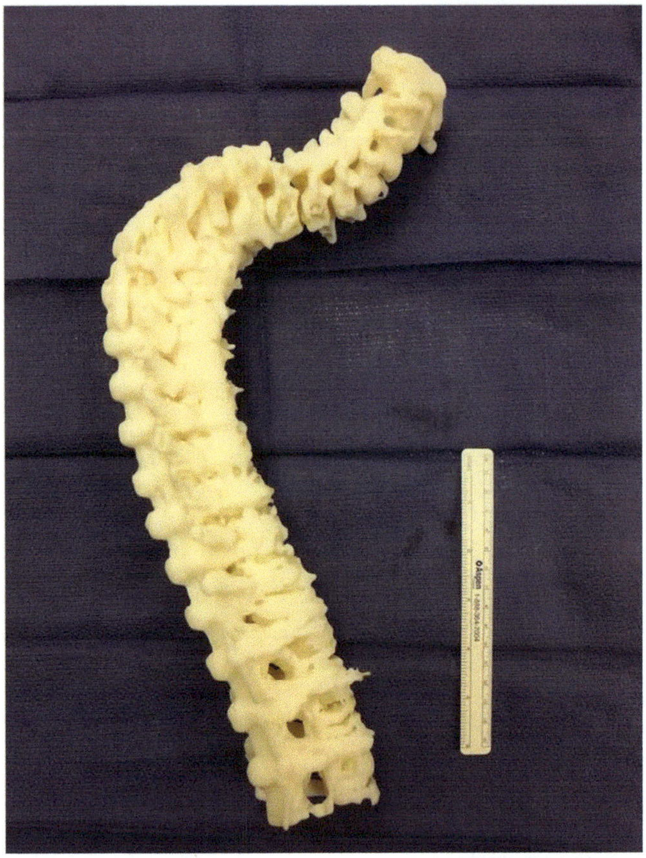

Fig. 8.3 A full-sized three-dimensional printed model may serve as a preoperative planning tool in cases with severe spinal deformity.

minimal traction is continued intraoperatively, and no countertraction is used so as to avoid overdistraction of the spinal cord during this dissociative shortening procedure. Bony prominences are well padded, and the patient is positioned prone on a radiolucent Jackson frame. Careful attention is placed on avoiding excessive pressure points and peripheral nerve traction injuries. In very small patients and when the dissection extends into the cervical spine, the arms are placed on the side. Multimodal spinal cord monitoring is imperative for completion of the procedure.

Preventive measures must be pursued to minimize blood loss during a PVCR. A loading and maintenance dose of tranexamic acid is used as an intraoperative antifibrinolytic agent. Thorough subperiosteal dissection exposing the posterior elements of the spine is achieved. A 3D printed model of the spine is useful in preoperative planning and in identifying intraoperative pathoanatomy during dissection and instrumentation. Following exposure, the spine is thoroughly irrigated and vancomycin antibiotic is spread through the soft tissues. Posterior ligament release and inferior facetectomies are performed followed by posterior column osteotomies (PCOs) as needed. These may aid in apical screw placement along the concavity of the coronal deformity by direct palpation of the medial pedicle wall, especially in patients with a prior fusion mass. In patients with severe angular kyphotic deformities, concave pedicle screws are placed along with a temporary rod before performing the periapical PCOs since, with this bony release, the posterior column elongates, which can in turn cause inadvertent spinal cord stretching. Pedicle screw fixation is obtained using the freehand technique as described by Kim et al,[35] proceeding from caudal to cranial aspects of the exposed spine. The use of multiaxial reduction screws is recommended along the apical concave region of the scoliosis as well as adjacent to the planned VCR. These aid in the efficient placement of temporary rods and prevent any vertebral subluxation once the spine is destabilized. In the thoracic spine, bilateral costotransversectomies are performed at the level to be resected, removing approximately 3 to 5 cm of the medial rib. This is done prior to commencing the laminectomy to avoid unintentional canal intrusion. The rib fragments are saved and eventually used as autograft spanning the VCR site posteriorly. A wide laminectomy is performed at the level of the planned VCR and is extended from the inferior aspect of the pedicle above, to the superior aspect of the pedicle below, completely visualizing the thecal sac. This permits adequate visualization of the dura during closure of the osteotomy. In previously fused deformities, placement of hooks over the fusion mass above and below the osteotomy site is helpful as an adjuvant for osteotomy closure and stability.

After the laminectomy, a subperiosteal dissection of the lateral pedicle wall and vertebral body is performed using Penfield elevators, pushing the soft tissues and segmental vessels anteriorly. In the thoracic spine, the convex nerve root of the level to be resected may be sacrificed to gain access to the vertebral body. Prior to cutting the nerve root at its exit from the dural sac, we recommend temporarily clamping the nerve root for 5 to 10 minutes while continuous spinal cord monitoring is performed to ensure there is no deterioration in the spinal cord blood supply. If neuromonitoring remains stable, the nerve root is ligated and transected. In the lumbar spine, both nerve roots are preserved. Temporary stabilizing rods are placed spanning at least two to three levels proximal and caudal to the resection site. Typically, a unilateral stabilizing rod is required, except in patients with severe angular kyphosis, where dual stabilizing rods are used during anterior column resection to avoid spinal column subluxation. The concave pedicle is encircled and resected first since it is usually located in a more ventral-dependent position where blood can accumulate, making later visualization difficult. Removing the concave pedicle also decreases the tension on the spinal cord by allowing it to drift away further medially once this pedicle is removed. A high-speed bur is carefully used to remove the concave pedicle since it is often completely sclerotic and cortical. In scoliotic deformities, the majority of the vertebral body is removed from the convex side. A malleable or "spoon" retractor is placed circumferentially around the body to protect the pleura and ventral structures. The vertebral body is accessed through the lateral pedicle-body entrance and is entirely resected except for a thin shell of the anterior wall attached to the anterior longitudinal ligament, which is kept intact for fusion purposes. Diskectomies above and below are performed with the use of curets, making sure not to violate the end plates, where structural interbody cages may rest. The last portions of the body to be removed are the posterior wall and the posterior longitudinal ligament (PLL), which have been kept in place until this point to protect the spinal cord during anterior body resection. The thecal sac is circumferentially freed from the epidural vessels, PLL, and bony prominences. Using a reverse-angle curet, specialized posterior

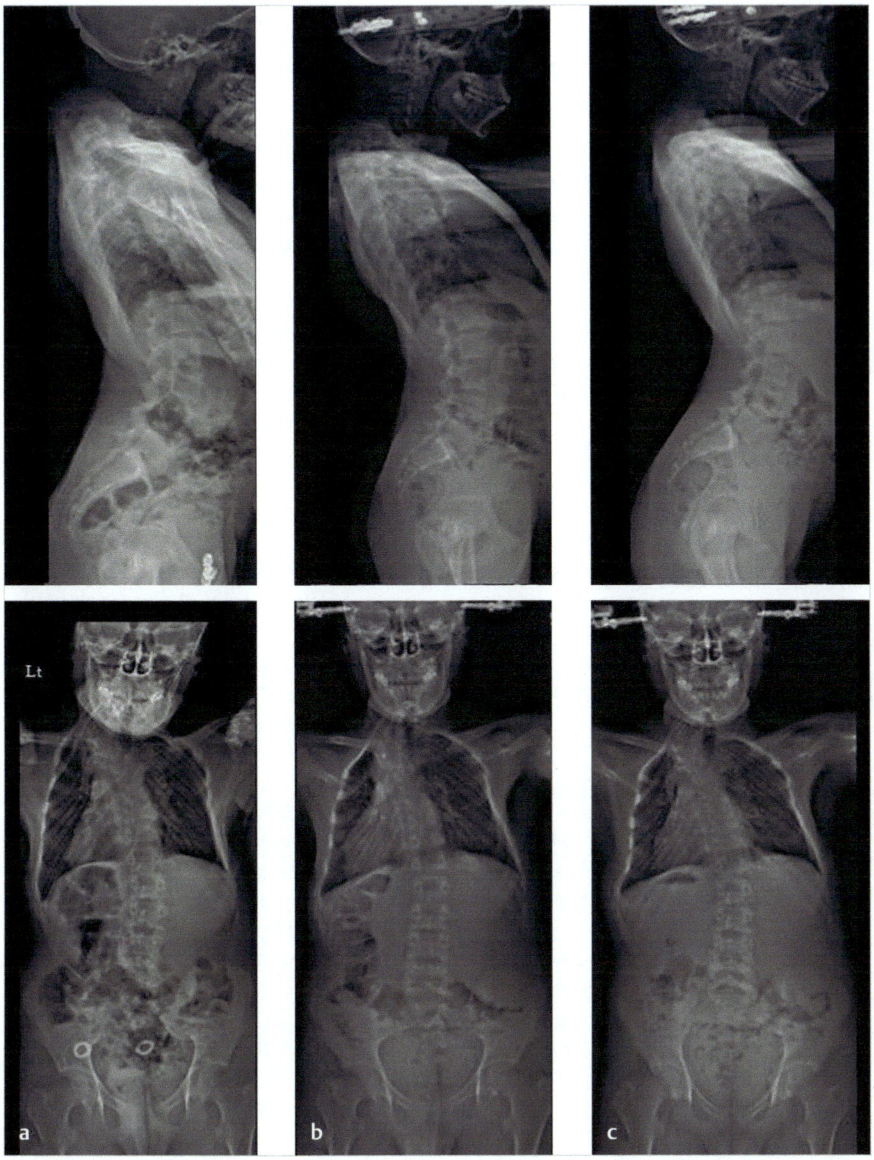

Fig. 8.4 Posteroanterior and lateral radiographs of a 17-year-old patient with a history of neurofibromatosis and severe kyphoscoliosis treated with preoperative halo traction.
(a) Prior to halo placement, **(b)** at 1 week, and **(c)** 3 weeks after halo traction.

wall impactor, Kerrison rongeurs, or Woodson elevators the posterior body wall is then impacted into the ventral defect.

After complete resection of the vertebral body(ies), closure of the osteotomy is begun. The main corrective force is compression over the convexity of the deformity, thereby shortening the spine. In cases with adequate bone stock, this compression can be done directly through the pedicle screws, otherwise a construct-to-construct or hook–rod construct closure mechanism can be used. For example, using domino connectors along the apex of the resected area and distributing forces through multiple levels is an effective construct-to-construct closure mechanism. It is crucial to monitor the thecal sac during this corrective maneuver to avoid inadvertent dural impingement. Correction continues slowly in a stepwise manner guided by the contralateral stabilizing rod, which prevents vertebral subluxation. In kyphotic deformities, an anteriorly based structural cage is placed before compression to act as a hinge for kyphosis correction and prevent spinal cord overshortening. Once closure of the resection site is complete, the contralateral stabilizing rod is replaced with a permanent rod, and the ipsilateral temporary rod or construct-to-construct rods are replaced with a final rod. Further corrective maneuvers are implemented as needed. A circumferential check of the exposed dura is done to determine that there is no residual impingement. Adequate alignment is confirmed with intraoperative posteroanterior and lateral full-spine radiographs. Decortication and bone graft placement are completed. The laminectomy defect is covered with the previously harvested rib fragments from the costotransversectomy and held in place by sutures or a crosslink. The rib fragments may be split longitudinally, exposing the cancellous surface, and placed against the decorticated laminar surface, acting as a structural posterior-based graft while protecting the dura. Final implant security is checked, and wound closure over drains is completed. An intraoperative wake-up test is performed prior to extubation.

8.5 Spinal Cord Monitoring

Multimodal neurophysiologic spinal cord monitoring is crucial during PVCR. The spinal cord monitoring team should be attentive during all stages of the procedure and maintain open-ended communication with the surgeon and the rest of the team at all times. We utilize intraoperative somatosensory evoked potentials (SSEPs) and transcranial motor evoked potentials (TcMEPs) or neurogenic mixed evoked potentials. TcMEPs allow direct evaluation of the corticospinal motor tracts as well as peripheral nerves, and, in combination with SSEPs, we can achieve global monitoring of spinal cord function. The use of free-running electromyography (EMG) during spinal cord monitoring allows for real-time information of nerve root irritation during surgical manipulation. Triggered EMG (TrgEMG) stimulation is used for pedicle screws placed from levels T6 to S1. This helps assess any potential medial pedicle wall violation. In an animal study with a clinical correlation, Lenke et al[36] determined the threshold for TrgEMG stimulus intensity in the lumbar spine with pedicle screw instrumentation. Screws with threshold intensities > 8 milliamperes (mA) were found to be entirely within the pedicle. Lumbar pedicle screws with intensities between 4 and 8 mA demonstrate a potential pedicle wall defect, and intensities < 4 mA indicate a strong likelihood of pedicle wall defect with potential contact with neurologic structures. In a prospective study of 90 patients and 512 screws, Glassman et al evaluated the accuracy of intraoperative TrgEMG pedicle screw stimulation in the lumbar spine and its correlation with postoperative CT scan confirmation.[37] In their study a threshold > 15 mA reliably indicated adequate screw position with an accuracy of 98%.[37] Raynor et al retrospectively evaluated 1,078 spinal surgical procedures with 4,857 lumbar pedicle screws placed. In their study medial breach rates for EMG thresholds > 8.0 mA, 4–8.0 mA, 4.0 mA, and 2.8 mA were 0.33%, 17.4%, 54.2%, and 100%, respectively. They concluded that the probability of a medial pedicle breach being detected by TrgEMG stimulation in the lumbar spine increases with decreasing thresholds, and that this technique should always be used in conjunction with direct probe palpation and radiographic evaluation of safe pedicle screw placement.[38] In the thoracic spine TrgEMG threshold results vary.[39,40,41] Using a porcine model with intercostal recordings, Lewis et al could not determine a specific threshold range to predict adequate placement of thoracic pedicle screws.[40] Raynor and Lenke et al[41] prospectively evaluated the sensitivity of TrgEMG recorded in the rectus abdominis to assess adequate thoracic pedicle screw placement. In 92 consecutive patients 677 thoracic pedicle screws were studied. They recommended that TrgEMG thresholds < 6.0 mA, in addition to values 60 to 65% less than the average of the rest of the screws in a given patient, should alert the surgeon to a potential medial wall pedicle screw breach and should be followed by further tactile and radiographic evaluation.

Loss of intraoperative spinal cord monitoring data during PVCR is not uncommon. In previous studies, the senior author (LGL) has reported loss or degradation of spinal cord data in 8%, 18%, and 16.7% of patients[17,18,42] during PVCR. In all cases data returned after prompt intervention, including elevation of mean arterial pressure, anterior cord decompression, correction of subluxation, or reduction of intraoperative traction. Other authors have reported an incidence of intraoperative data changes or complete loss during PVCR to be from 6.7 to 22%.[20,43,44,45] A predictive risk factor for these data changes or losses in all of these studies can be attributed to significant preoperative kyphosis.

8.6 Vertebral Column Resection for Progressive Myelopathy

PVCR remains the most challenging spine surgery procedure to date. The advantage of this complex technique over other less corrective osteotomies, such as posterior column or pedicle subtraction osteotomy, is that it completely dissociates adjacent spinal segments, thereby permitting multiplanar translation of the spinal column and providing extensive correction of the deformity. Multiple studies have reported excellent coronal and sagittal deformity correction with this technique.[14,15,16,17,18] The overall transient postoperative neurologic deficit during PVCR has been reported to be from 2 to 13.8%, whereas permanent neurologic complications have been reported to be up to 6.3%.[14,15,16,17,18,19,20,46,47] In patients with progressive myelopathy this percentage could be higher.[22] Risk factors for postoperative neurologic deficit following a PVCR include lack of intraoperative neuromonitoring data, preexisting myelopathy, preoperative neurologic deficit, previous anterior thoracic or intrathecal surgery, severe kyphosis, total deformity angular ratio ≥25, sagittal deformity angular ratio > 15, resection of two or more vertebrae, and increased intraoperative blood loss, among others.[14,15,16,17,18,19,20,21,22,23,44,46,48]

Intraoperative neuromonitoring is frequently unobtainable in patients with preexisting myelopathy, which increases the risk for neurologic deficit after a PVCR.[18,22,48] It is important to discuss this possibility preoperatively with patients and recognize that if there is persistent lack of preoperative neuromonitoring data, frequent intraoperative wake-up tests will be performed. Once the lack of spinal cord monitoring data is identified, the first wake-up test is done immediately after positioning. Subsequent tests are then performed after exposure, following instrumentation, after vertebral resection and corrective maneuvers, before closure, and before extubation.

A recent retrospective analysis of 112 consecutive adult and pediatric patients undergoing a PVCR found that the incidence of unobtainable intraoperative spinal cord monitoring signals was 17.9%.[22] Of the 20 patients with no detectable spinal cord data, 9 (45%) had a diagnosis of progressive myelopathy associated with the severe spinal deformity, whereas the 4 (20%) patients that developed transient postoperative paraplegia each had a preoperative diagnosis of severe progressive myelopathy located at the apex of their angular deformity. Three of the four patients who developed transient postoperative paraplegia were revision cases who had had a previous anterior spinal fusion with ligation of segmental vessels. Anecdotal experience from the senior author has suggested that patients with prior anterior thoracic fusion and severe kyphotic deformity, as well as those with previous intradural surgery, are at a higher risk of major postoperative neurologic complication following a PVCR.[21] Altering the configuration of the spine in these patients may diminish the already tenuous blood flow to the cord, predisposing them to further neurologic injury. Sharp angular deformities in the thoracic spine can also produce spinal cord compression at more than one level. Each deformity needs to be addressed sequentially with frequent evaluation of neuromonitoring signals because changes or loss of data may be caused by cord compression at more than one site. Spinal cord shortening by means of a PVCR may also help in relieving the tension on the spinal cord.

8.7 Case Illustration

The patient is a 23-year-old man with history of neurofibromatosis and severe progressive thoracic kyphoscoliosis. The patient was complaining of increasing back pain, shortness of breath, and lower extremity weakness. On physical examination he was found to be myelopathic with hyperreflexic knee and ankle reflexes, bilateral ankle clonus, and 4/5 strength in all lower-extremity muscle groups. Upright posteroanterior and lateral radiographs (▶ Fig. 8.5) demonstrate a 100-degree proximal thoracic, 115-degree main thoracic, and 30-degree lumbar scoliosis curve; 180 degrees of thoracic kyphosis; and severe rib-on-pelvis deformity. Preoperative CT 3D reconstructions (▶ Fig. 8.6) show the complexity of the kyphotic deformity, and the short distance between the upper thoracic and upper lumbar spine. T2-weighted images reveal signal intensity changes within the thoracic spinal cord as well as multiple neurofibromas along the exiting thoracic nerve roots and a dorsally located plexiform neurofibroma compressing the spinal cord along the sharp angular kyphotic deformity (▶ Fig. 8.7, ▶ Fig. 8.8). Preoperative pulmonary function tests demonstrated severe restrictive lung disease with a 38% predicted FVC and a 31% predicted forced expiratory volume. The patient was placed in halo gravity traction for approximately 8 weeks with improvement of his sagittal alignment (▶ Fig. 8.9). During this traction period his nutritional and pulmonary status was

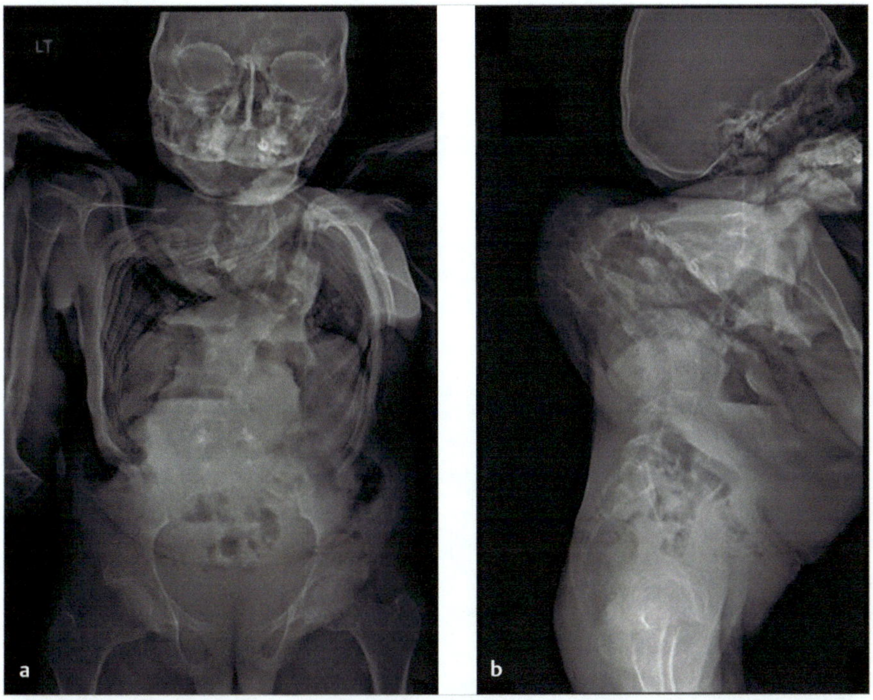

Fig. 8.5 (a) Posterioanterior and **(b)** lateral radiographs demonstrating kyphoscoliosis with rib-on-pelvis deformity.

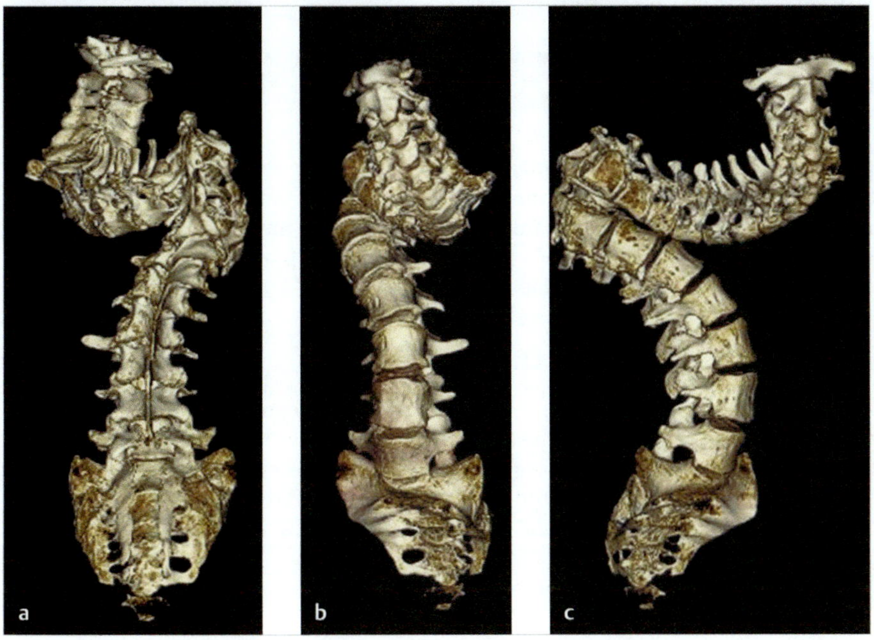

Fig. 8.6 (a–c) Three-dimensional reconstructions showing severe upper thoracic kyphoscoliosis. Notice the narrow distance between the upper thoracic and upper lumbar vertebrae.

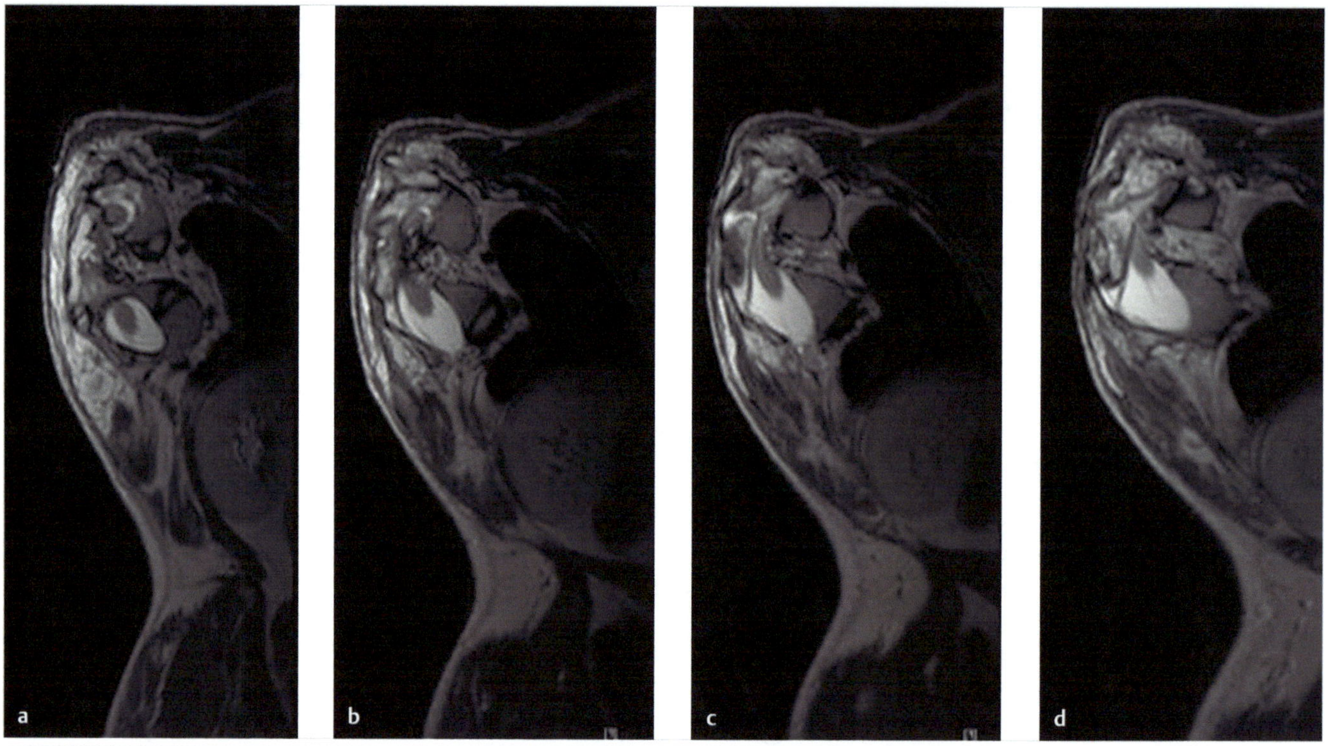

Fig. 8.7 (a–d) Sagittal T 2-weighted MRI scans showing spinal cord compression along the apex of the kyphotic deformity with signal intensity changes.

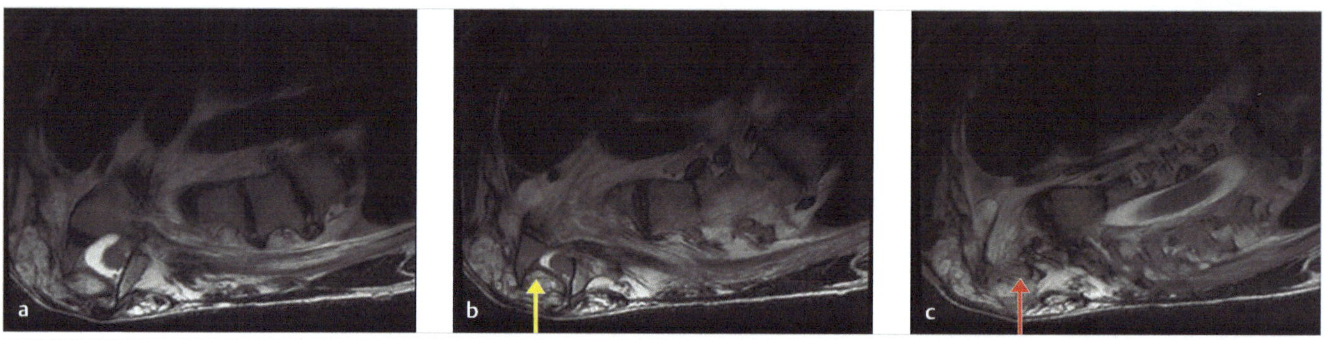

Fig. 8.8 (a–c) Axial T 2-weighted MRI scans demonstrating compression of the spinal cord (*red arrow*) by a large plexiform neurofibroma (*yellow arrow*) along the apex of the kyphotic deformity.

optimized, and he had a weight gain of approximately 12 lb. The traction weight goal was achieved on day 24. On traction day 44, the patient began to develop acute myelopathic symptoms with progressive left lower extremity weakness (2/5) and difficulty ambulating. Traction was immediately decreased, mean arterial pressures were optimized, and intravenous steroids were administered. MRI was repeated with no new evidence of cord compression. There was minimal improvement in his lower extremity motor function, and the decision was made to proceed with the surgery earlier than anticipated. A posterior spinal instrumentation and fusion from T 1 to L 4 with a T 7–T 9 VCR was performed and achieved excellent coronal and sagittal correction. The patient regained baseline motor function by postoperative day 2. Full strength and complete resolution of ankle clonus and hyperreflexia were noted at 4 months. Approximately 50% correction of the kyphotic deformity was obtained (▶ Fig. 8.10, ▶ Fig. 8.11), and the patient gained 5 inches in height postoperatively.

8.8 Conclusion

Treating patients with myelopathy and neurologic deficits rendered at the apex of severe angular spinal deformities are some of the most challenging deformities encountered. Our approach has been consideration for preoperative halo-gravity traction to improve the deformity along with the overall health of the

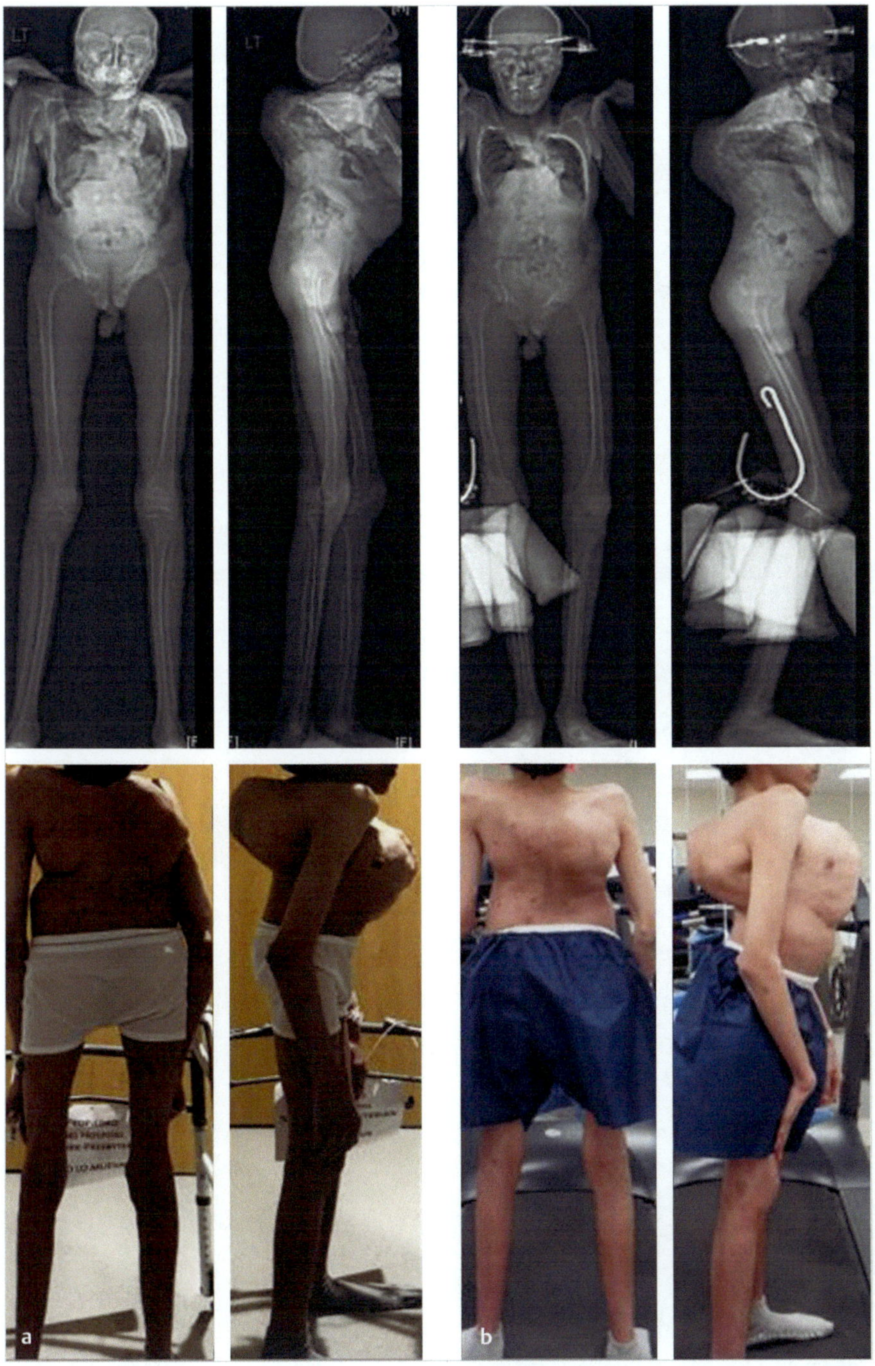

Fig. 8.9 **(a)** Posteroanterior (PA) radiographs and clinical pictures before traction was started and **(b)** after 7 weeks of halo gravity traction. Notice the improvement of the chest wall volume on the PA radiograph **(b)** and the increase in distance between the occiput and the apex of the kyphosis on the sagittal profile after 7 weeks of traction.

patient, followed by a single- or multiple-vertebrae PVCR for spinal cord decompression and deformity correction. This approach is ideal in that it accomplishes all of the required goals of the condition through a posterior-only operation; however, the pathology renders these surgeries extremely high risk, especially from a neurologic perspective. Although we have seen neurologic deterioration with this approach, most patients have gone on to make a full motor recovery (in the senior author's experience all patients except for one, who had had prior intradural surgery as a child at the level of a fixed angular kyphotic deformity and developed severe myelopathy into adulthood that rendered him wheelchair bound preoperatively). Certainly these surgeries are quite challenging and extensive; therefore, the surgeon, along with the entire operating team, needs to be able to take care of these types of patients to ensure an optimal outcome.

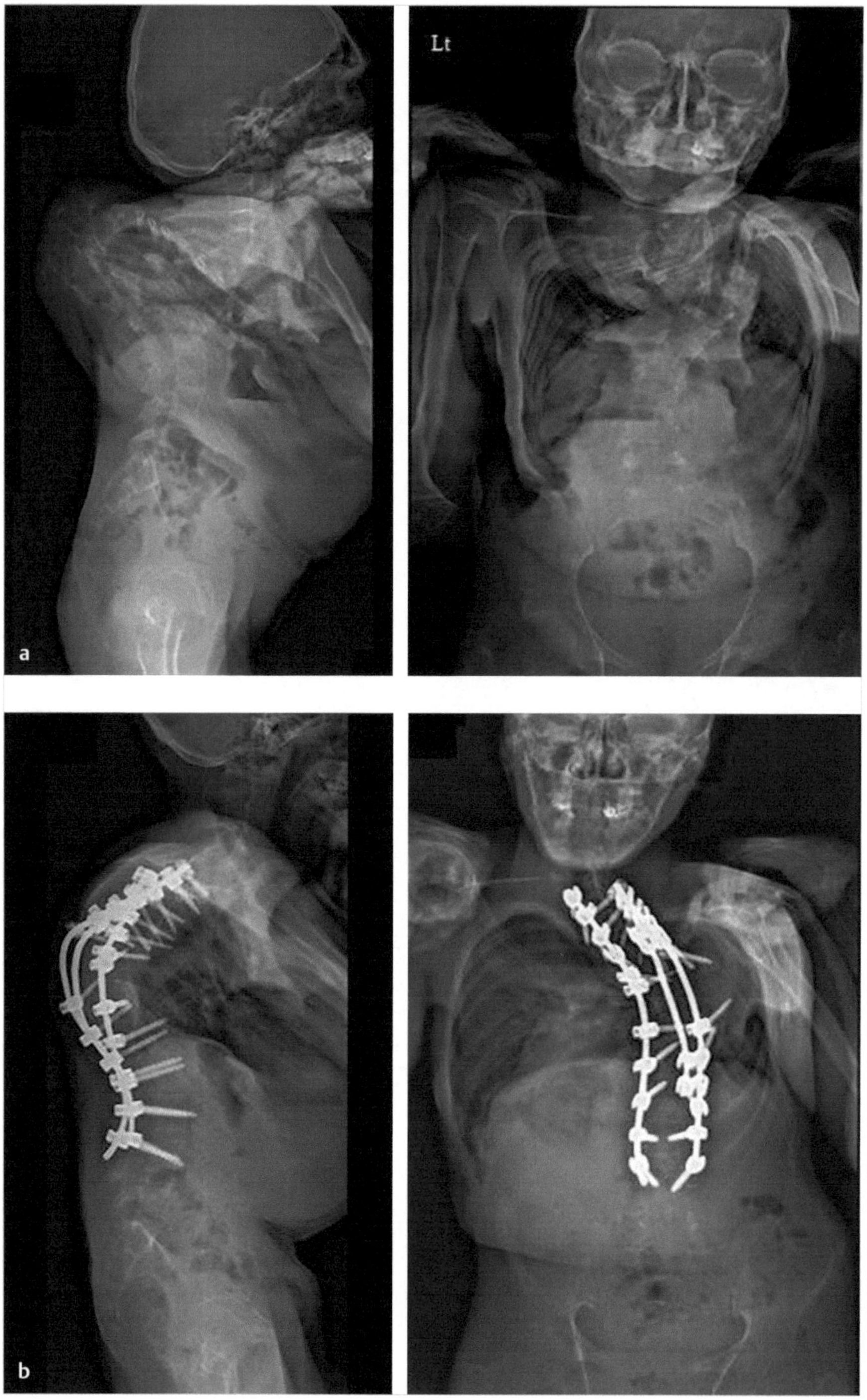

Fig. 8.10 **(a)** Preoperative and **(b)** 4 months postoperative posteroanterior and lateral radiographs demonstrating significant improvement in the sagittal alignment as well as coronal deformity. Notice the expansion and volume increase in the thoracic cavity postoperatively **(b)**.

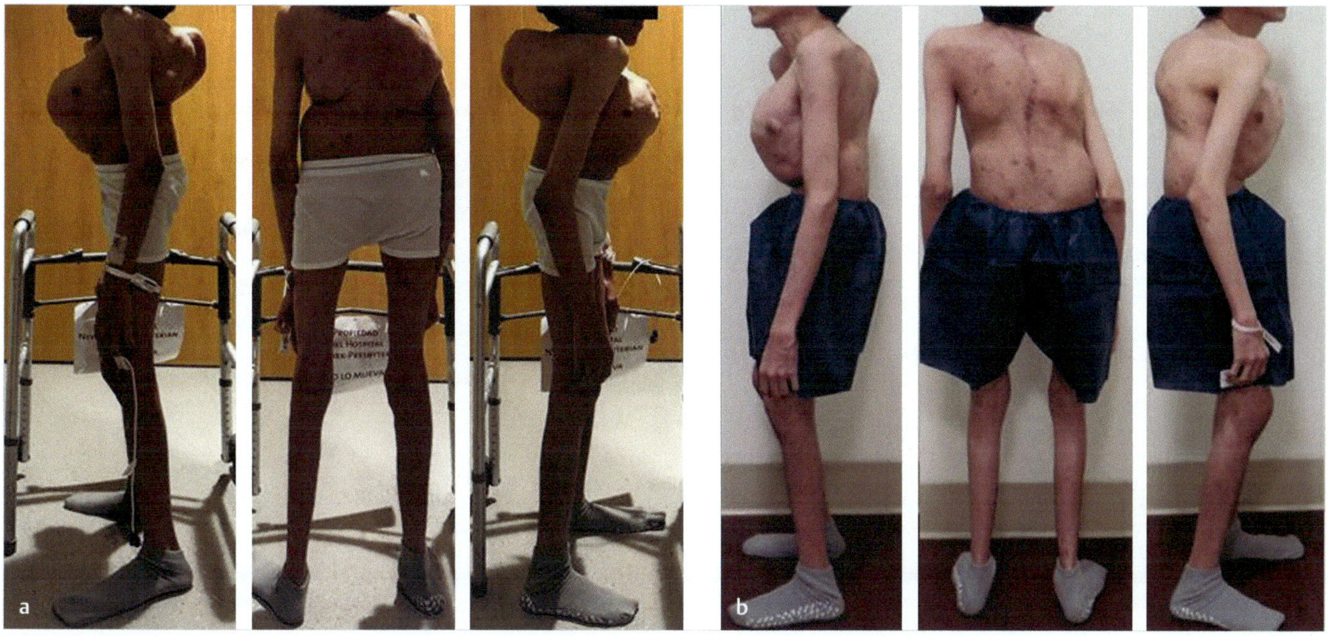

Fig. 8.11 (a) Preoperative and **(b)** 4 months postoperative clinical images showing improvement in both coronal and sagittal alignment. The thoracic prominence has significantly decreased. The patient gained 5 inches in height and has noticed improvement in his respiratory mechanics.

References

[1] MacLennan A. Scoliosis. BMJ. 1922; 2:864–866

[2] Leatherman KD, Dickson RA. Two-stage corrective surgery for congenital deformities of the spine. J Bone Joint Surg Br. 1979; 61-B(3):324–328

[3] Leatherman KD. Resection of vertebral bodies. J Bone Joint Surg Am. 1969; 51A:206

[4] Bradford DS. Vertebral column resection. Orthop Trans. 1987; 11:502

[5] Bradford DS, Boachie-Adjei O. One-stage anterior and posterior hemivertebral resection and arthrodesis for congenital scoliosis. J Bone Joint Surg Am. 1990; 72(4):536–540

[6] Boachie-Adjei O, Bradford DS. Vertebral column resection and arthrodesis for complex spinal deformities. J Spinal Disord. 1991; 4(2):193–202

[7] Wong CA, Cole AA, Watson L, Webb JK, Johnston ID, Kinnear WJ. Pulmonary function before and after anterior spinal surgery in adult idiopathic scoliosis. Thorax. 1996; 51(5):534–536

[8] Graham EJ, Lenke LG, Lowe TG, et al. Prospective pulmonary function evaluation following open thoracotomy for anterior spinal fusion in adolescent idiopathic scoliosis. Spine. 2000; 25(18):2319–2325

[9] Kim YJ, Lenke LG, Bridwell KH, Cheh G, Sides B, Whorton J. Prospective pulmonary function comparison of anterior spinal fusion in adolescent idiopathic scoliosis: thoracotomy versus thoracoabdominal approach. Spine. 2008; 33(10):1055–1060

[10] Lonner BS, Auerbach JD, Estreicher MB, et al. Pulmonary function changes after various anterior approaches in the treatment of adolescent idiopathic scoliosis. J Spinal Disord Tech. 2009; 22(8):551–558

[11] Vedantam R, Lenke LG, Bridwell KH, Haas J, Linville DA. A prospective evaluation of pulmonary function in patients with adolescent idiopathic scoliosis relative to the surgical approach used for spinal arthrodesis. Spine. 2000; 25(1):82–90

[12] Gitelman Y, Lenke LG, Bridwell KH, Auerbach JD, Sides BA. Pulmonary function in adolescent idiopathic scoliosis relative to the surgical procedure: a 10-year follow-up analysis. Spine. 2011; 36(20):1665–1672

[13] Pehrsson K, Danielsson A, Nachemson A. Pulmonary function in adolescent idiopathic scoliosis: a 25 year follow up after surgery or start of brace treatment. Thorax. 2001; 56(5):388–393

[14] Suk SI, Kim JH, Kim WJ, Lee SM, Chung ER, Nah KH. Posterior vertebral column resection for severe spinal deformities. Spine. 2002; 27(21):2374–2382

[15] Suk SI, Chung ER, Kim JH, Kim SS, Lee JS, Choi WK. Posterior vertebral column resection for severe rigid scoliosis. Spine. 2005; 30(14):1682–1687

[16] Suk SI, Chung ER, Lee SM, Lee JH, Kim SS, Kim JH. Posterior vertebral column resection in fixed lumbosacral deformity. Spine. 2005; 30(23):E703–E710

[17] Lenke LG, O'Leary PT, Bridwell KH, Sides BA, Koester LA, Blanke KM. Posterior vertebral column resection for severe pediatric deformity: minimum two-year follow-up of thirty-five consecutive patients. Spine. 2009; 34(20):2213–2221

[18] Lenke LG, Sides BA, Koester LA, Hensley M, Blanke KM. Vertebral column resection for the treatment of severe spinal deformity. Clin Orthop Relat Res. 2010; 468(3):687–699

[19] Lenke LG, Newton PO, Sucato DJ, et al. Complications after 147 consecutive vertebral column resections for severe pediatric spinal deformity: a multicenter analysis. Spine. 2013; 38(2):119–132

[20] Papadopoulos EC, Boachie-Adjei O, Hess WF, et al. Foundation of Orthopedics and Complex Spine, New York, NY. Early outcomes and complications of posterior vertebral column resection. Spine J. 2015; 15(5):983–991

[21] Auerbach JD, Lenke LG, Bridwell KH, et al. Major complications and comparison between 3-column osteotomy techniques in 105 consecutive spinal deformity procedures. Spine. 2012; 37(14):1198–1210

[22] Cho SK, Lenke LG, Bolon SM, et al. Progressive myelopathy patients who lack spinal cord monitoring data have the highest rate of spinal cord deficits following posterior vertebral column resection surgery. Spine Deform. 2015; 3(4):352–359

[23] Wang XB, Lenke LG, Thuet E, Blanke K, Koester LA, Roth M. Deformity angular ratio describes the severity of spinal deformity and predicts the risk of neurologic deficit in posterior vertebral column resection surgery. Spine. 2016; 41 (18):1447–1455

[24] Bumpass DB, Lenke LG, Bridwell KH, et al. Pulmonary function improvement after vertebral column resection for severe spinal deformity. Spine. 2014; 39 (7):587–595

[25] Ohshio I, Hatayama A, Kaneda K, Takahara M, Nagashima K. Correlation between histopathologic features and magnetic resonance images of spinal cord lesions. Spine. 1993; 18(9):1140–1149

[26] Koller H, Zenner J, Gajic V, Meier O, Ferraris L, Hitzl W. The impact of halo-gravity traction on curve rigidity and pulmonary function in the treatment of severe and rigid scoliosis and kyphoscoliosis: a clinical study and narrative review of the literature. Eur Spine J. 2012; 21(3):514–529

[27] Garabekyan T, Hosseinzadeh P, Iwinski HJ, et al. The results of preoperative halo-gravity traction in children with severe spinal deformity. J Pediatr Orthop B. 2014; 23(1):1–5

[28] Yang C, Wang H, Zheng Z, et al. Halo-gravity traction in the treatment of severe spinal deformity: a systematic review and meta-analysis. Eur Spine J. 2017; 26(7):1810–1816

[29] Sink EL, Karol LA, Sanders J, Birch JG, Johnston CE, Herring JA. Efficacy of perioperative halo-gravity traction in the treatment of severe scoliosis in children. J Pediatr Orthop. 2001; 21(4):519–524

[30] Rinella A, Lenke L, Whitaker C, et al. Perioperative halo-gravity traction in the treatment of severe scoliosis and kyphosis. Spine. 2005; 30(4):475–482

[31] Janus GJ, Finidori G, Engelbert RH, Pouliquen M, Pruijs JE. Operative treatment of severe scoliosis in osteogenesis imperfecta: results of 20 patients after halo traction and posterior spondylodesis with instrumentation. Eur Spine J. 2000; 9(6):486–491

[32] Wilkins C, MacEwen GD. Cranial nerve injury from halo traction. Clin Orthop Relat Res. 1977(126):106–110

[33] Ginsburg GM, Bassett GS. Hypoglossal nerve injury caused by halo-suspension traction. A case report. Spine. 1998; 23(13):1490–1493

[34] Bouchoucha S, Khelifi A, Saied W, Ammar C, Nessib MN, Ben Ghachem M. Progressive correction of severe spinal deformities with halo-gravity traction. Acta Orthop Belg. 2011; 77(4):529–534

[35] Kim YJ, Lenke LG, Bridwell KH, Cho YS, Riew KD. Free hand pedicle screw placement in the thoracic spine: is it safe? Spine. 2004; 29(3):333–342, discussion 342

[36] Lenke LG, Padberg AM, Russo MH, Bridwell KH, Gelb DE. Triggered electromyographic threshold for accuracy of pedicle screw placement. An animal model and clinical correlation. Spine. 1995; 20(14):1585–1591

[37] Glassman SD, Dimar JR, Puno RM, Johnson JR, Shields CB, Linden RD. A prospective analysis of intraoperative electromyographic monitoring of pedicle screw placement with computed tomographic scan confirmation. Spine. 1995; 20(12):1375–1379

[38] Raynor BL, Lenke LG, Bridwell KH, Taylor BA, Padberg AM. Correlation between low triggered electromyographic thresholds and lumbar pedicle screw malposition: analysis of 4 857 screws. Spine. 2007; 32(24):2673–2678

[39] Danesh-Clough T, Taylor P, Hodgson B, et al. The use of EMG in detecting misplaced thoracolumbar pedicle screws. Spine. Phila Pa. 1976; 2001(26):1313–1316

[40] Lewis SJ, Lenke LG, Raynor B, Long J, Bridwell KH, Padberg A. Triggered electromyographic threshold for accuracy of thoracic pedicle screw placement in a porcine model. Spine. 2001; 26(22):2485–2489, discussion 2490

[41] Raynor BL, Lenke LG, Kim Y, et al. Can triggered electromyograph thresholds predict safe thoracic pedicle screw placement? Spine. 2002; 27(18):2030–2035

[42] Cho SK, Lenke LG, Bolon SM, et al. Can intraoperative spinal cord monitoring reliably help prevent paraplegia during posterior vertebral column resection surgery. Spine Deform. 2015; 3(1):73–81

[43] Zhang HQ, Li JS, Liu SH, et al. The use of posterior vertebral column resection in the management of severe posttuberculous kyphosis: a retrospective study and literature review. Arch Orthop Trauma Surg. 2013; 133(9):1211–1218

[44] Xie JM, Zhang Y, Wang YS, et al. The risk factors of neurologic deficits of one-stage posterior vertebral column resection for patients with severe and rigid spinal deformities. Eur Spine J. 2014; 23(1):149–156

[45] Spiro AS, Rupprecht M, Stenger P, et al. Surgical treatment of severe congenital thoracolumbar kyphosis through a single posterior approach. Bone Joint J. 2013; 95-B(11):1527–1532

[46] Kim SS, Cho BC, Kim JH, et al. Complications of posterior vertebral resection for spinal deformity. Asian Spine J. 2012; 6(4):257–265

[47] Hamzaoglu A, Alanay A, Ozturk C, Sarier M, Karadereler S, Ganiyusufoglu K. Posterior vertebral column resection in severe spinal deformities: a total of 102 cases. Spine. 2011; 36(5):E340–E344

[48] Thuet ED, Padberg AM, Raynor BL, et al. Increased risk of postoperative neurologic deficit for spinal surgery patients with unobtainable intraoperative evoked potential data. Spine. 2005; 30(18):2094–2103

9 Osteotomies in Syndromic Patients

Dino Colo, René M. Castelein

Abstract

Treating rigid spinal deformities in a syndromic population is not only a challenge in executing a demanding surgical technique, but also in dealing holistically with an often seriously compromised population. Many syndromes lead to a disturbance of normal spinal growth and development: Examples are spina bifida, spinal muscular atrophy, Rett syndrome, Duchenne's muscular dystrophy, 22q-11 deletion syndrome, Marfan's syndrome, and many more. Each of them requires a careful multi-disciplinary approach, including in most cases, pediatricians, anesthesiologists, ICU specialists, rehab specialists, and sometimes a number of others, depending on the specific condition. Expectations of the patient, the parents, and the caregivers should be an essential part of the pre-operative work-up.

In this chapter, the options of different spinal osteotomies for a rigid spinal deformity in the presence of a syndromic condition are addressed. Depending on the underlying syndromic condition and the patients' mental and physical abilities, different goals of the procedure can be defined. In all cases, prevention of progression of the deformity, stabilization of the trunk in a balanced position, prevention of cardiopulmonary decline, and avoidance of complications will be paramount. Different osteotomies, as categorized by Schwab, can be performed in this patient group to obtain the required outcome. Special attention must be given to problems of general health, nutrition, blood management during and after the procedure, infection prevention, and rehabilitation.

Keywords: rigid deformity, osteotomies, syndromes, multidisciplinary approach, complications

9.1 Introduction

The development of different types of vertebral osteotomies has contributed significantly to spinal deformity surgery and its advancement over recent decades. Osteotomies have become powerful tools enabling the surgeon to achieve more correction, especially in rigid deformities. This, together with improved anesthetic techniques, more stable, sophisticated, pedicle-based instrumentation techniques, as well as comprehensive intraoperative neuromonitoring, enables restoration of spinal alignment in cases that were previously considered impossible. Current fixation constructs, mostly posterior-based, providing multisegmental three-column spinal fixation through pedicle screws, combined with posterior osteotomies, offer the surgeon the possibility to address spinal deformities through a posterior-only approach, although the more traditional anterior approaches still have their place. Despite the enormity of these procedures, spinal osteotomies have been described to be life-saving for certain indications.[1] Surgical treatment of rigid deformities in syndromic patients is often a challenge due to their complex and multidisciplinary surgical as well as medical problems. There are four ultimate goals of applying osteotomies in the rigid syndromic spine:

1. Prevent further deterioration of balance, cardiopulmonary function, and sometimes cosmesis.
2. Correct the deformity.
3. Achieve spinopelvic sitting and/or standing balance in both the coronal and sagittal planes.
4. Minimize postoperative complications.

9.2 Definition, Classification, and Indication

Osteotomies are indicated for severe rigid coronal and sagittal plane deformities. Their common feature is that they are difficult to correct; bending and traction radiographs usually show no more than 50% correction.[2] Careful assessment of the type of deformity (scoliosis/kyphosis/lordosis) and associated coronal, sagittal, or combined imbalance enables the surgeon to choose the appropriate type and extent of osteotomy.[1] If possible, depending on the patient's ambulatory status, full-spine upright anterior–posterior and lateral radiographs, or, when available, EOS studies with low-dose radiation exposure, are required.[3] The type of deformity can generally be classified as being in one of two categories: predominantly a sagittal imbalance, or both a coronal and sagittal imbalance. Usually the deformity is not limited to one anatomical plane but affects the spine in a multiplanar fashion. Bridwell classified the coronal plane deformity as flexible, partially flexible, or rigid, with flexible deformities requiring no osteotomy, and rigid deformities usually requiring osteotomy.[4] Shoulder and pelvic balance are important parameters for the patient. In the coronal plane, type I deformity according to Bridwell, has a high right shoulder and low right pelvis, which can be corrected by shortening the right side of the spine, for example, with an asymmetric pedicle subtraction osteotomy (PSO). Type II deformities represent a more complex relationship between shoulder and pelvic balance and cannot be corrected by a simple osteotomy: they may require a vertebral column resection (VCR).[1,4] Sagittal imbalance, as determined by the position of the C 7 plumb line (C 7PL) relative to the midsacral line, can also be classified as type I and type II deformities, aiding the surgeon in choosing the type of osteotomy. Type I is a segmental imbalance (C 7PL within 5 cm of a vertical line going through the sacrum), in which a part of the spine is hyperkyphotic, but the patient is still able to maintain balance by hyperextending segments above and below. This can be treated with multiple Smith–Petersen osteotomies (SPO) or sometimes a PSO. Type II is a more global sagittal imbalance in which the patient cannot balance the hyperkyphosis by hyperextending adjacent segments. This usually requires a PSO or VCR. Short angular kyphotic deformities may benefit more from a PSO or VCR, whereas long, sweeping kyphoses may be more amenable to multiple SPOs.[1]

9.3 Rigid Deformities in Syndromic Patients

There is no clear classification of rigid spine deformities in syndromic patients, despite the fact that spinal deformities are highly prevalent, in some cases up to 100%, in neuromuscular or syndromic patients, and, especially when neglected or left untreated, these curves can become very rigid and lead to compression of the lung and abdominal organs.[5,6] Certain syndromes such as Duchenne muscular dystrophy (DMD) or spinal muscular atrophy (SMA), due to their neurologic consequences, may lead to poor axial trunk balance and muscle weakness and/or spasticity, which subsequently alter the coronal and sagittal balance, as already described in general. Furthermore, significant pelvic obliquity may be present, resulting in poor sitting balance, general discomfort, and in some cases decubitus ulcer points. Usually the indication for surgery for rigid deformities in syndromic patients depends on the extent of the curve, the presence of pain, the functional impairment and significant spinal decompensation with poor sitting balance, and the risk for even more progression. In these cases, aggressive and early surgery is a good approach and can prevent the need for more complex surgical procedures at a later stage when the patient is often in worse physical condition, since progression can often reliably be predicted.

Many syndromes are associated with the development of spinal deformities, and in some cases rigid curves. For example, Marfan syndrome (MFS) has an estimated spinal deformity prevalence of around 60%, and 12 to 50% of the patients will require a surgical correction.[7] Unlike in idiopathic scoliosis, there is often an accompanying kyphosis greater than 50 degrees, especially in the thoracolumbar area, as well as relatively frequent double thoracic and triple major curve patterns.[8] Although these patients are in general very flexible, curves can be so rigid that osteotomies may be required to correct the deformity. According to Jones et al, the average bending correction in their group of 26 MFS patients was 37.1%, with a range of 4 to 89%, indicating that a certain number of these curves can definitely be rigid. Often, the number of levels that need to be fused is higher in MFS.[7] Also, the amount of correction of the thoracolumbar kyphosis and sagittal imbalance is higher than that in adolescent idiopathic scoliosis,[8] suggesting that the spine in MFS can achieve more intraoperative correction. MFS patients experience more hardware complications, pseudarthrosis, dural leaks, and reoperations compared to idiopathic cases[7,8]; neurologic deficits and length of hospital stay are not significantly different.[8] Whether these patients show increased intraoperative blood loss is debatable as data differ between several studies.[7,8]

Another syndrome with a high prevalence (36–100%) of spinal deformities is Rett syndrome, a progressive neurodevelopmental disorder almost exclusively affecting females.[9] No exact numbers are available in the literature describing the prevalence of rigid curves and the result of applied osteotomies; however, these patients often have severe deformity at an early age with associated pelvic obliquity, requiring osteotomies to correct sitting balance. As is the case with MFS, patients with Rett syndrome have a high risk of complications after spinal surgery, not only surgical but also related to their pulmonary and gastrointestinal comorbidity.[9]

Neuromuscular conditions like SMA (up to 100%) (▶ Fig. 9.1) or DMD (68–89%)[10] are highly at risk for developing a spine deformity and can lead to rigid curves if not treated at the appropriate time, often when the curve is still rather small. If left untreated, a scoliosis in SMA can progress 5 to 15 degrees annually.[11] These patients ultimately become wheelchair bound, and most of the curves (95%) become progressive. Patients tend to develop significant contractures and decreased

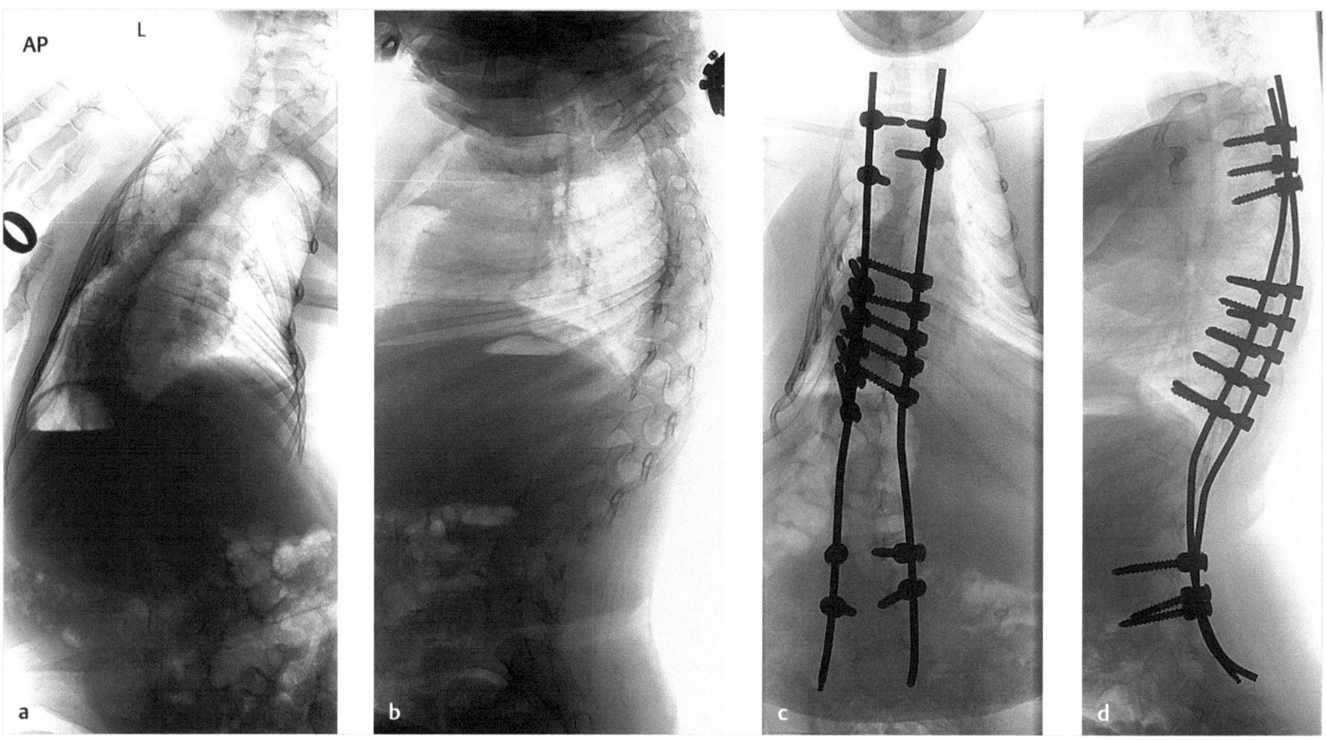

Fig. 9.1 (a) Posteroanterior (PA) and **(b)** lateral radiographs of an 8-year-old nonambulatory boy with spinal muscular atrophy type II and a progressive deformity. **(c)** Postoperative PA and **(d)** lateral radiographs show a satisfactory restoration of sitting balance after he was treated with multiple Ponte and Smith–Petersen osteotomies and a Shilla growth system from T2 to L4.

pulmonary function. These developments, combined with pelvic obliquity and loss of sitting balance, present a challenge for surgical treatment of the deformity.[10,11] Mehta et al suggested that the pelvis be included in the fixation if the pelvic obliquity exceeds 15 degrees.[10] Due to frequently present flexion contractures of the hips and knees, preserving the lumbar lordosis is important and is now easier to achieve with pedicle screw constructs, especially when combined with multiple Smith–Petersen or Ponte osteotomies in the lumbar area. An important complication in these severely handicapped patients, along with significant blood loss, is screw pullout related to osteopenia.[10] One should also realize that the trend in the literature appears to indicate that pulmonary function in SMA continues to decline after surgery, however, its rate is less marked.[12]

Cerebral palsy (CP) is another condition that can lead to a rigid spinal deformity interfering with gait in ambulatory patients, and with sitting balance in nonambulatory patients. It is one of the leading causes for neuromuscular scoliosis. The indication for surgery, estimated to be necessary in one in seven patients,[13] is commonly to restore the sitting balance by correcting the curve and pelvic obliquity, also relieving pain by allowing the concave ribs to be pulled out of the pelvis. Paralytic CP showed a significantly better Cobb angle correction compared to that for spastic CP, but no difference in pelvic obliquity correction has been observed.[6] Spinal surgery in CP has a high complication rate, varying from 8 to 33%, especially including deep infection, significant blood loss, increased hospital stay, proximal junctional kyphosis, and revision surgery.[13]

Another condition with an increased risk (around 15–20% prevalence) for spinal deformity is the 22q11 deletion syndrome, previously also referred to as velocardiofacial or DiGeorge syndrome.[14,15,16] These patients suffer from various comorbidities, such as cardiac, endocrine, and psychiatric disorders. These may, at times, obscure their spinal deformity, which, analogous to idiopathic scoliosis, may develop during the growth spurt in a relatively short time span and at an age that other disorders (e. g., psychosis) become more manifest, requiring intensive follow-up. Curves can rapidly progress into severe and rigid scoliosis, requiring spinal osteotomies. These children may initially not be recognized as having a syndrome, as many different organ systems can be affected. Moreover, they may have cervical instability, immune disorders, and a thrombocyte coagulopathy; thus the risk of intra- and postoperative complications, such as hypocalcemia and increased blood loss, especially during osteotomies, requires attention. Awareness of the syndrome, a multidisciplinary approach including a pediatrician, and an extensive preoperative workup should minimize these risks.[14,16]

A relatively new problem has arisen with the introduction of successful stem cell transplantation (SCT) for mucopolysaccharidoses (MPSs) such as Hurler's disease (MPS type I). Previously, this autosomal recessive lysosomal storage disease was lethal, often before early adolescence. With the introduction of SCT in the early 1980 s, survival rates have increased spectacularly.[17] Unfortunately, penetration of the donor enzyme through the SCT in the locomotor system is much less than optimal, leading to a number of previously unknown orthopaedic problems, also involving the spine, becoming clinically relevant. A majority (> 80%) of these patients develop an acute kyphosis at the thoracolumbar junction (usually the apex at the L 1–L 2 level), which is very difficult to treat (▶ Fig. 9.2).[17] Braces have been tried to prevent progression with varying success. Ultimately, this may lead to a dislocation at the thoracolumbar junction requiring surgery, including more or less extensive osteotomies (▶ Fig. 9.2c). Since not only the bone but also the ligaments around the spine are involved, and the posterior tension band of the longitudinal ligaments is insufficient, recurrence is a serious threat (▶ Fig. 9.2d, e). So far, many strategies have been attempted, but

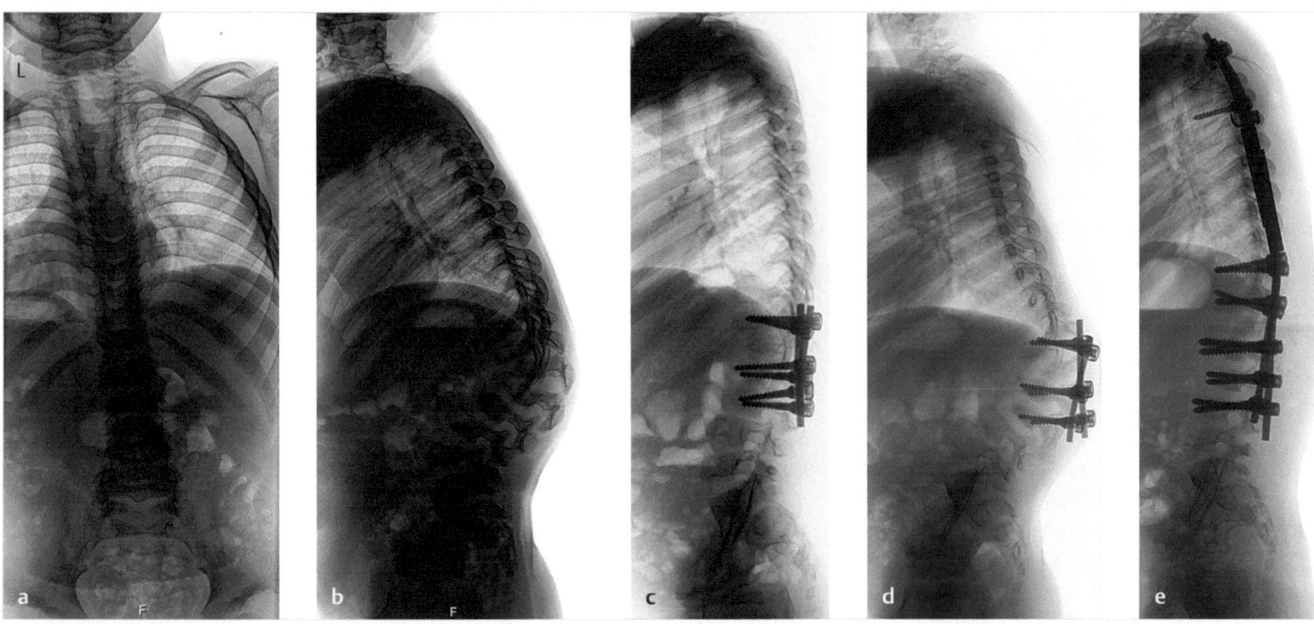

Fig. 9.2 **(a)** Posteroanterior and **(b)** lateral radiographs of a 6-year-old boy with mucopolysaccharidosis type I and a characteristic progressive thoracolumbar kyphosis. **(c)** The postoperative lateral radiograph shows a satisfactory result after he was treated with a pedicle subtraction osteotomy at L 1, a Smith–Petersen osteotomy at L 2, and a subsequent posterior spinal fusion from T 12 to L 3. **(d)** One and a half years later the kyphotic deformity recurred, and **(e)** he was treated with a growing rod from T 3 to T 11, and posterior spinal fusion from T 11 to L 4.

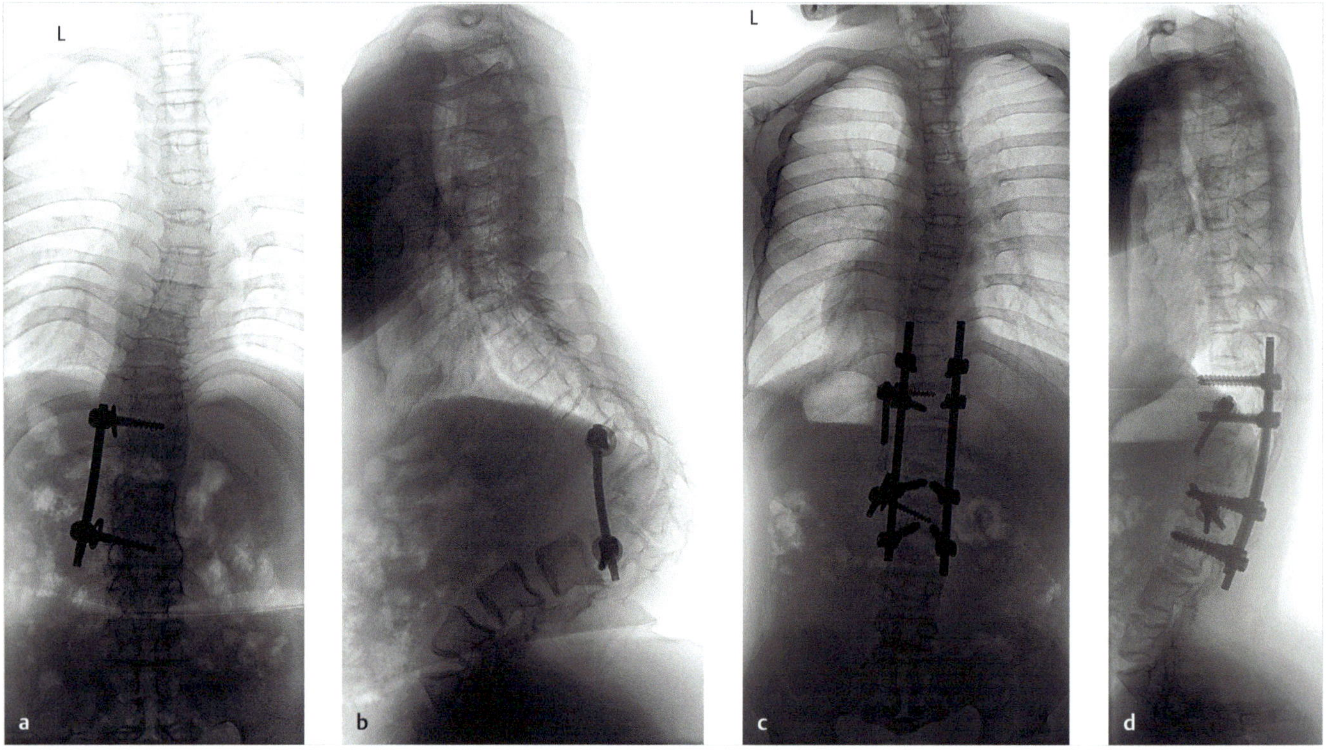

Fig. 9.3 (a) Posteroanterior and **(b)** lateral radiographs of a 16-year-old boy with achondroplasia, referred to us after being treated for his thoracolumbar kyphosis with an anterior spinal fusion at age 3 years. **(c)** Because of progression, he underwent a vertebral column resection of L 1 followed by **(d)** a posterior spinal fusion from T 10 to L 3.

no definitive procedure has been proven to be superior to the other. Similarly, but usually less severe, kyphosis at the thoracolumbar junction may develop in patients with achondroplasia. Usually, these cases are more amenable to less aggressive surgery, but osteotomies may be required (▶ Fig. 9.3).

There are many other syndromes and neuromuscular conditions, sometimes with congenital vertebral failures of formation or segmentation, which can result in rigid spinal deformities, requiring extensive posterior releases and osteotomies to achieve a reasonable amount of correction and improved spinopelvic and sitting balance. Examples include neurofibromatosis, VACTERL association (vertebral defects, anal atresia, cardiac defects, tracheoesophageal fistula, renal anomalies, limb abnormalities), Shprintzen–Goldberg syndrome, Coffin-Lowry syndrome, other MPSs, arthrogryposis, and various osteochondrodystrophies.

9.4 Choice of Osteotomy: Type and Goal

The required type of osteotomy depends on the type of deformity, the curve magnitude and flexibility, its location, the presence of spinal cord compression, bone quality, previous spinal surgery, and the surgeon's experience and comfort level with the procedure.[1] Accordingly, it is important for the surgeon to have a discussion with the patient about the possible benefits of surgery, the associated complications and risks, and the patient's expectations.

Schwab et al proposed a comprehensive spinal osteotomy classification system in order to provide a more homogeneous nomenclature and use of these osteotomies.[18] The various types of osteotomies are described in greater detail in section 9.6 and are shown in ▶ Fig. 9.4.

The goal of performing osteotomies is to restore sagittal and coronal balance so that the patient can sit, and if possible, stand and ambulate erectly, without the need for flexing the hip and knees to maintain balance. Combined with a solid fusion mass, further progression will be prevented, the pain reduced, a horizontal gait established, and the cosmetic appearance improved.[1] In nonambulatory patients, restoration of the sitting balance and pelvic obliquity is the most important goal, decreasing pain and risk of pressure sores, thereby increasing comfort level and ease for the caregivers.

9.5 Preoperative Workup

These are intrinsically complex patients, usually both for their orthopaedic condition but often even more so for their underlying disease. The decision to operate always has to be part of a shared decision making process that involves the patient, the parents and care givers, and other medical and paramedical disciplines involved in the care of the patient.

9.5.1 Patient History and Physical Findings

A comprehensive multidisciplinary preoperative evaluation, including input from pediatricians, anesthesiologists, cardiologists, neurologists or neurosurgeons, rehabilitation specialists, physical

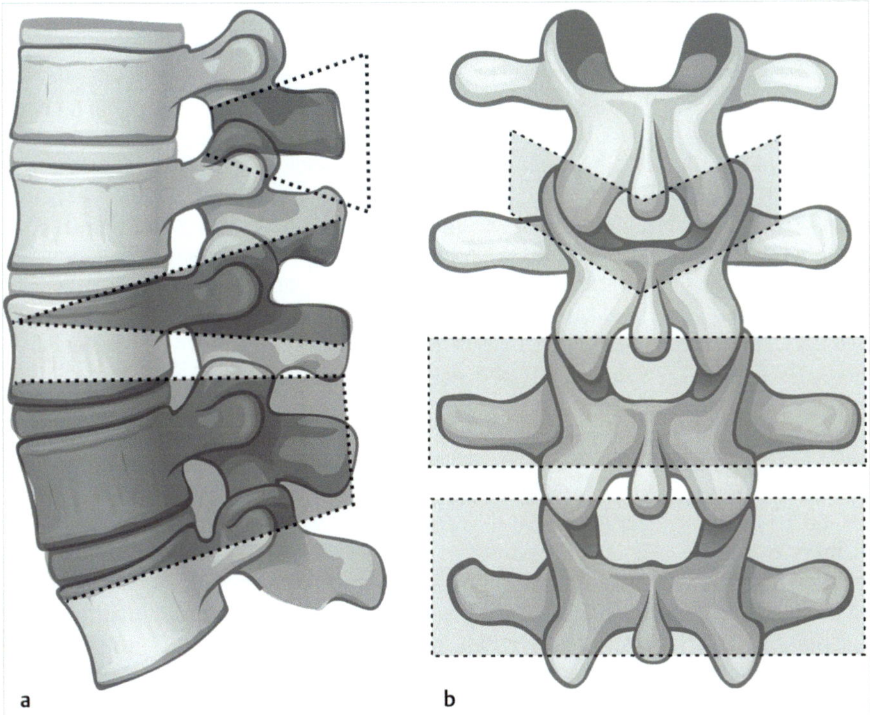

Fig. 9.4 Schematic overview of the various osteotomies. (**a**) Lateral view. (**b**) Coronal view as seen from posteriorly.

therapists, and nursing personnel often helps to achieve the best result. A thorough discussion with the patient and family about the goals of the planned procedure, their and the surgeon's expectations, and the potential risks is mandatory. In these complex patients and procedures, the surgical risks (e.g., infection, excessive bleeding, neurological damage, intensive care admission, persistent ventilator dependency) are usually high but depend on the condition and should be discussed as such.

A detailed cardiovascular and pulmonary function examination is important, evaluating a possible history of known cardiac and/or pulmonary disease, especially because some patients with severe rigid curves and an associated syndrome may have restrictive pulmonary disease. For example, patients with MFS have an increased chance of cardiac anomalies and should be screened preoperatively by a cardiologist. Patients with DMD, on the other hand, experience an annual decline of 3 to 10% in their vital lung capacity, which increases the complication risk of spine surgery.[19] Careful preoperative evaluation may also help in identifying those at risk for increased intraoperative bleeding: It is well known that neuromuscular patients are more susceptible to this due to a decreased coagulation reserve, changes in vascular smooth muscle cells (such as in DMD), increased fibrinolytic activity, and sometimes the use of antiepileptic medication that can cause increased bleeding time. Osteopenia may be a concern and should be screened for, sometimes requiring an adaptation of the surgical strategy. Sublaminar wires or (broader) bands can be used to augment screws, just like bone cement, if indicated.

General nutritional assessment is important, both to decrease postoperative wound healing and infectious complications as well as to identify those patients who might benefit from peri- or postoperative parenteral nutrition as early as possible.

For the nonambulatory patient, sitting balance is paramount. Good balance frees the arms for daily tasks, including professional and recreational activities, and it prevents pressure sores, especially in patients with disturbed sensation, such as in spina bifida. This can be best assessed in the wheelchair, but a more general examination looking for hip and knee contractures, skin irritation, previous scars in the operating area (e.g., in spina bifida), neurologic function, the presence and site of feeding tubes (important for positioning during surgery), requires the patient to be undressed on the examination bench in both the prone and the supine positions. The overall trunk balance, head control, flexibility, and pressure points due to pelvic obliquity are evaluated. Patients with fixed deformities may compensate by flexing their hips and knees to maintain balance, which can lead to significant back pain, fatigue, and increased energy consumption during walking for those who are ambulatory. In ambulatory patients, gait can be disturbed by spinal imbalance, and cosmetic concerns may play a role. A detailed neurologic history (e.g., seizures, deficits) and examination is key to detect any abnormalities that may point to spinal cord involvement, such as tethered cord, split cord, syringomyelia, and Arnold–Chiari malformations, which can complicate the surgery and lead to aggravation of the symptoms postoperatively, especially in the case of extensive osteotomies.

9.5.2 Imaging Studies

Radiographic evaluation should include long films of the whole spine in the coronal and sagittal planes, either standing, sitting, or supine, depending on the ambulatory status, with posteroanterior and lateral views, ideally including the cervical spine and both femoral heads. Measuring global coronal and sagittal spinopelvic parameters in ambulatory patients, such as sagittal vertical axis (C7PL), thoracic kyphosis, lumbar lordosis, pelvic incidence, pelvic tilt, and sacral slope, can guide the surgeon in the amount of correction needed to achieve a balanced spine.

Bending or traction (under general anesthesia) radiographs provide additional information, in both ambulatory and nonambulatory cases, about the stiffness of the main deformity and accompanying compensatory curves.

As deformities may reduce in supine positions, supine radiographs may help to determine sagittal flexibility if the spine corrects significantly in this position, thereby identifying rigid but also more flexible, compensatory parts of the spine.[2] The use of a bolster in the supine position can assist in determining the flexibility of a localized kyphotic deformity. Similarly, supine bending radiographs may help in assessing the correctability of curves.[2]

Advanced imaging techniques, such as MR and CT scans with three-dimensional reconstruction, are helpful in further understanding the local anatomy and aid in planning the resection and instrumentation. In congenital vertebral malformations, myelomeningocele, and neurofibromatosis, as well as when the neurologic history and examination suggest intraspinal abnormalities, such as tethering, split cord, or Arnold–Chiari malformations, these imaging techniques are mandatory in preoperative planning. MRI also provides information about the integrity of the disks and disk spaces in planned noninstrumented areas. CT provides valuable information about the bone quality and stock, the exact morphology of congenital anomalies or areas of bony destruction (e. g., in neurofibromatosis or MFS due to dural ectasia), and ankylosed regions of the spine, and it may assist in preoperative planning of screw placement. In extreme cases, CT-based three-dimensional printing of a model of the spine can be extremely helpful in studying the exact morphology from all sides.

Bone densitometry is useful for assessing bone quality if there are any doubts regarding this topic, either due to related syndromic disorders or otherwise. MFS and certain dystrophies (DMD, SMA) are known to have a lower bone mineral density, complicating screw fixation.[7]

9.6 Surgical Aspects and Technique

Very often in these patients, surgery will have to be extensive in order to re-align the spine, improve sitting balance and prevent further deterioration of the condition.

9.6.1 Positioning and Perioperative Measures

Positioning can be problematic in patients with extensive contractures, such as in CP. Therefore extreme care must be given to padding and continuously monitoring potential pressure points. Once positioned, patients should have a secure airway that can be sustained through many hours of operating and manipulating, be in a neutral alignment, and be protected from pressure, with special attention given to the eyes. For a posterior approach, the patient is placed in a prone position on the operative frame, either a four-poster frame or a Jackson frame. Bolsters under the patient's thigh may help to achieve better lumbar lordosis.

Perioperative prophylactic antibiotics are mandatory and most commonly include cefazolin (intravenous administration). Vancomycin powder sprinkled in the wound at the end of the procedure has become more or less standard in these cases.[20] Intraoperative blood loss can be minimized by both pre- and intraoperative strategies. Antifibrinolytics, such as tranexaminic acid, have been shown to decrease surgical blood loss, and their use has been shown to be safe, including in the pediatric population.[2] The preoperative use of recombinant human erythropoietin has been shown to decrease blood loss and the need for homologous blood transfusion.[21] Additionally, intraoperative careful packing with cottonoids and use of bone wax, topical hemostatic agents, autologous blood transfusion techniques (cell saver conservation), and controlled hypotensive anesthesia can prevent the need for allogeneic blood transfusions. The mean arterial pressure can be maintained at 50 to 60 mm Hg, increasing it to 80 mm Hg just before the correction maneuvers and when the risk of neurologic injury is greatest. Therefore, these patients require an experienced anesthetic team during surgery as well as comprehensive postoperative intensive care unit (ICU) monitoring for providing optimal care.[21]

Neuromonitoring, consisting of bimodal signal detection (transcranial motor evoked potentials and somatosensory evoked potentials), is essential in spine surgery, unless the neurological situation of the patient is such that no reliable monitoring can be performed: no osteotomy should be performed without it. Close collaboration with the anesthetic team is again important to maintain the optimal hemodynamic parameters (e. g., hemoglobin, clotting factors, and spinal cord oxygenation) without compromising neuromonitoring by the use of certain anesthetic agents. Usually, the surgeon notes changes in blood coagulation in the wound before changes in laboratory parameters can be detected, and the anesthetic team should be ready to react to the surgeon's observations.

9.7 Surgical Technique

9.7.1 Smith–Petersen Osteotomy and Ponte Osteotomy

The Smith-Peterson Osteotomy (SPO) was first described in 1945, initially as a one- or two-level osteotomy mainly for correcting rigid sagittal plane deformity, such as in ankylosing spondylitis with an ossified anterior longitudinal ligament.[22] Subsequently, many authors advocated multilevel SPOs for kyphosis correction, and this is considered to be a relatively safe procedure with a reduction in operative time, blood loss, and neurological complications compared to other osteotomies.[1] Ponte described a more extensive procedure for surgical correction and instrumentation of Scheuermann's kyphosis.[1] The surgical indication and extent of the osteotomy is in fact the main difference between an SPO and a Ponte osteotomy, as well as that the Ponte osteotomy is considered to be performed polysegmentally. Although Ponte's description of a multilevel posterior column wedge-shaped osteotomy probably represents the current practice more accurately, the names are sometimes interchangeable. The Smith–Petersen osteotomy qualifies as a Schwab type 1 procedure, however, whereas the true Ponte osteotomy is a type 2 procedure according to Schwab. Both SPOs and the true Ponte osteotomy relies on an anterior mobile disk space and is performed by resecting performed by resecting the spinous process and supraspinous ligaments, parts of the lamina, the interspinous ligaments, the ligamentum flavum, and the facet joints. This will expose the foramen, allowing removal of any soft tissue that may hamper nerve roots when closing the osteotomy site. By asymmetrically performing and closing the osteotomy one can achieve correction in both the sagittal and the coronal plane. Although not developed for this, these procedures can also allow for lengthening the posterior elements to re-create kyphosis.

Type I sagittal deformities, characterized by a local segmental imbalance, in contrast to the more global type II sagittal deformities, are usually a good indication for these type of osteotomies, as well as for performing these osteotomies around the apex of a coronal curve, mainly thoracic. One degree of correction can be achieved per millimeter of bone resected. Usually this yields around 10 degrees of correction per level.[1] These osteotomies are thus mainly used for cases that are relatively mobile. The majority fuse without the need for anterior grafting or reconstruction, except if the amount of posterior shortening leads to excessive anterior disk opening, necessitating additional anterior grafting.

9.7.2 Pedicle Subtraction Osteotomy

Initially, pedicle subtraction osteotomies (PSOs) were used for fixed sagittal imbalance or kyphotic deformities; however, as is the case with the previous osteotomies, its indications have continued to widen since its original description by Scudese in 1963. They now include coronal deformities as well as primary and revision surgeries.[1] PSOs, a type 3 osteotomy according to Schwab, are surgically more challenging than the type 1 and 2 osteotomies, but they surpass their limitation because no anterior lengthening may occur, stretching the cauda equina and vascular structures. PSOs can achieve bigger corrections by performing a transpedicular wedge (V-shaped) osteotomy through all three columns of the spine, resecting the posterior elements and both pedicles, down to the anterior aspect of the vertebral body, closing the osteotomy by hinging it on the anterior cortex. Before the osteotomy is performed, pedicle screws are placed in the adjacent levels, and temporary rods should be used to stabilize the spine, especially in the thoracic area. Subsequently, the posterior elements are removed from pedicles above and below the planned PSO level. The medial wall of the pedicle should initially be preserved to act as an internal nerve root protector while the rest of the pedicle is resected together with the body, after removal of the transverse process. Rongeurs, osteotomes, curets, and a high-speed bur can be used to remove the bone of the vertebral body to the anterior cortex, which should be preserved to act as a hinge and prevent translation during closure. The osteotomy line should be well planned and executed to avoid translation. The posterior wall of the canal is carefully removed underneath the dura, protecting it and controlling epidural bleeding with bipolar coagulation, bone wax, or hemostatic agents, such as foam or matrix. Lastly, the osteotomy can be closed, which should always start with compression on the rod, shortening the posterior elements, rather than in situ bending, which would lengthen the canal and thus put traction on the neural structures. After closing the osteotomy, dural buckling, nerve root impingement, or subluxation of the spine should be checked both visually and with fluoroscopy. Well placed and solid screws, multiple anchors, temporary rods, and domino connectors may assist in obtaining stable fixation of the osteotomy.

Type II sagittal deformities, especially those with a significant positive sagittal balance (>10 cm), a sharp angular kyphosis, and multilevel circumferential fusions are ideal indications for PSOs.[1] Similarly to Ponte's, coronal imbalance can be corrected at the same time by performing an asymmetrical osteotomy. The amount of possible correction ranges from 25 degrees in the thoracic spine up to 35 degrees in the lumbar spine.[1] Because of the larger pedicles, PSOs in the lumbar spine provide more correction per level than in the thoracic spine.

9.7.3 Bone–Disk–Bone Osteotomy

The bone–disk–bone osteotomy (BDBO) is performed by resecting the disk with its adjacent end plate.[1] The procedure is similar to a PSO but slightly more extensive, which makes it a grade 4 osteotomy according to Schwab. The wedge, including the disk is removed, and the osteotomy is closed bone-to-bone.

This osteotomy type is used in cases where the disk represents the apex of the deformity or in severe sagittal deformities needing a correction exceeding the amount a PSO can yield. Theoretically, a correction varying from 35 to 60 degrees can be achieved.

9.7.4 Vertebral Column Resection

Vertebral column resection (VCR) is an osteotomy technique that was initially described as a combined anterior and posterior procedure in 1922 by McLennan.[1] Suk later introduced a posterior-only approach, the posterior vertebral column resection (PVCR), which has been shown to have at least the same amount of correction and to reduce the pulmonary complication rate and ICU hospitalizations compared to a combined approach.[5,23] It is a very powerful corrective tool that enables shortening of the spinal canal, and thus avoids tension on an already compromised spinal cord. The technique involves complete removal of one or more vertebral segments with the posterior elements, entire vertebral body, and adjacent disks. This is called a grade 5 osteotomy. Often, in the thoracic spine, exposure can be improved by sacrificing one or two roots, but one should be aware that some vascularization of the cord may go along with the root. Special care should be taken in revision cases; it is advisable to use temporary clamping of the root and observe neuromonitoring changes for a few minutes.

First, pedicle screws are placed in the levels above and below the segment to be resected, which are then connected by a contoured unilateral (usually firstly concave) rod without performing any deformity correction. Wide laminectomies and foraminotomies of the level above and below the resection are done to prevent cord and nerve impingement. After removal of the adjacent disks, transverse processes, lateral wall, anterior wall, and posterior wall of the canal, the rod is moved to the other side and tightly locked with slight compression. The same procedure is repeated on the opposite side, and a second rod is placed. Anteriorly a cage filled with local bone and allograft is positioned to prevent excessive shortening of the spine, which would put the dura and spinal cord at risk for injury. Final compression completes the procedure.

PVCR is indicated for rigid, decompensated multiplanar deformities with no or very limited flexibility, sharp angulations, and resection of congenital anomalies (hemivertebrae).[1] Although technically the most demanding among all osteotomy types, with the highest neurologic complication rate and blood loss, it is considered to be a safe and effective procedure if performed by an experienced spine surgeon under close neuromonitoring. Nevertheless the reported rates of overall complications and neurologic complications (subluxation, dural buckling, cord compression due to residual bone or soft tissue) are 8–34% and 2–17%, respectively. A PVCR provides better correction than any other osteotomy without the need for anterior procedures with all their related morbidities. The amount of correction for the sagittal plane ranges from 45 to 72%, and 51 to 69% for coronal deformity.[1,5,23]

9.8 Postoperative Care

Usually these syndromic patients will have to spend some time in an ICU after this type of surgery. Sponseller et al reported an average ICU stay of 6 days in neuromuscular rigid deformity patients, followed by a hospital stay of 14 days.[5] The length of ICU stay or hospitalization did not differ between a rigid scoliosis, kyphosis, or combined deformity. Modi et al reported that 13 of 26 patients with rigid neuromuscular deformities required ICU care for an average of just more than 1 day.[24] Six of them required postoperative ventilation (all had undergone PVCR). The average length of hospitalization was 24 days.

Usually drains are required to prevent postoperative hematoma formation, possibly decreasing the risk of late-onset infection. We give antibiotics (usually cefazolin) for 24 hours in three doses, but this varies among institutions, countries, and continents. Adequate multimodal analgesia, while avoiding the use of morphine as much as possible, is key to a quick recovery and mobilization. We normally apply one or two epidural catheters for pain relief during the first postoperative days, but adequate neurological examination should still be possible.

Once the patient is stabilized, early mobilization is key to preventing complications, such as deep venous thrombosis, pneumonia, wound breakdown, and decubitus ulcers. The use of spinal orthoses depends on the surgeon's preference; in our experience, it is rarely indicated. Furthermore, applying a brace in children with psychomotor retardation can be a challenge. Patients who can understand it are advised to avoid strenuous activities, heavy lifting, and excessive bending and twisting for 4 to 6 months postoperatively. In nonambulatory patients, this is less of a concern.

9.9 Complications

Not surprisingly, spinal osteotomies carry a significant risk of complications. Spinal deformity surgery itself involves blood loss; with the addition of osteotomies the risks increase significantly, especially in the more extensive osteotomies, such as multiple PSOs or VCR.[21]

Sponseller et al reported that 6 of 23 patients (26%) had major complications.[5] Neurological complications, included intraoperative neuromonitoring changes in 3 cases, and none experienced postoperative neurological deficits. Two other patients did have neurological deficits postoperatively; 1 had numbness in the superficial peroneal nerve distribution, likely due to positioning. The other experienced motor and sensory loss of the lower extremities due to screw misplacement. The screw was removed immediately and reinstrumented later. Both patients fully recovered and did not have any permanent deficits.

In some syndromic patients, neuromonitoring can be problematic. It can be argued that in cases of very deficient function in the extremities, monitoring should perhaps not be attempted. Our policy is that in cases where there is any functional motor control, including bowel and bladder function, monitoring is performed. Our team usually succeeds in obtaining useful signals. If, however, no reliable signals can be obtained and neurological function is a concern, traditional wake-up tests can still be used, sometimes multiple times during one procedure.[5] As in all cases, the response to changes in neuromonitoring signals should include optimization of vital parameters, and blood pressure, and mean arterial pressure should be raised, blood loss compensated for, temperature normalized, implant position checked both visually and fluoroscopically, and correction reduced in the hope of a recovery of the signals. If no improvement occurs while all parameters are known to be satisfactory, we administer dexamethasone and the correction procedure is abandoned. If the spine is destabilized, a temporary rod without any correction can be implanted; we have not had any permanent sequelae with this policy. After stabilization of the patient, the procedure can often be resumed without further complications 5 to 7 days later. Neuromonitoring change alerts during three-column osteotomies (PSO or VCR) are known to be more common in neuromuscular or syndromic patients, as shown by Jarvis et al (13 of 21 alerts were in syndromic/neuromuscular cases).[25] Suh et al had only 1 motor evoked potentials (MEP)-change in their 13 neuromuscular patients with rigid curves, which recovered by reversing the correction and later carefully reapplying and instrumenting the spine.[6] Two patients experienced pneumonia (anteroposterior VCR, [AP-VCR]), one pancreatitis (AP-VCR), one deep wound infection (AP-VCR), one pleural effusion requiring tube insertion, and one revision due to a prominent iliac screw. They did not report any infection or pseudarthrosis; however, they describe screw loosening intraoperatively, especially in DMD and SMA patients due to their osteoporosis.[6]

Significant blood loss has been linked inherently to neuromuscular spine surgery as well as to osteotomies. Edler et al reported an almost sevenfold higher risk of losing 50% of their total blood volume (TBV) compared to other types of scoliosis.[26] Sponseller et al reported a significant blood loss in 23 neuromuscular patients, with a mean estimated blood loss (EBL) of 1,785 mL (range 250–6,000 mL). The mean percent EBL per TBV was 76%, with seven cases having >100% EBL per TBV.[5] There was a significant association with the magnitude of coronal and sagittal correction, as well as body weight, but not with the VCR approach type. Suh et al reported an average blood loss of 3,356 mL in their 13 patients,[6] which is less than that reported by Modi et al.[24] They reported an average EBL of 4,535 mL in their seven PVCR patients compared to 2,123 mL for non-PVCR patients diagnosed with various neuromuscular disorders. An increased EBL has been reported, specifically in MFS, Rett syndrome, CP, and DMD.[10] If the blood loss appears to be greater than estimated before destabilizing the spine, a two-staged procedure, if necessary with the use of temporary rods, may be considered.[5]

Other complications of posterior-based osteotomies include the following:

- Stretching of the cauda equina and vascular complications, which could theoretically result in rupture of the aorta or vena cava inferior due to anterior lengthening.[2] The aim of these procedures should, however, be posterior shortening.
- Intraspinal hematoma.
- Pseudarthrosis.
- Infection.
- Pneumonia, pulmonary embolus.
- Intestinal obstruction due to prolonged inactivity and medication.

9.10 Outcome

Sponseller et al reported a multicenter outcome of VCR in 23 consecutive neuromuscular patients (mean age 15.4 years) with a severe rigid deformity due to different diagnoses (CP, Rett syndrome, myelomeningocele, myopathy, etc.).[5] They classified the deformity in three groups: (1) severe scoliosis, (2) severe kyphosis, and (3) kyphoscoliosis. Of the 16 primary and 7 revision surgeries, 20 were performed using a posterior-only approach, and 3 with a combined anterior–posterior one. They reported a mean coronal, sagittal respectively pelvic obliquity correction per deformity group: 66%, 45%, 67% (group 1); 51%, 54%, 60% (group 2); and 55%, 57%, and 46% (group 3). There was no difference in correction magnitude between the combined anterior-posterior or posterior-only approaches.[5] Suh et al reported similar percentages of coronal and sagittal correction.[6] Modi et al showed similar correction rates of rigid curves > 90 degrees in 7 patients with CP, SMA, and DMD.[24]

9.11 Conclusion

Surgical treatment of rigid spinal deformities is challenging, and more so in syndromic patients. The indication for surgery may also differ from other forms of scoliosis: Besides restoring spinopelvic balance, especially in standing, ambulatory patients, improving sitting balance and pelvic obliquity is a major goal in the majority of syndromic patients with rigid spine deformities. Posterior-based osteotomies are widely used to achieve major correction. Their use, however, comes with an increased risk of complications in an already compromised population. Therefore, a thorough preoperative discussion with the patient and the family; a detailed, multidisciplinary preoperative assessment, a meticulous surgical technique, and proper postoperative care are all essential to achieving the desired result.

References

[1] Enercan M, Ozturk C, Kahraman S, Sarıer M, Hamzaoglu A, Alanay A. Osteotomies/spinal column resections in adult deformity. Eur Spine J. 2013; 22 Suppl 2:S254–S264

[2] Gupta MC, Kebaish K, Blondel B, Klineberg E. Spinal osteotomies for rigid deformities. Neurosurg Clin N Am. 2013; 24(2):203–211

[3] Somoskeöy S, Tunyogi-Csapó M, Bogyó C, Illés T. Accuracy and reliability of coronal and sagittal spinal curvature data based on patient-specific three-dimensional models created by the EOS 2D/3D imaging system. Spine J. 2012; 12(11):1052–1059

[4] Bridwell KH. Decision making regarding Smith-Petersen vs. pedicle subtraction osteotomy vs. vertebral column resection for spinal deformity. Spine. 2006; 31(19) Suppl:S171–S178

[5] Sponseller PD, Jain A, Lenke LG, et al. Vertebral column resection in children with neuromuscular spine deformity. Spine. 2012; 37(11):E655–E661

[6] Suh SW, Modi HN, Yang J, Song HR, Jang KM. Posterior multilevel vertebral osteotomy for correction of severe and rigid neuromuscular scoliosis: a preliminary study. Spine. 2009; 34(12):1315–1320

[7] Jones KB, Erkula G, Sponseller PD, Dormans JP. Spine deformity correction in Marfan syndrome. Spine. 2002; 27(18):2003–2012

[8] Gjolaj JP, Sponseller PD, Shah SA, et al. Spinal deformity correction in Marfan syndrome versus adolescent idiopathic scoliosis: learning from the differences. Spine. 2012; 37(18):1558–1565

[9] Gabos PG, Inan M, Thacker M, Borkhu B. Spinal fusion for scoliosis in Rett syndrome with an emphasis on early postoperative complications. Spine. 2012; 37(2):E90–E94

[10] Mehta SS, Modi HN, Srinivasalu S, et al. Pedicle screw-only constructs with lumbar or pelvic fixation for spinal stabilization in patients with Duchenne muscular dystrophy. J Spinal Disord Tech. 2009; 22(6):428–433

[11] Fujak A, Raab W, Schuh A, Kreß A, Forst R, Forst J. Operative treatment of scoliosis in proximal spinal muscular atrophy: results of 41 patients. Arch Orthop Trauma Surg. 2012; 132(12):1697–1706

[12] Chng SY, Wong YQ, Hui JH, Wong HK, Ong HT, Goh DY. Pulmonary function and scoliosis in children with spinal muscular atrophy types II and III. J Paediatr Child Health. 2003; 39(9):673–676

[13] Hasler CC. Operative treatment for spinal deformities in cerebral palsy. J Child Orthop. 2013; 7(5):419–423

[14] Colo D, Kruyt MC, Timmers-Raaijmaakers BC, Castelein RM. Scoliosis in children with chromosome 22q11.2 deletion syndrome [in Dutch]. Ned Tijdschr Geneeskd. 2012; 156(4):A4298

[15] Bassett AS, Chow EW, Husted J, et al. Clinical features of 78 adults with 22q11 Deletion Syndrome. Am J Med Genet A. 2005; 138(4):307–313

[16] Tsirikos AI, Khan LA, McMaster MJ. Spinal deformity in patients with DiGeorge syndrome. J Spinal Disord Tech. 2010; 23(3):208–214

[17] van der Linden MH, Kruyt MC, Sakkers RJ, de Koning TJ, Oner FC, Castelein RM. Orthopaedic management of Hurler's disease after hematopoietic stem cell transplantation: a systematic review. J Inherit Metab Dis. 2011; 34 (3):657–669

[18] Schwab F, Blondel B, Chay E, et al. The Comprehensive Anatomical Spinal Osteotomy Classification. Neurosurgery. 2013

[19] Mills B, Bach JR, Zhao C, Saporito L, Sabharwal S. Posterior spinal fusion in children with flaccid neuromuscular scoliosis: the role of noninvasive positive pressure ventilatory support. J Pediatr Orthop. 2013; 33(5):488–493

[20] Lemans JVC, Öner FC, Wijdicks SPJ, Ekkelenkamp MB, Vogely HC, Kruyt MC. The efficacy of intrawound vancomycin powder and povidone-iodine irrigation to prevent surgical site infections in complex instrumented spine surgery. Spine J. 2019;19(10):1648–1656.

[21] Diab MG, Franzone JM, Vitale MG. The role of posterior spinal osteotomies in pediatric spinal deformity surgery: indications and operative technique. J Pediatr Orthop. 2011; 31(1) Suppl:S88–S98

[22] Smith-Petersen MN, Larson CB, Aufranc OE. Osteotomy of the spine for correction of flexion deformity in rheumatoid arthritis. Clin Orthop Relat Res. 1969; 66(66):6–9

[23] Suk SI, Kim JH, Kim WJ, Lee SM, Chung ER, Nah KH. Posterior vertebral column resection for severe spinal deformities. Spine. 2002; 27(21):2374–2382

[24] Modi HN, Suh SW, Hong JY, Yang JH. Posterior multilevel vertebral osteotomy for severe and rigid idiopathic and nonidiopathic kyphoscoliosis: a further experience with minimum two-year follow-up. Spine. 2011; 36(14):1146–1153

[25] Jarvis JG, Strantzas S, Lipkus M, et al. Responding to neuromonitoring changes in 3-column posterior spinal osteotomies for rigid pediatric spinal deformities. Spine. 2013; 38(8):E493–E503

[26] Edler A, Murray DJ, Forbes RB. Blood loss during posterior spinal fusion surgery in patients with neuromuscular disease: is there an increased risk? Paediatr Anaesth. 2003; 13(9):818–822

10 Rigid Spine Deformities in Early-Onset Scoliosis

Pooria Hosseini, Behrooz A. Akbarnia

Abstract

Early-onset scoliosis (EOS) treatment in general is a challenge; the rigid pediatric deformity treatment is even more challenging. Lack of a clear definition of rigid spine in EOS adds to the complexity of stiff curve management in the pediatric population. Most authors rather borrow the definition of rigid curves in adolescent idiopathic scoliosis (AIS) and apply it to EOS patients. Consequently, there is a paucity of data on the management of rigid curve in EOS. This chapter discusses currently available management options for rigid spine. Treatment options ranging from nonoperative to operative managements with or without spinal fusion, anterior release, and growth-friendly techniques, including distraction-based, compression-based, and growth-guided options, are discussed in this chapter. Furthermore, this chapter discusses the procedures that are not normally used for the treatment of a simple EOS, but are usually required in the management of rigid cases. Extra measures can include preoperative halo-gravity traction, surgical release of soft tissues, temporary internal distraction rods (TIDR), and osteotomies. Pediatric rigid curve management is at its early stages of development and multicenter study groups can certainly contribute to its advancement by sharing their experiences with their novel techniques.

Keywords: early-onset scoliosis, stiff curves, temporary distraction, halo-gravity traction, MCGR

10.1 Introduction

Early-onset scoliosis (EOS) is present in the first 10 years of life, whereas adolescent scoliosis is found in those between the ages of 10 and 18. Historically Dickson categorized scoliosis into two groups: (1) EOS for those diagnosed under 5 years, and (2) late-onset scoliosis for those 5 to 10 years of age.[1] Recently a system of comprehensive classification of EOS has been introduced and is shown in ▶ Table 10.1.[2] This classification is based largely on etiology and curve magnitude as well as sagittal alignment. It may be safe to assume that congenital and syndromic scoliosis may be more rigid compared with the two other groups. However, this has yet to be well documented, and if left untreated all categories can become rigid deformities.

Resolution of EOS has been reported in the idiopathic group, but many curves will progress and if left untreated can cause cardiopulmonary complications, which can be fatal. The treatment of progressive spine deformities in very young children has proven to be difficult since these patients are young and have an increased growth velocity. Also, the treatment goals are not only curve correction and maintenance of curve correction (as in adults) but also preserving thorax and pulmonary growth, thereby preventing pulmonary compromise. The rigid curve management will be even more challenging since conventional management options will not be adequate and extra measures may be required.

Spinal rigidity in adolescent idiopathic scoliosis (AIS) is described using various terminology (e. g., rigid, stiff, stuck, fixed curve) in the literature. Luk et al[3] refer to flexibility of less than 50% on the fulcrum bending radiograph as a stiff spine, and those with more than 50% flexibility are labeled as flexible. Dobbs et al[4] define rigidity as a more than 70- to 80-degree residual side-bending curve. Arlet et al[5] define rigidity as side-bending films with a Cobb angle >65 degrees. Suk et al[6] consider spine flexibility of <25 degrees to be rigid, whereas Bullmann et al[7] accept flexibility of less than 30 degrees as rigid.

In addition, to the best of our knowledge, there is no consensus as to a definition for rigid spine in the EOS population, and all authors have used AIS rigid spine criteria for younger patients. Extending adult flexibility criteria to children is a questionable approach given that children naturally have a more flexible skeletal system. The authors believe that different criteria should be used for the pediatric rigid spine and that more research is required to define spinal rigidity, as well as its clinical significance and outcomes, in this specific population.

There is a paucity of data on the management of rigid spine in EOS. This chapter discusses some available options for management of rigid EOS.

10.2 Clinical and Radiographic Evaluation

10.2.1 History and Physical Examination

A thorough history and physical examination are mandatory initial steps. Curve flexibility can be assessed clinically by placing the child in a lateral position over the knee of the examiner, or the edge of the examining table, or by suspending the infant

Table 10.1 Early-onset scoliosis classification

Etiology	Cobb angle (major curve)	Maximum total kyphosis	Progression modifier (optional)
Congenital/structural	1: <20 degrees	(−): <20 degrees	P0: <10 degrees/y
Low-tone NM	2: 21–50 degrees	N: 21–50 degrees	P1: 10–20 degrees/y
High-tone NM	3: 51–90 degrees	(+): >50 degrees	P2: >20 degrees/y
Syndromic	4: >90 degrees		
Idiopathic			

Abbreviation: NM, neuromuscular.

under the arm by the examiner. A thorough examination of the head, pelvis, and lower extremities in rigid spine is the same as that for flexible EOS.[8]

10.2.2 Plain Radiographs

All patients should be evaluated with standing posteroanterior and lateral 14- by 36-inch radiographs covering the cervical spine to the femoral head and the iliac crest, which is helpful in estimation of skeletal maturity by Risser stages and triradiate cartilage as well as measurements of sagittal alignment and pelvic parameters.[9] It is of paramount importance that the patients do not use compensatory mechanisms, including unilateral or bilateral knee flexion, hyperextension of the cervical spine, and retroversion of the pelvis, during weight-bearing radiographs. In children who are too young to stand, supine radiographs are acceptable.[10] Rib vertebral angle difference (RVAD), which was first defined by Mehta in 1972, is used to predict the progression or resolution of the curve in the idiopathic group. An RVAD of <20 degrees indicates a curve that is likely to resolve, whereas angles of >21 degrees usually progress.[11]

Coronal spine left and right bending films, traction, or push prone images are used to assess coronal curve flexibility. Lateral hyperextension radiographs can be used to assess sagittal flexibility over a bolster in a young patient. Buchowski et al[12,13] recommended that traction radiographs taken in the side-bending, prone, hyperextension, and, in particular, supine position could be very helpful. It is suggested that if a large curve corrects by more than 50% on traction films, halo-gravity traction or temporary internal distraction rods (TIDRs) is unlikely to be necessary. Preoperative halo traction is more commonly used in the pediatric population both to evaluate how stiff a deformity is and to gain small increments of correction in a safe and gradual manner. In 1997, Cheung et al introduced fulcrum-bending radiographs for predicting the flexibility of thoracic adult idiopathic scoliosis, and in 2010 they extended the same technique to the cases that had pedicle screw fixation.[14] To achieve maximal preoperative correction, thoracic fulcrum-bending radiographs should be obtained for the main thoracic curves. However, side-bending views should still be used for both upper thoracic and thoracolumbar/lumbar curves.[15]

Bear in mind that unnecessary radiation should be avoided in EOS patients, and it is logical to wait 6 months between obtaining X-rays[12,13] or to consider using an EOS imaging system.

10.2.3 EOS Imaging System/Three-Dimensional Modeling Techniques

The EOS imaging system has been available since 2007.[16] It can produce high-quality images with less radiation than standard imaging techniques by adopting slot-scanning technology.[17] The EOS system also allows 3D spinal reconstructions in a functional standing position with reduced radiation, which is a certain advantage of this imaging system.[16] It allows physicians to observe the spinal distortions in 3D view, and thereby determine the best surgical procedures. However, given the cost, these modern technologies are not yet in common practice and not available in all centers. Some authors have questioned the cost-effectiveness of this technique at a national level.[17]

10.2.4 CT Scan

In addition to radiographs, thin-cut CT scans with sagittal reconstruction are very valuable in accurately identifying ankylosed regions of the spine. Based on the findings of a thin-cut CT scan, we can predict that patients with anterior column fusion are highly unlikely to benefit from multiple Smith–Petersen osteotomies (SPOs), making pedicle subtraction osteotomy (PSO) a better option in these cases. It is clear that a proper preoperative imaging study can change the entire treatment plan.

10.2.5 MRI

MRI has become the standard of care in evaluation of progressive spinal deformities in growing children. It has replaced more invasive and less accurate techniques, such as myelography and CT myelography in diagnosing intraspinal pathologies (e. g., syrinx, tethered cord, and tumor). In addition, progressive curves of more than 20 degrees may require MRI to assess for occult lesions of the central nervous system. In idiopathic EOS patients with a Cobb angle >20 degrees, even with a normal physical examination, a total spine MRI scan is indicated due to the high incidence of neural axis abnormalities.[18]

10.3 Treatment of Rigid Spine Deformities in EOS

If cases of progressive EOS are left untreated, the patients will face life-threatening cardiopulmonary complications. Less rigid curves can be managed nonoperatively or if progressive, by growth friendly techniques and simple distraction and correction by bringing the spine to an appropriately contoured rod and spine-based or rib-based foundation using pedicle screws or hooks as anchors. Patients with more rigid deformities, by contrast, frequently need additional preoperative or intraoperative techniques to achieve the desired correction, or they may need a growth friendly technique combined with a resection/fusion technique to achieve the desired correction. In these patients, the rigid curve can be transformed into a flexible curve by using apical osteotomies (i. e., SPO, PSO, or vertebral column resection [VCR]) followed by a growth-friendly distraction-based surgery to achieve the desired correction and spinal growth.

In this section, we examine the available techniques for the treatment of EOS and discuss whether they are applicable to the treatment of rigid spine deformities. In addition, we discuss the procedures that are not normally used for the treatment of a simple EOS but are usually required in the management of rigid cases.

10.3.1 Nonoperative Treatments

The treatment plan for children with EOS is based on the possibility or proof of curve progression. Active treatment should be initiated when curve progression is >10 degrees.

For example, idiopathic EOS curves with a Cobb angle between 20 and 35 degrees and an RVAD of >20 degrees are

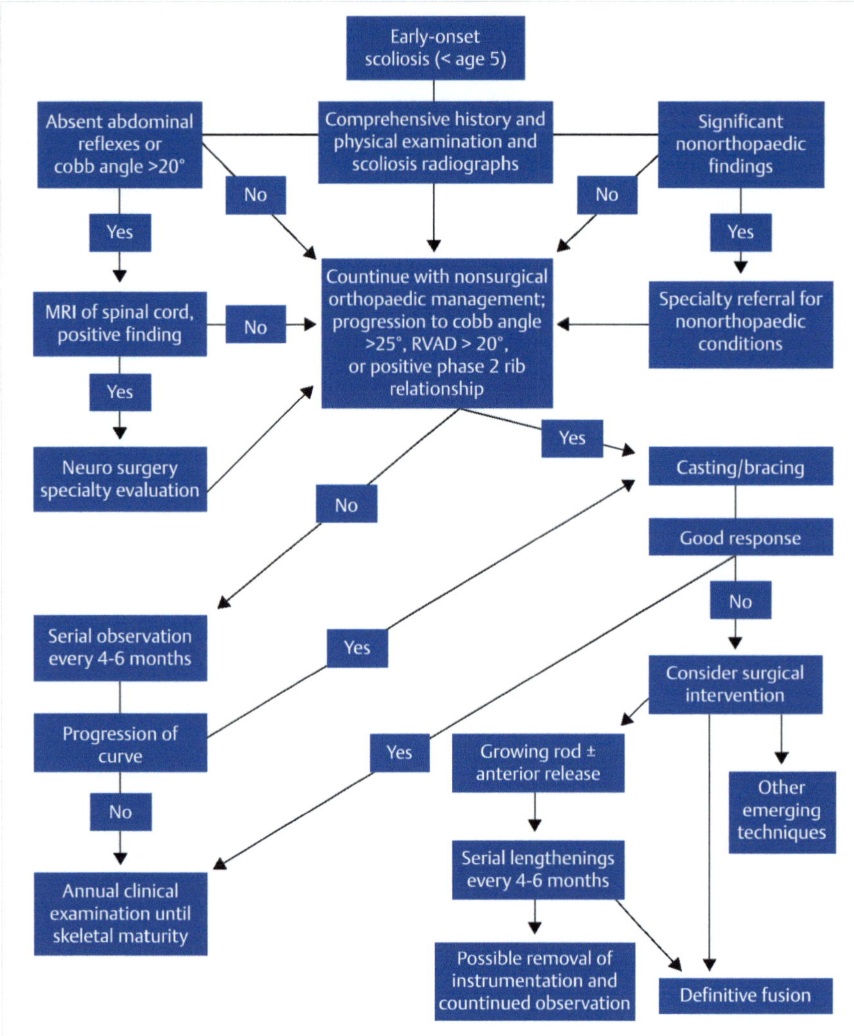

Fig. 10.1 Treatment algorithm for idiopathic early-onset scoliosis. Adapted from Gillingham BL, Fan RA, Akbarnia BA. Early onset idiopathic scoliosis. J Am Acad Orthop Surg.[19]

highly likely to progress. They should be observed every 4 to 6 months, and if any progression is seen active treatment should be initiated. The comprehensive treatment plan for idiopathic EOS is shown in ▶ Fig. 10.1.[19]

Casting and Bracing

Serial casting in EOS can result in improved curve correction in young patients with curves <60 degrees. Casting in larger curves and in older patients can still improve the deformity and delay the timing of definitive surgery. However, we should bear in mind that the nonoperative treatment should not compromise the patient's cardiopulmonary function.

If casting is the treatment option, it usually begins with application of a molded body cast under general anesthesia. The cast should be changed every 6 to 12 weeks until maximum correction is achieved followed by intermittent bracing until there is no further evidence of progression.

Although casting or bracing may seem to be harmless forms of treatment, skin breakdown can be problematic to the point of discontinuing care in severe cases. Another complication that may limit cast application is its effects on the growth of the thorax and its contents.

10.3.2 Operative Treatments

Operative managements are considered when bracing and casting are not indicated or fail to arrest curve progression. The type of operative management is highly dependent on the patient's diagnosis and age, the severity of the deformity, and flexibility of the curve.

Options for surgical treatment are definitive spinal fusion with or without excision and nonfusion or growth-friendly techniques. The growth-friendly techniques can be classified into three subgroups[20] (▶ Table 10.2):

1. Distraction-based techniques, for example growing rods (GRs), magnetically controlled growing rods (MCGRs), and vertical expandable prosthetic titanium ribs (VEPTRs).
2. Compression-based techniques, such as vertebral staples and tethers. (Note: These techniques are not commonly used for the treatment of rigid spines. They can be helpful in older children with mild curves but certainly are not an option in very young children with rigid curves, so we will not cover them in this chapter.)
3. Growth-guided techniques, such as hemiepiphysiodesis, Shilla, and Luque trolley.

Spinal Fusion with or without Bony Excision

In rapidly growing children with both flexible and rigid EOS, an isolated posterior spinal fusion is not a good option due to the possibility of the crankshaft phenomenon. Even adding an anterior fusion will not improve the results, since it stops the patient's spinal growth. Spinal fusion is commonly used as the definitive treatment in patients whose thorax and pulmonary growth is no longer of concern. However, in some cases with a progressive neurologic deficit with associated cord compression and concerns of paralysis, the surgeon has no other option than early spinal fusion/resection to prevent increasing neurologic deficit (▶ Fig. 10.2a–h).

Table 10.2 Growth-friendly spinal implants classification

Classification of growth friendly spinal implants		
Type	**Mechanism of action**	**Example**
1. Distraction-based systems	Correct spinal deformities by mechanically applying a distractive force across a deformed segment with anchors at the top and bottom of the implants, which commonly attach to the spine, rib, and/or pelvis	• Spine-based or rib-based growing rods • Vertical expandable titanium rib prosthesis • Remotely expandable devices
2. Compression-based systems	Correct spinal deformities with a compressive force applied to the convexity of the curve, causing convex growth inhibition	• Vertebral staples • Tethers
3. Growth-guided systems	Correct spinal deformity by anchoring multiple vertebrae (usually including the apical vertebrae) to rods with mechanical forces, including translation at the time of the initial implant. The majority of the anchors are not rigidly attached to the rods, thus permitting longitudinal growth over time as the anchors slide over the rods	• Luque trolley • Shilla

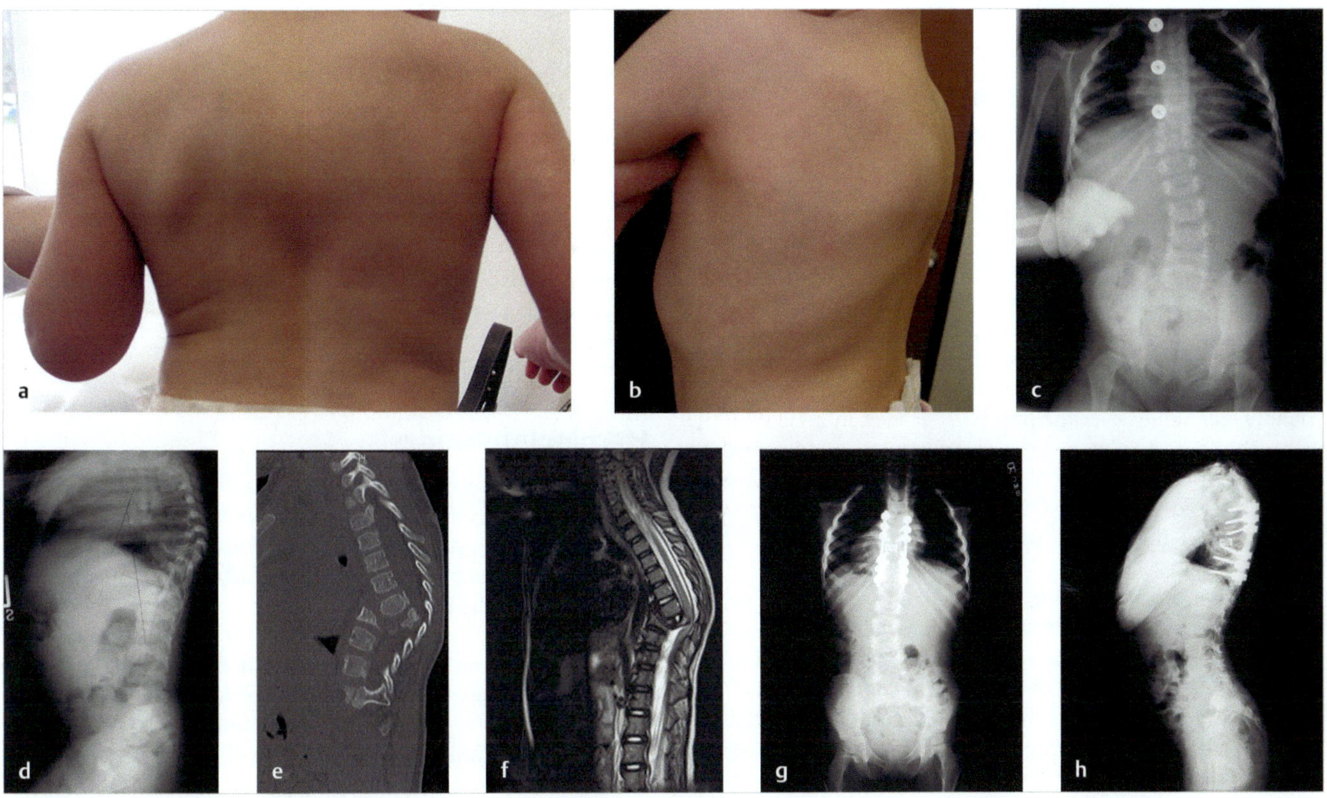

Fig. 10.2 (a, b) Posterior standing and lateral clinical photograph of a 2-year-old boy diagnosed with congenital rigid scoliosis and kyphosis. **(c–f)** Posteroanterior (PA) and lateral weight-bearing plain radiograph, CT scan, and MRI of the same patient showing an absent T 8–T 9 vertebral body and congenital dislocation of T 7 on T 10. Kyphosis increased from 25 to 40 degrees over 3 months, and neurologic function in the lower extremities deteriorated. Given the progressive neurologic deficit due to cord compression and concerns of paralysis, a definitive fusion through anterior approach with decompression of the spinal cord and fusion followed by posterior fusion and instrumentation was performed with successful results in terms of both curve correction and improvement of symptoms. **(g, h)** Last follow-up PA and lateral plain radiographs. In this case, the author modified the treatment plan based on the patient's needs and fused the spine (although short segments) at a very young age to prevent paralysis.

Spinal Fusion and Posterior Instrumentation with and without Anterior Release

Many severe deformities that were formerly treated in a staged anterior–posterior manner may now be corrected through a single-stage posterior-only approach.

Arlet et al[5] and Dobbs et al[4] similarly showed that the level of correction of rigid thoracic curves in the frontal plane using modern posterior instrumentation alone is similar to using combined approaches in adult idiopathic scoliosis. Their studies show that anterior release is not necessary for scoliosis of 70 to 90 degrees. Anterior release may be considered in curves >90 degrees or bending not <65 degrees (stiff).

Anterior release can only achieve 5.5-degree correction in each segment. Thus it should be done only in hyperkyphosis cases like Scheuermann kyphosis, coronal imbalance, or severe curves.[21] Having said that, this technique still has its advocates who feel that anterior release helps the correction of rigid curves. Cheung et al[14] showed an increase in fulcrum bending flexibility of 15 degrees (from 39 to 54 degrees) by thoracoscopic anterior spinal release in thoracic curves. They concluded that anterior release effectively improves the spinal flexibility. Similarly, Ruf advocates the anterior release technique, which addresses the imbalance of anterior and posterior spinal column length in AIS.[22] In addition, it can improve the results of posterior instrumentation and fusion in cases of marked rigidity and hypokyphosis.

Posterior Instrumentation without Fusion (Growing-Rod Instrumentation)

Harrington initially reported this technique in 1962 for the treatment of scoliosis. He proposed "progressive scoliosis in a child less than ten years old can be managed with the apparatus alone without fusion, whereas in a child more than ten years old fusion should usually be done at the time of initial correction."[23] Many pioneering surgeons, including Marchetti and Faldini,[24] Luque and Cardosa,[25] Pratt et al,[26] Mardjetko et al,[27] Klemme et al,[28] and Blakemore et al,[29] modified the growth-friendly techniques over the past five decades. In 2005 with the use of basic principles of Isola instrumentation described by Asher and dual rods described by McCarthy, Akbarnia et al developed and popularized the currently used dual growing rod technique that can be used submuscularly or subcutaneously[30] (▸ Fig. 10.3a–m).

If the goal of the growing rods, which is correction and/or maintenance of the deformity while allowing spinal growth, is not achievable, growing rods should be avoided. These include very rigid curves, older children with minimal remaining growth, and those in whom correction cannot be achieved (patients who are too young or those with very soft bones). Although there may be ways to increase flexibility in rigid cases and enhance bone quality in very soft bone, the procedure may still be very complex and require an expert surgeon.[10] Dual growing rods may not be an option when there is no further growth potential, or in patients with thoracic insufficiency syndrome and chest wall problems. In addition, the presence of kyphosis should raise a red flag for an undesirable outcome.

Magnetically Controlled Growing Rod

This novel technique is designed to gradually and noninvasively increase the length of growing rods in awake patients to prevent the risks of repeated surgeries and anesthesia and the possibility of neurologic complications. However, MCGRs can also be used as a means of temporary distraction before the definitive surgery. Prior to this novel technique, halo-gravity traction and TIDRs were in common practice to prevent complications. Cheung et al[31] reported the correction of kyphoscoliosis in a 12-year-old child who also had syringomyelia and Arnold–Chiari malformation, over a 2.5-month period without repeated operations and without neurologic complications by daily distraction of the MCGR in the ward.

TIDR can be an alternative to traction, but it still requires multiple operations and, in addition, it may lead to changes in motor evoked potential. In contrast MCGR can be performed even on an outpatient basis without the need for repeated surgeries, while the patient is fully awake and the neurologic status can be dynamically monitored. In addition, the outpatient lengthening procedure applies an external magnet, which is a noninvasive technique.

Retraction of the device is also possible if the patient feels any discomfort during the lengthening procedure.

Vertical Expandable Prosthetic Titanium Rib

VEPTR is a nonfusion technique that is applied mainly in patients with thoracic insufficiency syndrome (TIS) and fused ribs.[32] Astur et al[33] published the most recent report on the efficacy of VEPTR in the treatment of EOS in patients with arthrogryposis, which was the first study to characterize the use of VEPTR in treating scoliosis in children with arthrogryposis. Based on the results of 11 cases treated with VEPTR for EOS between 2006 and 2011, Qiu et al[34] claimed that the "VEPTR technique proves to be an effective way of preventing curve progression in early-onset scoliosis patients. Yet, indications for such a technique need to be strictly selected because of the relatively high complication rate."

Hemiepiphysiodesis

Hemiepiphysiodesis is based on the concept of convex growth retardation and continues to have supporters. It can be performed anteriorly and posteriorly. In 2003, Betz et al[35] reported the use of staples placed thoracoscopically in patients with AIS. This technique avoids fusion and thereby preserves the potential for future growth. However, this technique has not been attempted on any young patient with EOS. In addition, it is reported that the anterior and posterior hemiepiphysiodesis in patients with iatrogenic posterior element deficiency is a safe and efficient technique, particularly if it is combined with posterior pedicle screw instrumentation.[36]

Luque Trolley

Initially in 1977, Luque and Cardosa described the technique of fusionless treatment with segmental spinal instrumentation. Five years later, in 1982, Luque modified this technique and

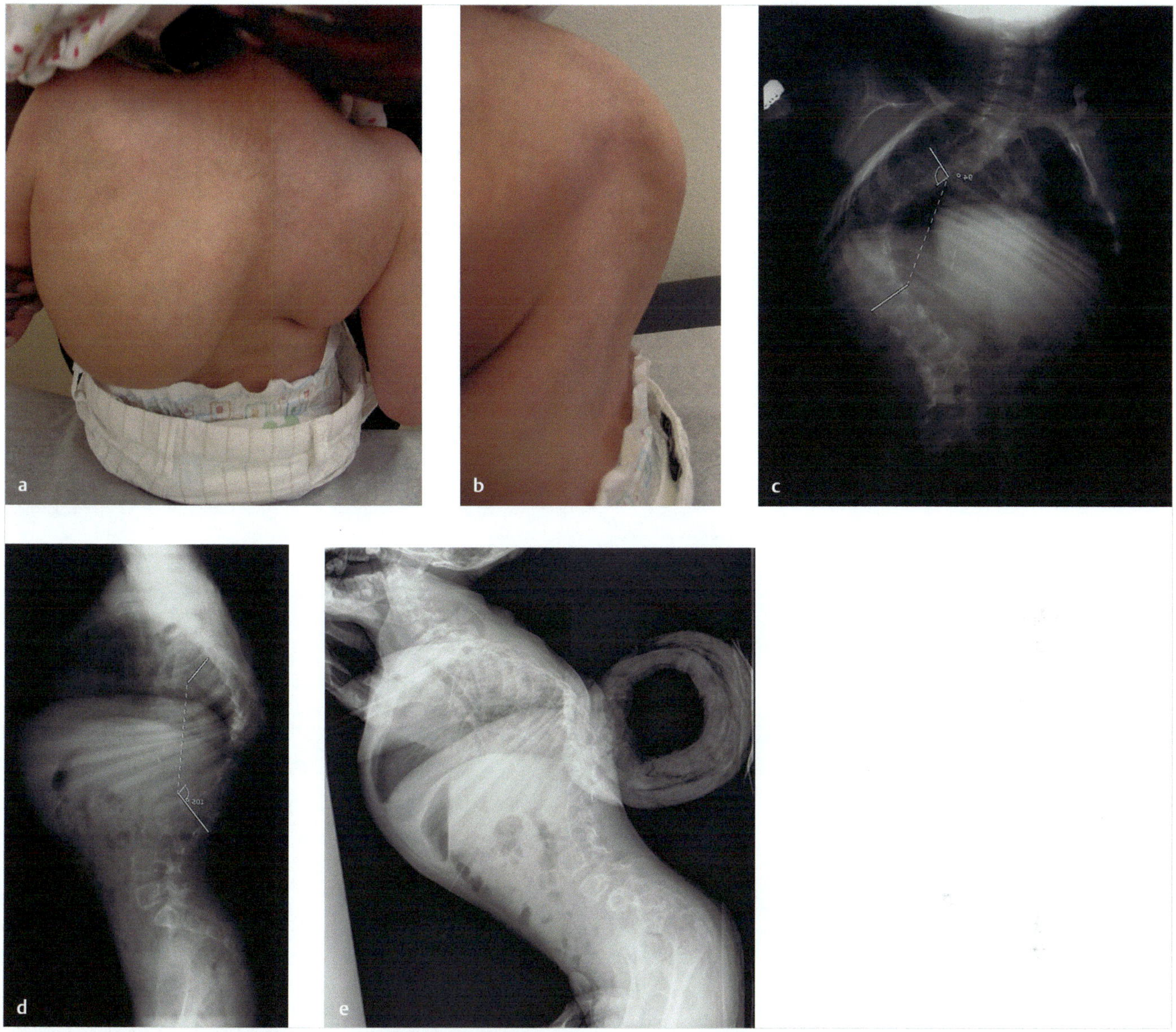

Fig. 10.3 (a, b) Posterior and lateral clinical image of a 7-year-old girl diagnosed with severe syndromic kyphoscoliosis. The patient had a past medical history of pyruvate dehydrogenase deficiency, normal pressure hydrocephalus, severe global developmental delays, bilateral hip dysplasia, renal insufficiency, and history of adrenal tumor, which was surgically removed. At the age of 6 she was noted to have a 70-degree scoliotic curve that had increased from approximately 40 degrees over the past 2 years. At the time of her visit to our clinic, the curve was 95 degrees. (c, d) Posteroanterior (PA) and lateral preoperative plain radiographs. (e) Preoperative radiograph assessing spine flexibility.

(Continued)

added sublaminar wires and replaced the Harrington rods with L-shaped rods. Later these rods were known as the Luque trolley.[37] However, this system became less popular after reports of scar tissue formation and weakening of the lamina, which made revision and final definitive fusion very difficult. Most recently, others have introduced new techniques using the Luque trolley but have not yet proven to be effective in rigid curves.

Shilla System

The precursor to the Shilla system was the Luque trolley, which did not provide reliable spinal growth or curve correction.[37] In the Shilla procedure, usually the multiplanar correction is obtained by pedicle fixation at the apex, which normally involves fusion of three to four segments. Then the Shilla gliding pedicle screws are placed at each end of the construct without subperiosteal exposure. The rods are left long at each end to allow gliding through screws by growth. Patients need to be in an orthosis for 3 months after the surgery.

In addition to the aforementioned procedures, a surgeon might need to consider extra measures to address rigid curves successfully. These extra measures differ based on the type of deformity. ▸ Table 10.3 presents these extra procedures in three groups. The explanation of each procedure follows here unless the procedure has already been covered earlier in the chapter.

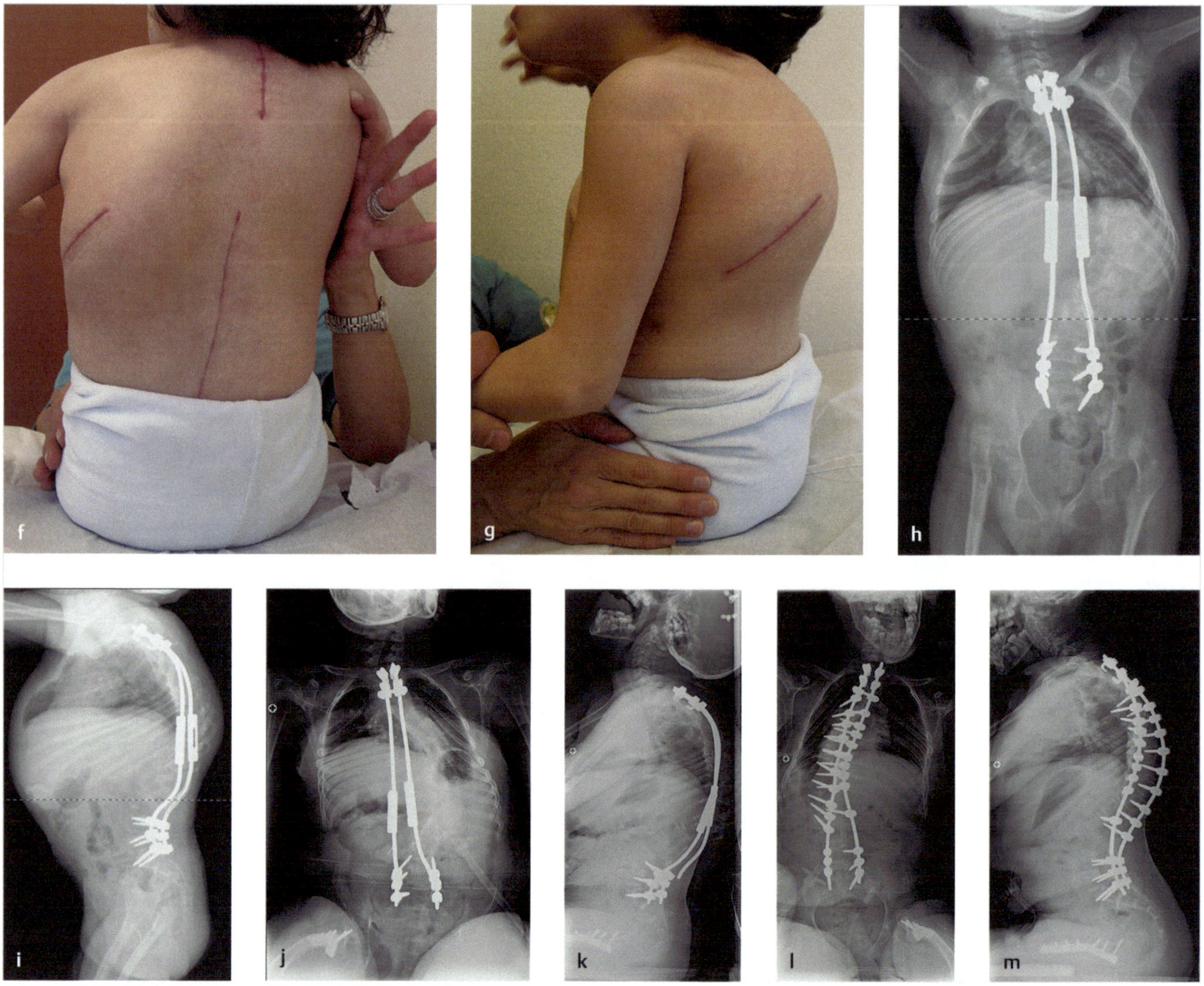

Fig. 10.3 (*Continued*) **(f–i)** Post-index surgery (multiple anterior annulotomies from T 5 to T 12, placement of growing rods from T 2 to S 1) clinical and plain radiographs. **(j, k)** PA and lateral plain radiographs before final fusion. The patient underwent five lengthening operations over 5 years and finally had the definitive spinal fusion operation in 2013. **(l, m)** The latest follow-up PA and lateral plain radiographs after definitive spinal fusion.

10.4 Extra Procedures Considered in the Treatment of Rigid Curves

10.4.1 Traction

The usual strategy for addressing severe rigid deformities includes halo-traction devices, mostly halo-gravity, to gradually lengthen the spine before definitive fusion surgery at a later time. Rapid correction of severe spinal curves increases the risk of neurologic complications. In addition, any patient with a history of intraspinal pathology, rigid kyphosis, or previous spinal surgery can be at increased risk of neurologic deficits after spinal stabilization. Halo-gravity traction, which was popularized by DeWald and Ray,[38] followed by Stagnara,[39] provides a safe and well-tolerated method of gradual and sustained traction to maximize postoperative correction in this difficult group of patients. If the traction is increased gradually to a maximum of 50% of the patient's body weight and daily neurological examinations are performed, the rate of complications decreases significantly.[40]

However, traction requires the patient to stay in the hospital for the duration of treatment. In addition, the use of bulky devices may not be pleasant for these patients. For these reasons some surgeons, including Skaggs and Cheung, have suggested newer techniques, such as TIDRs and MCGRs, respectively, which will be explained later in this chapter.[31]

Indications

The most common indication for preoperative halo traction is in a pediatric patient with a severe and stiff deformity and in whom we are considering a VCR. In these circumstances, halo traction provides a better assessment of spinal rigidity compared with plain imaging or physical examination.

Table 10.3 Extra procedures that might be considered in the treatment of rigid curves

Scoliosis	Kyphosis	Lordosis
1. Distraction techniques ∘ TIDR ∘ MCGR 2. Surgical release and resection (osteotomy) ∘ SPO ∘ VCR[a]	Surgical release and resection (osteotomy) • PSO[b] • VCR[c]	Segmental Pedicle Screw with multilevel posterior release with wide, multilevel SPOs

Abbreviations: MCGR, magnetically controlled growing rod; PSO, pedicle subtraction osteotomy; SPO, Smith–Petersen osteotomy; TIDR, temporary internal distraction rod; VCR, vertebral column resection.
[a]Works better in extremely stiff scoliotic curves.
[b]Works better in the lumbar region
[c]Works better in the thoracic region

Contraindications

Halo traction is contraindicated in cervical instability, kyphosis, or stenosis.[12] The only absolute contraindication to its use would be bone stock in the skull insufficient to gain halo purchase due to underlying diagnoses, such as osteogenesis imperfecta or fibrous dysplasia.

Otherwise, any patient with severe rigid deformity with or without kyphosis, actual or at risk of thoracic insufficiency syndrome, and osteopenia, is a candidate for halo-gravity traction as a primary step before other operative treatments to decrease the neurologic complications and improve respiratory function and suitability for anesthesia.

Other methods of halo traction other than halo-gravity, including halo-femoral and halo-tibial traction, require an extended period of bed rest, which is not tolerated by patients, especially in the pediatric population. Halo-pelvic traction allows patient mobility, but is not popular due to its long-term complications, including infection.

10.4.2 Surgical Release of Soft Tissues

Posterior soft-tissue release in many deformities is adequate to achieve an excellent correction. In curves of 50 to 70 degrees, soft tissue release is all the patients need. This procedure involves resection of the interspinous ligament, ligamentum flavum, and facet capsules. However, soft-tissue release does not necessarily need to be done posteriorly; it can also be achieved using an anterior approach as in multiple diskectomies and nucleotomy.

10.4.3 Temporary Internal Distraction Rod

Halo traction has been used for correcting severe, rigid scoliotic curves, but in cases of contraindications (explained under halo traction section) or due to its complications or prolonged hospital stay intolerance, TIDR, which consists of inserting a distraction rod in stage one of the operation and replacing it with the definitive implants about a week later, is now considered a viable alternative. The same as halo traction indications, rapid surgical correction of large, rigid curves can lead to neurologic injuries, especially if too much correction is attempted in one operation. ▶ Table 10.4 addresses some contraindications for TIDR.

Table 10.4 Contraindications for temporary internal distraction rods

Absolute contraindications	Relative contraindications
• Spinal cord abnormality that precludes deformity correction (e. g., syrinx, tethered cord) • Inability to achieve adequate fixation points to allow distraction • Medical comorbidities or poor nutritional status that make the patient a poor candidate for staged procedures	• Substantial rigid kyphoscoliosis may be considered as a relative contraindication

One of the advantages of TIDR is that it obviates the need for anterior release because correction through posterior resection is generally sufficient. On the other hand, the pitfall of this technique is that the cephalad and caudad fixation points may result in inadequate purchase of the final fixation points.[12]

10.4.4 Osteotomies

We can conclude from ▶ Table 10.3 that osteotomies play a very important roll in bringing flexibility to rigid spine deformities. However, since osteotomies have been covered in detail in other chapters of this book, we will not repeat them.

10.5 Discussion

Despite great advances in both diagnosis and treatment of spine deformities in recent years, rigid spine deformities in EOS have not been well studied. One of the reasons for seeing less than satisfactory outcomes with rigid curves in EOS can be attributed to poor preoperative recognition of the degree of rigidity, and consequently less than optimal surgical planning.

The current available operative and nonoperative treatments have been successful in management of EOS. However, rigid curves still need extra measures to be added to the routine treatment and still may not have successful outcomes as flexible curves. The authors believe that this failure is based on preoperative underestimation of curve rigidity. On the other hand, most surgeons prefer to apply less radical measures to achieve their goals, especially when it comes to the treatment of pediatric patients, even if less desirable outcomes are achieved.

Future studies should be aimed at defining what a rigid curve is in EOS, and what the clinical relevance is for different types of treatments. Multicenter studies in this group of patients are mandatory for finding answers to these questions.

References

[1] Dickson RA. Conservative treatment for idiopathic scoliosis. J Bone Joint Surg Br. 1985; 67(2):176–181

[2] Williams BA, Matsumoto H, McCalla DJ, et al. Development and initial validation of the Classification of Early-Onset Scoliosis (C-EOS). J Bone Joint Surg Am. 2014; 96(16):1359–1367

[3] Luk KD, Cheung KM, Lu DS, Leong JC. Assessment of scoliosis correction in relation to flexibility using the fulcrum bending correction index. Spine. 1998; 23(21):2303–2307

[4] Dobbs MB, Lenke LG, Kim YJ, Luhmann SJ, Bridwell KH. Anterior/posterior spinal instrumentation versus posterior instrumentation alone for the treatment of adolescent idiopathic scoliotic curves more than 90 degrees. Spine. 2006; 31(20):2386–2391

[5] Arlet V, Jiang L, Ouellet J. Is there a need for anterior release for 70–90 degrees masculine thoracic curves in adolescent scoliosis? Eur Spine J. 2004; 13(8):740–745

[6] Suk S-I, Chung E-R, Kim J-H, Kim S-S, Lee J-S, Choi W-K. Posterior vertebral column resection for severe rigid scoliosis. Spine. 2005; 30(14):1682–1687

[7] Bullmann V, Halm HFH, Schulte T, Lerner T, Weber TP, Liljenqvist UR. Combined anterior and posterior instrumentation in severe and rigid idiopathic scoliosis. Eur Spine J. 2006; 15(4):440–448

[8] Pawelek J, Varma V, Bagheri R. Clinical examination. In: Akbarnia BA, Yazichi M, Thompson G, eds. The Growing Spine. Berlin: Springer; 2011:63–69

[9] O'Shaughnessy BA, Kuklo TR, Hsieh PC, Yang BP, Koski TR, Ondra SL. Thoracic pedicle subtraction osteotomy for fixed sagittal spinal deformity. Spine. 2009; 34(26):2893–2899

[10] Akbarnia BA. Management themes in early onset scoliosis. J Bone Joint Surg Am. 2007; 89 Suppl 1:42–54

[11] Mehta MH. The rib-vertebra angle in the early diagnosis between resolving and progressive infantile scoliosis. J Bone Joint Surg Br. 1972; 54(2):230–243

[12] Buchowski JM, Skaggs DL, Sponseller PD. Temporary internal distraction as an aid to correction of severe scoliosis. Surgical technique. J Bone Joint Surg Am. 2007; 89 Suppl 2 Pt.2:297–309

[13] Buchowski JM, Bhatnagar R, Skaggs DL, Sponseller PD. Temporary internal distraction as an aid to correction of severe scoliosis. J Bone Joint Surg Am. 2006; 88(9):2035–2041

[14] Cheung WY, Lenke LG, Luk KDK. Prediction of scoliosis correction with thoracic segmental pedicle screw constructs using fulcrum bending radiographs. Spine. 2010; 35(5):557–561

[15] Klepps SJ, Lenke LG, Bridwell KH, Bassett GS, Whorton J. Prospective comparison of flexibility radiographs in adolescent idiopathic scoliosis. Spine. 2001; 26(5):E74–E79

[16] Ilharreborde B, Dubousset J, Le Huec J-C. Use of EOS imaging for the assessment of scoliosis deformities: application to postoperative 3D quantitative analysis of the trunk. Eur Spine J. 2014; 23 Suppl 4:S397–S405

[17] McKenna C, Wade R, Faria R, et al. EOS 2D/3D X-ray imaging system: a systematic review and economic evaluation. Health Technol Assess. 2012; 16 (14):1–188

[18] Dobbs MB, Lenke LG, Szymanski DA, et al. Prevalence of neural axis abnormalities in patients with infantile idiopathic scoliosis. J Bone Joint Surg Am. 2002; 84-A(12):2230–2234

[19] Gillingham BL, Fan RA, Akbarnia BA. Early onset idiopathic scoliosis. J Am Acad Orthop Surg. NaN. 2006; 14(2):101–112

[20] Skaggs DL, Akbarnia BA, Flynn JM, Myung KS, Sponseller PD, Vitale MG, Chest Wall and Spine Deformity Study Group, Growing Spine Study Group, Pediatric Orthopaedic Society of North America, Scoliosis Research Society Growing Spine Study Committee. A classification of growth friendly spine implants. J Pediatr Orthop. 2014; 34(3):260–274

[21] Hempfing A, Ferraris L, Koller H, Rump J, Metz-Stavenhagen P. Is anterior release effective to increase flexibility in idiopathic thoracic scoliosis? Assessment by traction films. Eur Spine J. 2007; 16(4):515–520

[22] Ruf M, Letko L, Matis N, Merk HR, Harms J. Effect of anterior mobilization and shortening in the correction of rigid idiopathic thoracic scoliosis. Spine. 2013;38(26):E1662–1668.

[23] Harrington PR. Treatment of scoliosis: correction and internal fixation by spine instrumentation. June 1962. J Bone Joint Surg Am. 2002; 84-A(2):316

[24] Marchetti PG, Faldini A. End fusions in the treatment of some progressing or severe scoliosis in childhood or early adolescence. Presented to the scoliosis research society. 1978;2:271–275

[25] Luque ER. Segmental spinal instrumentation for correction of scoliosis. Clin Orthop Relat Res 1982;163:192e8

[26] Pratt RK, Webb JK, Burwell RG, Cummings SL. Luque trolley and convex epiphysiodesis in the management of infantile and juvenile idiopathic scoliosis. Spine. 1999; 24(15):1538–1547

[27] Mardjetko SM, Hammerberg KW, Lubicky JP, Fister JS. The Luque trolley revisited. Review of nine cases requiring revision. Spine. 1992; 17(5):582–589

[28] Klemme WR, Denis F, Winter RB, Lonstein JW, Koop SE. Spinal instrumentation without fusion for progressive scoliosis in young children. J Pediatr Orthop. 1997; 17(6):734–742

[29] Blakemore LC, Scoles PV, Poe-Kochert C, Thompson GH. Submuscular Isola rod with or without limited apical fusion in the management of severe spinal deformities in young children: preliminary report. Spine. 2001; 26(18):2044–2048

[30] Akbarnia BA, Marks DS, Boachie-Adjei O, Thompson AG, Asher MA. Dual growing rod technique for the treatment of progressive early-onset scoliosis: a multicenter study. Spine. 2005; 30(17) Suppl:S46–S57

[31] Cheung JP-Y, Samartzis D, Cheung KM-C. A novel approach to gradual correction of severe spinal deformity in a pediatric patient using the magnetically-controlled growing rod. Spine J. 2014; 14(7):e7–e13

[32] Campbell RM, Jr, Smith MD, Hell-Vocke AK. Expansion thoracoplasty: the surgical technique of opening-wedge thoracostomy. Surgical technique. J Bone Joint Surg Am. 2004; 86-A Suppl 1:51–64

[33] Astur N, Flynn JM, Flynn JM, et al. The efficacy of rib-based distraction with VEPTR in the treatment of early-onset scoliosis in patients with arthrogryposis. J Pediatr Orthop. 2014; 34(1):8–13

[34] Qiu Y, Sun X, Wang B, et al. Early outcome of vertical expandable prosthetic titanium rib technique in treating early-onset scoliosis [in Chinese]. Zhonghua Wai Ke Za Zhi. 2012; 50(10):883–888

[35] Betz RR, Kim J, D'Andrea LP, Mulcahey MJ, Balsara RK, Clements DH. An innovative technique of vertebral body stapling for the treatment of patients with adolescent idiopathic scoliosis: a feasibility, safety, and utility study. Spine. 2003; 28(20):S255–S265

[36] Uzumcugil A, Cil A, Yazici M, et al. The efficacy of convex hemiepiphysiodesis in patients with iatrogenic posterior element deficiency resulting from diastematomyelia excision. Spine. 2003; 28(8):799–805

[37] Luque ER. Paralytic scoliosis in growing children. Clin Orthop Relat Res. 1982 (163):202–209

[38] Dewald RL, Ray RD. Skeletal traction for the treatment of severe scoliosis. The University of Illinois halo-hoop apparatus. J Bone Joint Surg Am. 1970; 52 (2):233–238

[39] Stagnara P. [Cranial traction using the "Halo" of Rancho Los Amigos]. Rev Chir Orthop Repar Appar Mot. 1971; 57(4):287–300

[40] Rinella A, Lenke L, Whitaker C, et al. Perioperative halo-gravity traction in the treatment of severe scoliosis and kyphosis. Spine. 2005; 30(4):475–482

11 Secondary Correction of Rigid Spinal Deformity after Failed Instrumentation

Meric Enercan, Azmi Hamzaoglu

Abstract

Revision surgeries can be significantly more challenging than primary deformity cases. Compared to primary cases, revision adult spinal deformity surgery has a higher risk of surgical complications and requires a longer hospital stay. Careful preoperative assessment and detailed preoperative surgical planning are essential for successful revision deformity surgery. Among all other osteotomy types, posterior vertebral column resection (PVCR) provides the greatest amount of correction with circumferential subperiosteal exposure of vertebral body and complete resection of one or more vertebral segments. Different correction techniques must be used to achieve ideal correction for scoliosis, kyphoscoliosis, lordoscoliosis deformity, and rigid pelvic obliquity following PVCR. Revision deformity surgery can be staged in order to lower the risk of complications related to longer operation time. Complications can be minimized and satisfactory results can be achieved with meticulous surgery and appropriate correction technique following PVCR.

Keywords: revision surgery, posterior vertebral column resection, three-column osteotomy, scoliosis, kyphoscoliosis, lordoscoliosis

11.1 Introduction

Revision surgeries can be significantly more challenging than primary deformity surgery due to the health, functional, and psychosocial conditions of the patients. Compared to primary surgery, revision deformity surgery carries a higher risk of surgical complications and a longer hospital stay. Successful treatment requires a comprehensive history and physical examination supplemented with carefully chosen confirmatory diagnostic tests. Preoperative careful assessment to determine the exact cause of symptoms and detailed preoperative planning are essentials in revision deformity surgery.[1,2,3]

The goals of revision surgery are to obtain a satisfactory balance in both sagittal and coronal planes, attain a solid fusion with a balanced spine, relieve pain, improve neurologic deficits if present, and prevent further deformity.[1,2] Adult spinal deformities requiring revision surgery can be managed with only posterior surgery with or without osteotomy or combined anterior–posterior surgery. Posterior osteotomy options are posterior-column osteotomy (Ponte) or three-column osteotomies. Options for three-column osteotomies include pedicle subtraction osteotomy (PSO), bone–disk–bone osteotomy (BDBO), and posterior vertebral column resection (PVCR) osteotomy.[4] Combined anterior–posterior revision spine deformity surgery is becoming less frequently utilized because of the versatility of three-column posterior osteotomies. PVCR is the most extreme posterior-only-approach osteotomy that is currently preferred by revision surgeons for severe and rigid spinal deformity. The PVCR osteotomy provides the most complete mobilization of the spine for deformity correction in all planes and is useful for deformities with very significant sagittal or coronal imbalance.[4,5,6,7,8]

Indications for the PVCR include the following:

- Gradual multilevel rigid deformity due to multilevel pseudarthrosis.
- Malunion following posterior or combined surgery.
- Severe decompensation and severe pelvic obliquity in neglected congenital scoliosis with intraspinal anomaly having had previous surgery.
- Flat back syndrome.
- Previous combined surgery for spinal deformity.
- Crankshaft phenomenon due to previous posterior surgery.
- Proximal or distal junctional failure due to adjacent vertebra fracture or fracture-dislocation.
- Postlaminectomy–posttraumatic severe sharp angular kyphosis.
- Decompensation or add-on phenomenon due to previous surgery for spinal deformity.

11.2 Preoperative Evaluation

Preoperative evaluation includes a careful medical history, detailed physical examination, and comprehensive radiologic assessment.

11.2.1 History

Review of medical records, reports of previous surgeries, and assessment of the medical history, especially evaluation of any medications and narcotic abuse; review of the patient's history, including work history and motivation for return to work; and involvement in litigation can identify comorbidities. History of smoking is important in differentiation between neurogenic and vascular claudication. Depression is common, especially in patients with multiple previous surgeries. Factors such as feelings of despair, sleep disturbance, loss of appetite, loss of sexual desire, irritability, and inability to make decisions can predict the functional outcome of revision surgeries. Addressing these psychological factors prior to revision surgery improves the outcomes.[1,2]

11.2.2 Physical Examination

1. **Neurologic examination:** The neurologic examination should include sensory examination, motor power, deep tendon reflexes, nerve root tension signs, and gait pattern. The patient should be observed undressed while standing and walking. Video recording of the gait from the front, back, and sides will provide more detail about the gait pattern, and also enable a comparison with the postoperative gait. Photographs should be taken from the front, back, and sides in the standing position for preoperative coronal and sagittal plane balance analyses. Flexion contractures of the hips and knees indicate sagittal balance problems.

2. **Sagittal balance:** Clinical evaluation of sagittal balance starts with an examination of the patient while standing with the knees fully extended to eliminate any compensatory knee flexion that may mask a severe sagittal plane deformity. The patient is then examined in the sitting position; if the trunk appears with good balance in relation to the pelvis, then a hip flexion contracture may be the cause of sagittal imbalance, and this can be demonstrated with the Thomas test. If forward displacement of the cervical spine in relation to the pelvis remains in the sitting position, the patient is then assessed in the supine position. When the deformity is localized to the lumbar spine, the patient will be able to lie with the shoulders on the table. If the head and upper thoracic spine remain elevated from the table, a fixed deformity in the cervical or thoracic spine or both is likely.
3. **Peripheral vascular examination:** Patients should be referred to a vascular surgeon if there is any concern regarding the peripheral circulation.
4. **Hip and knee joints:** Deformity and range of motion should be evaluated to rule out the hip or knee as the primary pain generator. Intra-articular local anesthetic injections may help to distinguish the primary source of pain.
5. **Pain:** Assessment of a detailed history and physical examination should be performed to rule out nonspinal causes and to identify the primary pain generator.

11.2.3 Imaging Studies

1. **Radiologic assessment of the sagittal and coronal balance:** This study includes standing anteroposterior and lateral full-length spine X-rays. Full extension of the hips and knees is important to eliminate any compensatory flexion that may mask a severe deformity. Sagittal and coronal spinal parameters should be measured. Any global or local imbalance, shoulder imbalance, and pelvic obliquity should be noted.
2. **Pelvis plain radiography:** Hip joint pathology can be assessed with plain X-rays.
3. **Flexion-extension radiography:** Flexion-extension images should be assessed for evidence of instability, pseudarthrosis, screw loosening, hardware failure, and adjacent-segment disease.
4. **CT:** Coronal and sagittal reconstructions of fine-cut CT provide the best imaging study for determining the fusion status. The CT will accurately assess any laminectomy defect and demonstrate any iatrogenic pars defect or the extent of a previous facetectomy. Three-dimensional (3D) reconstructions of high-resolution CT images in the coronal and sagittal planes are very important and helpful in preoperative planning, and will provide additional information for deformity correction. Three-dimensional reconstructions are essential when PVCR is considered for deformity correction.
5. **CT myelography:** This is indicated for patients in whom the MRI scan is difficult to evaluate due to metal artifacts due to previous instrumentation. Cobalt-chrome rods and multiple rod fixations cause excessive metal artifacts. CT myelography is also useful to evaluate the spinal cord when MRI could not provide sufficient imaging due to significant angulation of the deformity, as in severe kyphoscoliosis. CT myelography can also be performed when MRI is contraindicated due to a cardiac pacemaker.
6. **MRI with and without gadolinium enhancement:** Enhancement with gadolinium results in increased signal in vascularized tissues, especially epidural scarring. Comparing enhanced and nonenhanced sequences can accurately distinguish epidural scarring from a nonenhancing recurrent disk herniation. In addition, gadolinium enhancement in the intervertebral disk and vertebral bodies will demonstrate the presence of postoperative infection.
7. **Selective spinal angiography of the spinal artery:** It is very important to identify the great anterior radiculomedullary artery (artery of Adamkiewicz), which is the most important feeding artery of the thoracolumbar spinal cord. In revision deformity cases, if the planned PVCR level is at the same level as the previous anterior spinal surgery, identifying the branching level and the side of the Adamkiewicz artery is crucial for surgical planning in order to avoid any iatrogenic neurologic deficits due to vascular supply injury of the spinal cord.

11.3 Surgical Technique

In the surgical technique, once previous instrumentation is removed and the pseudarthrosis is evaluated, the pedicle screws are inserted segmentally at least three levels above and below the osteotomy level. In the presence of osteopenia or osteoporosis, cement-augmented fenestrated pedicle screws, expandable screws, or double-threaded pedicle screws should be used in order to provide adequate rigid fixation. In revision cases, when anatomical landmarks are not clear due to the previous surgeries and fusion mass, surgical exposure and new instrumentation may take longer and may cause more bleeding than a primary case. In these situations, surgery can be planned as a staged procedure, and osteotomy and deformity correction can be performed in the second stage.[6,7]

Following instrumentation, a temporary stabilizing rod, which is contoured to the shape of the deformity, is placed at the convex side prior to the initiation of the osteotomy. Wide laminectomy, including one level above and one level below the resection level, should be performed in order to decompress the neural elements and prevent any iatrogenic neurologic deficit and neural impingement after correction. In the thoracic spine, the exposed nerve roots can safely be sacrificed bilaterally to facilitate exposure and osteotomy, but nerve roots below T11, especially the T11 and T12 nerve roots, must be preserved for abdominal muscle innervation. Special care must be taken not to ligate or injure any segmentary artery during nerve root sacrifice. Ligating the segmentary arteries on both sides may disturb the spinal cord blood supply.[6,7]

The corresponding rib heads are resected bilaterally to expose the lateral wall of the pedicles. Careful subperiosteal dissection should be carried out to follow the lateral wall of the vertebral body until the anterior aspect is easily palpable. The disks above and below the planned resection level are then removed, followed by resection of the pedicle and vertebral body on the working side using osteotomies and a high-speed drill. A thin shell of bone at the anterior part along with the anterior longitudinal ligament is preserved to protect translation. A reverse curet is usually used to remove the thin shell of the posterior bone at the working side and below the dural sac.

After resection of the posterior wall on the working side, another temporary rod is inserted at this side. The temporary rod on the opposite side is then removed to allow resection of the remaining vertebra. The same sequence of resection is performed on the remaining vertebra. After completion of the resection, the second rod is placed at this side. A final evaluation of the spinal canal is then performed to confirm that there is no residual bone or disk tissue anterior to the dural sac.[6,7]

Different correction techniques must be used for each scoliosis, kyphoscoliosis, and lordoscoliosis deformity following PVCR.

11.3.1 Correction of Scoliosis Deformity

Following PVCR, a temporary rod is placed on the convex side to avoid any translation, and a temporary mesh cage is placed from the concave side. The height of the mesh cage should be approximately equal to the amount of the gap between end plates on the concave side. The scoliosis deformity will be corrected with repeated gradual compression maneuvers from the convex side. In situ bending of the rod on the concave side in both the coronal and the sagittal plane corrects the scoliosis deformity and restores thoracic kyphosis. The mesh cage will be changed as the gap on the concave side increases with the correction. Finally, a mesh cage of the proper size is placed from the concave side in order to prevent dural buckling and iatrogenic neurologic deficit and provide a secure correction (▶ Fig. 11.1). The final correction should be confirmed with an intraoperative X-ray. Neuromonitoring is mandatory during the correction procedure.

Another correction technique that can be used for the scoliosis correction is the cantilever technique. Following PVCR, the pedicle screws located two or three levels above and below the osteotomy level on the concave side should be changed with reduction (long-arm) screws. A temporary rod is placed on the convex side to avoid any translation during correction. A rod with the ideal sagittal contour is placed on the concave side and locked distally at the exact sagittal plane. Then the rod is placed in the long arms close to the osteotomy level with a cantilever maneuver. The deformity is corrected by translation over the long-arm screws segment by segment. Placing a mesh cage that is smaller than the gap size during the cantilever maneuver will prevent sudden shortening and dural buckling and thus prevent iatrogenic neurologic deficit. The correction should be checked and confirmed with an intraoperative X-ray. The final correction will be achieved with segmental compression and distraction maneuvers according to the intraoperative anteroposterior and lateral X-rays (▶ Fig. 11.2, ▶ Fig. 11.3).

11.3.2 Correction of Kyphoscoliosis Deformity

The correction of the kyphoscoliosis deformity is technically different than correction of the scoliosis. Correction of the kyphosis component is more important than scoliosis component. Following PVCR, a temporary rod is placed on the convex side, and a temporary cage in the size of the anterior gap is placed on the concave side. Following compression from the convex side, the temporary cage is removed, and a lamina spreader is placed anteriorly at the osteotomy site on the concave side. The anterior gap is lengthened using the lamina spreader on the concave side. A larger temporary cage is placed in the distracted anterior gap, and additional compression is applied on the convex side to achieve more correction. When kyphosis is corrected by more than 50%, the temporary cage on the concave side is removed and replaced with an expandable

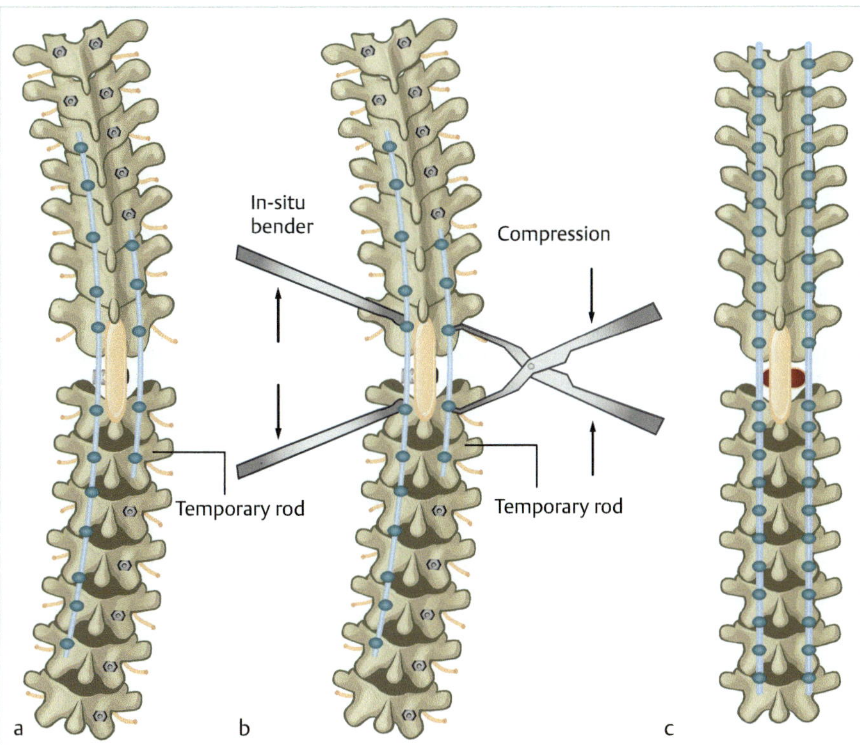

Fig. 11.1 (a–c) Scoliosis correction using in situ rod benders on the concave side.

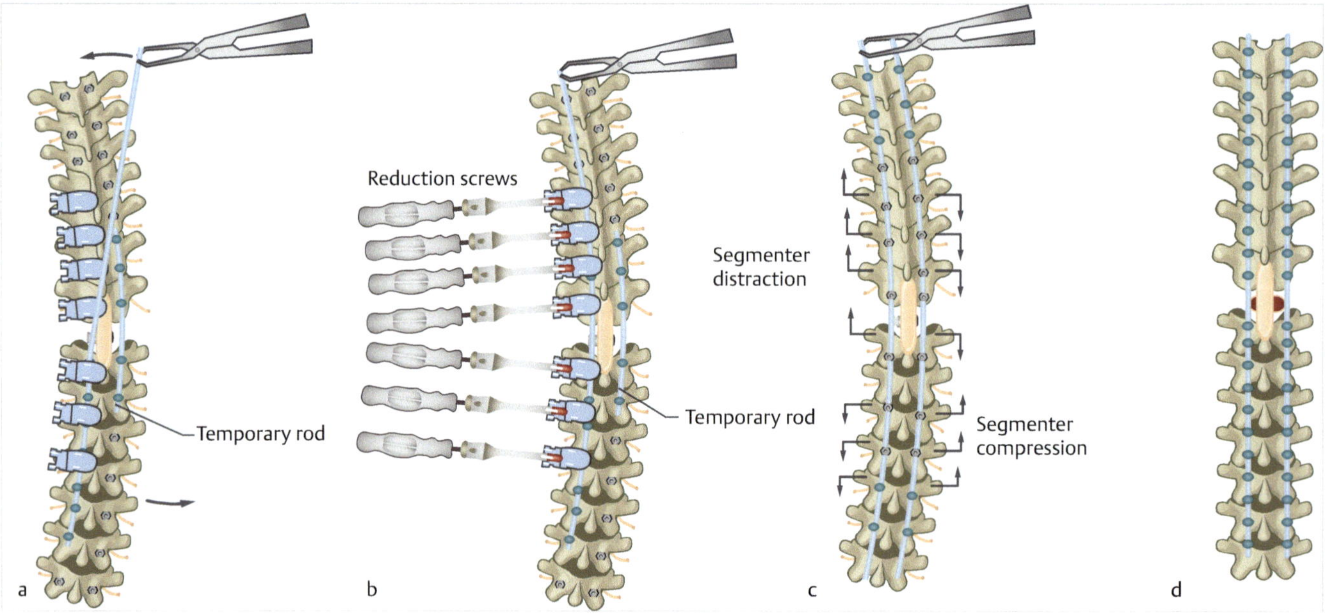

Fig. 11.2 (a–d) Scoliosis correction with a cantilever technique using reduction screws.

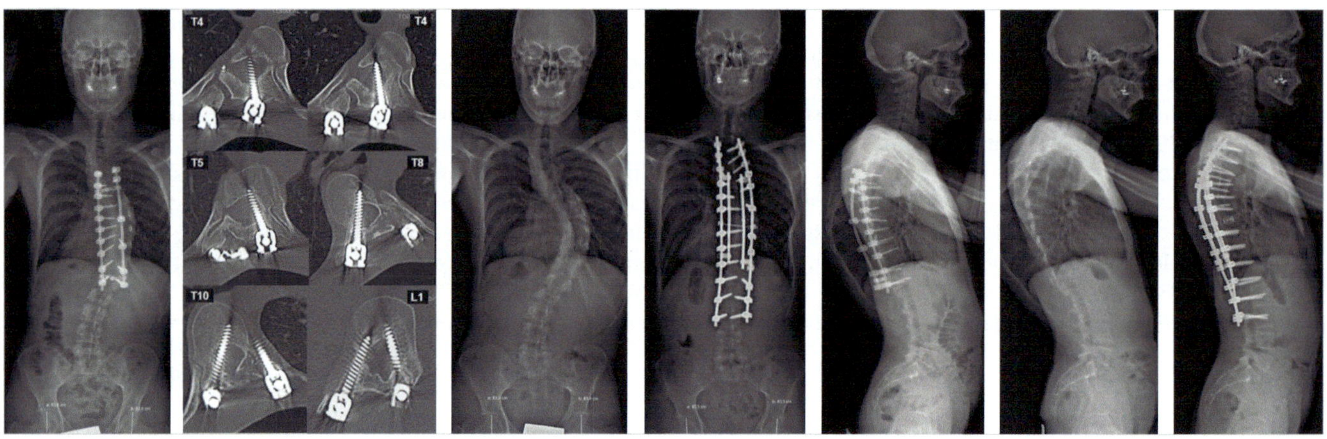

Fig. 11.3 A 22-year-old man with previous scoliosis surgery. Following the removal of the implants, multilevel posterior vertebral column resection (T 8–T 9) was performed for deformity correction as a staged surgery.

cage. The expandable cage is expanded, and the anterior column is lengthened from the concave side while posterior gradual compression is applied from the convex side. The compression maneuvers from the convex side simultaneously provide both scoliosis and kyphosis correction (▶ Fig. 11.4). The final coronal and sagittal alignment should be confirmed with intraoperative X-rays, and additional correction can be performed if needed (▶ Fig. 11.5).

11.3.3 Correction of Kyphosis Deformity

Following PVCR, a temporary mesh cage is placed anteriorly in the size of the gap between the anterior cortexes. Compression is applied over the rods on both sides for correction. Placing a temporary cage will prevent sudden shortening, dural buckling, and iatrogenic neurologic deficit. When the sharp angular kyphotic deformity is corrected by 30 to 50%, the temporary mesh cage is removed and replaced with the lamina spreader. The osteotomy site is distracted and lengthened anteriorly with the lamina spreader while simultaneous compression is applied posteriorly. When the anterior gap is lengthened by 50% compared to the initial status, an expandable cage is placed anteriorly at the osteotomy site. The expansion of the expandable cage provides additional anterior lengthening, and final correction is achieved by posterior compression maneuvers[9] (▶ Fig. 11.6). Final sagittal alignment is confirmed by an intraoperative lateral X-ray. Anterior lengthening and posterior compression will be continued until the ideal sagittal alignment is achieved (▶ Fig. 11.7).

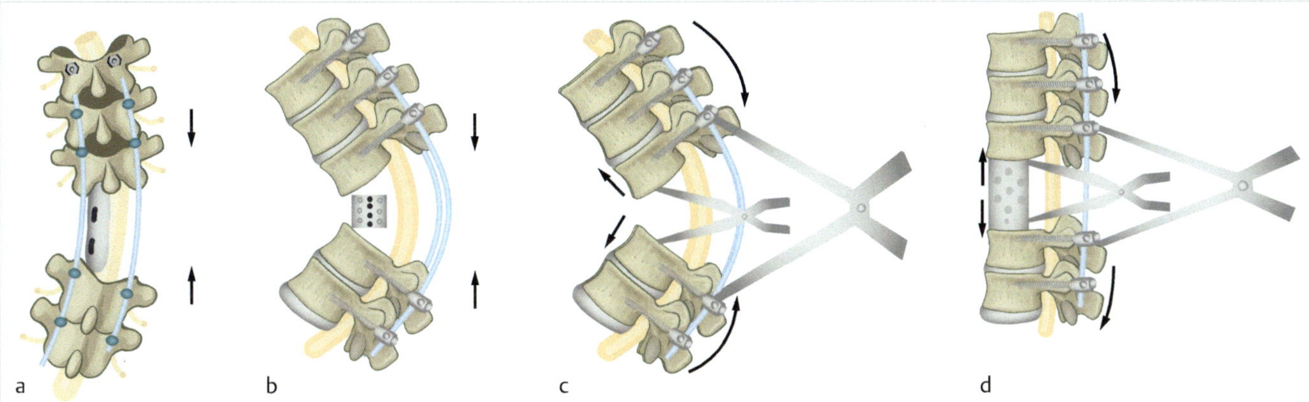

Fig. 11.4 (a–d) Kyphoscoliosis correction with anterior lengthening and posterior compression from the convex side.

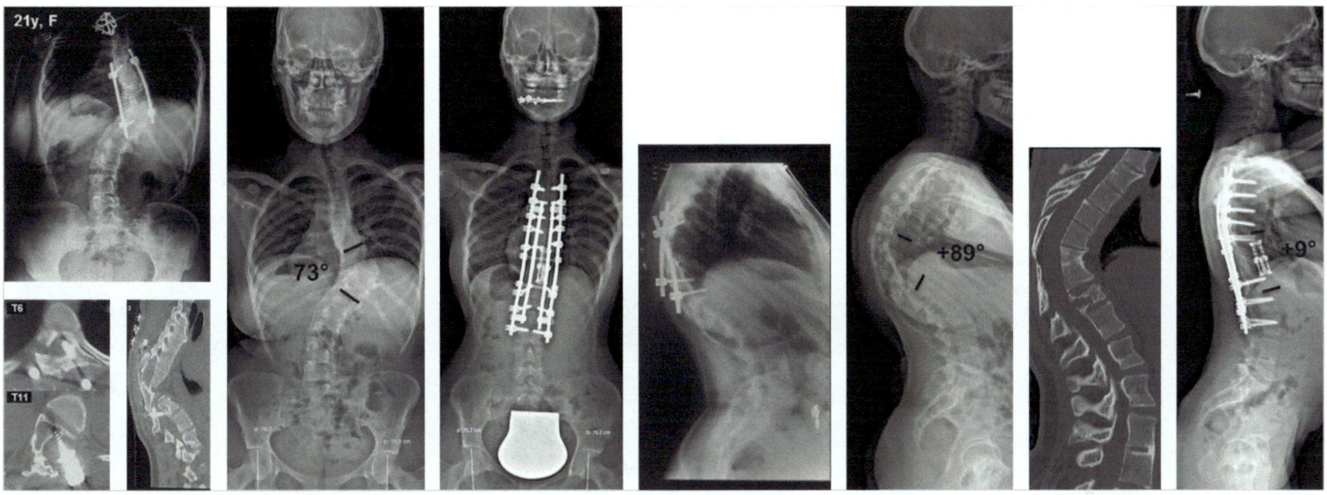

Fig. 11.5 A 21-year-old woman with previous deformity surgery. Multilevel posterior vertebral column resection (T 10–T 11–T 12) was performed for deformity correction.

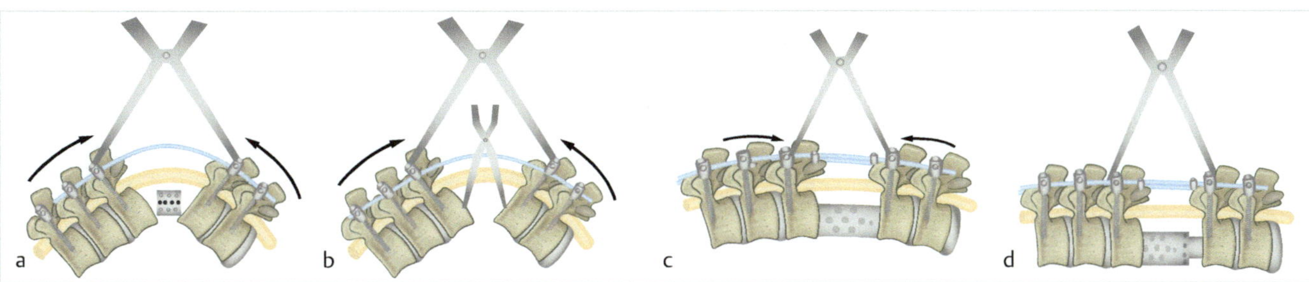

Fig. 11.6 (a–d) Kyphosis correction with sequential posterior compression and a simultaneous anterior column lengthening technique.

11.3.4 Correction of Lordosis/ Lordoscoliosis Deformity

PVCR must be performed at the apex of the lordosis or lordoscoliosis, and generally deformity correction requires more than one-level resection to restore physiologic thoracic kyphosis. The major technical challenge in lordoscoliosis is the resection of corresponding rib heads to mobilize the vertebral column. Due to severe thoracic lordosis, the costovertebral joints are located deep anterolaterally, and resection of rib heads may be challenging. Following PVCR, pedicle screws should be changed with reduction (long-arm) screws on both the concave and the convex sides to facilitate restoration of kyphosis. If reduction screws are instrumented before the osteotomy, they will obstruct the surgical view and working space of the osteotomy site and make it difficult to perform PVCR. Following osteotomy and instrumentation of the reduction screws, hyperkyphotic rods are placed during the first attempt at correction on both

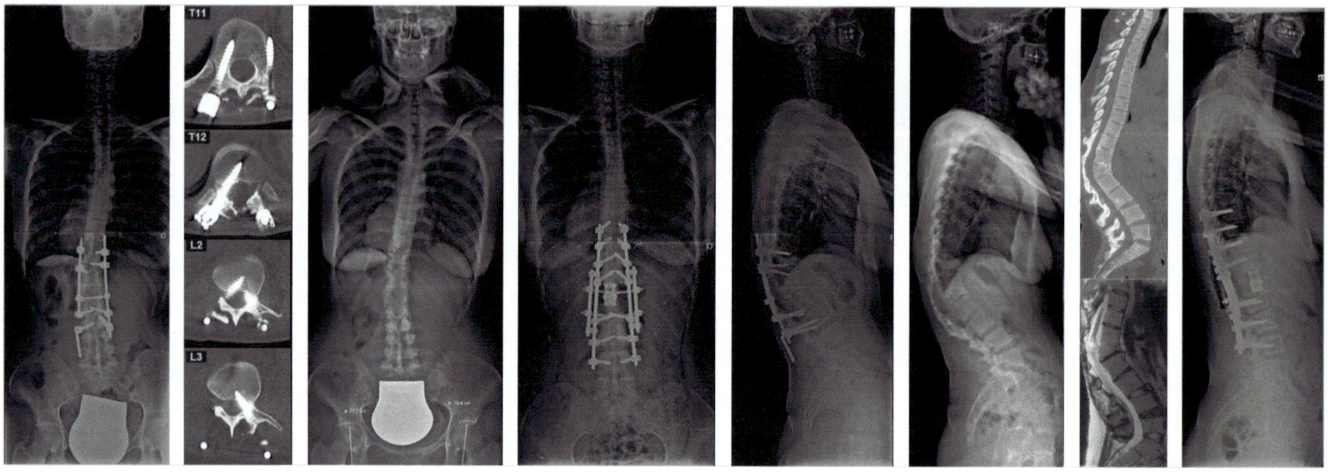

Fig. 11.7 A 31-year-old woman with posttraumatic kyphosis. She had a previous failed instrumented surgery. Following L 1 posterior vertebral column resection, sequential posterior compression and simultaneous anterior column lengthening were performed for deformity correction.

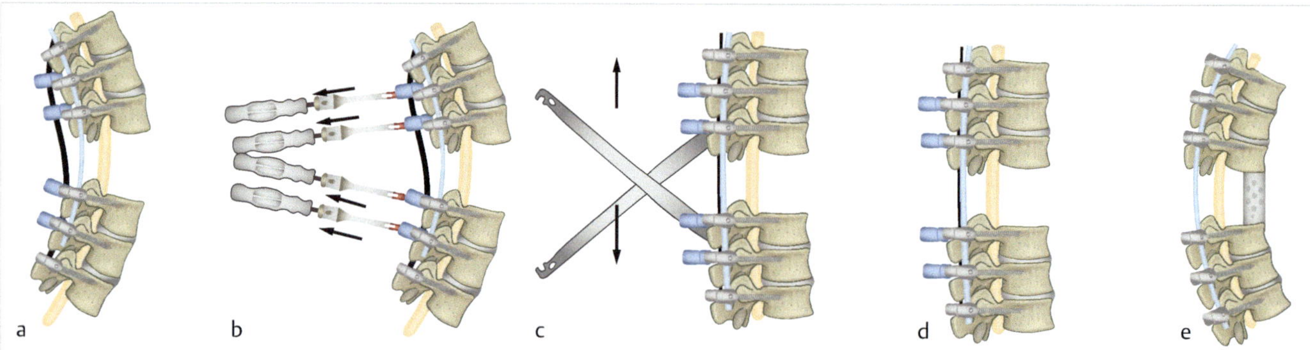

Fig. 11.8 (a–e) Lordoscoliosis correction using reduction screws.

the concave and the convex sides. Initial correction starts gradually from the concave side at the proximal and distal screws closest to the osteotomy level. This maneuver provides lordosis and scoliosis correction at the same time. The rods are changed at least two times with new, more kyphotic contoured rods until adequate kyphosis reduction is achieved. Additional kyphosis can be achieved with in situ benders. During correction, if bone to bone closure is achieved before satisfactory thoracic kyphosis restoration, additional vertebral resection should be performed to achieve the ideal kyphosis restoration. Following lordoscoliosis correction, if there is any residual gap at the osteotomy site, a mesh cage is placed to reconstruct the anterior column[10] (▶ Fig. 11.8, ▶ Fig. 11.9). Although performing PVCR for lordoscoliosis deformity is technically more challenging than that for scoliosis or kyphoscoliosis deformity, there is less risk of neurologic deficit because dural buckling is less common during correction of lordoscoliosis.

11.3.5 Correction of Severe Rigid Pelvic Obliquity in Neglected Congenital Scoliosis

It is possible to correct rigid, severe pelvic obliquity and significant trunk shift due to neglected congenital scoliosis with or without intraspinal anomaly with PVCR. The amount and level of resection are important in the surgical planning. When vertebrectomy of more than one level is performed with PVCR below T 12–L 1 level, rigid pelvic obliquity can be corrected. In the surgical technique, following PVCR, a temporary rod is placed on the concave side to avoid any translation. A mesh cage is placed on the concave side of the osteotomy site to avoid dural buckling and iatrogenic neurologic deficit. In the first step of the correction, distal rods are fixed and pelvic obliquity is corrected with a cantilever maneuver. The residual pelvic obliquity is corrected with gradual compression and in situ bending maneuvers from the lower side of the pelvis (▶ Fig. 11.10). Correction of the pelvic obliquity is confirmed with an intraoperative X-ray. If additional correction is needed after the initial correction, it can be achieved with more bone resection. Correction of the pelvic obliquity will also provide correction of coronal and sagittal plane deformity[11] (▶ Fig. 11.11a, b).

11.3.6 Reconstruction Laminectomy Defect following Posterior Vertebral Column Resection

The authors prefer to reconstruct the laminectomy defect using the femoral strut allograft. The H-shaped femoral strut allograft

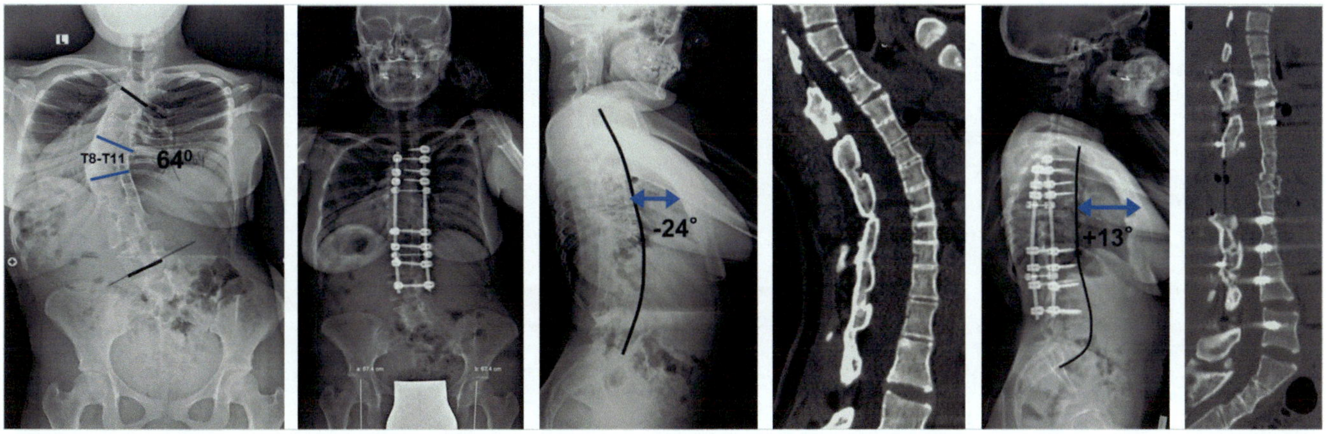

Fig. 11.9 A 20-year-old woman with two previous deformity surgeries. Multilevel posterior vertebral column resection was performed between the T 8 and T 11 levels to restore thoracic kyphosis.

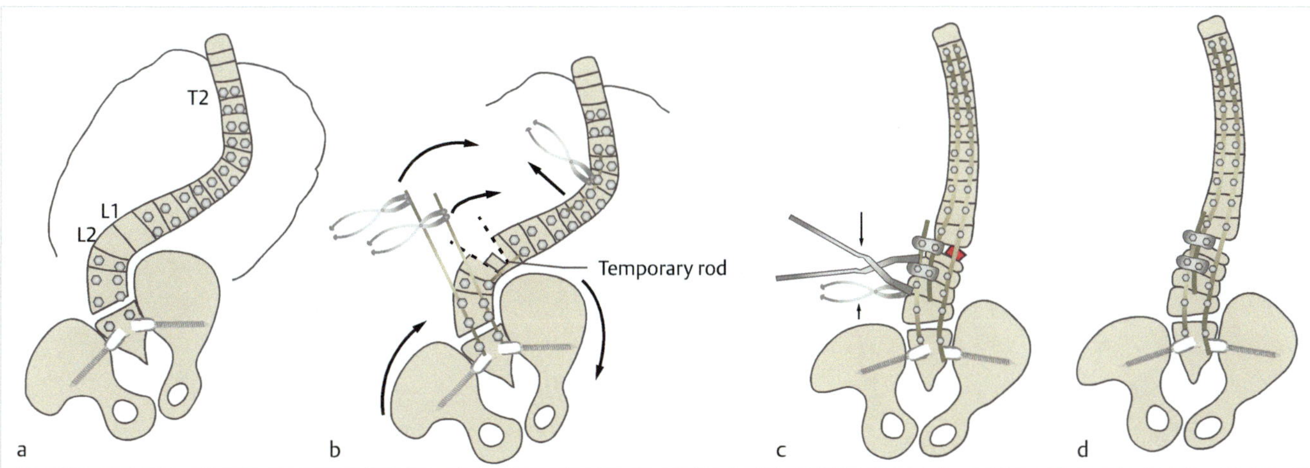

Fig. 11.10 (a–d) Correction of severe rigid pelvic obliquity in neglected congenital scoliosis.

is placed between the intact spinous processes above and below the laminectomy defect. The cross-bars placed between the rods and over the strut graft increase the stability and prevent the dislodgment of the graft. Local autografts are placed underneath and over both ends to promote fusion. The femoral strut allograft provides a rigid barrier over the dura, and prevents spinal cord compression due to hematoma and scar tissue formation[4,12] (▶ Fig. 11.12).

11.4 Complications

Revision deformity surgery is technically more challenging than that for primary cases and is prone to complications. Various studies reported a more than 60% overall complication rate, with a 9.6% reoperation rate for PVCR following adult spinal deformity surgery.[1,2,3,4,5,13,14,15] A major complication rate of 34.3% was reported for revision adult deformity surgery. Older age (> 60), body mass index greater than 30 kg/m^2, number of comorbidities greater than 2, estimated blood loss over 2000 mL, and increased thoracic kyphosis were the risk factors for major complications.[13] The most common reported complications were neurologic complications, pulmonary and urinary complications, intraoperative excessive bleeding, dural tears, pseudarthrosis, implant failure, infection, deep venous thrombosis (DVT), and pulmonary embolism (PE).[1] The neurologic complications, which were mostly transient, occurred in 6.3 to 15.8% of patients.[3,5] Patients with preoperative neurologic deficit had a higher risk for a postoperative permanent deficit. Intraoperative blood loss is a common problem in revision spine surgeries, and estimated blood loss (EBL) ranged from 0.8 to 7 L in several studies.[1,3,4] The incidence of a dural tear during revision spine surgery ranged from 0.3 to 17%.[2] Pseudarthrosis and implant failure are reported in 7.2 to 17.8% of revision spine deformity patients.[1] Postoperative infections are another risk of revision surgeries, and longer operative times or greater blood loss during surgery predisposes the patient to higher rates of wound infection. Wound infection rates between 4.1 and 9.7% have been reported following PVCR.[5] DVT and PE are potentially devastating complications in the postoperative follow-up period. The overall thromboembolic disease rate was 13.6%, and higher risk was associated with higher intraoperative blood loss. The reported rates for DVT were between 1.4 and 9.1%, and for PE were between 2 and 7.6% in adult spine deformity.[1]

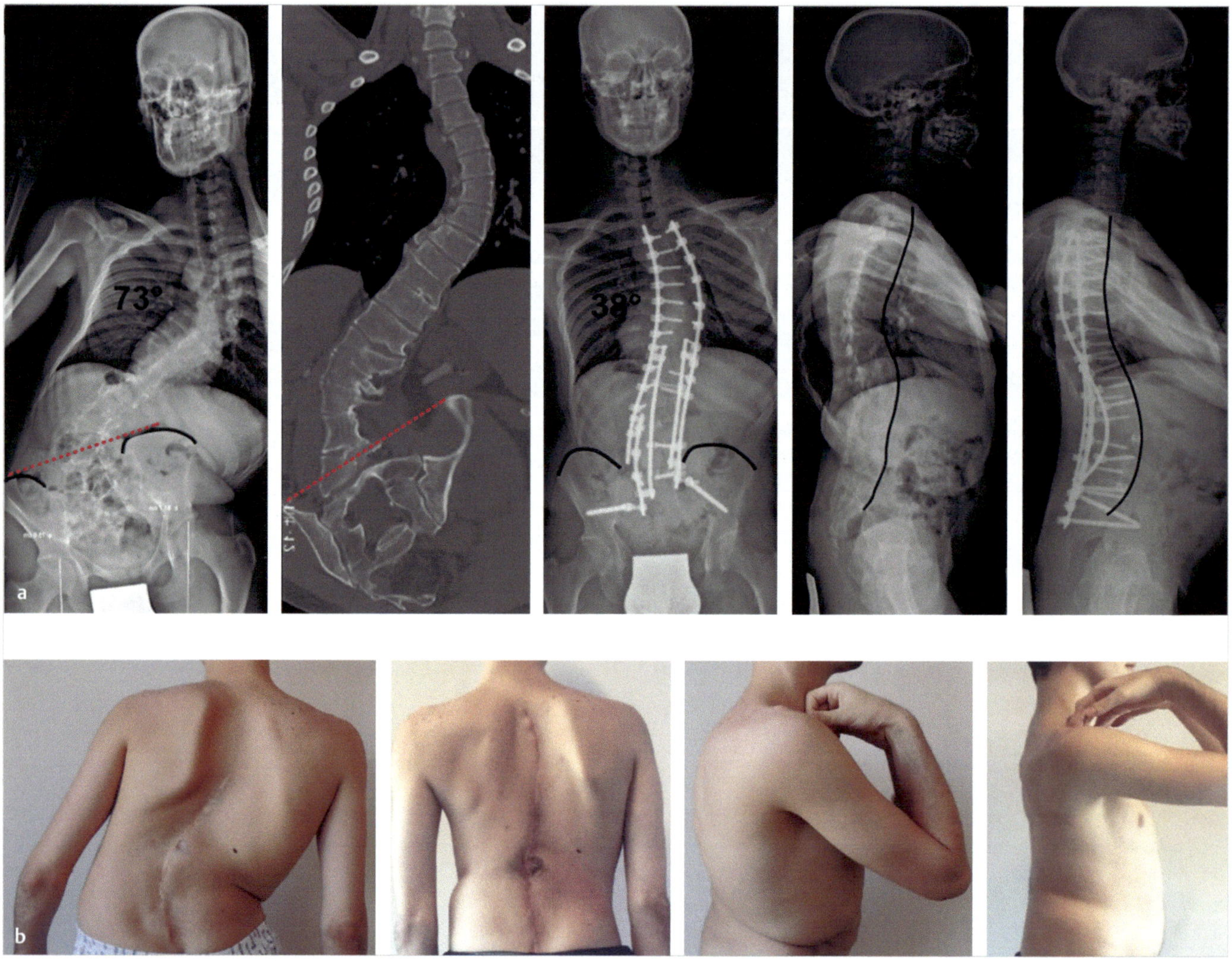

Fig. 11.11 (a) 20-year-old male patient with severe rigid pelvic obliquity and trunk shift due to neglected scoliosis. He had a previous tethered cord surgery. Multilevel PVCR (L2&L3) was performed for deformity correction without untethering procedure. (b) Preoperative and postoperative clinical photographs revealing the restoration of coronal and sagittal alignment.

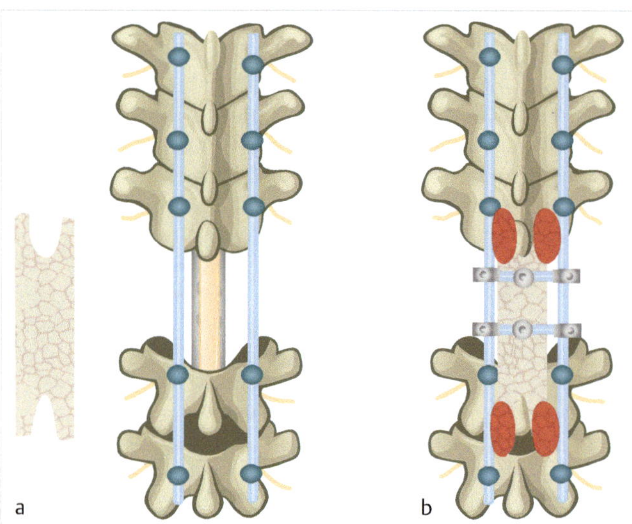

Fig. 11.12 (a–b) Reconstruction of the laminectomy defect with an H-shaped femoral strut allograft following posterior vertebral column resection.

According to the authors' clinical experience, 186 revision deformity cases were treated with PVCR. The most common complication was incidental dural tear (14.6%). When dural tear was observed intraoperatively, it was repaired primarily and a cerebrospinal fluid drainage catheter was used for 5 to 7 days postoperatively in order to prevent cerebrospinal fluid leakage. The rates of DVT and PE were 7.8% and 2.4%, respectively. One patient (0.053%) was revised for pseudarthrosis, and one for superficial infection (0.053%), which was treated with surgical debridement. There was no deterioration in the neurologic status of any patients. All patients with preoperative neurologic deficits showed improvement postoperatively.

11.5 Conclusion

Careful preoperative surgical planning is essential for obtaining satisfactory results. The assessment of the primary cause of the patient's symptoms is the key in preoperative planning. According to the primary source of pain, revision deformity cases can be managed by posterior surgery only, with or without osteotomy or combined anterior–posterior surgery. Posterior osteotomy options are posterior-column osteotomy (Ponte), or three-column osteotomies (PSO, BDBO, and PVCR). In recent years, PVCR has become a very popular technique. As experience in PVCR increases, it can be performed as multilevel resections. Some revision deformity cases may require an additional three-column osteotomy (PSO or BDBO), which will be performed at a different level than the PVCR to restore coronal and sagittal imbalance. Different techniques must be used to achieve ideal correction for scoliosis, kyphoscoliosis, and lordoscoliosis deformity following PVCR. Severe rigid pelvic obliquity with congenital scoliosis can also be treated with PVCR.

In patients with previous anterior spinal surgery, the Adamkiewicz artery must be identified preoperatively with selective spinal angiography. The surgical technique and location of the osteotomy can change according to the Adamkiewicz artery's location.

It is generally hard to distinguish the anatomical landmarks used for routine posterior instrumentation due to the previous surgery. Intraoperative CT-guided navigation systems can facilitate and provide accurate posterior instrumentation for revision cases. Revision deformity surgeries should be performed at centers with sufficient surgical equipment and the appropriate intraoperative imaging setup.

In complex revision cases, surgical exposure and reinstrumentation may take longer than primary cases due to multiple previous surgeries. For these cases, osteotomy and deformity correction can be planned as a second stage. This strategy will also lower the risk of complications. Relative to primary cases, revision adult spinal deformity cases carries a higher risk of surgical complications. The most common complication in revision cases is incidental dural tear. When fusion is extended down to the sacrum, augmentation of the lumbosacral region with multirod fixation will lower the implant failure rate. All surgical steps of revision deformity surgery must be performed under intraoperative neuromonitoring.

References

[1] Cunningham ME, Boachie-Adjei O. Revision surgeries for adult spinal deformity. In: Bridwell KH, DeWald RL, eds. The Textbook of Spinal Surgery. 3rd ed. Philadelphia, PA: Lippincott Williams & Wilkins; 2011:970–981

[2] Elgafy H, Vaccaro AR, Chapman JR, Dvorak MF. Rationale of revision lumbar spine surgery. Global Spine J. 2012; 2(1):7–14

[3] Iyer S, Nemani VM, Kim HJ. A review of complications and outcomes following vertebral column resection in adults. Asian Spine J. 2016; 10(3):601–609

[4] Enercan M, Ozturk C, Kahraman S, Sarıer M, Hamzaoglu A, Alanay A. Osteotomies/spinal column resections in adult deformity. Eur Spine J. 2013; 22 Suppl 2:S254–S264

[5] Saifi C, Laratta JL, Petridis P, Shillingford JN, Lehman RA, Lenke LG. Vertebral column resection for rigid spinal deformity. Global Spine J. 2017; 7(3):280–290

[6] Ozturk C, Alanay A, Ganiyusufoglu K, Karadereler S, Ulusoy L, Hamzaoglu A. Short-term X-ray results of posterior vertebral column resection in severe congenital kyphosis, scoliosis, and kyphoscoliosis. Spine. 2012; 37(12):1054–1057

[7] Hamzaoglu A, Alanay A, Ozturk C, Sarier M, Karadereler S, Ganiyusufoglu K. Posterior vertebral column resection in severe spinal deformities: a total of 102 cases. Spine. 2011; 36(5):E340–E344

[8] Suk SI, Kim JH, Kim WJ, Lee SM, Chung ER, Nah KH. Posterior vertebral column resection for severe spinal deformities. Spine. 2002; 27(21):2374–2382

[9] Karadereler S, Kahraman S, Sever C, et al. Surgical Correction of the Rigid Sharp Angular Kyphotic Deformity with Gradual Sequential Posterior Compression and Simultaneous Anterior Column Lengthening Technique After PVCR. Paper presented at: Annual Meeting and Course of the Scoliosis Research Society (SRS); September 8, 2017; Philadelphia, PA, USA

[10] Enercan M, Kahraman S, Hamzaoglu A. Treatment of congenital lordoscoliosis with posterior vertebral column resection. In: Gupta MC, Vaccaro AR, Gupta S, eds. Complex Spine Cases: A Collection of Current Techniques. New Delhi, India: Jaypee Brothers Medical Publishers; 2015:161–166

[11] Kaya O, Karadereler S, Kahraman S, et al. Surgical correction of the severe rigid pelvic obliquity with PVCR in neglected congenital scoliosis. Paper presented at: Annual Meeting of the 23rd International Meeting on Advanced Spine Techniques (IMAST); July 13, 2016; Washington, DC, USA

[12] Enercan M, Kahraman S, Mutlu A, et al. Reconstruction of wide laminectomy defects with femoral strut allograft (FSA) following three-column osteotomies (3CO). 21st International Meeting on Advanced Spine Techniques (IMAST), July 16–19, 2014; Valencia, Spain

[13] Cho SK, Bridwell KH, Lenke LG, et al. Major complications in revision adult deformity surgery: risk factors and clinical outcomes with 2- to 7-year follow-up. Spine. 2012; 37(6):489–500

[14] Hassanzadeh H, Jain A, El Dafrawy MH, et al. Clinical results and functional outcomes of primary and revision spinal deformity surgery in adults. J Bone Joint Surg Am. 2013; 95(15):1413–1419

[15] Diebo BG, Passias PG, Marascalchi BJ, et al. Primary Versus Revision Surgery in the Setting of Adult Spinal Deformity: A Nationwide Study on 10,912 Patients. Spine. 2015; 40(21):1674–1680

12 Kyphectomy in Patients with Myelomeningocele

Josh Schroeder, Leon Kaplan

Abstract

There is a high rate of spinal deformities in patients with myelomeningocele (MMC); the rate of congenital kyphosis increases if the MMC is a thoracic one. Thoracic MMC leads to severe thoracolumbar kyphosis. As the deformity progresses, a gibbus appears, leading to skin breakdown and a chronic pressure sore over the gibbus. As children with this deformity are frail, continued aggravation at the gibbus site causes difficulty in sitting and increased secondary complications. Surgical treatment of gibbus, kyphectomy, requires removal of several vertebrae in order to reduce the gibbus and strengthen the spine. It requires an open ventriculoperitoneal (VP) shunt and proper proximal and distal fixation, allowing anchoring of the spine in its new position. Patient preparation is key for surgical success; it includes involvement of a plastic surgeon and metabolic preparation. They are both important to achieve proper skin healing in this scarred area. There is a high rate of complication with kyphectomy; however, it allows balanced seating, and most children have improved ambulation and better lung functions.

Keywords: MMC, myelomeningocele, kyphosis, gibbus, kyphectomy

12.1 Introduction

Myelomeningocele (MMC) and other forms of spina bifida cystica are dystrophic disorders of the neural arch. MMCs are caused by the absence of proliferation of neuroectodermal cells after migration is finished.[1,2] There are three types of defects of the posterior elements of the spine. The first, spina bifida occulta, the occult form, without neurologic deficit, is estimated to have an incidence of up to 5% and is often seen as an incidental finding on imaging of the lumbar spine.[3,4] The second kind of defect, meningocele, is the least common form of spina bifida. In this form, the vertebrae develop normally, but the meninges protrude through gaps between the posterior elements of the vertebrae. As the nervous system remains undamaged, individuals with meningocele are unlikely to suffer long-term health problems, although cases of tethered cord have been reported. In MMC, there is a complete failure of formation of the posterior elements of the spine, with the myelin and the covering meninges protruding from the body given the lack of posterior elements of the spine.[5] This type of MMC creates complete paraplegia from the level of the MMC (the level of the neurosegment defect) downward. MMC occurs in 0.005% of live births. Surgery to close the sac and the early commencement of hydrocephalus has to be done prenatally or early after birth to prevent infections or complications of hydrocephalus.[6] If treated in a timely fashion, the life expectancy of patients with MMC has reached nearly 40 years.[7] As the child with MMC grows, more and more problems concerning the skeletal system arise, leading to difficulty in mobility and compromising nursing care. The clinical appearance of the MMC is dominated by the neurosegmental level of the lesion.[1]

The incomplete formation of the posterior elements of the spine, absence of a posterior tension band of the spine, and an imbalance of paraspinal musculature attached anterior to the instantaneous axis of rotation, led by the powerful psoas muscle, create a progressive kyphosis of the spine in 12 to 28% of children with MMC.[8,9] This type of kyphosis is referred to as congenital kyphosis and is malignant and progressive in nature. The lesions are mostly thoracic, and the kyphosis is most commonly present distal to the lesion. In parallel, many children with MMC suffer from a paralytic type of kyphosis that is more benign in nature. Scoliosis has been reported in patients with MMC, varying according to the functional level of the spinal dysraphism.[8] Between 83 and 100% of patients with thoracic-level dysraphisms have been noted to develop scoliosis, whereas only 5% of lumbosacral-level dysraphisms have been associated with scoliosis.[10]

Congenital kyphosis appears when the MMC is at the thoracic level.[11] The gibbus, however, usually develops in MMCs at lumbar levels between L2 and L5.[12,13] The gibbus creates pressure points in these sitting children, which contribute to epidermal ulceration, decubitus ulcers, and chronic nonhealing wounds leading to secondary infections. The gibbus also creates a functional impairment, making it harder for the child to sit and forcing the child to use his or her hands when sitting ("dependent sitting"); decreases abdominal volume creates respiratory compromise, and causes severe back pain, which makes it impossible for the child to lie in the supine position and prevents standard sitting. Casting, bracing, and wheelchair inserts provide little help in controlling this deformity.

The kyphosis progresses at a faster rate when the curve exceeds 90 degrees.[13] This is most common in the congenital kyphosis form. As the child grows, the deformity becomes aesthetically and functionally unacceptable.[11] These children are often small, with low body weight and impaired metabolic intake, leading to secondary failures of the soft tissues, which is most pronounced in the creation and healing of pressure sores. Because the child is severely malnourished, surgery is not advocated as it leads to increased complications.[14]

As conservative measures to control the gibbus are not effective, once the gibbus becomes apparent, the child needs to undergo corrective surgery. The gibbus is resected with the rudimentary cord, with proximal and distal fixation, allowing fusion in a stable position to allow balanced sitting and proper patient care.

12.2 Kyphectomy

Kyphectomy was first reported by Sharrard et al[15] in 1968. Over the years, the procedure developed from in situ fusion with spica casting of the patient to instrumented fusions. However, the surgery has a high rate of complications.

There are several prerequisites for considering the patient for surgery. First, the skin on the back has to be healed from any wounds or abrasions; these wounds, often over the apex of the gibbus, can be slow to heal. The lesions are often pressure sores

Table 12.1 Checklist prior to surgery on patients with myelomeningocele

Check	Improve
1. Skin condition	Make sure no open wounds are present; if so, refer patient to a plastic surgeon for wound management and possibly for skin grafting for wound closure.
2. Nutritional status	Evaluate albumin, protein, and white blood cell levels; have the patient be seen by a dietitian. If needed, place a percutaneous endoscopic gastrostomy tube to improve parenteral feeding.
3. Respiratory functions	Obtain a baseline reading of pulmonary function; improve the baseline with respiratory-based physical therapy. If the pulmonary function values are too low, the patient may not be able to undergo surgery.
4. Ventriculoperitoneal shunt	Make sure the shunt is working; if not, involve a neurosurgical team.
5. Urinary cultures	These patients are permanent catheter users and have recurrent urinary tract infections (UTIs). It is not advisable to operate on the child with an acute UTI; treat the patient with antibiotics prior to surgery.
6. Wheelchair preparation	Prior to surgery make sure the wheelchair has no pressure points and place silicon padding where needed.
7. Team conversation with parents	Have a team-based conversation with the parents; discuss the treatment plan, complication risks, and the need for a supportive brace after surgery. The parents are part of the team, and their compliance is critical for the success of surgery.

with large skin and soft tissue defects reaching the underlying bone. Plastic surgery and assistance from dermatology may be required to deal with these slow-healing wounds, which may require skin grafting at times. In addition, nutritional status is one of the most important conditions needed for these children and must be optimized to allow wound and bone healing. A joint evaluation with a nutritionist is needed for increasing caloric and intact protein intake to allow proper healing, and at times the children need parenteral feeding to improve albumin levels. The ventriculoperitoneal shunt (VPS) has to be patent and functioning to prevent an acute rise in cerebrospinal fluid (CSF) pressure when the sack is ligated, which may lead to herniation of the cerebellar tonsils and sudden death during the surgery. Patient, family, and caretakers must be briefed regarding the surgery and possible complications (▶ Table 12.1).

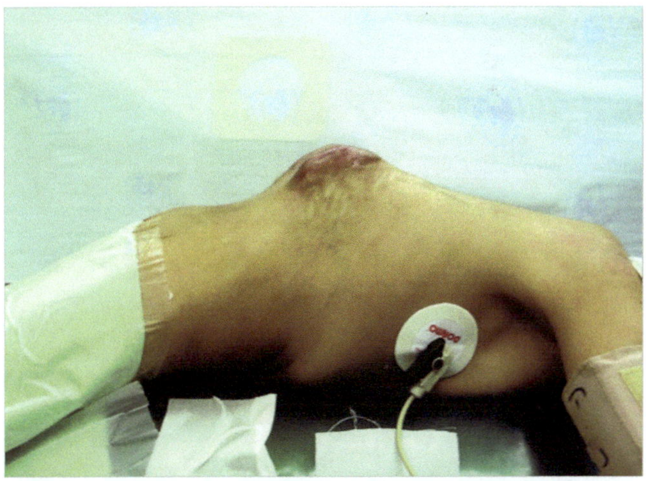

Fig. 12.1 Preoperative image of a child on the operating table; note two silicon rolls lowering pressures from the chest.

12.3 Surgical Technique

Several packed cell units must be ready prior to surgery as intense bleeding may be encountered when removing the gibbus from the osteoporotic bone and large vertebrobasilar veins. A cell saver and the use of aminocaproic acid should be used as well to minimize blood loss.

The entire room needs to be talc free and latex free as up to 40% of children are allergic and can develop a reaction during surgery.[16] The patients are intubated and placed on specialized silicon cushions (▶ Fig. 12.1) to minimize pressure points, In addition, because the children are quite small, proper holding devices are placed to prevent motion during surgery.

Patients should be warmed at all times as hypothermia is almost inevitable in these small patients. Draping of the entire spine is needed to allow proper exposure. The patient's spine is prepared for a posterior approach, and antibiotics are given. A posterior longitudinal incision is executed through the scarred tissue. The dissection of the soft tissue flap is kept as thick as possible to allow adequate coverage of the wound after resection, since after resection of the gibbus the skin and soft tissues are in excess, proper care of the tissues is mandatory to prevent long-term breakdown and skin necrosis. The spine proximal and distal to the kyphosis is identified and exposed, allowing multiple fixation points both proximal and distal to the osteotomy. The distal dissection must reach the sacrum to allow proper sacral fixation. The rudimentary dural sac is released from the adjacent tissue, ligated with a nonabsorbable suture, cut, and removed at the level of the MMC, exposing the vertebrae of the gibbus. An open VPS is critical for this step because, in its absence, the acute increase in the CSF pressure can lead to sudden death from acute hydrocephalus followed by tonsillar herniation through the foramen magnum.

Slow dissection alongside the vertebrae is performed with a blunt instrument in order to identify the anterior border of the vertebrae, covered by the anterior longitudinal ligament. Care must be taken not to penetrate the abdominal cavity, the kidneys, or any of the large vessels that lie anteriorly to the vertebrae in the retroperitoneal space. Slow channeling along the anterior aspect of the vertebrae is carried out with a blunt instrument, staying as close as possible to the anterior aspect of the vertebrae. Once the anterior aspect is exposed, a surgical pad can be passed from one side of the spine to the other and be used to release the vertebrae from all retroperitoneal structures and to safeguard against iatrogenic damage during resection. Two cuts are performed in the vertebrae above the gibbus, removing the lordotic part of the gibbus. Three to five vertebrae can be removed, but overresection can make it difficult to align both sides of the osteotomy. The kyphectomy is performed (▶ Fig. 12.2), and the bones are kept for local bone grafting.

At this time, the surgeon should see that both sides of the osteotomy can be connected with minimal defect. Fixation with sublaminar wires is performed with a 1.6 millimeter galvanized metal wire. Fixation should be started at least four or five segments proximal to the beginning of the deformity to spread the load over the spine, starting at the lordotic section of the thoracic spine. The distal fixation should be attached to all the everted lamina through the neuroforamina (▶ Fig. 12.3, ▶ Fig. 12.4, ▶ Fig. 12.5) and continued down to the sacrum. The nonfunctional rootlets in the neuroforamina are resected.

The rods (Luque 5 mm rods) are bent in a 90-degree angle and placed in the sacrum through the sacroiliac joints into the pelvis using the Galveston technique.[17] The wires are connected to the rods in a gradual fashion to allow slow reduction of the deformity and prevent wire cutout. The local bone graft is added to sides of the spine to induce fusion and fill in any defect in the osteotomy site. The best results of the kyphectomy are achieved with long posterior fixation and multiple points of attachment (segmental fixation).

Diligent closure is mandatory to reduce the chances of wound breakdown. Patients should be placed in a tailor-made jacket until bony fusion is evident to reduce the chances of hardware failure. Wound inspection should be routine as the scarred skin of the former gibbus is a slowly healing area. The tailor-made jacket worn by the patient reduces the strain on the rods and adjacent soft tissues, thus decreasing persistent skin breakdown.

There have been several modifications of this technique, with the use of pedicle screws, hybrid constructs, or other types of sacral fixation. But the principal concepts are the same—with

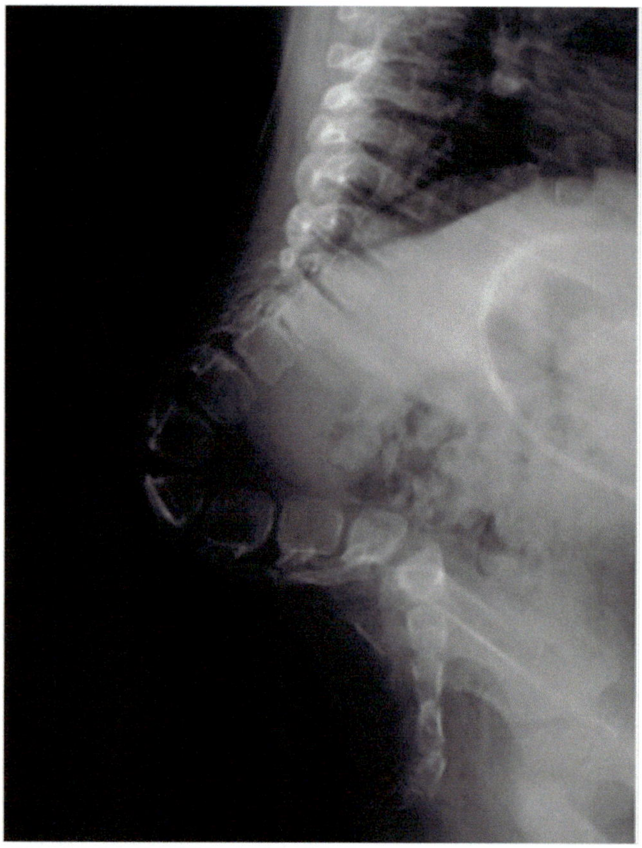

Fig. 12.2 Preoperative X-ray of the spine in the gibbus.

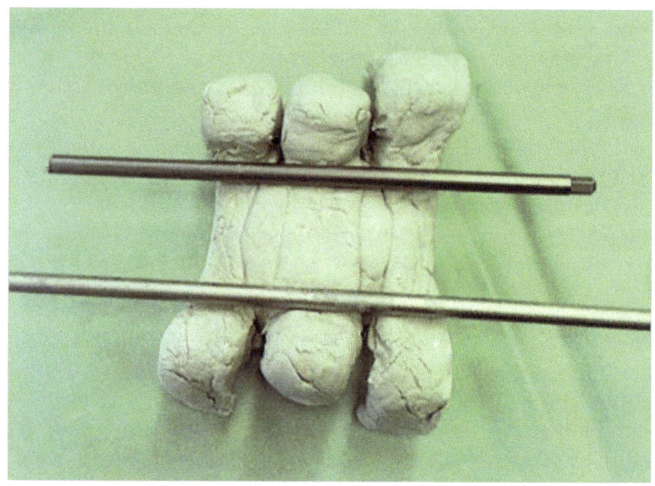

Fig. 12.3 Model showing placement of rods.

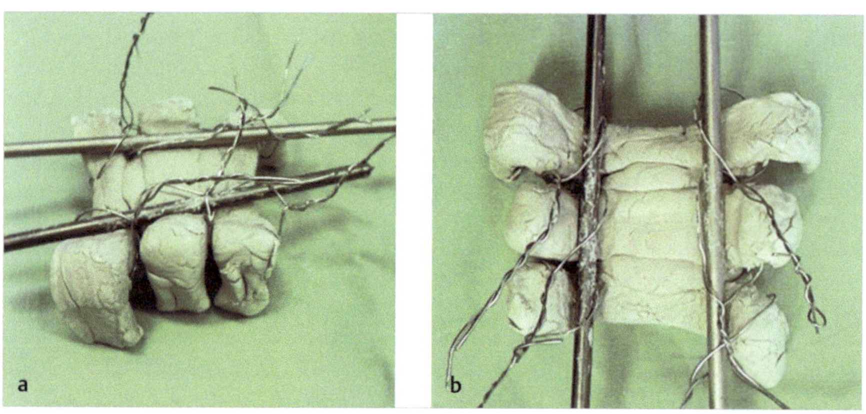

Fig. 12.4 (a, b) Tightening of the wires on the everted lamina.

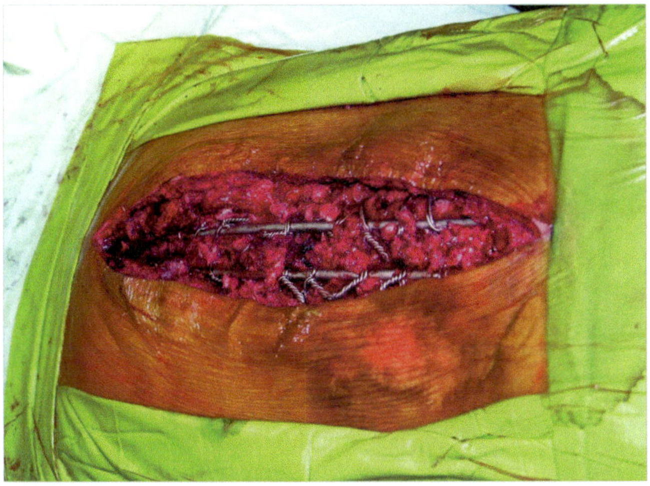

Fig. 12.5 The spine with the rods and wires after resection of the gibbus.

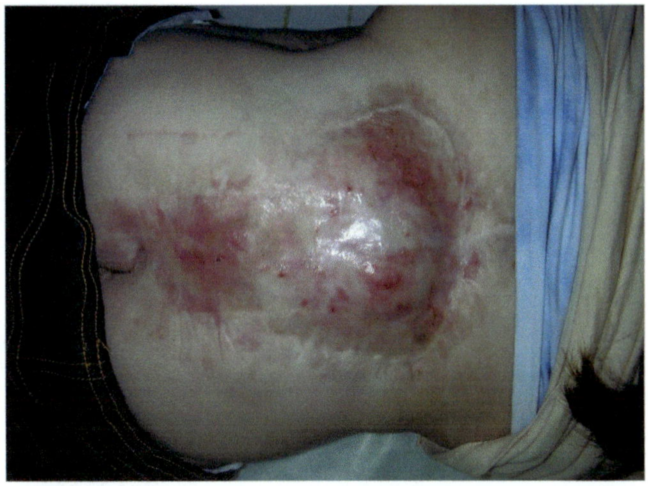

Fig. 12.6 The back of a 9-year-old girl after the wound was closed with a skin graft—the large necrosis occupied most of her spine.

proper dissection and resection, allowing healing in a favorable setting. No statistical influence of the technique of fusion and instrumentation on the occurrence of infections could be found.[18,19,20,21] This large, posterior-based resection eliminates the need for an anterior approach and reduces the morbidity of surgery.[22]

It is critical to keep the instrumentation as low a profile as possible in order to reduce pressure on the soft tissues and the skin.

12.4 Outcome

Kyphectomy allows great correction of the deformity; patients have a stable, balanced, and fused spine allowing balanced sitting, free mobilization, and proper nutrition.[11] Wound checks and standard X-rays should be performed every 6 to 8 weeks to evaluate skin healing, and spinal fusion, and to make sure no hardware-related complications are present.

This correction affects not only the children but also their parents and caretakers, with an improvement in activities of daily living (ADLs) and a subjective improvement in social status and self-image. A study performed by the authors of this chapter,[11] which included 18 patients who underwent kyphectomy for MMC, found that solid fusion was achieved in 70% of patients, with a mean time to fusion of 12 months. Patients improved in their ADLs and were all independently sitting after surgery.

Follow-up durations from reported series have ranged from 27 to 133 months (in our series the follow-up was 10 years). Because the children are operated on at a young age, long-term follow-up is needed to rule out secondary complications, which reached close to 40% in our series. Progression of the kyphosis varies in different studies, and ranges from 8 to 33.7 degrees, with a mean progression of 10 degrees over time. Further analysis or interpretation is of limited value because the variation in surgical technique and instrumentation type prohibits the forming of reliable conclusions.[1,12,13,15,22]

The complication rate of this surgery in MMC patients is high and can exceed 50% of the cases[14] in several small series (in the series published by the authors of this chapter, the complication rate was 38%). Hardware-related problems, pseudarthrosis,

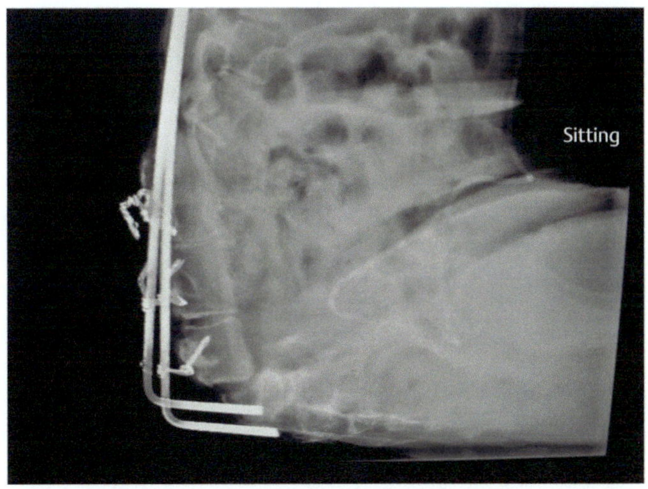

Fig. 12.7 The spine of an 11-year-old boy 2 years after the initial fixation, with the distal pullout of the hardware and the newly formed kyphosis at the sacral level.

infection, and loss of correction and wound breakdown are the common complications reported. However, patient death is rare but can occur if the VPS is not patent, or if during the anterior dissection any of the major organs is injured. Mortality is a risk that should be discussed with all families of the patients who are undergoing kyphectomy. Other complications that arise due to the magnitude of the surgery or the fragility of the patients include rhabdomyolysis, excessive blood loss, epidural hematoma, meningitis, acute respiratory distress syndrome, pneumonia, wound breakdown, skin necrosis, hardware pullout, infection, CSF leakage, and urinary tract infections.

In the series collected by the authors of this chapter, there were several complications: a patient presented with wide skin necrosis due to metal prominence (▶ Fig. 12.6) and was treated with recurrent debridements and a wound vacuum until the soft tissue coverage allowed wound closure with a skin graft.

A second patient developed a Charcot joint (neuropathic joint) through his sacrum (▶ Fig. 12.7) that was accompanied by

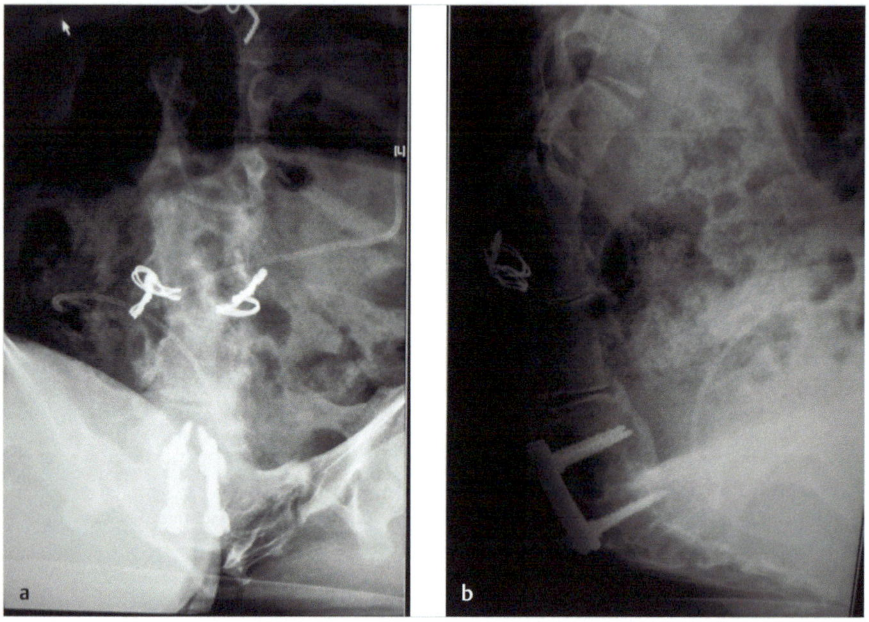

Fig. 12.8 (a, b) Two-year follow-up imaging of the spine after the hardware was removed, and a single-level fusion was performed, using pedicle screws and rods.

a pullout of the hardware, leading to the development of a distal unstable sacral kyphosis. The patient was taken to the operating room, where the joint was removed, and a ring bone graft was placed in the area of the joint. Low-profile pedicle screws (Solera, Medtronic Sofamor Danek) were placed above and below the joint with a good outcome (▶ Fig. 12.8).

The rate of nonunion and hardware-related complications in patients with MMC is high. Masur et al[23] reported 20% hardware failure and 33% pseudarthrosis if the Harrington rod was used. Bonnett et al[24] reported 34% hardware problems, and Kumar and Townsend[25] 26% pseudarthrosis or hardware problems. In the largest series reported (77 patients)[26] the hardware-related complication was 29.8% with a 22% rate of screw loosening and pseudarthroses. In that series, a combined anterior and posterior approach was performed in several of the patients; adding the anterior instrumentation reduced the incidence of hardware-related complications to 15%. Proximal junctional kyphosis has been reported as well.

As hardware loosens, a secondary loss of correction happens; this can affect 30 to 76% of these patients.[26] It is not clear that the anterior instrumentation increases fusion rates, but fusion rates change in series reported for anterior instrumentation.

Infection rates are high, ranging from 20 to 43%.[14,26] Wound complication rate is high as well and can occur in over half of patients. This may necessitate a removal of the instrumentation that will cause secondary loss of fixation. McMaster[27] reported that 2 of his 10 patients (treated with a variety of surgical techniques) had superficial wound necrosis after kyphectomy, which healed with nonoperative treatment, and three other patients had ulcerations over prominent hardware requiring hardware removal for wound healing. Ko et al[28] reported 7 of 9 patients with wound healing issues after kyphectomy. Eventually 6 of their 7 patients required implant removal. Niall et al[29] reported 19 of 24 patients with wound complications. Thirteen of these patients had issues with primary wound healing, with 11 of these patients eventually having chronic issues with hardware exposure. Six patients had delayed wound breakdown as a result of hardware prominence and ulceration.

In order to reduce such complications, we made sure not to cut through the scarred tissue, leaving 5 cm from the edge of the scar. In addition, flaps were deep and in one plane. If skin breakdown occurs, we propose using local wound care until healing has been obtained; if the area is larger the use of a vacuum-based dressing should be used.

Deep infection is a common severe complication in this patient population. It mandates debridement and suppression of the infection with long-term antibiotics to delay removal of the implants until a solid posterior fusion has developed. However, if implants are removed, after a presumed solid fusion, patients can still develop recurrent deformity distal to the fusion. Therefore, if no implants can be placed with a posterior approach, an anterior approach with anterior-based fusion can be performed.

In conclusion, despite having a high rate of complications and nonunions, the correction of a gibbus in MMC via a kyphectomy is a good solution and provides children with a stable, balanced spine.

References

[1] Swank M, Dias L. Myelomeningocele: a review of the orthopaedic aspects of 206 patients treated from birth with no selection criteria. Dev Med Child Neurol. 1992; 34(12):1047–1052

[2] Herman JM, McLone DG, Storrs BB, Dauser RC. Analysis of 153 patients with myelomeningocele or spinal lipoma reoperated upon for a tethered cord. Presentation, management and outcome. Pediatr Neurosurg. 1993; 19(5):243–249

[3] Whiteman D, Murphy M, Hey K, O'Donnell M, Goldacre M. Reproductive factors, subfertility, and risk of neural tube defects: a case-control study based on the Oxford Record Linkage Study Register. Am J Epidemiol. 2000; 152 (9):823–828

[4] Werler MM, Mitchell AA. Neural-tube defects. N Engl J Med. 2000; 342 (15):1135–1136, author reply 1136–1137

[5] Adzick NS, Thom EA, Spong CY, et al. MOMS Investigators. A randomized trial of prenatal versus postnatal repair of myelomeningocele. N Engl J Med. 2011; 364(11):993–1004

[6] Moldenhauer JS. In utero repair of spina bifida. Am J Perinatol. 2014; 31 (7):595–604

[7] Davis BE, Daley CM, Shurtleff DB, et al. Long-term survival of individuals with myelomeningocele. Pediatr Neurosurg. 2005; 41(4):186–191

[8] Guille JT, Sarwark JF, Sherk HH, Kumar SJ. Congenital and developmental deformities of the spine in children with myelomeningocele. J Am Acad Orthop Surg. 2006; 14(5):294–302
[9] Hoppenfeld S. Congenital kyphosis in myelomeningocele. J Bone Joint Surg Br. 1967; 49(2):276–280
[10] Müller EB, Nordwall A. Prevalence of scoliosis in children with myelomeningocele in western Sweden. Spine. 1992; 17(9):1097–1102
[11] Schroeder JE, Barzilay Y, Hasharoni A, Kaplan L. Long-term outcome of surgical correction of congenital kyphosis in patients with myelomeningocele (MMC) with segmental spino-pelvic fixation. Evid Based Spine Care J. 2011; 2 (1):17–22
[12] Smith JT, Novais E. Treatment of Gibbus deformity associated with myelomeningocele in the young child with use of the vertical expandable prosthetic titanium rib (VEPTR): a case report. J Bone Joint Surg Am. 2010; 92 (12):2211–2215
[13] Torode I, Godette G. Surgical correction of congenital kyphosis in myelomeningocele. J Pediatr Orthop. 1995; 15(2):202–205
[14] Hatlen T, Song K, Shurtleff D, Duguay S. Contributory factors to postoperative spinal fusion complications for children with myelomeningocele. Spine. 2010; 35(13):1294–1299
[15] Sharrard WJ. Spinal osteotomy for congenital kyphosis in myelomeningocele. J Bone Joint Surg Br. 1968; 50(3):466–471
[16] Ausili E, Tabacco F, Focarelli B, Nucera E, Patriarca G, Rendeli C. Prevalence of latex allergy in spina bifida: genetic and environmental risk factors. Eur Rev Med Pharmacol Sci. 2007; 11(3):149–153
[17] Benson ER, Thomson JD, Smith BG, Banta JV. Results and morbidity in a consecutive series of patients undergoing spinal fusion for neuromuscular scoliosis. Spine. 1998; 23(21):2308–2317, discussion 2318
[18] Kocaoğlu B, Erol B, Akgülle H, Gasimov E, Yalçin S. Combination of luque instrumentation with polyaxial screws in the treatment of myelomeningocele kyphosis. J Spinal Disord Tech. 2008; 21(3):199–204
[19] Laing AJ, Walsh A, O'Grady P, Nelligan M, McCormack D. Short segment posterior locking cervical plate fixation after kyphectomy for myelomeningocoele-associated kyphosis. J Spinal Disord Tech. 2006; 19(4):292–294
[20] Nolden MT, Sarwark JF, Vora A, Grayhack JJ. A kyphectomy technique with reduced perioperative morbidity for myelomeningocele kyphosis. Spine. 2002; 27(16):1807–1813
[21] Christofersen MR, Brooks AL. Excision and wire fixation of rigid myelomeningocele kyphosis. J Pediatr Orthop. 1985; 5(6):691–696
[22] Shimode M, Kojima T, Sowa K. Spinal wedge osteotomy by a single posterior approach for correction of severe and rigid kyphosis or kyphoscoliosis. Spine. 2002; 27(20):2260–2267
[23] Mazur J, Menelaus MB, Dickens DR, Doig WG. Efficacy of surgical management for scoliosis in myelomeningocele: correction of deformity and alteration of functional status. J Pediatr Orthop. 1986; 6(5):568–575
[24] Bonnett C, Brown JC, Perry J, et al. Evolution of treatment of paralytic scoliosis at Rancho Los Amigos Hospital. J Bone Joint Surg Am. 1975; 57(2):206–215
[25] Kumar SJ, Townsend P. Posterolateral spinal fusion for the treatment of scoliosis in myelodysplasia. J Pediatr Orthop. 1982; 2(5):514–520
[26] Geiger F, Parsch D, Carstens C. Complications of scoliosis surgery in children with myelomeningocele. Eur Spine J. 1999; 8(1):22–26
[27] McMaster MJ. Anterior and posterior instrumentation and fusion of thoracolumbar scoliosis due to myelomeningocele. J Bone Joint Surg Br. 1987; 69 (1):20–25
[28] Ko AL, Song K, Ellenbogen RG, Avellino AM. Retrospective review of multilevel spinal fusion combined with spinal cord transection for treatment of kyphoscoliosis in pediatric myelomeningocele patients. Spine. 2007; 32(22):2493–2501
[29] Niall DM, Dowling FE, Fogarty EE, Moore DP, Goldberg C. Kyphectomy in children with myelomeningocele: a long-term outcome study. J Pediatr Orthop. 2004; 24(1):37–44

13 Pitfalls and Difficulties in the Surgical Management of Severe Adolescent Idiopathic Scoliosis

Mario Di Silvestre

Abstract

Different strategies have been used for surgical treatment of severe adolescent idiopathic scoliosis (AIS). It is risky for these patients to undergo aggressive operations, such as combined anterior-posterior surgery or posterior vertebral column resection. A posterior-only approach with less aggressive osteotomies is preferable, but a gradual preoperative period of traction is necessary. Preoperative halo traction is one method available, but there are controversies over its efficacy.

A two-staged posterior surgery using a magnetically controlled growing rod (MAGEC; Ellipse Technologies, Inc.) (MCGR) has been adopted in the last few years by the author. Its use has been preferred for gradual and safe correction of deformity. The MCGR is an internal distraction device, and hence a major advantage over halo traction.

The first surgery consists of a posterior aggressive release with Ponte osteotomies at many levels with high density pedicle screw instrumentation; an MCGR is implanted on the concavity of the scoliotic curve. A distraction is applied postoperatively to obtain gradual correction of the curve. The correction is performed over a series of distractions of the implanted device using an external magnet. In the second posterior surgery, the magnetic rod is removed and the definitive rods (generally three or four) are applied for definitive correction and fusion.

Keywords: severe adolescent idiopathic scoliosis, two-staged posterior correction, Ponte osteotomy

13.1 Definition of Severe Idiopathic Scoliosis

The definition of severe scoliosis is still controversial. O'Brien et al[1] consider a curve as severe when the Cobb angle is ≥70 degrees. Other authors[2] defined as severe a curve >80 degrees. Greiner[3] concluded that scoliosis is severe when the Cobb angle is >60 degrees, because significant respiratory symptoms are not present until the curve is around 60 degrees. It seems a more pragmatic definition of severe scoliosis is a curve with a Cobb angle > 80 degrees. In fact, the surgical procedure presents different and more demanding aspects: typically, it is a rigid deformity of the spine, with a low flexibility index on bending films (about 30%).

13.1.1 Preoperative Study

Surgical treatment requires accurate clinical and radiological evaluation of an adolescent with severe scoliosis.

The physical examination must be focused on excluding *non-idiopathic* cases of scoliosis, which generally require a different surgical approach to the deformity. Young age (>10 years) at onset of scoliosis, rapid progression of the curve, and mostly neurologic symptoms are important criteria used to differentiate the scoliosis from idiopathic cases. Neurologic deficits are not commonly found in the physical examination of severe adolescent idiopathic scoliosis; however, they should be tested and may be indicative of underlying neurologic problems. In severe scoliosis, deformity is also seen in the chest wall, resulting in poor pulmonary function. This is especially the case in curves >100 degrees, where pulmonary function is seriously decreased and presents higher risks for corrective surgery. Patients present with a low body mass and require nutritional supplements before surgery, as advised by a developmental pediatrician and a dietician.[4] Both the surgeon and the anesthesiologist must evaluate the cardiac system, which can be secondarily affected: a preoperative cardiac study must include electrocardiography, echocardiography, and stress testing.

The radiological study with standard standing X-rays is used to quantify the scoliosis curvature and to assess the flexibility of the deformity using traction films (generally the flexibility index is low, ≤30% in severe curves). It is also used to evaluate the extension of the arthrodesis and identify the presence of associated spondylolisthesis. The X-ray study must include the entire spine, including the cervical spine, for those patients who are going to be placed in preoperative traction. A CT scan of the entire spine is mandatory for studying pedicle anatomy and to assess for screw placement. Reconstruction of the axial images clarifies the complex anatomy of the scoliotic curve and allows the surgeon to visualize the levels of planned vertebral osteotomies or resections.[4] A CT scan can provide a three-dimensional (3D) study of the curved spine (▶ Fig. 13.1). An

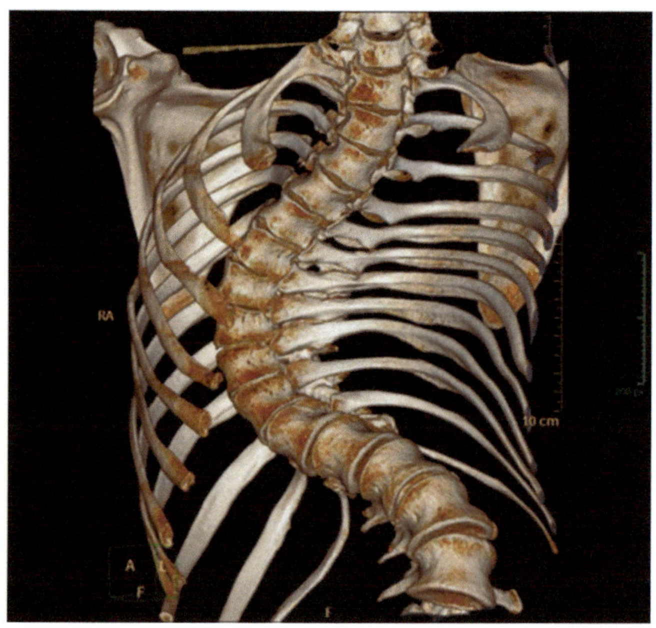

Fig. 13.1 A CT scan provides a three-dimensional study of the curved spine.

MRI scan is fundamental to assessing the neural axis, especially for those patients who are undergoing a large operative correction. It is important to exclude or to evaluate whether syrinx or Chiari malformations are present, as well as any stenosis or cord impingement secondary to severe deformity. If spinal stenosis is identified, some surgeons use CT myelography to understand the specific levels of compression. It is possible to have cord compression on the concave pedicle, which may require a resection of that pedicle with the remaining body. In cases of a planned aggressive osteotomy (e.g., a pedicle subtraction osteotomy), the blood flow to the spinal cord over the planned level of resection must be evaluated. In the future, MRI, contrast-enhanced gradient echo, and 3D pulse sequence may have a role in these patients.[4]

13.1.2 Preoperative Halo Traction

Traction can be utilized both before and immediately following anterior release and fusion, being removed after definitive posterior spinal fusion (▶ Fig. 13.2). It is now commonly used before posterior spinal fusion without anterior release. Halo traction represents the usual preoperative strategy employed to manage severe deformities to gradually straighten the spine before surgery. To prevent neurologic compromise after acute corrective maneuvers, the use of halo-gravity traction is advocated to allow for gradual curve correction and monitoring of neurologic function in the awake patient, which reduces the risk of permanent neurologic deficits.[5]

Preoperative traction has evolved considerably. After the halo-plaster vest, Stagnara[6] popularized halo-gravity traction utilizing a wheelchair for treatment of severe spinal deformity, noting some limitations to its use in cervical kyphosis and significant ligamentous laxity. Halo-gravity traction remains an often-used method and is safer than halo-femoral and halo-pelvic traction, which have a higher incidence of complications, such as hip subluxation or dislocation and sometimes femur fractures. Halo-gravity traction has the advantage in that it is transferable between the hospital bed, wheelchair, and walker (▶ Fig. 13.3).

Patients underwent local anesthesia for application of the halo ring, secured with eight pins. The initial traction force is about 2 kg and increased subsequently by 1 kg every day until the goal of 30% body weight is achieved. Daily neurologic control is performed. The patient is controlled for headache and motor and sensory function in all peripheral nerve distributions (including the cranial nerves). Traction is reduced at night, with the bed positioned in a slight reverse Trendelenburg position. Antibiotics are used in cases of pin-site infection. Every 5 to 6 days, X-rays are obtained in traction: possible overdistraction of the cervical spine must be avoided (▶ Fig. 13.3). The duration of traction is about 3 weeks. In the days immediately before surgery, traction is gradually reduced, and the patient will arrive at the operating room with a low traction of 2 kg. The halo is removed before surgery after induction of general anesthesia.

There are two mechanisms at work in correction of a scoliosis curve under traction.[7] The initial correction is due to the elastic properties of tissues: the elastic deformation is followed by a creep phase where most of the correction is achieved; this period of primary creep lasts for about 2 to 4 hours, with important correction. A secondary creep period allows a more gradual reduction of the spinal deformity, such that near maximal curve correction can be obtained after about 10 to 12 days. For this reason, the maximum scoliosis correction can be obtained after only 2 weeks of correction.[8]

However, the role of halo-traction and its safety and efficacy are actually the objects of discussion. For Koptan and ElMiligui,[7] traction increased curve flexibility compared to the curve seen in the supine side-bending films performed before traction. In the study by Sponseller et al,[9] there was no statistically significant difference between traction and control groups in coronal or sagittal curve correction, spinal length gain, blood loss, operating time, or complications; however, the patients who had halo traction less frequently had a vertebral body resection but achieved comparable and less demanding deformity correction. In our experience, halo

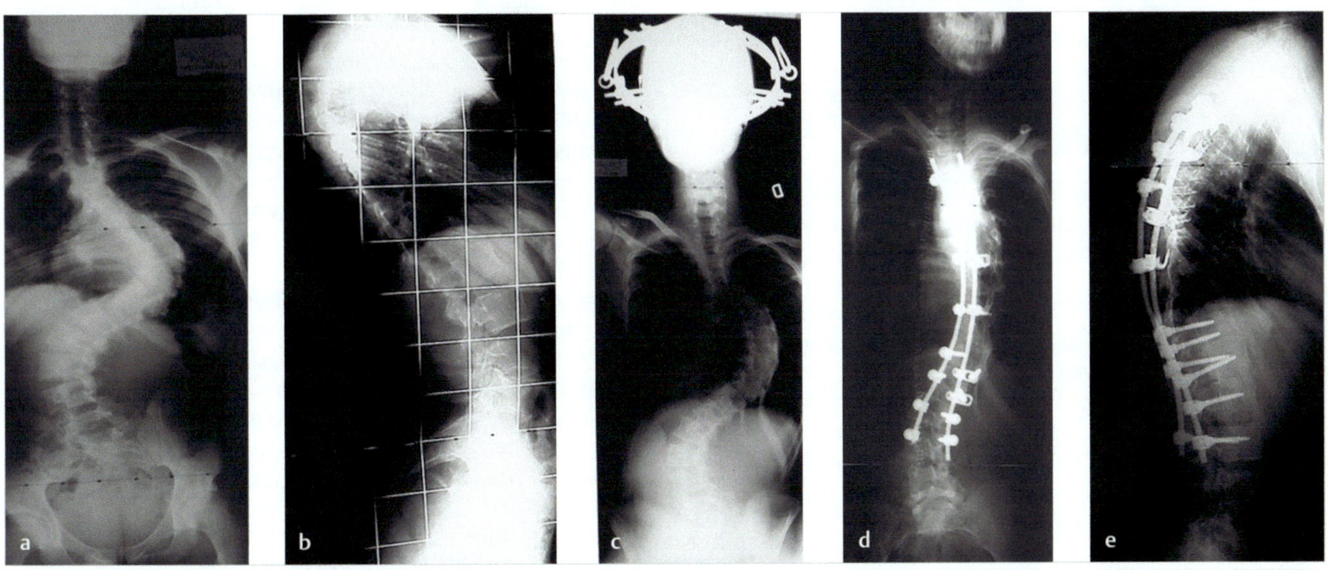

Fig. 13.2 A 17-year-old boy, **(a, b)** with severe idiopathic scoliosis treated years ago with **(c)** an anterior release and fusion (by a thoracotomy) and a post-operative period of halo traction. **(d, e)** Second surgery after removal of halo-traction consisted of posterior fusion with instrumentation (hybrid constructs with hooks and screws).

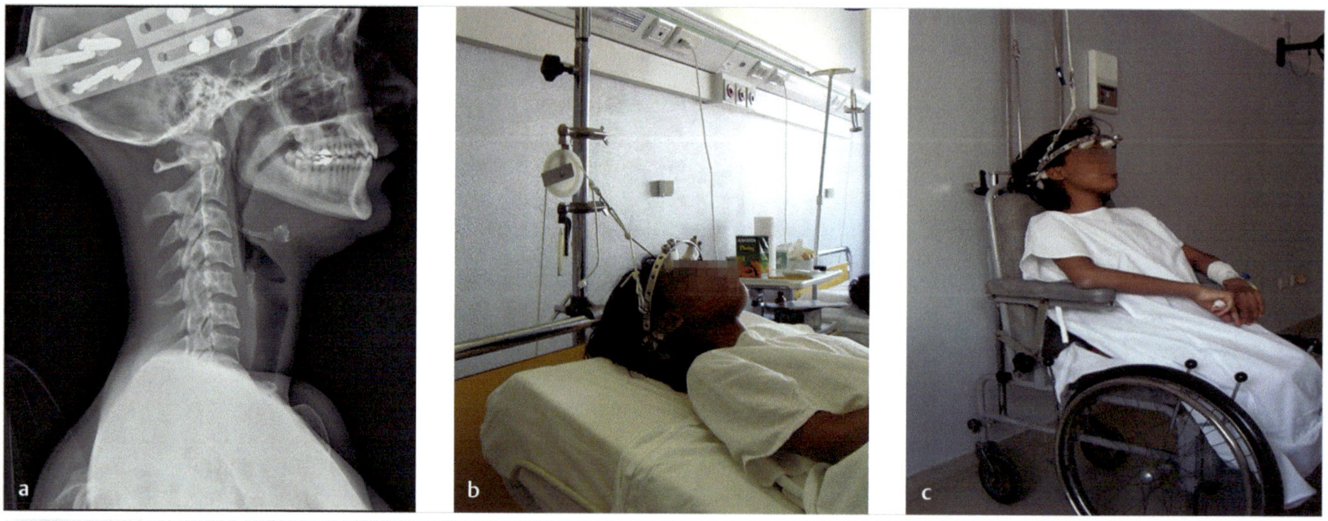

Fig. 13.3 Halo-gravity traction. (a) X-ray of the cervical spine: possible overdistraction of the cervical spine must be avoided. (b) A girl in traction in bed and (c) in the wheelchair.

traction resulted in a safer correction of the scoliosis, increasing the flexibility of the spine and of the chest, and improving pulmonary function. However, it had numerous problems, such as difficulties in daily activities, and possible complications, such as cranial nerve injuries or temporary brachial plexus palsies.

In conclusion, halo traction has been largely used in patients who have severe pulmonary dysfunction, severe spinal deformity, especially when previous surgery has been performed, and severe chest wall deformities and constriction. It is generally contraindicated with congenital kyphosis, with previous spinal cord tumor resections, with residual neurologic deficits, and when cord tethering is present. It is true, however, that traction without spinal release presents no advantage in comparison with immediate spinal fusion with instrumentation.

13.2 Surgical Treatment

Different surgical strategies have been used for severe adolescent idiopathic scoliosis (AIS).

13.2.1 Introduction

Originally, treatment consisted of posterior spinal fusion with Harrington instrumentation, combined with a prolonged period of preoperative halo-traction and respiratory rehabilitation.[10,11]

Later, the most common treatment was anterior release with an open thoracotomy,[12,13,14] followed by a posterior instrumented fusion (▶ Fig. 13.2). Halo-traction was often applied in the time period between the anterior release and posterior instrumentation (▶ Fig. 13.2, ▶ Fig. 13.3).[15] Sometimes, in highly rigid scoliosis, this combined program was preceded by an additional posterior release.[12] The correction rate of severe idiopathic curves with the combined treatment was about 45 to 47%, using Harrington instrumentation[13] or a multiple-hook construct[16]; 52% using Zielke instrumentation with a Harrington rod,[17] and up to 67% using anterior instrumentation and a posterior hybrid construct.[12] The combined anterior and posterior procedure was performed in one- or two-stage surgery according to different authors with different outcomes. Shufflebarger et al[16] found decreased hospital stay and operating time, fewer complications, and better correction in the continuous group compared to the staged group; instead Shen et al[18] concluded that there was no significant difference in safety or efficacy between the one- or two-stage groups. Additional anterior surgery requires increased time for general anesthesia and may have a negative impact on pulmonary function. Kim et al[19] reported that an open anterior approach may have a deleterious effect on pulmonary function for as long as 5 years postoperatively, after surgical treatment of adolescent idiopathic scoliosis. Video-assisted thoracoscopy, used for the anterior release, followed by posterior instrumentation for scoliosis treatment,[20,21,22] can minimize, but not eliminate, the negative effect on pulmonary function, as reported by Newton et al.[22]

Combined anterior and posterior vertebral column resection has been used more often to treat severe congenital and rigid scoliosis, and more rarely, idiopathic curves. This demanding procedure was used by Bradford and Tribus[23] for seven patients with severe idiopathic curves (mean Cobb angle 91 degrees) and achieved an average scoliosis correction of 59%. Suk et al[24] presented the results of vertebral column resection at the apex of the deformity performed through a single posterior approach in 16 cases (six of them with idiopathic curves) in curves >80 degrees, and with a flexibility of less than 25%; the procedure obtained a scoliosis curve mean correction of 59%, with complications in 4 cases, one of the four patients had permanent complete paraplegia. Since these studies were published, the use of vertebral column resection has increased. Recently Lenke[25] presented a paper on his large experience using this procedure, concluding that, when the deformity or imbalance is so severe that other osteotomies cannot correct the deformity, vertebral column resection offers the greatest potential correction.

13.3 Posterior-Only Procedures

The use of thoracic pedicle screws made it possible to reassess the role of posterior-only fusion as treatment for severe.

13.3.1 Pedicle Screws

Previous studies used posterior-only instrumentation with multiple hooks[26] or hybrid construct.[27,28] Burton et al used a varied combination of hooks, wires, and screws[28] in their treatment of patients with adolescent idiopathic scoliosis and thoracic curves between 70 and 90 degrees: They achieved an average curve correction of 64%, and concluded that these curves do not need anterior release to achieve acceptable results. The hybrid construct (thoracic hooks and lower screws) has been used by Arlet et al[27] in cases with thoracic scoliosis between 70 and 90 degrees and has achieved 54% correction.

However, the use of thoracic pedicle screws increased the interest for posterior-only fusion in deformity correction of large-magnitude scoliosis. Luhmann et al[29] compared combined treatment (anterior and posterior fusion) versus posterior fusion only in severe idiopathic scoliosis: they concluded that the patients treated with pedicle-screw-only instrumentation provided results similar to those obtained in patients with combined treatment (60.7% vs. 58.5%), without the negative effects of an anterior release on pulmonary function. Chang[30] used only posterior pedicle screw instrumentation in cases with thoracic scoliosis between 75 and 135 degrees, achieving a correction of 67%. Kuklo et al,[31] used 352 thoracic screws to correct idiopathic scoliosis >90 degrees, and achieved a 68% correction. The scoliosis correction rate of these two studies[30,31] adopting pedicle screws was surprisingly high, similar to that achieved by Bullmann et al,[12] using a combination of anterior instrumentation and a posterior hybrid construct. Most of the literature on the surgical treatment of severe idiopathic thoracic curves shows more contained values, generally lower than 60% regardless of the technique used.[2,17,23,24,27] In severe thoracic scoliosis the aim should not be to maximize the curve correction but to obtain an acceptable balance of the spine and reduce levels of fusion. Furthermore, the risks of a too aggressive posterior-only correction not preceded by an anterior release should not be underestimated. Overdistraction should be avoided, given the risk of spinal cord ischemia (▶ Fig. 13.4).[32] It has been reported that an intraoperative correction exceeding the preoperative bending correction was one of the factors related to an increased risk for spinal cord injury.[33]

Thoracic screw fixation can be potentially dangerous in the surgical treatment of scoliosis.[34,35] The technical difficulties in scoliotic deformities have been emphasized. In severe scoliosis, placement of thoracic screws may present further difficulties. However, the biomechanical advantages associated with their use make screws the ideal construct in large curves.[31] Thoracic screws on the concavity are the crucial anchor points for better scoliosis correction and restoring thoracic kyphosis.[36] Instead, the use of hooks at the apex of severe scoliosis has been shown to be both unreliable and dangerous; they are inside the canal and are thus invasive. It has been found that canal intrusion of a medially placed screw (with a 3-mm breach) is less invasive than a perfectly positioned pediatric laminar hook.[37] Therefore, hooks can sometimes be more dangerous than screws because of their position and can themselves cause complications.[38] Furthermore, hooks ensure a less rigid fixation, which can lead to dislocation during correction maneuvers or, subsequently, due to hook pullout with laminar fractures.

Neurologic complications are rarely reported in the literature in thoracic scoliosis treatment with pedicle screws,[39,40] although medially positioned thoracic screws are quite commonly reported.[41] Kuklo et al[31] reported screw accuracy of 96.3% in severe scoliosis by postoperative CT scanning: 10 screws had a breach of between 2 and 4 mm (three medial and seven lateral), whereas in 3 screws, the breach was 4 mm (two medial and one lateral). The two medial screws (0.57%) were the only ones removed, although there were no neurologic complications. Although the authors claimed that these screws would not be removed by today's standards, their acceptability remains controversial. According to some authors,[42] medial wall penetration ≤ 2 mm is well tolerated, and the screws can be considered acceptably positioned. Other authors[41] have hypothesized a 4-mm "safe zone" of medial encroachment (2 mm of epidural space and 2 mm of subarachnoid space). Still others[43] hypothesize a "definite safe zone" within 2 mm, a "probable safe zone" within 2 and 4 mm, and a "questionable safe zone" of 4 to 8 mm of medial encroachment. Recently, however, Liljenqvist et al[44] showed with MRI that the width of the epidural space was <1 mm at the thoracic apical level on the concave side. This means that there is no safety zone on the concavity; therefore, screw placement, especially at this level, should be very precise.

13.3.2 Posterior Staged Technique

Hui-Min et al[45] used temporary internal distraction as an aid in the correction of severe scoliosis as an alternative for situations in which halo traction is contraindicated. In their report, a temporary internal distraction procedure was performed.

The concept of using an internal distraction rod to correct the coronal and sagittal planes before definitive posterior fusion was suggested by Buchowski et al.[46] The authors implanted conventional growing rods in patients with severe curves and used two distraction procedures to perform a staged correction of the deformities. The use of growing rods for temporary internal distractions could facilitate curve correction by stretching the soft tissues safely. The results showed that only modest correction was found in the second distraction procedure. This phenomenon could be caused by progressive stiffness of the spine because of sudden and forceful distractions at irregular intervals. The main drawback of this procedure is the requirement of patients to undergo multiple operations for distraction of the implanted device. This can lead to high anesthetic risks, wound infection, and other surgical risks. Cheng et al[47] similarly employed two stages for the corrective procedure, first on the concave side by internal distraction of pedicle screws and rods through intramuscular tunnels in the first operation, followed by respiratory function exercises and improving nutritional status during the intervening period, and finally by additional posterior correction, ultimate instrumentation, and spinal fusion in the second operation.

13.4 Preferred Operative Technique

Correction of severe spinal deformities presents a very high incidence of risks related to neurologic deficits and to compromised

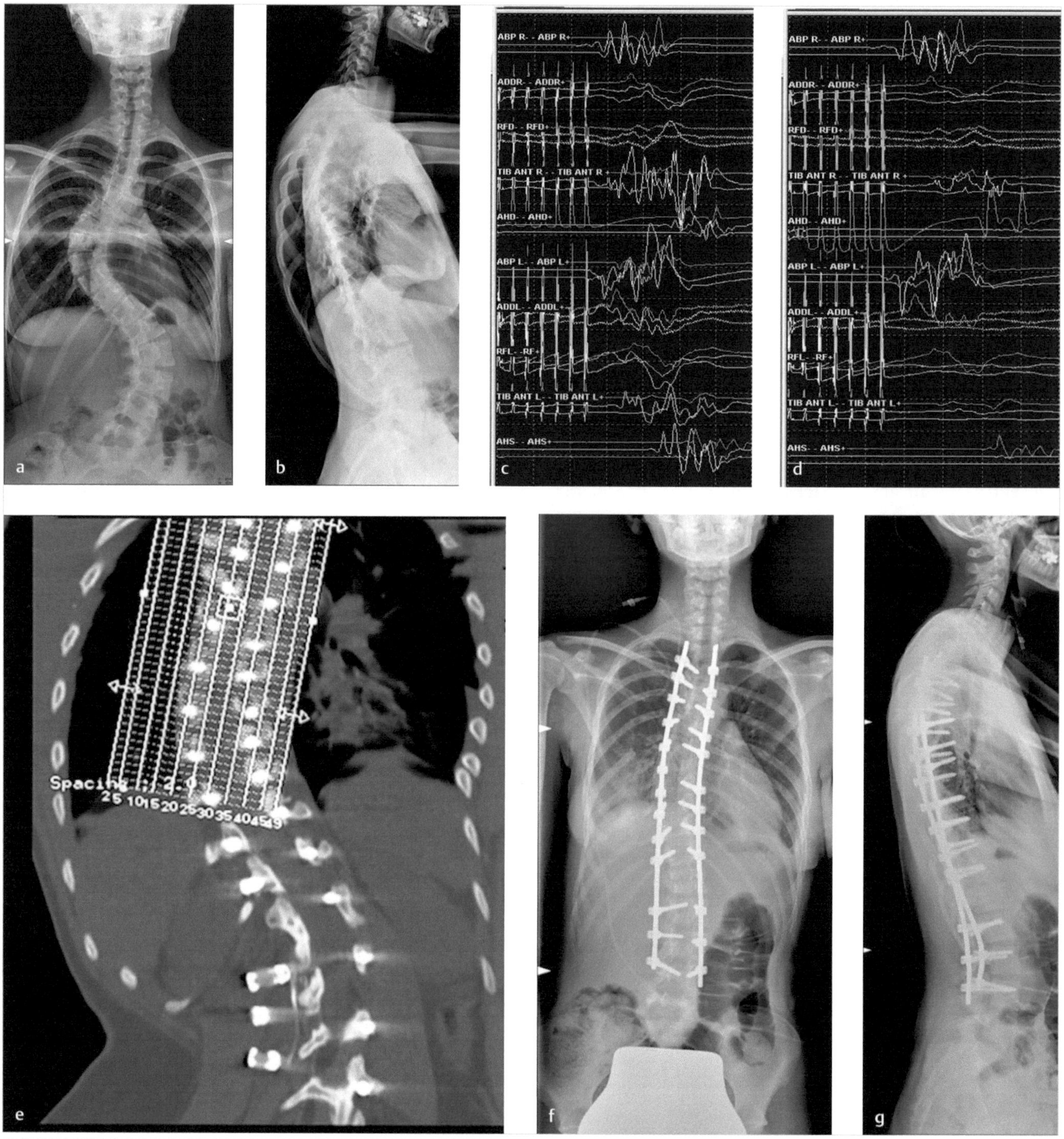

Fig. 13.4 (a, b) A 16-year-old girl underwent posterior correction without having undergone prior halo-traction. **(c, d)** Intraoperatively, there was a persistent and severe reduction in amplitude of somatosensory and motor-evoked potentials after scoliosis correction. The rods were removed immediately. The wake-up test resulted in a return to normal, and there was no deficit at the end of surgery. The surgery was terminated with the screws left inside. **(e)** CT scan done on the postoperative day confirmed the correct placement of the screws. **(f, g)** After a week a new surgery was performed for definitive correction without problems.

pulmonary function and malnutrition. It is, therefore, risky for these patients to undergo aggressive operations, such as combined anterior–posterior surgery and vertebral column resection. A posterior-only approach to the deformity with less aggressive osteotomies seems to be preferable for the patient. Similarly a posterior-only one-stage procedure can expose the patient to neurologic complications without a gradual period of traction. In severe scoliosis, our preferred strategy in recent years has consisted of a period of halo-gravity traction followed by posterior-only surgery (aggressive release with Ponte osteotomies at many levels and instrumented fusion) (▶ Fig. 13.5, ▶ Fig. 13.6). Preoperative halo traction is one method available, but there are

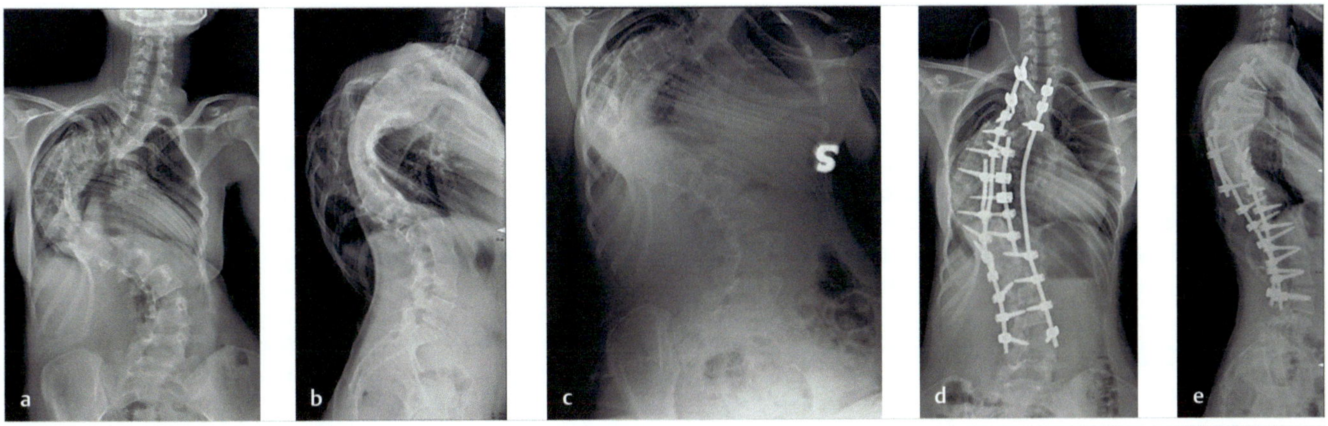

Fig. 13.5 A 15-year-old girl with severe scoliosis **(a–c)** treated with preoperative halo-traction: (X-ray after 21 days of traction). **(d, e)** Treatment consisted in a posterior instrumented fusion with aggressive posterior release and thoracoplasty.

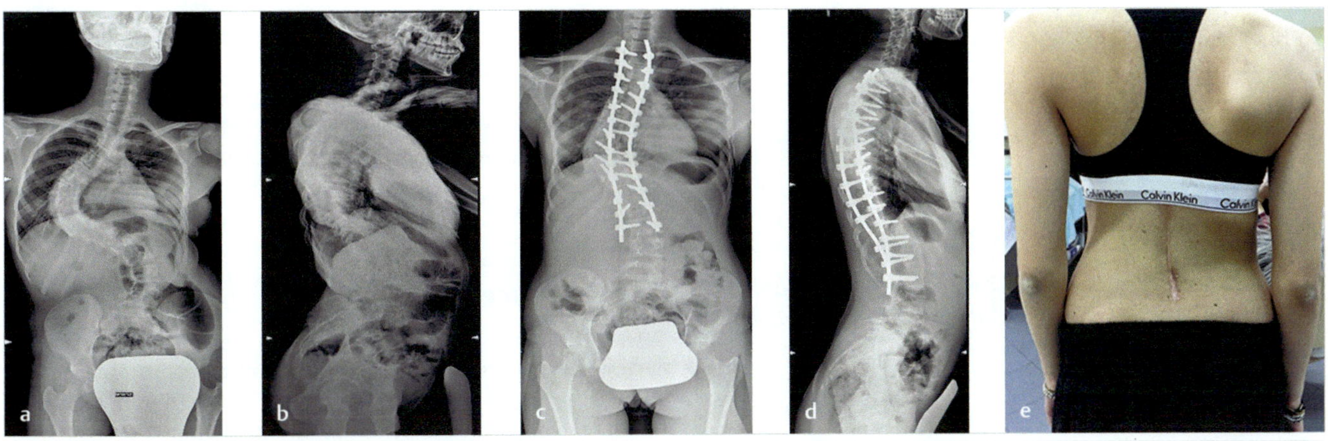

Fig. 13.6 A 14-year-old girl with **(a, b)** severe idiopathic scoliosis treated with preoperative halo-traction, and **(c, d)** posterior instrumented fusion with multilevel posterior release and thoracoplasty, with **(e)** a good clinical result.

controversies regarding its efficacy when compared with the non–halo traction group.[9]

To optimize surgical correction and minimize operative risks and complications, a two-stage posterior-only approach is safer for treatment of severe scoliosis. Internal distraction devices have been proposed for deformity correction. Some have adopted the use of conventional growing rods, and others have used intraoperative skeletal traction. These procedures can allow staged correction of deformities but may require multiple surgeries. In addition, intraoperative traction has been shown to lead to changes in the motor evoked potential (MEP).

13.4.1 Magnetically Controlled Growing Rod

The use of an MCGR(MAGEC; Ellipse Technologies, Inc.) has been proposed for gradual and safe correction of deformities. The correction is performed over a series of distractions of the implanted device using an external magnet.[48] This device has been studied in animals,[49] and it has been used in human subjects.[50] Cheung et al[48] report on the case of a girl with severe kyphoscoliosis and concurrent syringomyelia and Arnold–Chiari type 1 malformation treated with this novel approach, using the MCGR for gradual daily correction of the deformity. Although the original indication for the use of this device is to correct scoliosis deformities while allowing for spinal growth, it has been extended to gradual correction of severe spinal deformities by applying the technology of noninvasive distraction.

The MCGR is an internal distraction device and hence a major advantage over halo traction and growing rods because it can potentially be performed on an outpatient basis, thereby limiting the patients' hospitalization time, the time away from work for parents, and the number of operations required with the associated anesthetic and surgical risks.[48] In addition, the distraction is manually controlled and can be applied with the patient awake, which provides the best form of neurologic monitoring. Daily distraction procedures were performed to avoid progressive stiffness or autofusion of the spinal segments associated with growing rods. Preliminary clinical results of the MCGR in early-onset scoliosis have been published, and the results are promising.[51]

The procedure adopted by the author as the preferred method in the last years for problems related to the use of halo-gravity: a two-staged posterior surgery, using MCGR correction, was preferred.

The first surgery is a posterior aggressive release with Ponte osteotomies at many levels with screws implanted. A magnetic expanding rod is implanted on the concavity of the scoliotic curve. Later, in the postoperative period, a distraction is applied obtaining gradually correction of the curve. A CT study is used to evaluate the screws. In the second posterior surgery, the magnetic rod is removed and the definitive rods (in general three or four) are applied for definitive correction. The procedure is completed by thoracoplasty, and the bone chips obtained from resected ribs are used for definitive fusion.

13.4.2 Intraoperative Monitoring of Spinal Cord Function

Intraoperative monitoring of spinal cord function is mandatory in all patients by recording somatosensory evoked potentials (SSEPs) and transcranial electric stimulation–motor evoked potentials (TES-MEPs). A neurophysiologic change was defined as relevant when it consisted of a persistent unilateral or bilateral reduction in amplitude of 50% for SSEPs and of 65% for TES-MEPs compared with baseline. The wake-up test is performed intraoperatively in only a limited number of cases due to particular technical difficulties in acquiring the evoked responses.

13.4.3 First Posterior Surgery

The first posterior surgery is characterized by exposure of the posterior elements of the spine. In this first procedure, the surgical steps are placement of screws, aggressive release (Ponte osteotomies) and sometimes thoracic pedicle subtraction osteotomy at the apical vertebra, and implantation of the MCGR.

Screw Placement

The use of thoracic pedicle screws has become increasingly widespread in the treatment of scoliosis and has led to a significant improvement in deformity correction, even in large-magnitude curves. However, the use of thoracic screws in scoliosis remains controversial because of the technical difficulties and the risk of complications.[34] Various techniques are used to make thoracic pedicle screw placement safer, from guide pins inserted into the pedicles[40] to the C-arm intensifier,[52] from triggered electromyography[53] to image-guided systems based on CT.[54] Electromyographic monitoring appeared to be of limited value in the thoracic spine: in the study by Reidy et al[53] postoperative CT showed that 8.8% of screws had breached the walls of the pedicle; thus the monitoring had not significantly improved the reliability of safe thoracic screw placement. Computer-assisted screw pedicle installation permitted increased accuracy in placing screws and thus decreased the incidence of misplaced screws,[54] but the method entails preoperative CT scanning, high costs, and a longer operative period.

Safe methods for thoracic screw placement include the "anatomical" techniques, such as the freehand method[55] and the open-lamina technique[56]: the latter provides direct visualization of the medial wall of the pedicle. A method similar to the open-lamina technique that is more economical in resecting the lamina is the mini-laminotomy,[57,58] which allows palpation of the borders of the thoracic pedicles with a spatula inside the canal. This procedure, combined with the freehand technique, is very safe for apical vertebra on the concavity. For the other levels a simple freehand technique is preferred.

Mini-laminotomy Technique

A mini-laminotomy is performed in the cephalad part of the lamina.[58] After excision of the spinous process, the ligamentum flavum is completely removed with a small portion of the lamina in the upper part. This technique allows for inspection with a spatula inside the canal of the superior, medial, and inferior borders of the pedicle, and is the first portion of the posterior release, which is then completed more laterally, once all screws have been placed. Gelfoam is applied to control bleeding from the canal.

Pedicle Entry Point

Besides the probe inside the canal, to determine the pedicle entry point, the well-known anatomical landmarks are used.[40] The entry point at T11 and T12 is checked at the junction of the bisected transverse process and lamina at the lateral aspect of the pars; for the vertebrae of the midthoracic region, the entry point is more medial and cephalad, whereas above the midthoracic vertebrae, the entry point tends to be slightly lateral and caudad.[40]

Screw Placement

The presumed pedicle entry point was prepared with a rongeur. The pedicle was entered using a small curet: the instrument was inserted by applying mild pressure for 30 mm in the proximal thoracic pedicles, for 35 mm in the midthoracic region, and for 40 to 45 mm for the lower thoracic pedicles, directed along the axis of the pedicle in the frontal and sagittal plane. The screw tract inside the pedicle was checked with a pedicle probe to palpate distinct bony borders. Pedicle screws were inserted with a slow and gentle force using a screw diameter corresponding to about 80% of the pedicle diameter. In severe scoliosis, a preoperative CT can be useful to evaluate diameter and morphology of the concave pedicle. The screw length was chosen to be about 70% of the vertebral body on lateral fluoroscopy. The direction of the screw is more convergent medially in the upper thoracic spine, whereas it was convergent in the midthoracic spine and quite straight at T11 and T12. Screw placement must be confirmed by fluoroscopy using the anteroposterior, lateral, and oblique views. The oblique view permits a further check for screw placement inside the pedicle and also for the tip of the screw and the anterior border of the vertebral body. That way, if the tip of the screw is beyond the anterior border of the body, it is immediately removed, its tract is palpated, and a new screw is inserted with the appropriate shorter length.

There is no consensus of opinion in the literature as to the criteria for determining which asymptomatic malpositioned screws must be revised and which must be observed. With regard to lateral malpositioned screws, they should be prophylactically revised, despite being asymptomatic, if they are in direct proximity to the thoracic aorta (<5 mm), due to the risk of possible subsequent vascular lesions; otherwise, malposi-

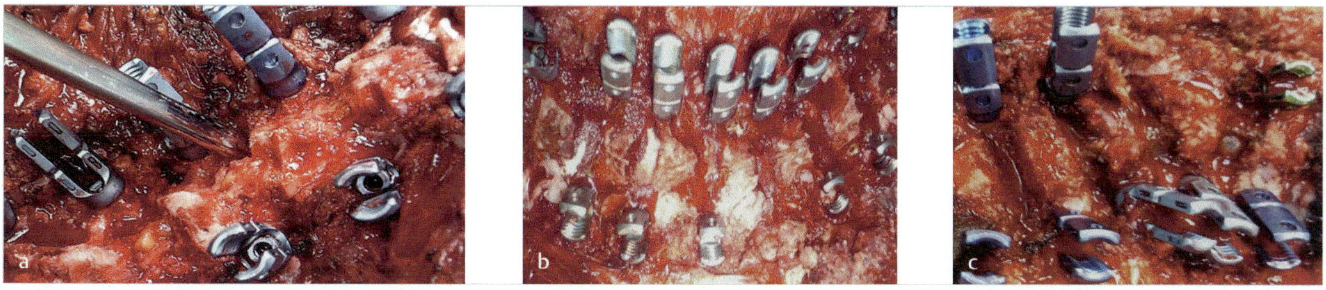

Fig. 13.7 Ponte osteotomy: **(a–c)** It is a generous posterior resection of the superior and inferior part of the lamina with the ligamentum flavum, with the complete resection of the superior and inferior facets bilaterally. Previously during exposure of the spine, spinous process and interspinous ligaments have been removed. At each level of a Ponte osteotomy, a gap of at least 6 mm is created.

tioned screws with moderate lateral cortical perforation (range, 3–6 mm) can be left where they are. On the contrary, long screws must always be removed. Medial wall penetration of 2 mm would appear well tolerated and the screws can be considered acceptably positioned, although in one study,[44] MRI revealed that the width of the epidural space was <1 mm at the thoracic apical level on the concavity. Our previous study[58] reviewed 115 consecutive patients who underwent posterior instrumented fusion in our department (1999–2001) performed by three different surgeons using 1,035 transpedicular thoracic screws. Eighteen screws (1.7%) were misplaced in 13 patients (11.3%). Postoperative CT was performed, however, in 25 of the 115 patients (21.7%) when standard and oblique postoperative radiographs raised well-founded doubts regarding the positioning of 30 screws. Therefore, compared with the 311 screws examined by CT, these 18 misplaced screws represented instead 5.7% (i.e., a much higher rate).

Posterior Release

After screw placement, the posterior release is realized using Ponte osteotomies at many levels (▶ Fig. 13.7). Ponte osteotomies are posterior shortening procedures introduced for Scheuermann kyphosis[59] treatment and subsequently used in the treatment of scoliosis. The procedure is realized through a generous posterior resection of the superior and inferior lamina with the ligamentum flavum as well as the complete resection of the superior and inferior facets bilaterally. Previously, during exposure of the spine, spinous process and interspinous ligaments have been removed at each level, leaving them in place for just the first three upper levels of fusion to avoid junctional problems. Thus, at each level of a Ponte osteotomy, a gap of at least 6 mm is created. On the concavity, during bone resection, a spatula must be insert to protect the cord. Large undercutting of the lamina is crucial to prevent spinal cord compression when the gaps created are closed during correction of scoliosis.

Pedicle Subtraction Osteotomy

A pedicle subtraction osteotomy (▶ Fig. 13.8) is performed at the apical vertebra of severe scoliosis presenting a main thoracic curve with a Cobb angle >100 degrees[60]: the procedure was preferred to apical vertebral resection, which involves the resection of one or more vertebral levels and presents higher risks for complications.

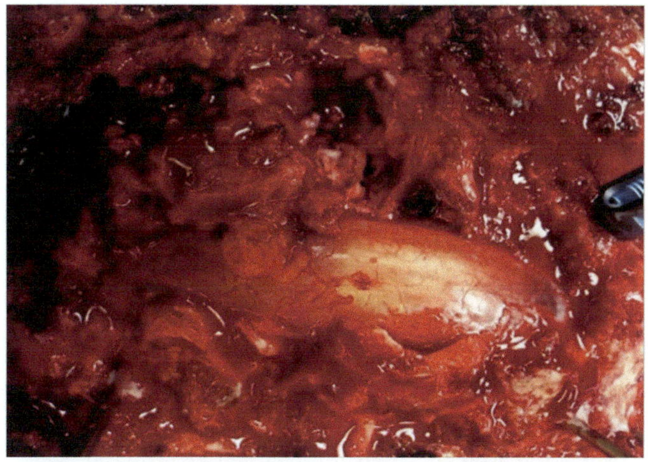

Fig. 13.8 Thoracic pedicle subtraction osteotomy. A pedicle subtraction osteotomy is performed at the apical vertebra of scoliosis presenting a main thoracic curve with a Cobb angle >100 degrees. A wide laminectomy is performed over the apical level with the entire lamina of the cephalad and caudal vertebrae being removed. The spinal cord and the emergence of the corresponding roots must be well exposed. It is better to remove both pedicles, not only the pedicle on the convex side, to provide a more effective correction.

A wide laminectomy is performed over the apical level with the entire lamina of the cephalad and caudal vertebrae being removed. The spinal cord and the emergence of the corresponding roots must be well exposed. Then the pedicles to be resected are encircled, and removal of the vertebral body is started (more aggressive on the convexity of the curve) by means of straight and curved curets through a lateral pedicle-body entrance. It is better to remove both pedicles, not only the pedicle on convex side, to provide a more effective correction. Finally a posterior-based closing wedge osteotomy is performed, quite similar to a lumbar osteotomy used for sagittal imbalance of the spine. It is very important to minimize epidural and osseous blood loss during this surgery, not only with careful subperiosteal stripping of the posterior vertebral elements, but also with the continuous use of adjunctive hemostatic agents. Before starting bone resection of the osteotomy, two short rods are implanted to stabilize above and below the level to be resected. Upon completion of the procedure, compression across the pedicle screws closes the osteotomy. The short rods can be left in the site.

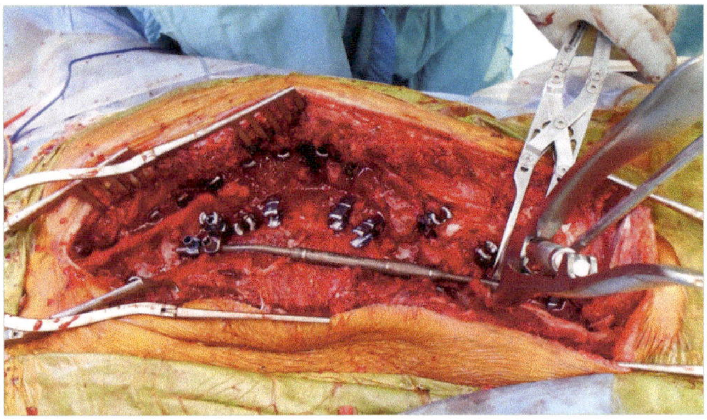

Fig. 13.9 A magnetically controlled growing rod is inserted on the concave side of the thoracic curve, in general between T 3–T 4 and L 1–L 2. A first distraction is performed intraoperatively. The other screws were preinserted for the later definitive correction.

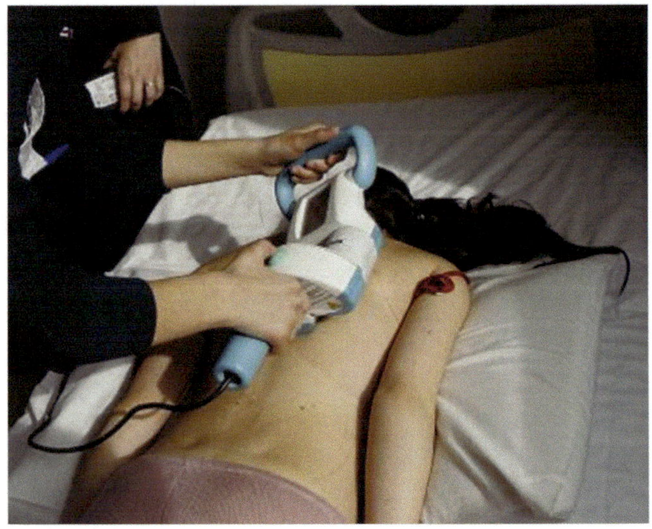

Fig. 13.10 Distraction of the magnetically controlled growing rod in the days after the first posterior surgery, using an external magnet.

Magnetically Controlled Growing Rod

Before implanting the MCGR, a very short convex rod (limited to the apical vertebra) is implanted in compression, in general in sites of multilevel aggressive release or eventually thoracic pedicle subtraction osteotomy (▶ Fig. 13.9). The other two short rods are implanted, one in the lumbar levels and the other in the upper thoracic site to align the spine.

The short convex rod is removed and the MGCR is inserted on the concave side of the thoracic curve, in general between T3-T4 and L1-L2. It is better not to prebend the rod to avoid harming the magnetic mechanism of the rod. Before implantation, it is necessary to distract the rod to confirm its effectiveness. A first distraction is performed intraoperatively. The other screws were preinserted for the later definitive correction. Surgery must be stopped for about 15 minutes to check MEPs and SSEPs, which must remain the same as baseline values. In cases of changed MEPs and SSEPs a wake-up test is performed prior to the end of surgery.

Distractions can start 3 days postsurgery (▶ Fig. 13.10). Distraction is started at 2 mm per day under screening using a CT control, at 7 days and again 14 days later. CT is also useful for controlling the correct screw insertion. At postoperative 2 weeks, 2 cm total distraction is obtained. In cases of back pain after distraction, the amount of daily distractions can be slowed to 1 mm distraction per day. The young patient is fully ambulant throughout all the distraction procedures and is able to perform the activities of daily living.

After postoperative 2 weeks, in general it is difficult to improve the scoliosis correction obtained and it is better to do the second phase of surgery: the advantage being a simple exposure of the spine. In general, the correction obtained after this program of distraction is around 40% of the scoliosis.

13.4.4 Second Stage of Posterior Surgery

The second surgery consists of removal of the MCGR and other temporary rods. The first step is to implant a short convex rod for a gentle maneuver of derotation. Then, the long concave rod and finally a long convex rod connected with the previous short rod are implanted. Again surgery must be stopped for about 15 minutes to check MEPs and SSEPs, which must remain at baseline values. In the case of changes, a wake-up test is performed before the end of surgery. After the definitive instrumentation and fusion of the instrumented area, a thoracoplasty is performed to improve the clinical result (▶ Fig. 13.11).

Derotation

In severe scoliosis it is also possible to use direct derotation maneuvers. The flexibility index must be around, but not less than, 40%. In the direct vertebral rotation introduced by Lee et al,[61] during or after the concave rod rotation, screw derotators, which are inserted into the juxta-apical screws on the concave and convex sides, are rotated to the opposite direction of rod rotation. On the contrary, the vertebral coplanar alignment proposed by Vallespir et al[62] used slotted tubes attached to monoaxial convex screws.

The rod must be short and limited to the convex apical vertebra only. The idea of Vallespir et al[62] to consider derotation on the convex side of the scoliosis can be very effective in these severe curves. The derotation is done with an en bloc maneuver applied to the apical screws only: the convex screws are not tightened. Concurrently, an assistant applies a force on the rib prominence. Once the maneuver has been completed, the set apical screws are tightened. The entire derotation procedure requires about 20 minutes. The procedure cannot avoid thoracoplasty because of the incomplete effect of derotation on the severe rib hump. The direct rotation can expose the patient to neurologic risks: the use of SSEPs and MEPs is strongly recommended and avoids neurologic deficits. Monoaxial screws can significantly improve the vertebral derotation effect, as other authors have maintained,[63] but in severe scoliosis during derotation maneuvers screw pullout is possible, so uniplanar screws could be better to use.

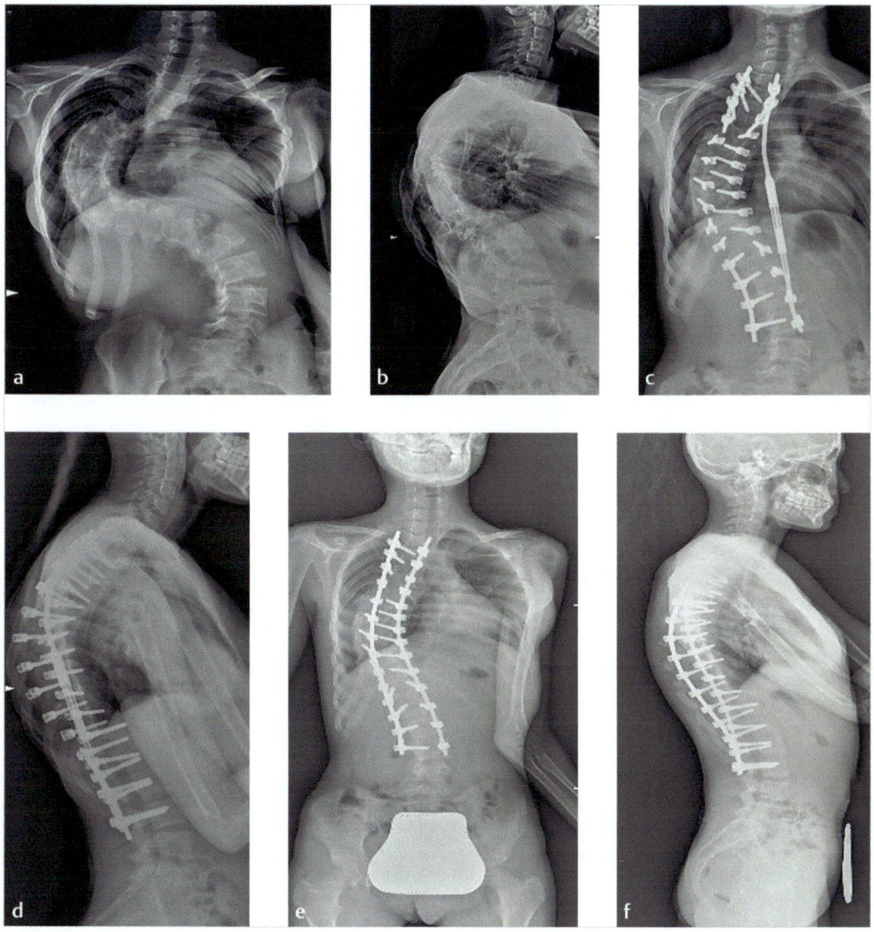

Fig. 13.11 **(a, b)** A 17-year-old boy with severe idiopathic scoliosis, treated with a two-staged posterior surgery using a magnetically controlled growing rod (MCGR). The first surgery consists of a posterior aggressive release with Ponte osteotomies at many levels with implantation of screws. **(c, d)** An MCGR is implanted on the concavity of the scoliotic curve: later, in the postoperative period, a distraction is applied obtaining gradual correction of the curve. **(e, f)** In the second posterior surgery, the MCGR is removed and definitive rods are applied for definitive correction, completing surgery with thoracoplasty.

Definitive Instrumentation

Generally the definitive rod alloy implanted is titanium. Polyaxial screws are used for severe scoliosis in periapical sites to reduce the difficulties of rod capture. For the concave rod a cobalt-chrome alloy is sometimes preferred as its inherent stiffness permits a better correction of scoliosis curve and thoracic hypokyphosis. Different rods are implanted. A short one is applied on the convex apical vertebrae. A long rod is applied on the concavity of the curve. And a third, long rod is applied on the convexity of the scoliosis, connected with the previous short one.

Thoracoplasty

Thoracoplasty completes the surgery. The skin incision is the same as that for the previous procedure. The thoracolumbar fascia needs to be incised and elevated. A finger is slipped between the fascia and the paravertebral muscles. The fascia is then retracted toward the convexity of the curve over the rib deformity. The single ribs are then palpated, and the muscle covering the rib is incised with electrocautery, through to the periosteum. In general, four to six ribs must be incised. The periosteum must be pulled off the surface of the rib completely (upper and inferior edge of the rib). After that the periosteum is stripped underneath the rib. A Doyen elevator is passed: the rib is completely free from the periosteum, and the rib is resected with a rib cutter. The rib resection is around, but not more than, 4 cm to avoid a concavity where the original rib deformity was. It is important to resect different ribs and to reduce the length of resection in proximal and distal ribs. The suture of the periosteum and paravertebral muscles must be very accurate. The water test (Valsalva maneuver three times to see air bubbles to look for a leak in the pleura) is not always mandatory. Pleural effusion may develop postoperatively, without a leak, as the result of trauma to the pleura. It is better to insert a chest tube in every patient immediately at the end of the suture to avoid a quite painful and frightening thoracentesis for young patients days after surgery.

Finally the procedure is finished. No braces are used in the postoperative weeks due to the stability of the applied screw instrumentation.

13.5 Conclusion

In conclusion, to optimize surgical correction and minimize operative risks and complications, a two-stage, posterior-only approach can be safer for treatment of severe adolescent idiopathic scoliosis. The first surgery is a posterior aggressive release with Ponte osteotomies at many levels with implantation of multiple pedicle screws: an MCGR is implanted on the concavity of the scoliotic curve. Later, in the postoperative period, a distraction is applied to obtain gradual correction of the curve. The correction is performed over a series of distractions of the implanted device using an external magnet. In the second posterior surgery, the magnetic rod is removed, and the definitive rods are applied for final correction and fusion. Generally, a thoracoplasty is performed to improve the clinical result.

References

[1] O'Brien MF, Lenke LG, Bridwell KH, Blanke K, Baldus C. Preoperative spinal canal investigation in adolescent idiopathic scoliosis curves > or = 70 °. Spine. 1994; 19(14):1606–1610

[2] Tokunaga M, Minami S, Kitahara H, Isobe K, Nakata Y, Moriya H. Vertebral decancellation for severe scoliosis. Spine. 2000; 25(4):469–474

[3] Greiner KA. Adolescent idiopathic scoliosis: radiologic decision-making. Am Fam Physician. 2002; 65(9):1817–1822

[4] Sucato DJ. Management of severe spinal deformity: scoliosis and kyphosis. Spine. 2010; 35(25):2186–2192

[5] Perry J, Nickel VL. Total cervicalspine fusion for neck paralysis. J Bone Joint Surg Am. 1959; 41-A(1):37–60

[6] Stagnara P. Cranial traction using the "Halo" of rancho los amigos. Rev Chir Orthop Repar Appar Mot. 1971; 57(4):287–300

[7] Koptan W, ElMiligui Y. Three-staged correction of severe rigid idiopathic scoliosis using limited halo-gravity traction. Eur Spine J. 2012; 21(6):1091–1098

[8] Clark JA, Hsu LCS, Yau AC. Viscoelastic behaviour of deformed spines under correction with halo pelvic distraction. Clin Orthop Relat Res. 1975(110):90–111

[9] Sponseller PD, Takenaga RK, Newton P, et al. The use of traction in the treatment of severe spinal deformity. Spine. 2008; 33(21):2305–2309

[10] Pellin B, Zielke K. Severe scoliosis in adults and older, adolescents. 41 operated cases [in French]. Rev Chir Orthop Repar Appar Mot. 1974; 60(8):623–633

[11] Savini R, Parisini P, Corbascio M, Prosperi L. Halo-traction associated with kinesitherapy in the corrective treatment of scoliosis with severe respiratory insufficiency [in Italian]. Chir Organi Mov. 1977; 64(4):353–360

[12] Bullmann V, Halm HFH, Schulte T, Lerner T, Weber TP, Liljenqvist UR. Combined anterior and posterior instrumentation in severe and rigid idiopathic scoliosis. Eur Spine J. 2006; 15(4):440–448

[13] Byrd JA, III, Scoles PV, Winter RB, Bradford DS, Lonstein JE, Moe JH. Adult idiopathic scoliosis treated by anterior and posterior spinal fusion. J Bone Joint Surg Am. 1987; 69(6):843–850

[14] Savini R, Parisini P. The surgical correction of severe vertebral deformities by combined anterior and posterior instrumentation. Prog Spinal Pathol. 1989; 4:211–221

[15] Rinella A, Lenke L, Whitaker C, et al. Perioperative halo-gravity traction in the treatment of severe scoliosis and kyphosis. Spine. 2005; 30(4):475–482

[16] Shufflebarger HL, Grimm JO, Bui V, Thomson JD. Anterior and posterior spinal fusion. Staged versus same-day surgery. Spine. 1991; 16(8):930–933

[17] Korovessis P. Combined VDS and Harrington instrumentation for treatment of idiopathic double major curves. Spine. 1987; 12(3):244–250

[18] Shen J, Qiu G, Wang Y, Zhang Z, Zhao Y. Comparison of 1-stage versus 2-stage anterior and posterior spinal fusion for severe and rigid idiopathic scoliosis–a randomized prospective study. Spine. 2006; 31(22):2525–2528

[19] Kim YJ, Lenke LG, Bridwell KH, Kim KL, Steger-May K. Pulmonary function in adolescent idiopathic scoliosis relative to the surgical procedure. J Bone Joint Surg Am. 2005; 87(7):1534–1541

[20] Arlet V. Anterior thoracoscopic spine release in deformity surgery: a meta-analysis and review. Eur Spine J. 2000; 9 Suppl 1:S17–S23

[21] Lenke LG. Anterior endoscopic discectomy and fusion for adolescent idiopathic scoliosis. Spine. 2003; 28(15) Suppl:S36–S43

[22] Newton PO, Marks M, Faro F, et al. Use of video-assisted thoracoscopic surgery to reduce perioperative morbidity in scoliosis surgery. Spine. 2003; 28 (20):S249–S254

[23] Bradford DS, Tribus CB. Vertebral column resection for the treatment of rigid coronal decompensation. Spine. 1997; 22(14):1590–1599

[24] Suk SI, Chung ER, Kim JH, Kim SS, Lee JS, Choi WK. Posterior vertebral column resection for severe rigid scoliosis. Spine. 2005; 30(14):1682–1687

[25] Saifi C, Laratta JL, Petridis P, Shillingford JN, Lehman RA, Lenke LG. Vertebral column resection for rigid spine deformity. Global Spine J. 2017; 7(3):280–290

[26] De Giorgi G, Stella G, Becchetti S, Martucci G, Miscioscia D. Cotrel-Dubousset instrumentation for the treatment of severe scoliosis. Eur Spine J. 1999; 8 (1):8–15

[27] Arlet V, Jiang L, Ouellet J. Is there a need for anterior release for 70–90 thoracic curves in adolescent scoliosis. Eur Spine J. 2004; 13:740–745

[28] Burton DC, Sama AA, Asher MA, et al. The treatment of large (> 70 degrees) thoracic idiopathic scoliosis curves with posterior instrumentation and arthrodesis: when is anterior release indicated? Spine. 2005; 30(17):1979–1984

[29] Luhmann SJ, Lenke LG, Kim YJ, Bridwell KH, Schootman M. Thoracic adolescent idiopathic scoliosis curves between 70 degrees and 100 degrees: is anterior release necessary? Spine. 2005; 30(18):2061–2067

[30] Chang KW. Cantilever bending technique for treatment of large and rigid scoliosis. Spine. 2003; 28(21):2452–2458

[31] Kuklo TR, Lenke LG, O'Brien MF, Lehman RA, Jr, Polly DW, Jr, Schroeder TM. Accuracy and efficacy of thoracic pedicle screws in curves more than 90 degrees. Spine. 2005; 30(2):222–226

[32] Delank KS, Delank HW, König DP, Popken F, Fürderer S, Eysel P. Iatrogenic paraplegia in spinal surgery. Arch Orthop Trauma Surg. 2005; 125(1):33–41

[33] Wilber RG, Thompson GH, Shaffer JW, Brown RH, Nash CL, Jr. Postoperative neurological deficits in segmental spinal instrumentation. A study using spinal cord monitoring. J Bone Joint Surg Am. 1984; 66(8):1178–1187

[34] Mulholland RC. Pedicle screw fixation in the spine. J Bone Joint Surg Br. 1994; 76(4):517–519

[35] Vaccaro AR, Rizzolo SJ, Allardyce TJ, et al. Placement of pedicle screws in the thoracic spine. Part I: Morphometric analysis of the thoracic vertebrae. J Bone Joint Surg Am. 1995; 77(8):1193–1199

[36] Suk SI, Lee CK, Min HJ, Cho KH, Oh JH. Comparison of Cotrel-Dubousset pedicle screws and hooks in the treatment of idiopathic scoliosis. Int Orthop. 1994; 18(6):341–346

[37] Polly DW, Jr, Potter BK, Kuklo T, Young S, Johnson C, Klemme WR. Volumetric spinal canal intrusion: a comparison between thoracic pedicle screws and thoracic hooks. Spine. 2004; 29(1):63–69

[38] Been HD, Kalkman CJ, Traast HS, Ongerboer de Visser BW. Neurologic injury after insertion of laminar hooks during Cotrel-Dubousset instrumentation. Spine. 1994; 19(12):1402–1405

[39] Papin P, Arlet V, Marchesi D, Rosenblatt B, Aebi M. Unusual presentation of spinal cord compression related to misplaced pedicle screws in thoracic scoliosis. Eur Spine J. 1999; 8(2):156–159

[40] Suk SI, Kim WJ, Lee SM, Kim JH, Chung ER. Thoracic pedicle screw fixation in spinal deformities: are they really safe? Spine. 2001; 26(18):2049–2057

[41] Belmont PJ, Jr, Klemme WR, Dhawan A, Polly DW, Jr. In vivo accuracy of thoracic pedicle screws. Spine. 2001; 26(21):2340–2346

[42] Liljenqvist UR, Halm HF, Link TM. Pedicle screw instrumentation of the thoracic spine in idiopathic scoliosis. Spine. 1997; 22(19):2239–2245

[43] Gertzbein SD, Robbins SE. Accuracy of pedicular screw placement in vivo. Spine. 1990; 15(1):11–14

[44] Liljenqvist UR, Allkemper T, Hackenberg L, Link TM, Steinbeck J, Halm HF. Analysis of vertebral morphology in idiopathic scoliosis with use of magnetic resonance imaging and multiplanar reconstruction. J Bone Joint Surg Am. 2002; 84-A(3):359–368

[45] Hui-Min H, Hua H, Hai-Ping Z, et al. The impact of posterior temporary internal distraction on stepwise corrective surgery for extremely severe and rigid scoliosis greater than 130°. Eur Spine J. 2012. DOI: 10.1007/s00586-015-4013-z

[46] Buchowski JM, Bhatnagar R, Skaggs DL, Sponseller PD. Temporary internal distraction as an aid to correction of severe scoliosis. J Bone Joint Surg Am. 2006; 88(9):2035–2041

[47] Cheng X, Ma H, Tan R, Wu J, Zhou J, Zou D. Two-stage posterior-only procedures for correction of severe spinal deformities. Arch Orthop Trauma Surg. 2012; 132(2):193–201

[48] Cheung JP-Y, Samartzis D, Cheung KM-C. A novel approach to gradual correction of severe spinal deformity in a pediatric patient using the magnetically-controlled growing rod. Spine J. 2014; 14(7):e7–e13

[49] Akbarnia BA, Mundis G, Salari P, et al. Innovation in growing rod technique; study of safety and efficacy of remotely expandable rod in animal model. J Child Orthop. 2009; 3:513–514

[50] Cheung KM, Cheung JP, Samartzis D, et al. Magnetically controlled growing rods for severe spinal curvature in young children: a prospective case series. Lancet. 2012; 379(9830):1967–1974

[51] Akbarnia BA, Cheung K, Noordeen H, et al. Next generation of growth-sparing techniques: preliminary clinical results of a magnetically controlled growing rod in 14 patients with early-onset scoliosis. Spine. 2013; 38(8):665–670

[52] Liljenqvist U, Lepsien U, Hackenberg L, Niemeyer T, Halm H. Comparative analysis of pedicle screw and hook instrumentation in posterior correction and fusion of idiopathic thoracic scoliosis. Eur Spine J. 2002; 11(4):336–343

[53] Reidy DP, Houlden D, Nolan PC, Kim M, Finkelstein JA. Evaluation of electromyographic monitoring during insertion of thoracic pedicle screws. J Bone Joint Surg Br. 2001; 83(7):1009–1014

[54] Amiot L-P, Lang K, Putzier M, Zippel H, Labelle H. Comparative results between conventional and computer-assisted pedicle screw installation in the thoracic, lumbar, and sacral spine. Spine. 2000; 25(5):606–614

[55] Kim YJ, Lenke LG, Bridwell KH, Cho YS, Riew KD. Free hand pedicle screw placement in the thoracic spine: is it safe? Spine. 2004; 29(3):333–342, discussion 342

[56] Xu R, Ebraheim NA, Ou Y, Yeasting RA. Anatomic considerations of pedicle screw placement in the thoracic spine. Roy-Camille technique versus open-lamina technique. Spine. 1998; 23(9):1065–1068

[57] Kabins MB. Point of view. Spine. 2004; 29:342

[58] Di Silvestre M, Parisini P, Lolli F, Bakaloudis G. Complications of thoracic pedicle screws in scoliosis treatment. Spine. 2007; 32(15):1655–1661

[59] Ponte A. Posterior column shortening for Scheuermann's kyphosis: An innovative one-stage technique. In: Haher TR, ed. Surgical Techniques for the Spine. New York: Thieme; 2003:107–113

[60] Bakaloudis G, Lolli F, Di Silvestre M, et al. Thoracic pedicle subtraction osteotomy in the treatment of severe pediatric deformities. Eur Spine J. 2011; 20 Suppl 1:S95–S104

[61] Lee SM, Suk SI, Chung ER. Direct vertebral rotation: a new technique of three-dimensional deformity correction with segmental pedicle screw fixation in adolescent idiopathic scoliosis. Spine. 2004; 29(3):343–349

[62] Vallespir GP, Flores JB, Trigueros IS, et al. Vertebral coplanar alignment: a standardized technique for three dimensional correction in scoliosis surgery: technical description and preliminary results in Lenke type 1 curves. Spine. 2008; 33(14):1588–1597

[63] Dalal A, Upasani VV, Bastrom TP, et al. Apical vertebral rotation in adolescent idiopathic scoliosis: comparison of uniplanar and polyaxial pedicle screws. J Spinal Disord Tech. 2011; 24(4):251–257

Further Reading

Pratt RK, Webb JK, Burwell RG, Cole AA. Changes in surface and radiographic deformity after Universal Spine System for right thoracic adolescent idiopathic scoliosis: is rib-hump reassertion a mechanical problem of the thoracic cage rather than an effect of relative anterior spinal overgrowth? Spine. 2001; 26(16):1778–1787

Chang MS, Lenke GL. Vertebral derotation in adolescent idiopathic scoliosis. Oper Tech Orthop. 2009; 19:19–23

14 Posttraumatic Spine Deformity

David B. Bumpass, Lawrence G. Lenke

Abstract

Posttraumatic spinal deformity is a challenging form of rigid spine deformity. A thorough understanding of acute spine fracture biomechanics as well as the chronic sequelae of spinal trauma is essential. Preoperative evaluation requires a careful history and physical examination, as well as comprehensive spinal imaging and bone density evaluation. Spinal flexibility should be assessed on physical examination and on recumbent imaging. Surgical approach will typically require some form of osteotomy; operative planning should focus on reconstructing the damaged columns of the spine in order to restore functional biomechanics, particularly in the sagittal plane. Frequently, these patients have had prior surgery, with retained implants and dural scarring being common challenges. There are substantial risks for perioperative complications, and extensive preoperative discussion should include shared decision-making with the patient.

Keywords: posttraumatic spinal deformity, spine fracture, kyphosis, sagittal imbalance, vertebral column resection

14.1 Introduction

Patients with posttraumatic spine deformity (PTSD) are increasing in prevalence and present unique challenges for the spine surgeon. PTSD patients often have long-standing inflexible deformities. Correction is made more difficult due to spinal canal stenosis, postinjury scarring around the dura, posttraumatic syrinxes, and osteonecrosis of the fractured vertebra. PTSD is often a vicious cycle of progression, as kyphosis exacerbates sagittal imbalance, which in turn causes the supporting structures of the spine to further weaken over time. Patients experience significant pain and disability, sometimes presenting with worsening neurologic function as well.

Treating PTSD requires restoration of biomechanical stability and alignment, particularly in the sagittal plane. The original injury pattern needs to be understood to determine the best surgical approach, instrumentation, and correction techniques. Complete decompression of the spinal canal is critical. While anterior approaches for decompression and instrumentation were most common into the 1990 s, surgical techniques for posterior-only PTSD correction have rapidly advanced and are now the mainstay method for treating these patients. Posterior spinal osteotomies can achieve significant corrections while also providing access to the anterior spine for decompression. Pedicle screw instrumentation provides sufficient stabilization to avoid concomitant anterior approaches in many patients.

Due to the complex nature of these deformities, PTSD patients are at high risk of neurologic and medical complications. Understanding the unique difficulties of treating this population is essential for surgeons to achieve safe and lasting outcomes.

14.2 Epidemiology

Thoracic and lumbar vertebral fractures are a common injury, although the exact incidence is difficult to pinpoint.[1] There are approximately 12,000 new spinal cord injuries (SCIs) in the United States annually, and many more spine traumas without SCI.[2] The number of thoracolumbar fractures, particularly those caused by motor vehicle collisions, may actually be increasing at a rate of up to 8% annually.[3] In addition, low-energy spine fractures secondary to osteoporosis are very common, and these injuries do not typically cause SCI. An estimated 700,000 osteoporotic vertebral fractures occur each year in the United States.[4,5]

The demographics of spinal injuries are changing as well. The mean age at injury of an SCI patient has increased from 29 years in the 1970 s to 43 years in 2010, and the percentage of SCI patients over age 60 at the time of injury has increased from 5 to 13% over the same period.[2,6] This may be due in part to improved survival of older patients after trauma and the general aging of the population. Together, these statistics suggest that PTSD will continue to be commonly encountered by spine specialists, particularly as these patients age and their deformities progress due to bone density loss.

The spectrum of injury severity with spine fractures is wide; many injuries are stable, whereas others are unstable and associated with a higher risk for neurologic injury. However, spine fractures of nearly any type can create spinal deformity. PTSD can occur in both the sagittal and coronal planes, and once the fractures heal these often become rigid deformities. Benli et al found that kyphosis about a thoracolumbar fracture averaged 46 degrees within 1 year of injury, and 65 degrees in patients who were still untreated more than 1 year after injury, with a statistically significant association between severity of kyphosis and time from injury.[7] Shen et al reported less severe initial kyphosis from thoracolumbar burst fractures, initially averaging 21 degrees and progressing by a mean of 4 degrees after 2 years in patients treated nonoperatively.[8] Yagi et al identified a 26% incidence of scoliosis in 214 adult SCI patients, with a mean magnitude of 29 degrees.[9] The risk of developing scoliosis was associated with a more severe cord injury, as graded by the American Spinal Injury Association (ASIA) system.

Even patients treated acutely with surgical fixation for vertebral fractures can have deformity progression. Numerous case series of patients treated with short-segment pedicle screw instrumentation, consisting of pedicle screws placed into one vertebra above and one vertebra below the fracture, have indicated that this technique can lead to progressive kyphosis over time. Loss of correction ranged from a mean of 6 to 10 degrees.[8,10,11,12,13,14,15] Complicating the minimal fixation used in these studies is the fact that the instrumentation was often removed and arthrodesis was not always performed. Anterior column support was not added in these series. Several studies investigated why this progression occurred; breakdown of the disks adjacent to a fractured vertebra seemed to drive much of the progression. However, residual vertebral wedging and height loss did predispose to increased risk of disk space collapse.[12,14]

14.3 Evaluation of Posttraumatic Deformity

Assessment of PTSD patients requires thorough integration of injury history, physical exam, imaging findings, and bone quality to achieve an optimal surgical plan.

14.3.1 Normal Thoracolumbar Alignment

In order to evaluate PTSD, normal sagittal alignment parameters must be understood. The thoracic spine, as measured from T 2 to T 12, usually has between 20 and 50 degrees of kyphosis. The thoracolumbar segment is generally measured from T 10 to L 2 and is essentially neutral. The lumbar spine typically has 40 to 80 degrees of lordosis from T 12 to S 1.[16]

The sagittal vertical axis (SVA) is used to assess sagittal balance. The SVA is a plumb line from the center of the C 7 body, which typically falls in line with the posterior-superior corner of S 1; a positive value indicates that the plumb line falls anterior to S 1, and a negative value means the plumb line is posterior to S 1.[17] Normal adults typically have an SVA of ± 3 cm.[18,19] Finally, sagittal pelvic parameters are critical to note as well. Pelvic incidence (PI) is a constant morphological parameter that relates the position of the acetabuli to the sacrum. Pelvic tilt (PT) does increase as the pelvis is retroflexed, and a high PI can indicate that a patient is attempting to compensate for kyphosis elsewhere in the spine to maintain a neutral sagittal balance. Normative values are 50 to 55 degrees for PI, and 10 to 15 degrees for PT.[18]

14.3.2 Classification

No classification exists specifically for PTSD, but several classification systems have been established that seek to guide treatment decisions for thoracolumbar fractures. A brief description of these can help to clarify the pathomechanics of postfracture deformity. The Denis classification divides the spine into three structural columns: anterior, middle, and posterior. The anterior column incorporates the anterior half of the vertebral body, the middle column encompasses the posterior half of the vertebral body and the posterior longitudinal ligament, and the posterior column consists of the facets, the interspinous ligament, and the other posterior elements.[20]

The modified Magerl/AO thoracolumbar classification categorizes fractures into three groups based on morphology and mechanism. Type A injuries are caused by axial compression, and the posterior elements remain intact (standard burst fractures are type A fractures). Type B injuries occur when the posterior constraining elements are compromised (Chance fractures are type B fractures). Type C injuries are the most severe; both anterior and posterior structures are disrupted, resulting in spinal displacement.[21] While patients with severe three-column or Magerl/AO type C injuries are most at risk for PTSD, patients with "minor" stable fractures, such as Magerl/AO type A fractures, which are typically treated nonoperatively, are still at risk for deformity progression over time.[16,22]

14.3.3 Biomechanics and Pathology

Deforming Forces

Axial loading and flexion are frequently the mechanisms of injury for spinal fractures. Thus the most common PTSD is kyphosis at the fractured level due to compressive failure of the anterior and middle columns. If the posterior ligaments are also injured, then patients have an even higher risk of developing a kyphotic deformity, as these structures serve as a tension band to reduce tensile forces and maintain upright posture. Focal kyphosis of more than 20 degrees suggests posterior column distractive injury, placing patients at greater risk of developing a progressive deformity.[16]

Posttraumatic kyphosis most frequently presents with thoracic and thoracolumbar fractures, as these regions of the spine naturally have kyphotic or neutral alignment. However, kyphosis is sometimes observed in lumbar fractures as well.[16] Risk of deformity progression is greater for thoracolumbar and lumbar fractures because there is not the stabilization conferred by the rigid rib cage. As the patient's center of gravity shifts forward, the posterior paraspinal muscles gradually weaken, creating a vicious cycle.[23,24] The anterior column fails due to progressive compressive force, and the posterior column fails due to progressive tensile force. Malcolm et al documented kyphosis progression in 46% of their PTSD patients, and half of the patients in their study had prior laminectomies at the injury level.[25] Laminectomies disrupt the posterior tension band, further disposing patients to kyphosis progression.

As focal deformity worsens, patients will compensate through uninjured portions of their spine and their pelvis in order to maintain a neutral sagittal balance. For example, a patient might stand with more lumbar lordosis and more pelvic retroversion to compensate for thoracic kyphosis from a T 8 fracture. However, deformity often continues to progress even when compensatory spinal mechanisms have been maximized. Patients then expend greater amounts of energy to stay upright, often altering their gate with a flex-kneed posture. Moreover, increased compensatory lumbar lordosis places additional strain on the lumbar facets and disks, often leading to progressive degenerative changes and pain below the injured level.[16,24]

PTSD can occur acutely as a direct result of the anatomical damage caused by the fracture. Late deformity can also occur, with a relatively well aligned fracture progressing over time. This can occur due to poor bone quality, such as patients with osteoporosis or renal osteodystrophy. Late deformity can also occur in patients who were initially treated with surgery who present with implant failure, pseudarthrosis, chronic wound infection, laminectomy, or short-segment or posterior-only fusions.[16,26]

Charcot Arthropathy of the Spine

In patients with SCIs that result in loss of protective sensation distal to the level of the fracture, a Charcot spine can develop.

Similar to neuropathic arthropathy in other joints, articular destruction and vertebral collapse can progress over a relatively short period of time (12–18 months), although decades may also pass after the initial neurologic injury before Charcot arthropathy develops.[27,28] Generally, the Charcot degeneration occurs distal to the level of the initial injury. The process begins with abnormal motion between insensate vertebrae, causing hypertrophic bone formation and facet instability. End plate fragmentation can eventually lead to extreme periosteal bone formation. The spine then becomes progressively unstable, even forming a ball-and-socket pseudarthrosis in advanced cases. Development of Charcot spine is strongly associated with prior thoracic or lumbar laminectomy.[27,28] Similar radiographic changes in the spine can be caused by neoplasms, infection, or, rarely, syphilis.[28] Effective surgical stabilization can be accomplished with anterior debridement of the hypertrophic bone with reconstruction of the anterior column, backed up with multilevel posterior instrumentation and fusion, although secondary levels of Charcot arthropathy can develop distal to a fusion.[29,30]

Kümmell Disease (Posttraumatic Vertebral Avascular Necrosis)

Kümmell disease is vertebral avascular necrosis, a phenomenon that can occur after relatively minor trauma to the spine, such as an osteoporotic compression fracture. Incidence has been documented to range from 7 to 37% of vertebral fractures and is more frequent in elderly patients. This condition can cause progressive spinal deformity as the affected vertebra collapses. Kümmell disease is diagnosed on imaging by visualization of intravertebral gas within a fracture cleft, as the collapse of the cancellous body creates a mobile pseudarthrosis. Persistent pain for more than 3 months may necessitate vertebroplasty; neurologic compression requires formal surgical decompression and stabilization.[5,16,31]

In some cases transudative fluid and gas from the necrosing vertebral body are pushed into the psoas, creating imaging findings that can be misdiagnosed as an abscess. Percutaneous biopsy can be helpful in ruling out infection in such cases.[5]

Syringomyelia and Tethering

Posttraumatic syringomyelia can occur as early as 3 weeks after spinal fracture; impaired flow of cerebrospinal fluid (CSF) at the fractured level seems to be important in pathogenesis.[32] Symptoms include pain, motor weakness, sensory disturbances, and spasticity correlating with a spinal level above the level of the initial injury.[33] Asano et al found that approximately 50% of patients who developed posttraumatic syrinxes experienced new neurologic deterioration.[34] The risk of developing syringomyelia after spinal fracture causing paraplegia is correlated with having 15 degrees or more of residual kyphosis and more than 25% canal stenosis.[35] Effective treatment of posttraumatic syringomyelia must address residual canal stenosis and deformity.[36]

Cord tethering can also develop, often in conjunction with syringomyelia. Lee et al found that simply untethering the spinal cord could dramatically reduce the size of the syrinx in up to 95% of patients with both pathologies, presumably by restoring normal CSF flow. Syringosubarachnoid shunting can reduce syrinx size in patients that do not have tethering or that do not respond to untethering alone, although as many as 50% of patients require shunt revision.[33,37]

14.3.4 Presentation and Physical Exam

Patients most commonly present with pain at or especially just below the apex of their deformity. Often they fatigue quickly while standing, particularly when they have significant sagittal imbalance.[25,38] There can be radiation of pain to the buttocks, and lying supine often alleviates the discomfort. Some patients may even describe a feeling of subjective spinal instability or crepitus.[25]

Many patients present with partial or complete neurologic deficits that resulted from their initial injury. However, new or progressive neurologic deficits are typically caused by either syringomyelia or progressive deformity.[16] Kostuik and Matsusaki reported progression of symptomatic spinal stenosis in 9 of 37 (24%) patients with posttraumatic kyphosis.[24] Malcolm et al observed that 27% of their patients had progressive neurologic deficits.[25]

To accurately determine the etiology of patients' pain and neurologic symptoms, a careful physical exam is essential. The patient should be examined while standing, walking, and lying both supine and prone. This will allow sagittal and coronal balance to be assessed, as well as the flexibility of the deformity. Patients with significant positive sagittal imbalance often stand with their knees flexed in order to maintain balance and an upright gaze. A flattened gluteal region suggests compensatory pelvic retroversion. Motor and sensory function in all extremities should be assessed, and signs of myelopathy such as clonus and a Babinski sign elicited. Incisions over the back or the anterior thoracoabdominal region should be noted to clarify the spine's previous surgical history.

14.3.5 Radiographic Evaluation

Standard radiographic evaluation should include standing full-spine frontal and lateral radiographs. Flexibility films, particularly a supine hyperextension lateral film with a bolster if kyphosis is present, should be obtained to determine the correctability of the deformity.[26] A supine anteroposterior film can provide better visualization of pedicles for instrumentation planning.

On standing lateral radiographs, the SVA should be measured. Pelvic parameters, specifically PI and PT, should also be determined.[39] Emerging evidence suggests that postcorrection lumbar lordosis should be within 10 degrees of the PI to effectively restore sagittal balance. A high PT ($\geq$25 degrees) indicates pelvic retroversion.[40,41]

Measuring the acute kyphosis based on the end plates of the fractured vertebra is often subject to variability due to distorted anatomy and has only moderate reliability. Using the Cobb technique by measuring the angle subtended by the superior end plate of the vertebra cephalad to the fracture and the inferior end plate of the vertebra caudad to the fracture is most reliable.[42]

Farcy et al proposed the sagittal index (SI) as a decision tool for surgical treatment of burst fractures. The lateral Cobb angle is measured from the inferior end plate of the vertebra just cephalad to the fracture to the inferior end plate of the fractured vertebra.[43] The normal sagittal contour is then subtracted from the measured angle; differences greater than 15 degrees suggest that the patient may be at risk of progressive kyphotic deformity.[44] The normal sagittal contour is defined as + 5 degrees for the thoracic spine, 0 degrees for the thoracolumbar junction, and −10 degrees of lordosis. While SI is a useful method to evaluate the amount of kyphosis that has resulted from a fracture, the cutoff value of 15 degrees has never been rigorously tested and thus is not a perfect predictor of which patients will eventually develop a progressive sagittal deformity.[43] However, an SI greater than 15 degrees has been associated with a greater likelihood of moderate to severe back pain.[12]

All PTSD patients considered to be surgical candidates should have both CT and MRI scans of the thoracolumbar spine. CT will provide the best information regarding the anatomy of the original fracture, which is often distorted. MRI is necessary to evaluate for syringomyelia, cord tethering, and spinal stenosis, all of which increase the risk of significant neurologic injury during deformity correction.[15,28] Also, MRI is critical to assess the integrity of the posterior ligamentous structures.[26] CT and MRI will help confirm that the original fracture has indeed healed, as a pseudarthrosis can be a chronic pain generator and cause of progressive deformity.[26] This is the case in some patients with Kümmell disease.[31]

Bone densitometry is another study that is essential to obtain prior to surgical intervention in patients who are age 50 or older. Because many patients with PTSD are elderly or minimally active, bone density is often poor. However, surgical correction requires good instrument purchase in the vertebrae. A patient with a T-score less than 2.0 should be referred to endocrinology for potential bisphosphonate or teriparatide therapy prior to surgery.

14.4 Nonoperative Management

Nonoperative treatment should first be attempted in PTSD patients who have stable radiographic alignment and do not have neurologic deficits. Physical therapy with extension exercises and core strengthening can be of some benefit. Facet injections are another potentially useful modality, as are transforaminal epidural corticosteroid injections for patients that have mild radiculopathy.

Continued observation of these patients is warranted to make sure that the deformity does not continue to progress or cause new neurologic symptoms. In patients with a relatively recent fracture, additional time may be needed for complete fracture healing. Osteoporotic patients in particular should be managed without surgery to the maximum extent possible.[38]

14.5 Operative Management

14.5.1 Surgical Indications and Planning

Indications for surgical management of PTSD include new neurologic deficits, increasing axial back pain, progressive deformity, pseudarthrosis, or degeneration of adjacent levels.[16,24,26] Focal kyphosis greater than 30 degrees or an SI greater than 20 degrees has been proposed as a threshold for surgical intervention.[26,39] In addition, a pelvic tilt that exceeds normal values by 20 degrees or more is a relative indication for surgery. Surgery should be considered only after all reasonable nonoperative treatments have failed.

Surgical planning must consider a number of variables related to the deformity in order to select the proper approach, instrumentation, and correction technique. Restoration of sagittal balance is the most important consideration for deciding how to correct PTSD.[45] Sagittal imbalance, particularly if caused by deformity in the thoracolumbar and lumbar spine, is strongly correlated with disability.[46] Buchowski et al proposed a decision tree that breaks PTSD into two basic types: type I is a focal deformity with normal sagittal balance, and type II is a deformity with sagittal imbalance. Type II patients require more aggressive correction techniques to restore sagittal balance.[16] Over the past decade, the understanding of treating sagittal imbalance has progressed significantly. While much of the work done in this area relates to treating iatrogenic "flatback syndrome" resulting from Harrington distraction instrumentation, many of the principles of evaluating and treating sagittal imbalance remain true for PTSD. Numerous studies have demonstrated that patients with sagittal imbalance whose balance is restored have much better long-term outcomes than those in whom balance is not effectively restored.[46,47]

Surgical planning must take into account previous surgical approaches and instrumentation.[45] The location of the kyphosis is also important; thoracic deformities are often less flexible due to the rigidity of the rib cage. Risk of spinal cord damage is higher with thoracic and thoracolumbar corrections, whereas the risk of nerve root injury is higher with lumbar corrections.

More than 20 years ago, Gertzbein and Harris noted the critical importance of determining the flexibility of the deformity to developing the proper treatment strategy.[48] This concept remains true and guides decision making regarding the use of osteotomies and the extent of instrumentation.[26] The Schwab osteotomy classification has now clarified terminology and orders osteotomies based on the extent of vertebral resection (▶ Table 14.1).[49] Deformities with some flexibility may not require any osteotomies or only posterior-column osteotomies (PCOs, or type I and II osteotomies) (▶ Fig. 14.1). However, stiffer deformities often require more extensive osteotomies to restore sagittal balance, such as a pedicle subtraction osteotomy (PSO, or type III/IV osteotomies) or vertebral column resection (VCR, or type V/VI osteotomies) (▶ Fig. 14.2).

Table 14.1 Schwab osteotomy classification[49]

Classification	Description
Type I osteotomy	Partial facet joint resection
Type II osteotomy	Complete facet joint resection
Type III osteotomy	Pedicle and partial body resection
Type IV osteotomy	Pedicle, partial body, and disk resection
Type V osteotomy	Complete vertebra and disk resection
Type VI osteotomy	Multiple adjacent vertebrae and disk resections

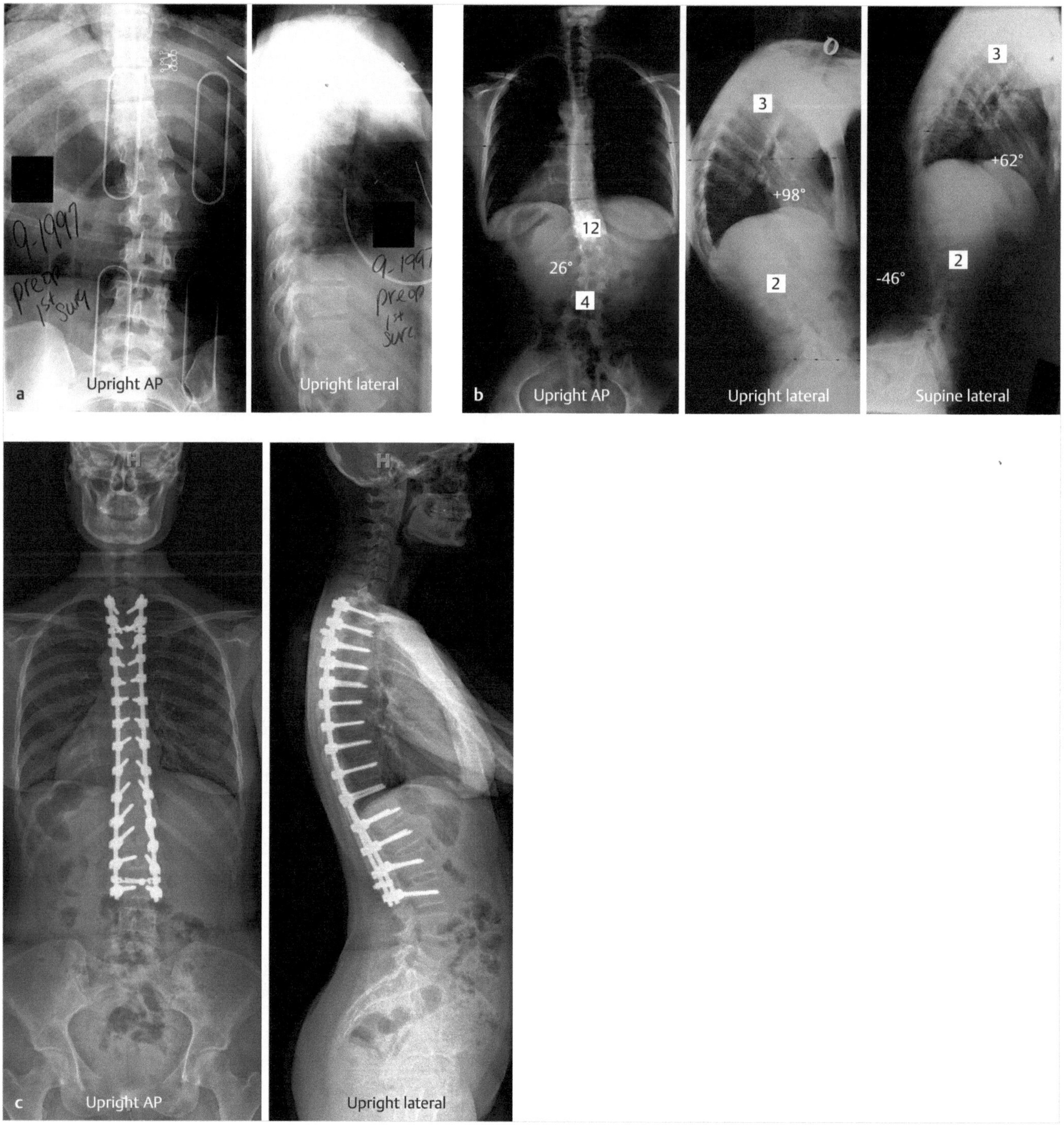

Fig. 14.1 **(a)** A 33-year-old woman who sustained a T 12 burst fracture from a falling tree at age 26. She initially underwent T 2–L 1 instrumented posterior fusion, and instrumentation was removed 1 year postoperatively. **(b)** She then presented with significant, progressive kyphosis with sagittal imbalance with diffuse back pain; her kyphosis did reduce when supine, and was not angular. She had pseudarthroses from T 2 to T 12 and underwent revision posterior spinal fusion from T 2 to L 3 with type II osteotomies at T 5–L 1. **(c)** Now 9 years postsurgery, she is doing well with minimal symptoms and excellent coronal and sagittal balance.

Surgical planning should be guided by an understanding of the injured structures and biomechanical derangement in each individual patient.[26] Injury to the posterior ligamentous tension band necessitates posterior instrumentation and fusion. Similarly, restoration of anterior column stability is critical for long-term maintenance of spinal balance.[23,50] Current treatment algorithms for thoracolumbar fractures incorporate these considerations, and CT and MRI studies should be reviewed in detail prior to surgery to understand the pathomechanics of each patient's deformity.[51]

Finally, the extent of neurologic injury from the initial injury should be incorporated into the treatment plan. Previous operations, as well as the traumatic injury itself, may have created scarring of the neural elements. Patients with spinal

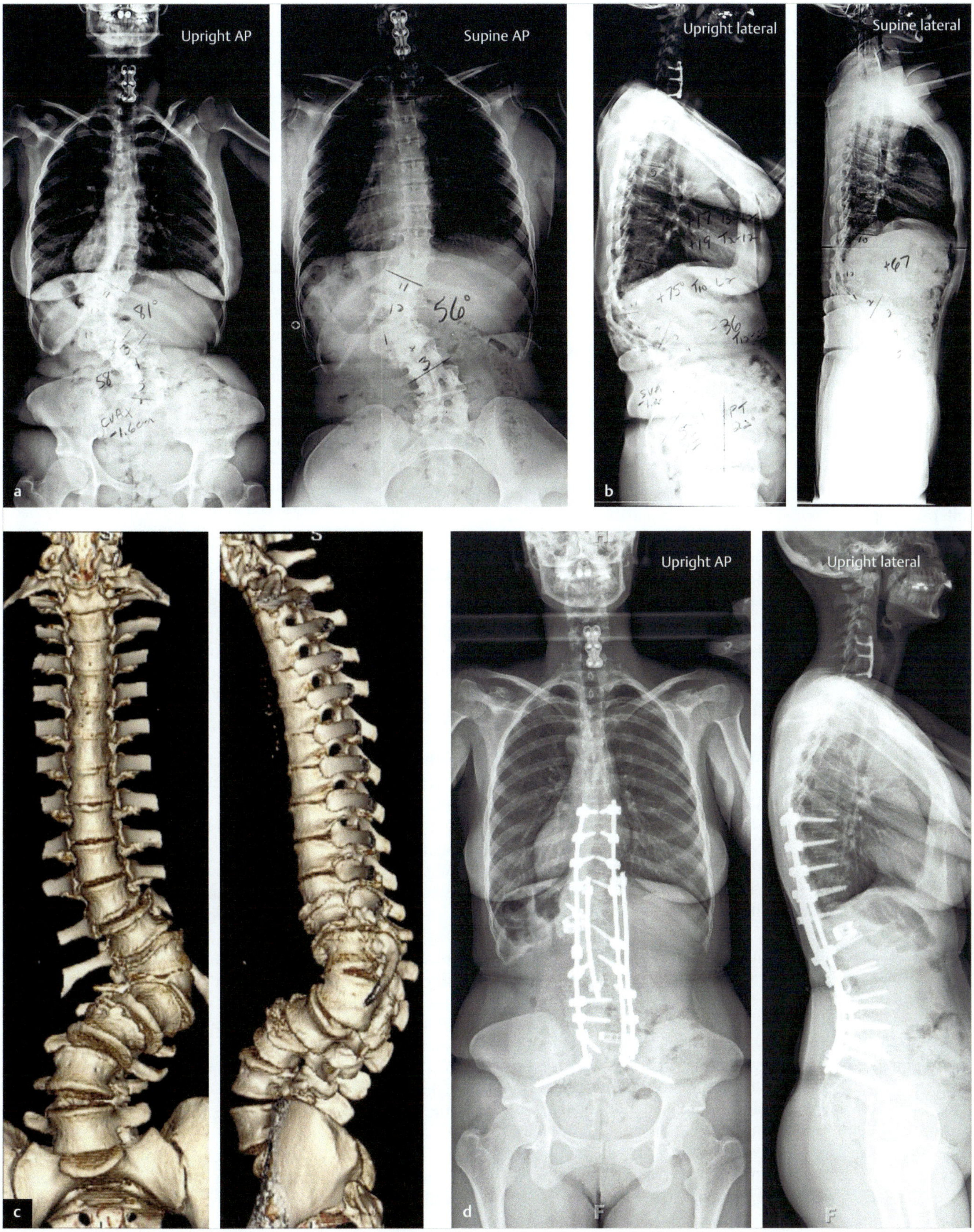

Fig. 14.2 A 43-year-old woman who had suffered an L 1 fracture 20 years prior. **(a–c)** She developed a progressive kyphoscoliosis and underwent a T 8–sacrum posterior spinal fusion with iliac fixation using S 2 alar iliac screws. A vertebral column resection (type V osteotomy) of L 1 was performed, as were type II osteotomies at T 11–T 12 and L 2–L 3. **(d)** One year after surgery, she is doing well and has maintained her much-improved spinal alignment.

stenosis, especially those with progressive neurologic deficits, should be completely decompressed prior to any corrective maneuvers. The cause and extent of neurologic compression and canal stenosis can influence the choice of surgical approach. Typically, the anterior and middle columns are the cause of spinal cord compression in kyphosis cases. Thus this bone must be removed, either through a direct anterior approach or a posterior costotransversectomy approach. In a systematic review, Verlaan et al concluded that neurologic recovery correlated with the initial Frankel grade of neurologic injury, and that surgical approach did not have a significant effect.[15] Even years after an injury, patients can have significant reduction in pain as well as neurologic improvement after decompression.[52,53]

14.5.2 Anterior Surgical Approaches

PTSD can be approached anteriorly, posteriorly, or with combined approaches. As instrumentation and surgical techniques have changed, algorithms for the management of PTSD have evolved as well. In the 1960 s and 1970 s, Harrington rod instrumentation proved largely inadequate for correction and maintenance of sagittal deformity correction in these patients.[24] Thus anterior approaches with interbody fusion and instrumentation were initially the technique of choice. Anterior approaches allowed for direct decompression of the spinal canal by removing the fractured vertebral body and deformity correction by placing an interbody graft. In the setting of a new or progressive neurologic deficit in a PTSD patient, direct anterior decompression produced the best results for achieving neurologic improvement.[23,24]

In 1981, Malcolm et al reported a 50% failure rate with anterior fusion alone, but instrumentation was not used in these patients.[25] By modifying surgical technique to incorporate a vascularized rib strut graft, McBride and Bradford were able to improve anterior-only fusion rates to 100% in 7 patients with posttraumatic kyphosis ranging from 20 to 83 degrees, again without instrumentation.[54] Kostuik and Matsusaki reported on a series of 37 patients with posttraumatic kyphosis; all were treated with an anterior approach. Surgical technique consisted of corpectomy of the fractured level, interbody strut grafting, and anterior instrumentation. They experienced one pseudarthrosis and no neurologic complications.[24] Roberson and Whitesides achieved successful deformity correction and fusion in 17 of 18 patients with anterior-only surgery; of note, none of these patients had posterior spinal instability from their initial injuries.[23]

In 2007, Benli et al reported on 40 patients treated anteriorly for a minimum of 30 degrees of posttraumatic kyphosis.[7] Vertebrectomy was performed for decompression and correction in all patients; half were stabilized with dual rods and half with a plate system. No significant differences were seen at follow-up between treatment groups. All 24 patients who had neurologic deficits experienced some degree of neurologic improvement. Patients who had surgery within 1 year of injury had significantly greater correction (mean 92%) than those who had surgery more than 1 year after injury (mean 72%). Patients had significant improvement in their pain and functional assessment scores postoperatively, although improvement positively correlated with shorter time to operation and a less severe preoperative deformity.

14.5.3 Combined Anterior–Posterior Surgical Approaches

Been et al surgically treated 25 patients with PTSD after Magerl A fractures.[55] Ten patients were treated from an anterior approach, and 15 patients with combined anterior–posterior approaches. No significant differences were found in radiographic correction or back pain scores at a minimum of 6 years of follow-up. Chang reported on 17 patients with a mean thoracolumbar kyphosis of 39 degrees from fractures between T12 and L3.[50] Using a back-front-back technique, arthrodesis was achieved by instrumenting across only the two motion segments immediately above and below the fracture. He achieved a mean of 37 degrees of correction at final follow-up. Kostuik et al described a combined technique to correct iatrogenic flatback, with an anterior opening wedge osteotomy and a posterior closing wedge osteotomy.[56] In a series of 16 PTSD patients, Jodoin et al treated 6 patients with combined approaches. They noted no significant perioperative complications and minimal loss of kyphosis correction at a mean 3 years of follow-up.[57]

14.5.4 Posterior Surgical Approaches

In 1992, Gertzbein and Harris first described an all-posterior surgery for PTSD using a pedicle subtraction closing-wedge osteotomy.[48] Since that time, posterior deformity correction techniques have advanced with refinements in osteotomies and improved segmental pedicle screw instrumentation. Posterior-only approaches have largely obviated the need for separate anterior and posterior procedures, while still allowing the surgeon to decompress the anterior spinal cord and correct the deformity caused by the fractured anterior and middle columns. Importantly, posterior approaches also allow the surgeon to directly restore stability to the posterior column in the presence of ligamentous injury.

Lehmer et al performed three-column closing wedge osteotomies via an all-posterior technique in 38 patients, 21 of whom had PTSD. Mean correction of 35 degrees was maintained in 93% of patients.[58] Wu et al reported on posterior-only corrections on 13 patients by performing partial vertebral body decancellations, essentially PSOs.[59] They achieved mean correction of 40 degrees of preoperative kyphosis to 2 degrees, with good maintenance of this correction at 2-year follow-up. Short-segment pedicle screw constructs were used for instrumentation. All patients achieved fusion, and none experienced a neurologic injury from surgery.

Suk et al compared correction of posttraumatic kyphosis between a combined anterior–posterior technique (11 patients) and a posterior-only closing wedge osteotomy (15 patients).[60] Of note, all patients had fractures secondary to osteoporosis, typically from low-energy injuries; the average age was 63 years, an older population than many studies in which patients experienced high-energy trauma. The authors achieved shorter operating times, less blood loss, and fewer complications with the posterior-only osteotomy technique. A higher rate of neurologic improvement from preoperative deficits was achieved in the posterior-only group as well.

Kawahara et al report 7 cases of acute rigid thoracic kyphosis averaging 67 degrees that were corrected using a posterior-only approach; 5 of the cases were posttraumatic.[61] The authors first performed a closing-wedge VCR, then placed an intervertebral cage just anterior to the spinal cord to create a fulcrum to complete the correction. Placing the fulcrum in this position restored some length to the spinal column for the purpose of preventing dural buckling and overshortening of the spinal cord, given that they averaged 50 degrees of kyphosis correction. No neurologic complications were reported.

Lazennec et al performed PSOs on 13 patients with posttraumatic kyphosis.[62] They compared outcomes for the patients with PSOs in the thoracolumbar region against those in the lumbar spine, finding that anatomical alignment was better restored in the patients with thoracolumbar fractures. They attributed this difference to the fact that the normally lordotic lumbar disks adjacent to the lumbar fractures had collapsed and become kyphotic, possibly from disk injury from the initial trauma. Only the vertebrae immediately above and below the fracture were instrumented, and this limited fixation may have been inadequate to fully correct these lumbar deformities. Heary and Bono performed lumbar PSOs on three patients with PTSD, achieving more than 50 degrees of kyphosis correction with good pain and functional improvement.[63]

Recently, Chou et al reported two cases in which posterior-only PSO was effectively used to correct posttraumatic kyphosis at the thoracolumbar junction without incurring a neurologic injury.[38] They achieved between 20 and 50 degrees of correction in this fashion, instrumenting two to three levels above and below the osteotomy. In a 2011 multicenter study, El-Sharkawi et al prospectively followed 43 patients with posttraumatic kyphosis who were treated with PSO at the thoracolumbar junction.[64] In comparison to a historical cohort with a similar deformity treated with anterior corpectomy and plating, the PSO patients had greater correction, with a mean of 30 degrees of improvement. Mean patient-reported outcomes score differences between the two groups were significant but small in magnitude and favored the PSO group. The surgeons instrumented only a single level above and below the PSO in 29 patients, and two levels above and below in 14 patients; one implant failure was noted in an osteoporotic patient.

14.5.5 Technical Considerations

Anterior Approaches

If an anterior approach is used, particularly in the thoracic spine, caution must be exercised with lengthening the anterior column to restore alignment, as doing so can stretch the neural elements. Anterior decompressions at T5–T9 have been reported to have a higher risk for neurologic injury, possibly due to the watershed vascular zone of the spinal cord at these levels.[23,25] In order to achieve anterior column restoration, the end plates above and below the resected vertebral body must be left intact. However, thorough diskectomies should be done, carefully releasing the lateral annulus bilaterally as much as possible. If the patient is in the lateral decubitus position, the contralateral cortical shell of the vertebra can be left intact, and the corpectomy should proceed in an anterior-to-posterior fashion.[23] Regardless of interbody device selection (fixed cage, expandable cage, allograft), the amount of surface area contact with the end plates should be maximized.[39]

Posterior Approaches

Buchowski et al have proposed a decision tree for selection of osteotomies to achieve correction of PTSD with posterior-only approaches.[16] Multiple PCOs are often effective for thoracic angular kyphotic deformities, particularly if some flexibility is present. In the lumbar spine, focal kyphotic deformities can be addressed with a PSO at a single level or PCOs at multiple levels. Cho et al demonstrated that for fixed lumbar sagittal imbalance, three PCOs achieved kyphosis correction equivalent to that of a single PSO, although the PCOs were more likely to worsen coronal balance.[65]

PCOs can create iatrogenic foraminal stenosis, particularly in the lumbar spine, so the surgeon must be careful not to overcompress the closure of these osteotomies and must continually check central canal and foraminal patency as the osteotomies are closed. Also, PCOs do not shorten the anterior column; because the spinal cord is often draped over the apex of the deformity, thoracic PCOs in particular should be closed very slowly, with careful attention paid to any changes in neuromonitoring. PCOs require a flexible disk in order to create change in sagittal alignment, and this is sometimes not possible at the fractured level.[39] However, when properly performed, PCOs can yield 10 to 15 degrees of correction at a single level.[16]

Three-column osteotomies (3COs) include PSOs and VCRs. Unlike PCOs, 3COs do not lengthen the anterior column and provide a large surface area for osteotomy healing. Also, 3COs can be performed in an asymmetric or biplanar fashion to achieve correction in both sagittal and coronal planes. Performing a 3CO can yield more than 35 degrees of focal correction. When a 3CO is needed, the ideal level is at the apex of kyphosis.[39,66,67] If a 3CO is needed in the thoracic spine, a VCR is often preferable to a PSO because the VCR actually shortens the anterior column, minimizing the risk of a vascular insult to the cord from stretching during correction. In the lumbar spine, a PSO is frequently sufficient to re-create lordosis.

Longer operative times and more intraoperative blood loss should be expected when performing 3COs. Osteotomy closure must be done very slowly, with frequent assessment of dural impingement to ensure that decompression is adequate.[63] Typically a minimum of six points of fixation both above and below the osteotomy should be placed; pedicle screws provide the best fixation as well as a lever arm across all three columns of the spine. Placing three or more rods across a three-column osteotomy has been shown to reduce implant failure and pseudarthrosis.[68]

Transforaminal lumber interbody fusion (TLIF) is a useful technique that is now familiar to most spine surgeons. Polly et al described bilateral TLIF approaches for placing interbody grafts in the anterior column of the lumbar spine in PTSD patients. This technique provides anterior column stability and increases lordosis while avoiding difficult low lumbar anterior reconstructive approaches.[69] In addition, interbody fusion below a PSO has been linked to decreasing the risk of a pseudarthrosis of the PSO.[70]

14.5.6 Complications

PTSD correction carries with it a relatively high risk of complications. Case series have cited rates of neurologic injury up to 20%, and of infection up to 7% for PTSD patients.[16,26,58] PTSD patients often have long-standing stiff deformities surrounded by scar tissue from the initial injury. As the majority of PTSD patients have focal kyphosis, the spinal cord is often draped tightly over the apex. Moreover, many have had previous spine surgeries. These factors increase the likelihood of complications with PTSD correction, and patients should be counseled regarding this fact prior to surgery. Neuromonitoring should be used in each PTSD correction case to minimize the chance of permanent neurologic injury.

Both anterior and posterior approaches have inherent risks. Malcolm et al reported a complication rate of 40% with anterior approaches. Risk of new or worsened postoperative neurologic deficits was associated with older age, longer time from injury to deformity correction, midthoracic (higher risk than lower thoracic) deformity apex, and more intraoperative blood loss.[25] In 54 patients undergoing combined anterior–posterior approaches, Kostuik et al experienced injury to the great vessels in 5 patients and ureteral injuries in 2 patients. All of these patients had previous anterior fusions, demonstrating the high level of risk involved with revision anterior approaches for spine deformity.[56]

Posterior osteotomies can also cause complications, particularly neurologic injuries. The rate of all complications for 3COs approaches 50%, and the chance of a major complication is as high as 35%.[71,72] New neurologic deficits are present after almost 10% of 3COs.[72] Heary and Bono reported new lower extremity motor deficits 3 days after PSO, requiring emergent revision surgery to further decompress above and below the osteotomy.[63] Good implant fixation is critical in posterior-only surgery, and implant failure can lead to loss of correction.[62,64]

Other possible complications include superior mesenteric artery syndrome or abdominal compartment syndrome.[48,67] Because PTSD patients are often disabled and have frequently had multiple extended hospital stays, the surgeon must be vigilant for respiratory or urinary infections caused by hospital-acquired organisms.[26]

References

[1] Francis RM, Baillie SP, Chuck AJ, et al. Acute and long-term management of patients with vertebral fractures. QJM. 2004; 97(2):63–74

[2] Spinal cord injury facts and figures at a glance. National Spinal Cord Injury Statistical Center, February 2013. (Accessed September 16, 2014, at https://www.nscisc.uab.edu/PublicDocuments/fact_figures_docs/Facts%202 013.pdf.)

[3] Doud AN, Weaver AA, Talton JW, et al. Has the incidence of thoracolumbar spine injuries increased in the United States from 1998 to 2011? Clin Orthop Relat Res. 2015; 473(1):297–305

[4] Riggs BL, Melton LJ, III. The worldwide problem of osteoporosis: insights afforded by epidemiology. Bone. 1995; 17(5) Suppl:505S–511S

[5] Freedman BA, Heller JG. Kummel disease: a not-so-rare complication of osteoporotic vertebral compression fractures. J Am Board Fam Med. 2009; 22 (1):75–78

[6] DeVivo MJ, Chen Y. Trends in new injuries, prevalent cases, and aging with spinal cord injury. Arch Phys Med Rehabil. 2011; 92(3):332–338

[7] Benli IT, Kaya A, Uruç V, Akalin S. Minimum 5-year follow-up surgical results of post-traumatic thoracic and lumbar kyphosis treated with anterior instrumentation: comparison of anterior plate and dual rod systems. Spine. 2007; 32(9):986–994

[8] Shen WJ, Liu TJ, Shen YS. Nonoperative treatment versus posterior fixation for thoracolumbar junction burst fractures without neurologic deficit. Spine. 2001; 26(9):1038–1045

[9] Yagi M, Hasegawa A, Takemitsu M, Yato Y, Machida M, Asazuma T. Incidence and the risk factors of spinal deformity in adult patient after spinal cord injury: a single center cohort study. Eur Spine J. 2015; 24(1):203–208

[10] Knop C, Fabian HF, Bastian L, Blauth M. Late results of thoracolumbar fractures after posterior instrumentation and transpedicular bone grafting. Spine. 2001; 26(1):88–99

[11] McLain RF, Burkus JK, Benson DR. Segmental instrumentation for thoracic and thoracolumbar fractures: prospective analysis of construct survival and five-year follow-up. Spine J. 2001; 1(5):310–323

[12] Wang XY, Dai LY, Xu HZ, Chi YL. Kyphosis recurrence after posterior short-segment fixation in thoracolumbar burst fractures. J Neurosurg Spine. 2008; 8(3):246–254

[13] Lakshmanan P, Jones A, Mehta J, Ahuja S, Davies PR, Howes JP. Recurrence of kyphosis and its functional implications after surgical stabilization of dorsolumbar unstable burst fractures. Spine J. 2009; 9(12):1003–1009

[14] Andress HJ, Braun H, Helmberger T, Schürmann M, Hertlein H, Hartl WH. Long-term results after posterior fixation of thoraco-lumbar burst fractures. Injury. 2002; 33(4):357–365

[15] Verlaan JJ, Diekerhof CH, Buskens E, et al. Surgical treatment of traumatic fractures of the thoracic and lumbar spine: a systematic review of the literature on techniques, complications, and outcome. Spine. 2004; 29(7):803–814

[16] Buchowski JM, Kuhns CA, Bridwell KH, Lenke LG. Surgical management of posttraumatic thoracolumbar kyphosis. Spine J. 2008; 8(4):666–677

[17] Lafage V, Schwab F, Skalli W, et al. Standing balance and sagittal plane spinal deformity: analysis of spinopelvic and gravity line parameters. Spine. 2008; 33(14):1572–1578

[18] Schwab F, Patel A, Ungar B, Farcy JP, Lafage V. Adult spinal deformity-postoperative standing imbalance: how much can you tolerate? An overview of key parameters in assessing alignment and planning corrective surgery. Spine. 2010; 35(25):2224–2231

[19] Vedantam R, Lenke LG, Keeney JA, Bridwell KH. Comparison of standing sagittal spinal alignment in asymptomatic adolescents and adults. Spine. 1998; 23 (2):211–215

[20] Denis F. The three column spine and its significance in the classification of acute thoracolumbar spinal injuries. Spine. 1983; 8(8):817–831

[21] Reinhold M, Audigé L, Schnake KJ, Bellabarba C, Dai LY, Oner FC. AO spine injury classification system: a revision proposal for the thoracic and lumbar spine. Eur Spine J. 2013; 22(10):2184–2201

[22] Bohlman HH. Treatment of fractures and dislocations of the thoracic and lumbar spine. J Bone Joint Surg Am. 1985; 67(1):165–169

[23] Roberson JR, Whitesides TE, Jr. Surgical reconstruction of late post-traumatic thoracolumbar kyphosis. Spine. 1985; 10(4):307–312

[24] Kostuik JP, Matsusaki H. Anterior stabilization, instrumentation, and decompression for post-traumatic kyphosis. Spine. 1989; 14(4):379–386

[25] Malcolm BW, Bradford DS, Winter RB, Chou SN. Post-traumatic kyphosis. A review of forty-eight surgically treated patients. J Bone Joint Surg Am. 1981; 63(6):891–899

[26] Vaccaro AR, Silber JS. Post-traumatic spinal deformity. Spine. 2001; 26(24) Suppl:S111–S118

[27] Sobel JW, Bohlman HH, Freehafer AA. Charcot's arthropathy of the spine following spinal cord injury. A report of five cases. J Bone Joint Surg Am. 1985; 67(5):771–776

[28] Vialle R, Mary P, Tassin JL, Parker F, Guillaumat M. Charcot's disease of the spine: diagnosis and treatment. Spine. 2005; 30(11):E315–E322

[29] Suda Y, Shioda M, Kohno H, Machida M, Yamagishi M. Surgical treatment of Charcot spine. J Spinal Disord Tech. 2007; 20(1):85–88

[30] Brown CW, Jones B, Donaldson DH, Akmakjian J, Brugman JL. Neuropathic (Charcot) arthropathy of the spine after traumatic spinal paraplegia. Spine. 1992; 17(6) Suppl:S103–S108

[31] Wiggins MC, Sehizadeh M, Pilgram TK, Gilula LA. Importance of intravertebral fracture clefts in vertebroplasty outcome. AJR Am J Roentgenol. 2007; 188 (3):634–640

[32] Bains RS, Althausen PL, Gitlin GN, Gupta MC, Benson DR. The role of acute decompression and restoration of spinal alignment in the prevention of post-traumatic syringomyelia: case report and review of recent literature. Spine. 2001; 26(17):E399–E402

[33] Lee TT, Alameda GJ, Camilo E, Green BA. Surgical treatment of post-traumatic myelopathy associated with syringomyelia. Spine. 2001; 26(24) Suppl:S119–S127

[34] Asano M, Fujiwara K, Yonenobu K, Hiroshima K. Post-traumatic syringomyelia. Spine. 1996; 21(12):1446–1453
[35] Abel R, Gerner HJ, Smit C, Meiners T. Residual deformity of the spinal canal in patients with traumatic paraplegia and secondary changes of the spinal cord. Spinal Cord. 1999; 37(1):14–19
[36] Perrouin-Verbe B, Lenne-Aurier K, Robert R, et al. Post-traumatic syringomyelia and post-traumatic spinal canal stenosis: a direct relationship: review of 75 patients with a spinal cord injury. Spinal Cord. 1998; 36(2):137–143
[37] Batzdorf U, Klekamp J, Johnson JP. A critical appraisal of syrinx cavity shunting procedures. J Neurosurg. 1998; 89(3):382–388
[38] Chou D, Wang VY, Storm PB. Pedicle subtraction osteotomies for the correction of post-traumatic thoracolumbar kyphosis. J Clin Neurosci. 2010; 17 (1):113–117
[39] Cecchinato R, Berjano P, Damilano M, Lamartina C. Spinal osteotomies to treat post-traumatic thoracolumbar deformity. Eur J Orthop Surg Traumatol. 2014; 24 Suppl 1:S31–S37
[40] Rose PS, Bridwell KH, Lenke LG, et al. Role of pelvic incidence, thoracic kyphosis, and patient factors on sagittal plane correction following pedicle subtraction osteotomy. Spine. 2009; 34(8):785–791
[41] Schwab F, Lafage V, Patel A, Farcy JP. Sagittal plane considerations and the pelvis in the adult patient. Spine. 2009; 34(17):1828–1833
[42] Kuklo TR, Polly DW, Owens BD, Zeidman SM, Chang AS, Klemme WR. Measurement of thoracic and lumbar fracture kyphosis: evaluation of intraobserver, interobserver, and technique variability. Spine. 2001; 26(1):61–65, discussion 66
[43] Farcy JP, Weidenbaum M, Glassman SD. Sagittal index in management of thoracolumbar burst fractures. Spine. 1990; 15(9):958–965
[44] Goutallier D, Louis R. Therapeutic indications in unstable fractures of the spine [in French]. Rev Chir Orthop Repar Appar Mot. 1977; 63(5):475–481
[45] Munting E. Surgical treatment of post-traumatic kyphosis in the thoracolumbar spine: indications and technical aspects. Eur Spine J. 2010; 19 Suppl 1: S69–S73
[46] Glassman SD, Bridwell K, Dimar JR, Horton W, Berven S, Schwab F. The impact of positive sagittal balance in adult spinal deformity. Spine. 2005; 30 (18):2024–2029
[47] Booth KC, Bridwell KH, Lenke LG, Baldus CR, Blanke KM. Complications and predictive factors for the successful treatment of flatback deformity (fixed sagittal imbalance). Spine. 1999; 24(16):1712–1720
[48] Gertzbein SD, Harris MB. Scoliosis Research Society. Multicenter spine fracture study. Spine. 1992; 17(5):528–540
[49] Schwab F, Blondel B, Chay E, et al. The comprehensive anatomical spinal osteotomy classification. Neurosurgery. 2014; 74(1):112–120, discussion 120
[50] Chang KW. Oligosegmental correction of post-traumatic thoracolumbar angular kyphosis. Spine. 1993; 18(13):1909–1915
[51] Vaccaro AR, Lehman RA, Jr, Hurlbert RJ, et al. A new classification of thoracolumbar injuries: the importance of injury morphology, the integrity of the posterior ligamentous complex, and neurologic status. Spine. 2005; 30 (20):2325–2333
[52] Bohlman HH, Kirkpatrick JS, Delamarter RB, Leventhal M. Anterior decompression for late pain and paralysis after fractures of the thoracolumbar spine. Clin Orthop Relat Res. 1994(300):24–29
[53] Transfeldt EE, White D, Bradford DS, Roche B. Delayed anterior decompression in patients with spinal cord and cauda equina injuries of the thoracolumbar spine. Spine. 1990; 15(9):953–957
[54] McBride GG, Bradford DS. Vertebral body replacement with femoral neck allograft and vascularized rib strut graft. A technique for treating post-traumatic kyphosis with neurologic deficit. Spine. 1983; 8(4):406–415
[55] Been HD, Poolman RW, Ubags LH. Clinical outcome and radiographic results after surgical treatment of post-traumatic thoracolumbar kyphosis following simple type A fractures. Eur Spine J. 2004; 13(2):101–107
[56] Kostuik JP, Maurais GR, Richardson WJ, Okajima Y. Combined single stage anterior and posterior osteotomy for correction of iatrogenic lumbar kyphosis. Spine. 1988; 13(3):257–266
[57] Jodoin A, Gillet P, Dupuis PR, Maurais G. Surgical treatment of post-traumatic kyphosis: a report of 16 cases. Can J Surg. 1989; 32(1):36–42
[58] Lehmer SM, Keppler L, Biscup RS, Enker P, Miller SD, Steffee AD. Posterior transvertebral osteotomy for adult thoracolumbar kyphosis. Spine. 1994; 19 (18):2060–2067
[59] Wu SS, Hwa SY, Lin LC, Pai WM, Chen PQ, Au MK. Management of rigid post-traumatic kyphosis. Spine. 1996; 21(19):2260–2266, discussion 2267
[60] Suk SI, Kim JH, Lee SM, Chung ER, Lee JH. Anterior-posterior surgery versus posterior closing wedge osteotomy in posttraumatic kyphosis with neurologic compromised osteoporotic fracture. Spine. 2003; 28(18):2170–2175
[61] Kawahara N, Tomita K, Baba H, Kobayashi T, Fujita T, Murakami H. Closing-opening wedge osteotomy to correct angular kyphotic deformity by a single posterior approach. Spine. 2001; 26(4):391–402
[62] Lazennec JY, Neves N, Rousseau MA, Boyer P, Pascal-Mousselard H, Saillant G. Wedge osteotomy for treating post-traumatic kyphosis at thoracolumbar and lumbar levels. J Spinal Disord Tech. 2006; 19(7):487–494
[63] Heary RF, Bono CM. Pedicle subtraction osteotomy in the treatment of chronic, posttraumatic kyphotic deformity. J Neurosurg Spine. 2006; 5(1):1–8
[64] El-Sharkawi MM, Koptan WM, El-Miligui YH, Said GZ. Comparison between pedicle subtraction osteotomy and anterior corpectomy and plating for correcting post-traumatic kyphosis: a multicenter study. Eur Spine J. 2011; 20 (9):1434–1440
[65] Cho KJ, Bridwell KH, Lenke LG, Berra A, Baldus C. Comparison of Smith-Petersen versus pedicle subtraction osteotomy for the correction of fixed sagittal imbalance. Spine. 2005; 30(18):2030–2037, discussion 2038
[66] Bridwell KH, Lewis SJ, Lenke LG, Baldus C, Blanke K. Pedicle subtraction osteotomy for the treatment of fixed sagittal imbalance. J Bone Joint Surg Am. 2003; 85-A(3):454–463
[67] Bridwell KH, Lewis SJ, Edwards C, et al. Complications and outcomes of pedicle subtraction osteotomies for fixed sagittal imbalance. Spine. 2003; 28 (18):2093–2101
[68] Hyun SJ, Lenke LG, Kim YC, Koester LA, Blanke KM. Comparison of standard 2-rod constructs to multiple-rod constructs for fixation across 3-column spinal osteotomies. Spine. 2014; 39(22):1899–1904
[69] Polly DW, Klemme WR, Shawen S. Management options for the treatment of posttraumatic thoracic kyphosis. Semin Spine Surg. 2000; 12:110–116
[70] Dickson DD, Lenke LG, Bridwell KH, Koester LA. Risk factors for and assessment of symptomatic pseudarthrosis after lumbar pedicle subtraction osteotomy in adult spinal deformity. Spine. 2014; 39(15):1190–1195
[71] Auerbach JD, Lenke LG, Bridwell KH, et al. Major complications and comparison between 3-column osteotomy techniques in 105 consecutive spinal deformity procedures. Spine. 2012; 37(14):1198–1210
[72] Kelly MP, Lenke LG, Shaffrey CI, et al. Evaluation of complications and neurological deficits with three-column spine reconstructions for complex spinal deformity: a retrospective Scoli-RISK-1 study. Neurosurg Focus. 2014; 36(5):E17

15 Osteoporotic Rigid Spinal Deformities

Marco Brayda-Bruno, Andrea Luca, Gabriele Ristori, Lisa Babbi, Alessio Lovi

Abstract

Osteoporotic vertebral fractures (VCFs) represent a major health problem and can lead to back pain, secondary spinal deformities, low quality of life, and increased mortality risk. In case of a failed conservative treatment, surgery could be necessary. In osteoporotic spine, mechanical stability and bone–metal integration are limited with a higher rate of complications. In this chapter, the authors describe their routine solutions to prevent loss of correction and implant failure.

A1 fracture (according to AO classification) can be treated by vertebroplasty or kyphoplasty. The authors recommend the use of high viscosity polymethylmethacrylate (PMMA). Unstable A3-A4 fractures or post-traumatic deformities need a more aggressive surgical treatment by posterior instrumented fusion or, in select cases, by anterior-posterior fusion. In order to improve screw stability, the use of cannulated and fenestrated large pedicle screws with PMMA augmentation is advisable. After meticulous assessment of the patient's balance, the authors' corrective strategy is based on several tricks, such as neural decompression (when needed), multilevel Ponte osteotomies (PCO), and multiple fixation points (including cranial hocks and sublaminar bands), with stable distal and proximal bilateral screw foundations and a 60 to 65% screw density at the remaining levels. Proximal rods kyphotic contour, proximal hybrid construct, careful preoperative sagittal profile, and BMD assessments are the specific features in the authors' strategy to reduce the most common complications after osteoporotic deformities surgical treatment, such as proximal junctional kyphosis (PJK), adjacent vertebral fractures, or adjacent level disease.

Keywords: osteoporotic vertebral fractures, post-traumatic deformities, bone–metal integration, corrective strategy, proximal junctional kyphosis, adjacent level disease

15.1 Introduction

Osteoporosis is a systemic bone disorder that leads to reduced bone mass and degradation of the skeletal microarchitecture. The result is increased bone fragility and susceptibility to fracture, with the spine, wrist, and hip being the most common parts of the skeleton that have an increased risk of fracture.[1]

15.2 Epidemiology and Etiology of Osteoporotic Deformities

The prevalence of osteoporosis in the population is age and sex related. In Europe approximately 6% of men and 21% of women aged 50 to 84 are affected by osteoporosis, which means a total of 27.6 million people are affected.[2]

Osteoporotic vertebral compression fractures (VCFs) constitute a major health problem because they commonly cause both acute and chronic back pain, substantial spinal deformity, functional disability, decreased quality of life, and high treatment costs. The mortality risk is also increased in these patients.

However, the incidence of vertebral fractures is underreported. The low rate of VCF diagnoses may be related in part to the lack of a traumatic event (only 25% of vertebral fractures result from falls); therefore the symptoms are often misinterpreted as muscle strain.[3]

A healthy, stable spine has a mechanical balance of forces acting on its axis of rotation, but in the presence of an osteoporotic fracture, the anterior spinal collapse increases the anterior lever arm, which cannot be effectively counteracted by the posterior column. This situation can be worsened by the further collapse of the fractured vertebral body, with a consequent overload on the anterior column. As a result, less force will be required to produce further adjacent fractures and a progressive kyphotic deformity.[4]

This is why osteoporotic fractures often occur during a low-energy traumatic event. They can also occur spontaneously. Usually, the main symptom is an acute onset of well localized pain, for which a radiological investigation (X-ray and MRI) is mandatory.

But a persistent, subacute, mechanical back pain that lasts for weeks should arouse suspicion for a neglected VCF. Imaging is required to assess for a nonunion with possible instability and progressive deformity. Again MRI is the exam of choice (particularly in a short tau inversion recovery [STIR] sequence) for detecting a recent bone edema or a chronic painful nonunion (▶ Fig. 15.1). Therefore patients at risk should be monitored carefully with repeated clinical controls.

15.3 Our Philosophy of Treatment in Osteoporotic VCFs and Related Kyphotic Deformities

The main treatment goals in osteoporotic VCFs are to reduce pain and to avoid new fractures, and then a possible consequent spinal deformity.[5] In most cases, these fractures are classified as type A1 (according to AO classification), and a conservative approach is then indicated, including short bed rest, analgesics, and bracing.[6]

Although most VCFs gradually heal in a few months, some patients experience long-lasting pain and disability and may require surgical treatment. In the last 20 years, the most common interventions are the percutaneous vertebroplasty (introduced in 1987 as a new way to treat spinal angiomas[7]) and the kyphoplasty, which itself evolved from the vertebroplasty.[8] More rarely, osteoporotic VCFs should be classified as unstable spinal fractures type A3 or A4. In these cases, a posterior instrumented fusion with a pedicle screw–rod construct is always necessary, and the anterior column defects often need to be stabilized (titanium mesh with bone graft is our technique of choice) to prevent loss of reduction and implant failure.

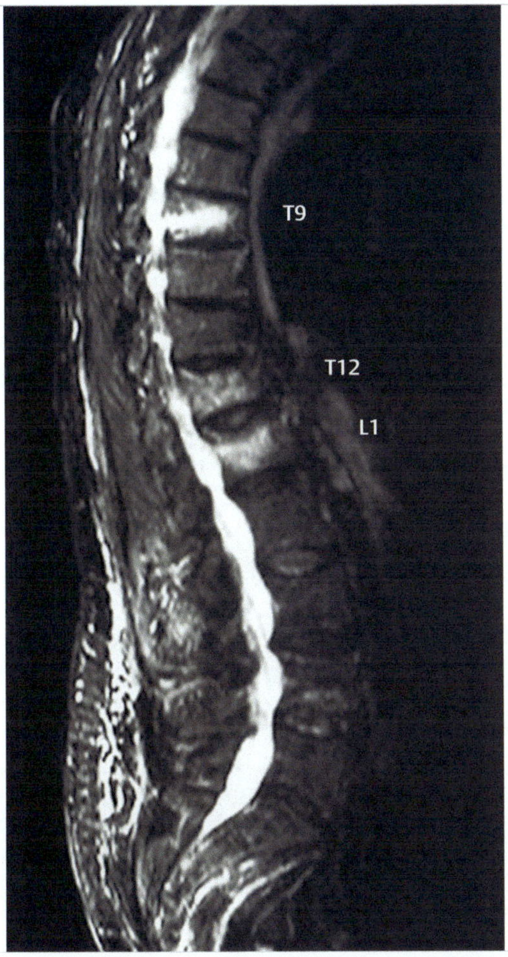

Fig. 15.1 MRI short tau inversion recovery (STIR) sequence showing bone marrow edema at three levels (T 9, T 12, L 1).

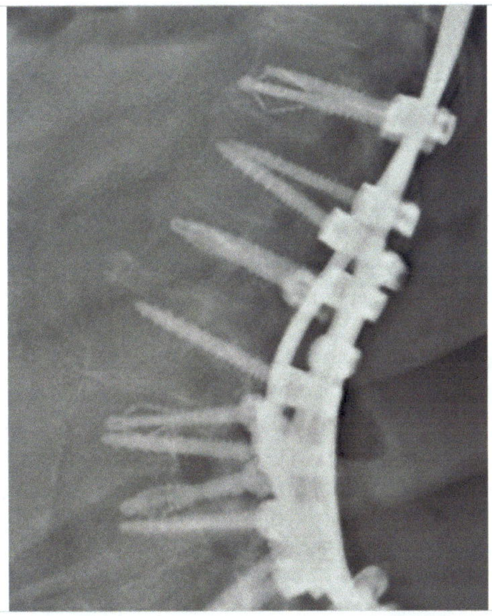

Fig. 15.2 Postoperative sagittal X-ray showing expandable pedicle screws at some levels.

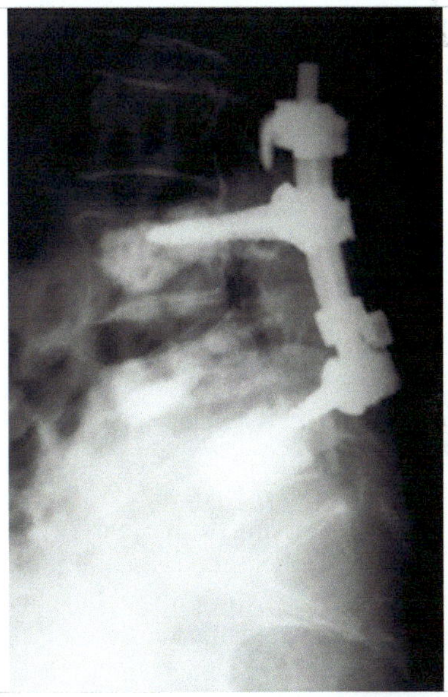

Fig. 15.3 Postoperative sagittal X-ray showing augmentation of pedicle screws with polymethylmethacrylate.

15.4 How to Improve Pedicle Screw Stability

In an osteoporotic vertebral body, mechanical stability and bone–metal integration are limited. Loosening of pedicle screws, the pullout phenomenon, and, finally, loss of stability with instrumentation failure are the possible consequences.[9,10]

Many strategies were described in the literature for improving the stability of pedicle screws.[11] The following are our routine solutions:

1. The first trick is to use the biggest screw diameter possible at each level: this solution has shown to be effective in improving pedicle screw stability; however, it must be carefully applied to avoid potential risks of pedicle breakage and vascular or neurologic complications.[12]Furthermore, substantial undertapping or no tapping is recommended.
2. Expandable pedicle screws have been used since 2000s for spinal surgical treatment in osteoporotic patients: the anterior third of these specific screws can be expanded after being inserted in the vertebral body.[13] Many biomechanical studies on osteoporotic human cadaver spines have shown a significantly improved resistance of these screws to pullout (▶ Fig. 15.2).
3. In the 2000 s, hydroxyapatite-coated titanium pedicle screws were introduced,[14] showing a 1.6-fold higher resistance to pullout forces than classic screws.[15] However, bony integration is not immediately achieved, and their primary stability is thus similar to that of classic screws.
4. In the last several years, polymethylmethacrylate (PMMA) augmentation of pedicle screws has been used with satisfactory results. PMMA injected immediately before screw insertion can increase their fixation in osteoporotic bone and allows better primary stability,[16] with an increased resistance to fatigue and to axial forces preventing pullout[17] (▶ Fig. 15.3). The more recent introduction of cannulated and

fenestrated screws has been an evident technical improvement,[18] because PMMA can be injected directly through the screw and can leak through its fenestrations inside the vertebral body. Cement injection can thus be better controlled, resulting in a reduced risk of cement leakage.

15.5 Osteoporotic Spine Deformity Correction

The assessment of sagittal and coronal global balance is of paramount importance to plan the degrees of correction needed. Long-standing anteroposterior and sagittal X-rays (possibly performed using an EOS machine) are mandatory for measuring pelvic and spinal parameters on the frontal and sagittal planes. Forced-extension X-rays over a bolster can give an idea of the correction achievable without a significant release.

A classical osteoporotic fracture type A is usually considered a stable fracture; nevertheless, if not correctly managed, it could lead to progressive deformity over a period of weeks or months as the fracture collapses and the posterior ligaments stretch.

Progressive kyphotic, or more rarely scoliotic, deformities can often produce persistent pain and eventually compression of the neural structures. In these cases an open surgical treatment is indicated. Moreover, a multilevel osteoporotic vertebral collapse, usually at the midthoracic and thoracolumbar spine, can induce an increased thoracic hyperkyphosis with loss of lumbar lordosis and positive sagittal imbalance that may require surgical correction.

This kind of surgery is of course very challenging, with a high rate of implant failure and complications. Several surgical techniques have been described.[19] Our corrective strategy is based on the following:

- Decompression of neural elements (if necessary).
- Release and correction of the deformity, often requiring a posterior column osteotomy (PCO) or pedicle subtraction osteotomy (PSO). We prefer PCOs (i. e., Ponte osteotomy) whenever possible, reserving the more risky PSO for very severe cases.[20] A correctly bent rod is then necessary, avoiding excessive correction and with a proximal kyphotic shape to help prevent proximal junctional kyphosis.
- Posterior instrumentation is done on multiple levels and with multiple fixation points (using the methods already described to strengthen the bone–screw interface) and fusion (frequently to the pelvis), to assure construct stability.[21]
- Several fixation options (i. e., pedicle screws, hooks, sublaminar bands, connectors) are important and available in modern instrumentations. Hooks and sublaminar bands are very resistant to failure, being fixed on the posterior arch, the most solid and resistant part of the osteoporotic vertebrae.[22] Nevertheless, PMMA pedicle screws are our first choice, showing good pullout resistance and the capacity to hold major deformity correction.[23]
- Strong and stable foundations are mandatory and are obtained by placing bilateral screws at a minimum of two distal levels of the instrumentation.[24] At the proximal end of the construct, we always prefer to instrument, bilaterally, the upper two to three levels in a hybrid manner (hooks/bands and screws), in a clamp configuration, and the rods are carefully shaped to be kyphotic. At the remaining levels, we insert one screw per level, based on our strategic planning for the correction (around 60–65% screw density), achieving a similar corrective power while reducing the surgical time, hardware costs, and potential complication of screw malpositioning.
- CoCr alloy rods are used except when some metal allergy is present; they are stiffer and more plastic, and allow in situ bending, otherwise not possible with the elastic titanium rods. Furthermore, CoCr rods have greater yield strength, which potentially allows maintenance of a larger correction in severe deformities. They are also less affected by notching and then less likely to break, therefore increasing construct longevity and time for fusion.[25,26]

15.6 Complications and Conclusions

A common complication in the treatment of osteoporotic deformities is screws loosening because of bone weakness. Fortunately, the cement-augmented screws had good results in many studies, significantly reducing peri-implant osteolysis.[16,17] The complications of cement leakage into the neural canal and/or segmentary vessels can also be reduced thanks to the injection of high-viscosity cement (▶ Fig. 15.4).

Vertebral body fractures adjacent to fusions are another frequent concern in osteoporotic patients.[27] Several studies have suggested that prophylactic vertebroplasty may reduce the risk of adjacent-level failure following extended spinal fusions.[28] For these reasons, we recommend adjacent-level augmentation of vertebrae proximal to the fusion (▶ Fig. 15.5).

Finally, proximal junctional kyphosis and adjacent segment disease are probably two of the most fearsome complications after adult deformity surgical treatment, occurring in up to 39%

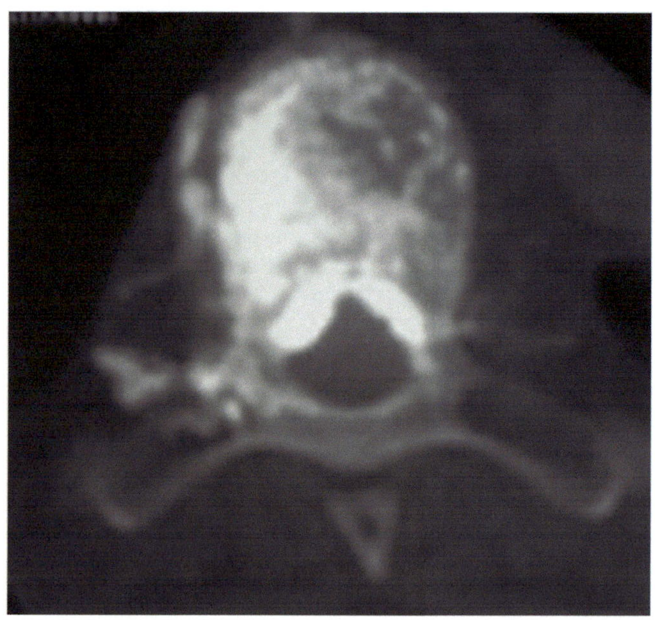

Fig. 15.4 Postoperative CT scan showing epidural, foraminal, and venous cement leakage.

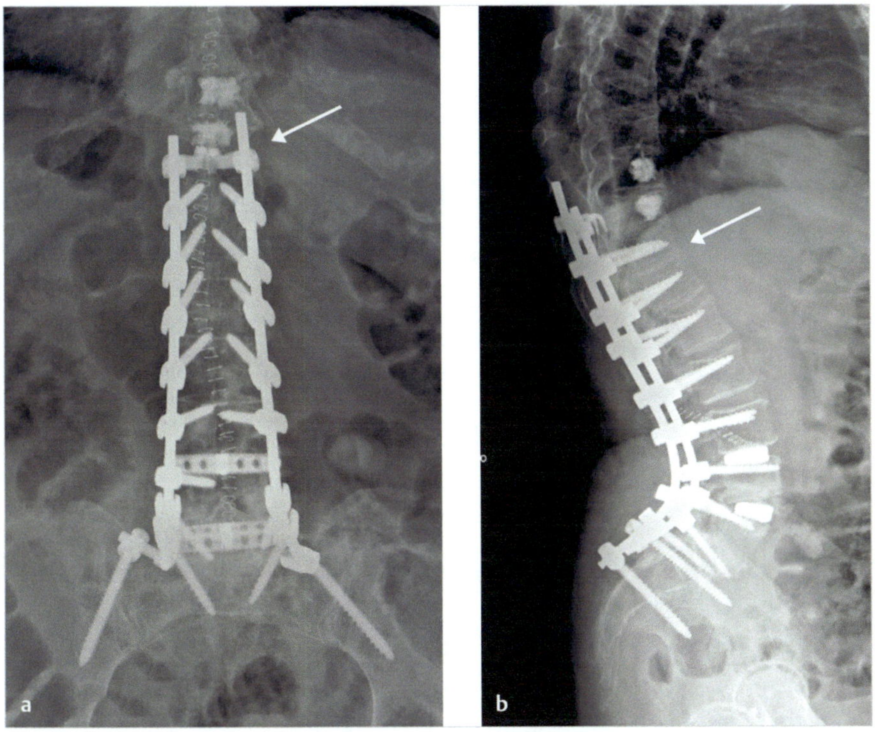

Fig. 15.5 (a) Postoperative anteroposterior and (b) sagittal X-ray showing prophylactic vertebroplasty at two cranial levels of a posterior thoracolumbar fusion (arrows).

of patients, most often within the first 6 to 8 weeks postsurgery. Age (patients over 55–60 years old), osteoporosis, and aggressive surgical approaches are still major risk factors.[29] No effective solution has yet been proposed to effectively reduce this complication.

The authors' strategy for preventing these complications, as described earlier in the chapter, is based on the routine use of proximal hybrid constructs, which are less stiff than screws alone, and on the proximal rods' kyphotic contour. But the authors believe that the best way to minimize the risk is to make a careful preoperative assessment of the sagittal profile and bone mass index: presurgical teriparatide treatment for 6 months and an individually correct sagittal contour of the instrumentation are crucial in their opinion, when addressing an osteoporotic spinal deformity with surgical treatment.

References

[1] Glaser DL, Kaplan FS. Osteoporosis. Definition and clinical presentation. Spine. 1997; 22(24) Suppl:12S–16S

[2] Hernlund E, Svedbom A, Ivergård M, et al. Osteoporosis in the European Union: medical management, epidemiology and economic burden. A report prepared in collaboration with the International Osteoporosis Foundation (IOF) and the European Federation of Pharmaceutical Industry Associations (EFPIA). Arch Osteoporos. 2013; 8:136

[3] Chin DK, Park JY, Yoon YS, et al. Prevalence of osteoporosis in patients requiring spine surgery: incidence and significance of osteoporosis in spine disease. Osteoporos Int. 2007; 18(9):1219–1224

[4] Keller TS, Harrison DE, Colloca CJ, Harrison DD, Janik TJ. Prediction of osteoporotic spinal deformity. Spine. 2003; 28(5):455–462

[5] Alexandru D, So W. Evaluation and management of vertebral compression fractures. Perm J. 2012; 16(4):46–51

[6] Malmivaara A, Häkkinen U, Aro T, et al. The treatment of acute low back pain–bed rest, exercises, or ordinary activity? N Engl J Med. 1995; 332 (6):351–355

[7] Galibert P, Deramond H, Rosat P, Le Gars D. Preliminary note on the treatment of vertebral angioma by percutaneous acrylic vertebroplasty [in French]. Neurochirurgie. 1987; 33(2):166–168

[8] Lovi A, Teli M, Ortolina A, Costa F, Fornari M, Brayda-Bruno M. Vertebroplasty and kyphoplasty: complementary techniques for the treatment of painful osteoporotic vertebral compression fractures. A prospective non-randomised study on 154 patients. Eur Spine J. 2009; 18 Suppl 1:95–101

[9] Cook SD, Salkeld SL, Stanley T, Faciane A, Miller SD. Biomechanical study of pedicle screw fixation in severely osteoporotic bone. Spine J. 2004; 4(4):402–408

[10] Halvorson TL, Kelley LA, Thomas KA, Whitecloud TS, III, Cook SD. Effects of bone mineral density on pedicle screw fixation. Spine. 1994; 19(21):2415–2420

[11] Goldstein CL, Brodke DS, Choma TJ. Surgical Management of Spinal Conditions in the Elderly Osteoporotic Spine. Neurosurgery. 2015; 77 Suppl 4:S98–S107

[12] Polly DW, Jr, Orchowski JR, Ellenbogen RG. Revision pedicle screws. Bigger, longer shims–what is best? Spine. 1998; 23(12):1374–1379

[13] Kettler A, Schmoelz W, Shezifi Y, et al. Biomechanical performance of the new BeadEx implant in the treatment of osteoporotic vertebral body compression fractures: restoration and maintenance of height and stability. Clin Biomech (Bristol, Avon). 2006; 21(7):676–682

[14] Sandén B, Olerud C, Petrén-Mallmin M, Larsson S. Hydroxyapatite coating improves fixation of pedicle screws. A clinical study. J Bone Joint Surg Br. 2002; 84(3):387–391

[15] Hasegawa T, Inufusa A, Imai Y, Mikawa Y, Lim TH, An HS. Hydroxyapatite-coating of pedicle screws improves resistance against pull-out force in the osteoporotic canine lumbar spine model: a pilot study. Spine J. 2005; 5 (3):239–243

[16] Choma TJ, Pfeiffer FM, Swope RW, et al. Pedicle screws design and cement augmentation in osteoporotic vertebrae. Spine. 2012; 26:e1628–e1632

[17] Frankel BM, D'Agostino S, Wang C. A biomechanical cadaveric analysis of polymethylmethacrylate-augmented pedicle screw fixation. J Neurosurg Spine. 2007; 7(1):47–53

[18] Yazu M, Kin A, Kosaka R, Kinoshita M, Abe M. Efficacy of novel-concept pedicle screw fixation augmented with calcium phosphate cement in the osteoporotic spine. J Orthop Sci. 2005; 10(1):56–61

[19] Behrbalk E, Uri O, Folman Y, Rickert M, Kaiser R, Boszczyk BM. Staged correction of severe thoracic kyphosis in patients with multilevel osteoporotic vertebral compression fractures. Global Spine J. 2016; 6(7):710–720

[20] Gill JB, Levin A, Burd T, Longley M. Corrective osteotomies in spine surgery. J Bone Joint Surg Am. 2008; 90(11):2509–2520

[21] Cho W, Mason JR, Smith JS, et al. Failure of lumbopelvic fixation after long construct fusions in patients with adult spinal deformity: clinical and radiographic risk factors: clinical article. J Neurosurg Spine. 2013; 19(4):445–453

[22] Coe JD, Warden KE, Herzig MA, McAfee PC. Influence of bone mineral density on the fixation of thoracolumbar implants. A comparative study of transpedicular screws, laminar hooks, and spinous process wires. Spine. 1990; 15 (9):902–907

[23] Hitchon PW, Brenton MD, Black AG, et al. In vitro biomechanical comparison of pedicle screws, sublaminar hooks, and sublaminar cables. J Neurosurg. 2003; 99(1) Suppl:104–109

[24] Tobias Pitzen M. Overview of surgical techniques and implants. In: Vieweg U, Grochulla F, eds. Manual of Spine Surgery. New York: Springer-Verlag; 2012:117–125

[25] Nguyen TQ, Buckley JM, Ames C, Deviren V. The fatigue life of contoured cobalt chrome posterior spinal fusion rods. Proc Inst Mech Eng H. 2011; 225 (2):194–198

[26] Yoshihara H. Rods in spinal surgery: a review of the literature. Spine J. 2013; 13(10):1350–1358

[27] Patil S, Rawall S, Singh D, et al. Surgical patterns in osteoporotic vertebral compression fractures. Eur Spine J. 2013; 22(4):883–891

[28] Chiang C-K, Wang Y-H, Yang C-Y, Yang BD, Wang JL. Prophylactic vertebroplasty may reduce the risk of adjacent intact vertebra from fatigue injury: an ex vivo biomechanical study. Spine. 2009; 34(4):356–364

[29] Kim YJ, Bridwell KH, Lenke LG, Glattes CR, Rhim S, Cheh G. Proximal junctional kyphosis in adult spinal deformity after segmental posterior spinal instrumentation and fusion: minimum five-year follow-up. Spine. 2008; 33 (20):2179–2184

16 Spinal Deformities in Patients with Parkinson's Disease

Stéphane Wolff, Peter Upex, Guillaume Riouallon

Abstract

Parkinson's disease is often associated with spinal deformity. Sometimes mild at the beginning of the disease, deformities mainly occur in advanced stages. At the most, the patient presents with camptocormia with a great imbalance. The treatment should be coordinated between the family doctor, neurologist, surgeon, and physiotherapist. Medical treatment, braces, and regular physiotherapy are efficient to limit the deformity. Surgery allows correction of the scoliosis, but with a high rate of general complication and mechanical failure. However, some patients who underwent a long fusion have stable results due to careful selection at an early stage, good technique with solid instrumentation, and restoration of a good shape of spine.

Keywords: Parkinson's disease, camptocormia, scoliosis, postoperative balance, suspension X-rays

16.1 Introduction

Parkinson's disease is often associated with spinal deformity. Sometimes a scoliosis has been followed since childhood, with successive X-rays. In other cases, the deformity occurs during the advanced stage of the neurologic disease. In the first case, the deformity is similar to an idiopathic scoliosis. In the second case, the deformity has a clearly neurologic pattern, with symptoms and imbalance variations throughout the day. The scoliosis will increase along with the neurologic impairment with progressive imbalance.[1,2,3,4,5] At an early stage, anterior and lateral imbalance is unspectacular, changing at different times, and fully reducible when the patient is lying supine. (▶ Fig. 16.1a–c).

The deformity will often change toward a huge imbalance and much less flexibility. Lumbar pain and sometimes sciatica aggravate the discomfort. Neurologic worsening, extrapyramidal tone disorders, and scoliosis lead to walking difficulties, and ultimately to the inability to walk.

When the trunk is fully bent down, the deformity is described as camptocormia (▶ Fig. 16.2a–d). Parkinson's disease is currently the leading cause of camptocormia.[6,7,8]

The weak and changing sagittal balance is caused by both trunk disorder and lower limb disorder. Falls are frequent. The deformity's treatment is, overall, medical. A modification of dopamine administration could lead to improved balance and walking ability. Regular physiotherapy should be proposed, at best, through group exercises. Brain surgery with neurostimulation is helpful to reduce the shaking but is less effective for muscular axial tone disorders and scoliosis.[9]

16.2 Surgical Considerations

Bracing is often used. It can provide pain relief and leads to improved balance. The heavier and older the patients are, the less they tolerate a brace. Also, it is very difficult to use bracing in patients with camptocormia.

Spine surgery in Parkinson's disease is known to have a high rate of complications and poor results. For laminectomy or a short arthrodesis, the functional results are reported as inferior to those for the general population.[10,11] In addition to the usual complications associated with spinal surgery, there is a risk of camptocormia in the short term. It is also not surprising that long fusions are not always successful (▶ Fig. 16.3).

A few publications have reported on a series of long fusion for Parkinson's deformities.[12,13,14,15,16,17,18] They have a high rate of mechanical failure, and major medical complications are also frequent. Bouyer et al reported on a large, multicenter series of 48 cases in which there was a 49% rate of mechanical failure and a reoperation rate of 42%.[13] Overall, except for patients who undergo multiple operations due to recurrent mechanical failure, the functional results have been acceptable[12,13,18]

There are, undoubtedly, excellent and stable results for some patients who had a worsening deformity. Patient selection is a key factor. We recommend operating at an early stage, as soon as evolution of the deformity has been proven. In these cases, one can easily achieve a good outcome after operating on a flexible spine. Examination in the supine position and suspension X-rays can confirm a satisfactory outcome. On the other hand, if the deformity is major with a low flexibility, frequent falls, and some comorbidity, we prefer to refrain from surgical intervention.

There are no written rules to guide us, and the decision is difficult, especially when the patient has hope that surgery will provide relief and recovery. A negative decision is traumatic in that the patient thereby realizes that he or she has reached an advanced stage and will never recover improved balance. We must consider the family's opinion as well as the neurologist's

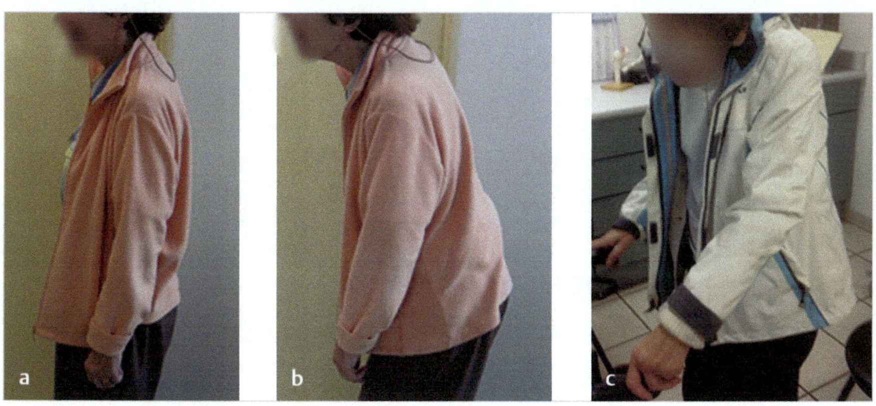

Fig. 16.1 **(a, b)** Variability of trunk position before surgery in a mild form. **(c)** Ten years postsurgery, the trunk remains straight, but the head is drooping, and the patient is using a walker.

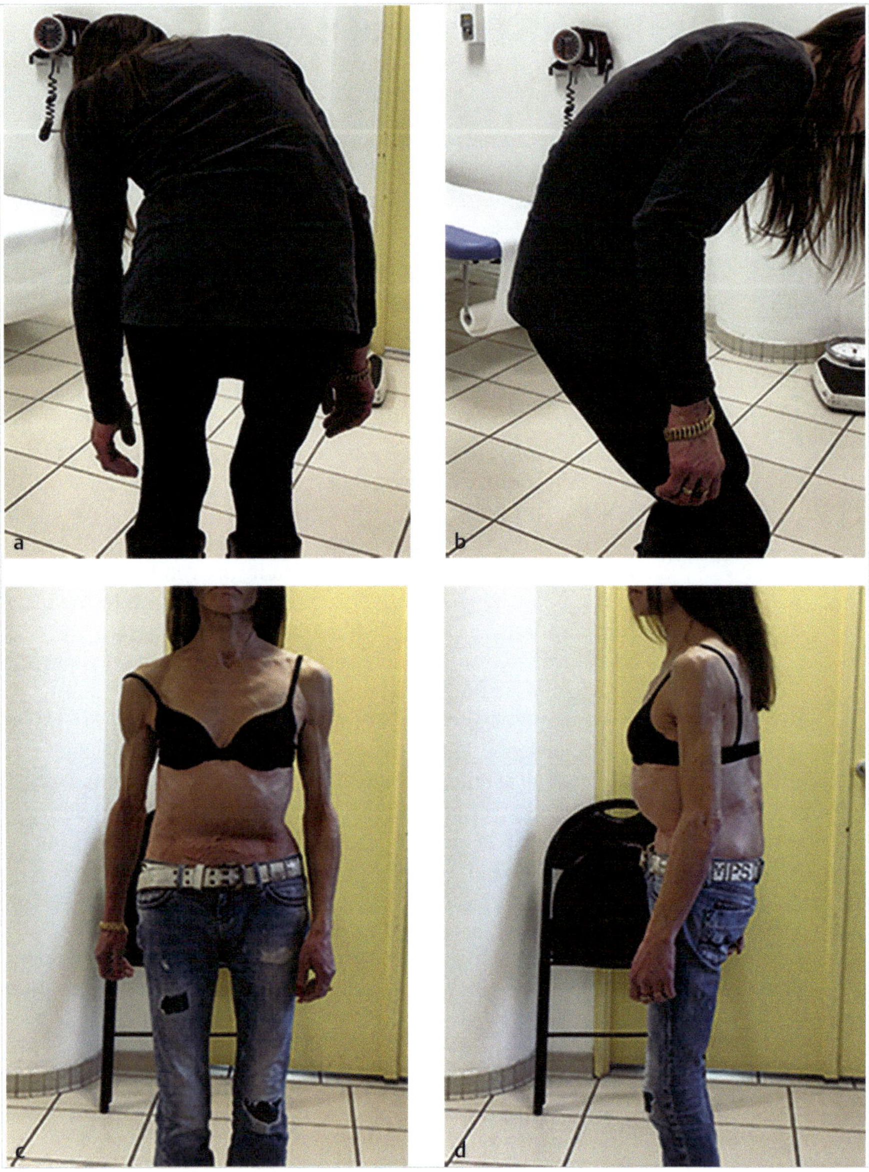

Fig. 16.2 (a, b) Camptocormia in Parkinson's disease before and **(c, d)** after surgery.

advice. The technique, benefits, and risks of complications must be clearly presented and discussed. It should be noted that patients more readily accept reoperation in cases of mechanical failure.

16.3 Surgical Technique

Once the surgery is planned, the decision must be made as to the preferred technique. The technique is not specific, being a long fusion, thoracic and lumbar. In cases of childhood scoliosis and with only slight neurologic impairment and no imbalance, the fusion can stop on L4 or L5. In these favorable situations, the recovery will be easier with a lower rate of pseudarthrosis. The risk of immediate imbalance is low. Moreover, when imbalance does occur, reoperation can be performed using a simple procedure at a later date.

In the majority of cases, the fusion including the pelvis is required. A good sagittal and frontal postoperative balance is an essential condition for success. However, it is unfortunately not a sufficient condition to avoid mechanical failure and other problems. We must understand that even with a good spinal shape, the trunk's balance will often be bad: the patient will remain bent in the hips, walking is not smooth, and every movement is performed in an inappropriate manner. Implants are put to severe testing.

The instrumentation should have a strong pelvic fixation. Depending on the surgeon's preference, sacral screws with iliac screws, iliosacral screws, and most recently sacral screws with S2-alar-iliac screws can be used.

Our current preference is to use iliosacral screws implanted with navigation.

During the follow-up, we don't use bracing, but the maximum effort is made to prevent falls, including medical treatment, nursing, and consideration of environmental conditions, as well as potentially constant surveillance.

16.4 Conclusion

Surgery has to be considered in the treatment of a Parkinson's deformity. At an early stage, the result can be very good, with

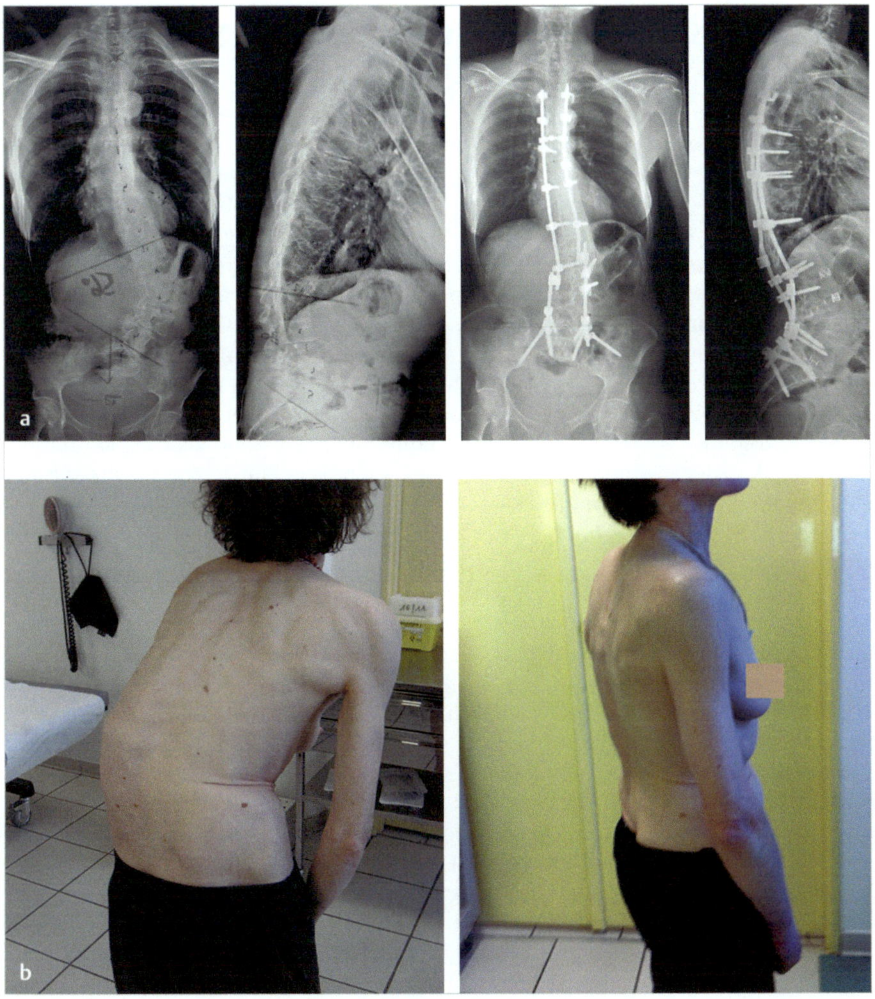

Fig. 16.3 **(a)** Deformation X-rays before and after a long fusion surgery, **(b)** photos before and after surgery.

long and strong instrumentation. The sagittal and frontal balance must be restored with all operative resources, including various osteotomies. At the stage of camptocormia, the principles of surgical treatment are the same, but complications are frequent, and the results are much less favorable. At advanced stages, the surgeon must abstain from surgical treatment, sometimes to the patient's dismay.

References

[1] Ye X, Lou D, Ding X, et al. A clinical study of the coronal plane deformity in Parkinson disease. Eur Spine J. 2017; 26(7):1862–1870

[2] Pandey S, Kumar H. Assessment of striatal & postural deformities in patients with Parkinson's disease. Indian J Med Res. 2016; 144(5):682–688

[3] Bissolotti L, Isacco-Grassi F, Orizio C, et al. Spinopelvic balance and body image perception in Parkinson's disease: analysis of correlation. Eur Spine J. 2015; 24 Suppl 7:898–905

[4] Bissolotti L, Donzelli S, Gobbo M, Zaina F, Villafañe JH, Negrini S. Association Between Sagittal Balance and Scoliosis in Patients with Parkinson Disease: A Cross-sectional Study. Am J Phys Med Rehabil. 2016; 95(1):39–46

[5] Choi HJ, Smith JS, Shaffrey CI, et al. Coronal plane spinal malalignment and Parkinson's disease: prevalence and associations with disease severity. Spine J. 2015; 15(1):115–121

[6] Margraf NG, Wrede A, Deuschl G, Schulz-Schaeffer WJ. Pathophysiological Concepts and Treatment of Camptocormia. J Parkinsons Dis. 2016; 6(3):485–501

[7] Tiple D, Fabbrini G, Colosimo C, et al. Camptocormia in Parkinson disease: an epidemiological and clinical study. J Neurol Neurosurg Psychiatry. 2009; 80 (2):145–148

[8] Lenoir T, Guedj N, Boulu P, Guigui P, Benoist M. Camptocormia: the bent spine syndrome, an update. Eur Spine J. 2010; 19(8):1229–1237

[9] Umemura A, Oka Y, Ohkita K, Yamawaki T, Yamada K. Effect of subthalamic deep brain stimulation on postural abnormality in Parkinson disease. J Neurosurg. 2010; 112(6):1283–1288

[10] Babat LB, McLain RF, Bingaman W, Kalfas I, Young P, Rufo-Smith C. Spinal surgery in patients with Parkinson's disease: construct failure and progressive deformity. Spine. 2004; 29(18):2006–2012

[11] Westermann L, Eysel P, Hantscher J, et al. The Influence of Parkinson Disease on Lumbar Decompression Surgery: A Retrospective Case Control Study. World Neurosurg. 2017; 108:513–518

[12] Koller H, Acosta F, Zenner J, et al. Spinal surgery in patients with Parkinson's disease: experiences with the challenges posed by sagittal imbalance and the Parkinson's spine. Eur Spine J. 2010; 19(10):1785–1794

[13] Bouyer B, Scemama C, Roussouly P, et al. Evolution and complications after surgery for spine deformation in patients with Parkinson's disease. Orthop Traumatol Surg Res. 2017; 103(4):517–522

[14] Upadhyaya CD, Starr PA, Mummaneni PV. Spinal deformity and Parkinson disease: a treatment algorithm. Neurosurg Focus. 2010; 28(3):E5

[15] Tabamo RE, Fernandez HH, Friedman JH, Lucas PR. Spinal surgery for severe scoliosis in Parkinson's disease. Med Health R I. 2000; 83(4):114–115

[16] Moon S-H, Lee H-M, Chun H-J, et al. Surgical outcome of lumbar fusion surgery in patients with Parkinson disease. J Spinal Disord Tech. 2012; 25 (7):351–355

[17] Sarkiss CA, Fogg GA, Skovrlj B, Cho SK, Caridi JM. To operate or not?: A literature review of surgical outcomes in 95 patients with Parkinson's disease undergoing spine surgery. Clin Neurol Neurosurg. 2015; 134:122–125

[18] Bourghli A, Guérin P, Vital J-M, et al. Posterior spinal fusion from T2 to the sacrum for the management of major deformities in patients with Parkinson disease: a retrospective review with analysis of complications. J Spinal Disord Tech. 2012; 25(3):E53–E60

17 Surgical Planning for En Bloc Resection of Spinal Tumors: Tailoring the Osteotomy to Tumor Extensions

Stefano Boriani, Alessandro Gasbarrini, Riccardo Ghermandi, Shifra Fraifeld, José E. Cohen, Eyal Itshayek

Abstract

En bloc resection of a spinal tumor, defined as removal of a tumor in its entirety, fully covered by a continuous shell of healthy tissue called the margin, may be indicated (1) in cases of aggressive (Enneking stage 3) primary tumors, or (2) in patients with spinal metastases that are refractory to radiation and/or chemotherapy, or that pose a risk of spinal instability or cord compression, or when en bloc resection of the spinal lesion offers the potential for a significant improvement in disease control and survival. Surgical planning should consider oncological staging, definition of the suggested margins and functional losses that may occur, and anatomical features and tumor extensions. The surgical approach should be designed to ensure visual control during release or resection of important anatomical structures to achieve the required margin. The authors propose use of the Weinstein-Boriani-Biagini (WBB) system for surgical staging of tumor extensions based on clear assessment of the layers of tissue involved in the tumor and the pattern of circumferential growth around the spinal cord. Six types of surgical strategies, including 10 combinations of approaches, are described, with clear illustration and discussion of the surgical steps.

Keywords: En bloc resection, oncological staging, osteotomy, spinal tumors, tumor extension, Weinstein-Boriani-Biagini (WBB) staging system

17.1 Introduction

Spinal metastases develop in 70% of patients with systemic cancers, and rates are expected to increase as oncology treatments advance.[1,2,3] Primary tumors of the spine are far less common, representing < 10% of spinal tumors.[4] The clinical manifestations of both primary and metastatic spinal tumors include pain, neurologic deficits, pathological fractures, spinal instability, and deformity. Techniques and indications for spine surgery in patients with both primary and secondary tumors have evolved significantly in the past two decades, led by the rapid evolution of imaging, surgical approaches, and spinal instrumentation, as well as understanding of spinal biomechanics in general and the importance of preservation and restoration of the sagittal balance in particular. These changes have enabled surgeons to perform more extensive operations that provide cord decompression and spinal column stabilization, as well as oncologically sound en bloc resection. En bloc resection is defined as removal of a tumor in its entirety, fully covered by a continuous shell of healthy tissue called the margin.[5]

From an oncological perspective, the treatment of metastatic disease is often palliative, a term that indicates that the quality of life is an important target to be achieved, together with local control when feasible. Conversely, in the treatment of primary tumors, the surgeon should focus on the goal of achieving local and systemic control and disregard the functional role of anatomical structures that are closely contiguous or infiltrated by the tumor. However, the decision to sacrifice a critical structure, for example, a nerve, nerve sheath, dura, thoracic duct, or major vessel, can only be made after carefully weighing the resulting functional loss against the risk of local recurrence and the impact on final outcome.[6,7] This decision will be strongly influenced by the biological aggressiveness of the tumor, the patient's prognosis and preoperative neurologic status, and the functional loss that the patient is willing to accept with the aim of gaining local control and possibly curing the disease.

Primary tumor aggressiveness can be graded according to the Enneking classification system,[5] a valid and reproducible tool for the surgical staging of bone and soft tissue tumors.[8] When a functional loss is anticipated, the patient and caregivers must be carefully apprised of the risks and benefits of radical surgery and must be prepared to accept the loss as necessary to achieve disease control. With this important caveat, the diagnosis of an aggressive benign or malignant primary tumor is an accepted indication for en bloc resection.[5]

When anatomically feasible, and with informed patient consent, en bloc resection is recommended in cases of aggressive (Enneking stage 3[5]) osteoblastomas and giant cell tumors of the thoracic and lumbar spine,[9,10] chordoma and chondrosarcoma,[11] osteosarcoma,[12,13] and Ewing sarcoma.[14] "Intralesional" resection occurs in cases where the surgeon incidentally or intentionally violates the tumor. Intentional intralesional resection may be an option in cases where obtaining a surgical margin requires resection of functionally relevant tissue that is closely contiguous to the tumor or has been infiltrated by the tumor; however, intentional violation of the tumor margins significantly worsens the prognosis.[15]

In patients with spinal metastases, surgery may be indicated in cases where tumors are resistant to radiation-based treatment and/or chemotherapy, or there is current or impending risk of spinal instability or cord compression.[16,17,18] The primary goal in these patients is generally to preserve or improve function and quality of life without unnecessary morbidity; thus, in principle, no functionally significant nerve root, for example, should be sacrificed when resecting a benign tumor or metastasis. En bloc resection with the primary goal of achieving complete local control should be performed only in selected cases of spinal metastases.[19,20,21] In the authors' experience, this decision may be appropriate in cases where there is full tumor control at the primary site; a single area of spinal involvement, with or without existing or impending spinal cord compression or destabilization; and/or severe pain that is refractory to medical management.[22] The key point in this decision is the lack of sensitivity to any another treatment; alternatively, less aggressive surgery could be combined with such treatments, reducing the surgical morbidity without reducing the possibility to cure.

This chapter discusses factors that influence surgical planning for en bloc resection, presents the Rizzoli Institute experience with these surgeries, and illustrates the techniques and

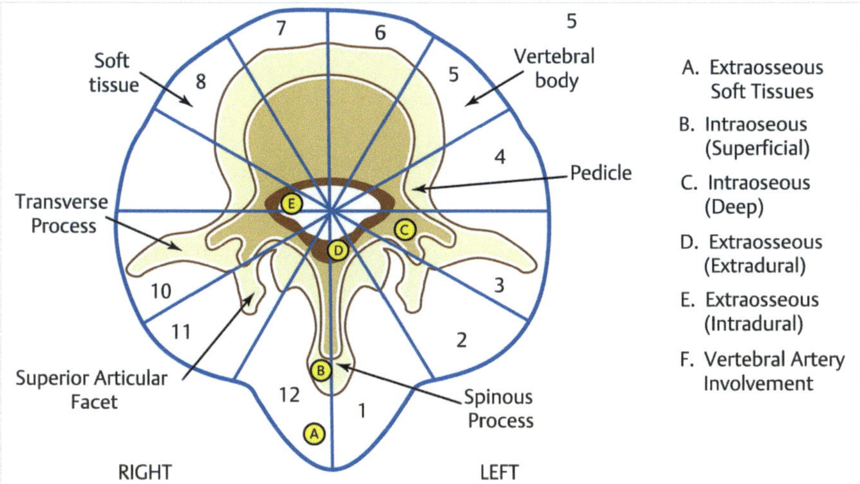

Fig. 17.1 The Weinstein-Boriani-Biagini (WBB) surgical system for staging extensions of primary bone tumors of the spine. The region of the spine is divided into compartments that may be involved in the tumor, ranging from A, which encompasses all extraosseous soft tissue surrounding the spinal column, to E, the extraosseous/intradural region, for tumors that have penetrated the dura. The letter *F* is used to connote vertebral artery involvement. In addition, 12 sectors are defined to describe circumferential extensions.

challenges in achieving stabilization with good sagittal alignment in these aggressive surgeries.

17.2 Planning En Bloc Resection

En bloc resection is a demanding procedure that requires careful planning. Infringement of oncological principles at this stage with intentional intralesional resection to preserve critical structures and improve functional outcome markedly reduces the possibility of local control. In addition, the rates of complications and tumor recurrence are significantly higher for revision surgery.[23] Nevertheless, planning must include a well-conducted decision-making process that includes extensive discussions to ensure that the patient and caregivers have a clear and correct understanding of the surgical goal, as well as the expected and potential morbidity. Fully informed consent is a precondition for the surgeon to undertake en bloc resection.

The Weinstein-Boriani-Biagini (WBB) surgical system for staging extensions of primary bone tumors of the spine (▶ Fig. 17.1) was proposed in 1997.[24] More recently, the WBB system has been validated by a multidisciplinary team of spine tumor experts,[8] and is currently used by many centers worldwide.[25] The planning process described here is based on the WBB system, with the goal of achieving the required oncological margin with the lowest possible morbidity. Seven different strategies based on four surgical approaches are proposed: anterior, posterior, anterior followed by posterior, and posterior followed by simultaneous anterior and posterior. These techniques, the proposed steps for surgical planning, and the criteria for surgery have evolved based on the experience of the Rizzoli Institute as well as reports from other centers.

17.2.1 Steps for Surgical Planning

- Oncological staging and definition of suggested margins.
- Definition of the functional implications of suggested surgical margins.
- Review of anatomical features.
- Review of tumor extension.

Oncological Staging

Based on tumor diagnosis and staging, the Enneking system suggests the required surgical margin.[5] In cases where the tumor is growing in the epidural space. The surgeon may consider resecting the dura together with the tumor to achieve a tumor-free margin at surgery.[26] Dura covering the scar is only expected when the epidural space is occupied by scar, a frequent finding in cases of tumor recurrence. In patients with de novo, previously unoperated tumors, tumor extension into the epidural space may be presumed to indicate contamination of a region extending from the skull to the sacrum, reducing the oncological validity of dura resection over the tumor, notably in cases of malignant tumors that have no capsule.

Functional Relevance of the Margins

A cost–benefit assessment is required in situations where diagnosis and staging indicate the need for a wide margin that includes a structure such as a nerve root whose sacrifice will result in functional or neurologic compromise. The patient must be fully informed regarding the expected functional loss as well as the risk of recurrence with intentional intralesional resection. In cases where the patient opts for preservation of the critical structure, adjuvant therapy is indicated. This careful planning becomes more and more important as the number of important extraspinal structures, major vessels, organs, and other structures involved increases. Oncological criteria and the probability of achieving good local control must be carefully weighed against expected morbidity, and the trade-offs discussed with the patient, as the surgery is planned.

Anatomical Features

It is a relatively simple task to release the vertebrae from the aorta in the upper thoracic spine (T1–T4) since no segmental arteries are closely connected to the vertebral bodies in this area. However, below T5 the intercostal arteries run around the vertebral bodies, and the aorta is closely related to bone; thus, careful retraction is required during en bloc resection via a posterior approach.

The pillars of the diaphragm can extend to T 12, increasing the difficulty of dissection via a posterior approach. An anterior approach may be required for a safe release.

Debate continues regarding the role of the Adamkiewicz artery (AKA) as an exclusive feeder to the anterior spinal artery. It would appear reasonable that cord vascularity is not solely dependent on a single artery, and there is evidence of multiple feeding arteries.[27] Earlier we relied on preoperative angiography to identify the radiculomedullary artery feeding the AKA, but after four cases where the AKA was sacrificed without damage to cord vascularity we consider this study less essential, and in most cases it does not affect surgical planning. Tomita and his group have concluded that the risk of cord ischemia is dependent on the number of contiguous radicular arteries sacrificed rather than loss of a single artery.[27,28,29,30,31]

Current evidence suggests that surgery should be planned with bilateral ligation and sacrifice of no more than three nerve roots in the thoracic spine.[28,29,31]

Tumor Extension

Surgical planning is primarily driven by the tumor's extensions. In cases of anterior growth into the mediastinum (compartment A in WBB staging, extracompartmental), an anterior approach is required for visualization of the tumor during surgery and preservation of a good surrounding margin. Only an anterior approach enables visual control during resection of the pleura, which is considered an appropriate margin; digital dissection will result in penetration of the anterior aspect of the tumor when surgery is performed via a posterior approach.[32,33]

17.2.2 Essential Surgical Criteria

- Visual control is essential to achieve the required margin.
- The most important anatomical structures must be released or resected under visual control.
- Combined simultaneous approaches are associated with higher morbidity and should be performed only when mandatory.
- Cord vascularity must be considered in multisegmental resections.
- Epidural bleeding can become a serious problem if underestimated.
- Removal of the specimen must be planned by the best approach to avoid tractions or torsions of the cord.

17.2.3 Surgical Tips and Techniques

When intralesional surgery is planned or the risk of penetrating the tumor during resection is significant, selective arterial embolization is mandatory; however, when the surgeon anticipates a good probability of successful en bloc resection with oncological margins, tumor ischemia following embolization may induce peritumoral vascularization with increased risk of bleeding. Hemostasis is essential; poorly controlled epidural bleeding increases the risk of cardiovascular failure at the last steps of such a long procedure. In cases where two separate approaches are essential, overnight staging may reduce the risk of complications, since increased tissue from larger open wounds may be associated with longer and more profuse bleeding.

17.2.4 Surgical Approach

Careful selection of the surgical approach and timing is essential to assure visual control throughout the procedure: while approaching the canal, releasing or resecting the dura, releasing the tumor from surrounding tissue, defining the margins, determining which critical structures will be preserved and which must be sacrificed, and gently removing the specimen while avoiding damage to the spinal cord. The traction, torsion, pushing, and shortening required to safely achieve this final step also require careful planning.

We propose six combinations of surgical approaches for en bloc resection of tumors of the spine: a single anterior approach (type 1); a single posterior approach, including three subtypes (types 2A, 2B, 2C); an anterior and then a posterior approach, with three subtypes (types 3A, 3B, 3C); a posterior approach, and then an anterior approach contralateral and ipsilateral to the tumor (type 4); anterior and then simultaneous anterior and posterior approaches (type 5); and an anterior approach on the contralateral side of the tumor, followed by a posterior approach, and then simultaneous anterior and posterior approaches (type 6). Ten different strategies result from consideration of tumor extensions and spinal location.

Type 1: Single Anterior Approach

A single anterior approach (▸ Fig. 17.2) enables en bloc resection only of small tumors of the thoracic and lumbar vertebral bodies. These must be enclosed inside sectors 8 to 5 and arise from compartment A and/or B, but not extend into compartment C. (In the case of extension into compartment C, a posterior approach is required to provide an appropriate margin under direct visual control by entering the canal and releasing the dura.)

Three Steps

First: Provide the appropriate margin over the anterior tumor growing by releasing the anterior structures from the tumor pseudocapsule or leaving the selected anatomical structures as margin. These are also the cases of direct bone invasion by contiguous tumor. Second: Perform an osteotomy between the tumor and the posterior wall. Third: Finalize the en bloc resection.

Type 2A: Single Posterior Approach

A single posterior approach is the obvious strategy for en bloc resection to remove a tumor arising in the posterior arch (▸ Fig. 17.3) in the cervical, thoracic, and lumbar spine. Criteria to achieve appropriate margins include complete removal of the tumor from sectors 9 and 4. If the tumor grows in layer D, resection will result in intralesional penetration during release from the dura.

Three Steps

First: Provide the appropriate margin over the tumor on its posterior aspect by resecting inside the posterior muscles covering the tumor mass if it is expanding in compartment A. Second: Perform piecemeal excision of sectors 9 and 4, or

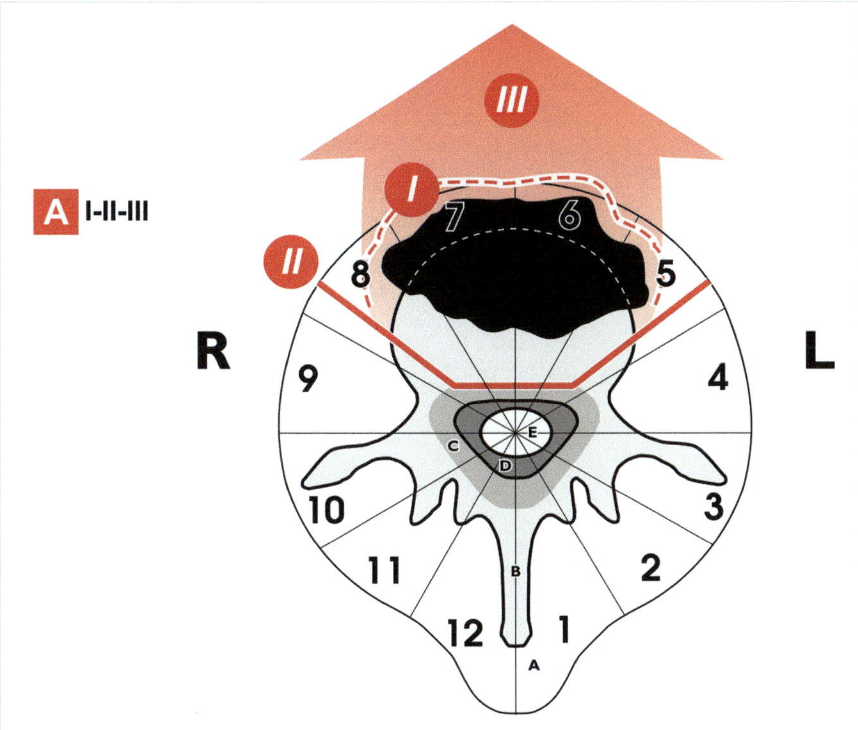

Fig. 17.2 Resection type 1: Single anterior approach (A) for en bloc resection of small tumors (*black highlighted area*) of the thoracic and lumbar vertebral bodies that arise from extraosseous soft tissues (compartment A) or superficial intraosseous tissue (compartment B), without extension to deep intraosseous tissue (compartment C). Tumors must be enclosed within sectors 5–8 to achieve en bloc resection under full visual control with this approach. Surgical steps I, II, and III are illustrated.

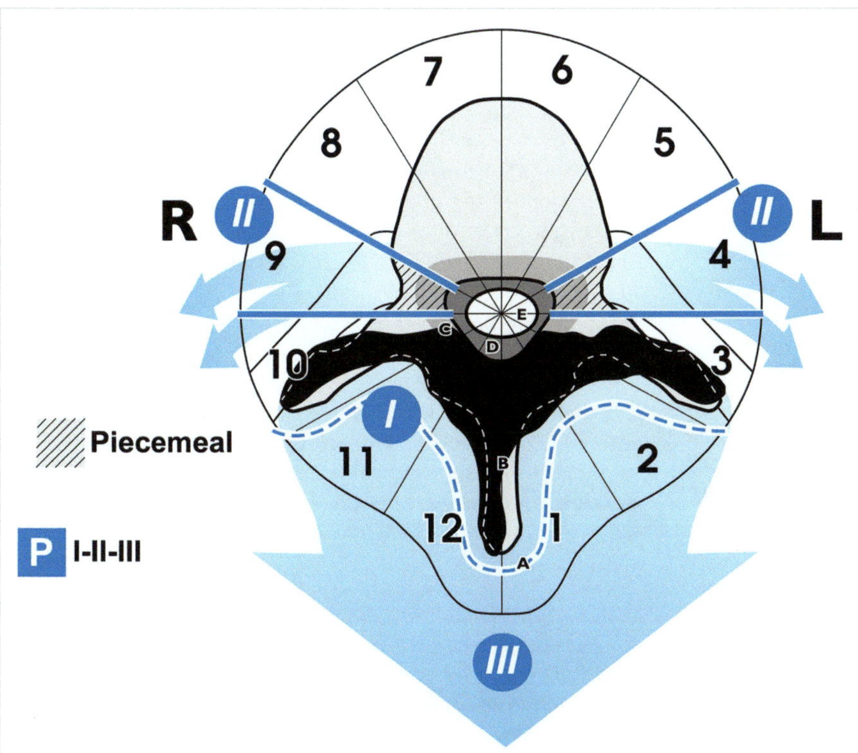

Fig. 17.3 Resection type 2A: Single posterior approach (P) for tumors arising in a posterior arch, in the cervical, thoracic, or lumbar spine. For en bloc resection under full visual control with this approach, the tumor must be absent from sectors 4–9. If the tumor has penetrated the extraosseous extradural tissue (compartment D), intralesional penetration will occur during release from the dura. Surgical steps I, II, and III are shown.

perform osteotomy using a wire, saw, chisel, high-speed bur, or ultrasound osteotome. This is obviously particularly delicate in the cervical spine, with a higher risk of incidental violation of the tumor margins. Third: a transverse laminotomy above and below the involved vertebra has been performed, the tumor is released from the dura, and the specimen is resected en bloc.

Type 2B: Single Posterior Approach with a Surgical Sequence

A single posterior approach with one of several surgical sequences enables en bloc resection of a tumor arising in the vertebral body of a thoracic vertebra (▶ Fig. 17.4). Criteria to achieve appropriate margins include complete removal of the

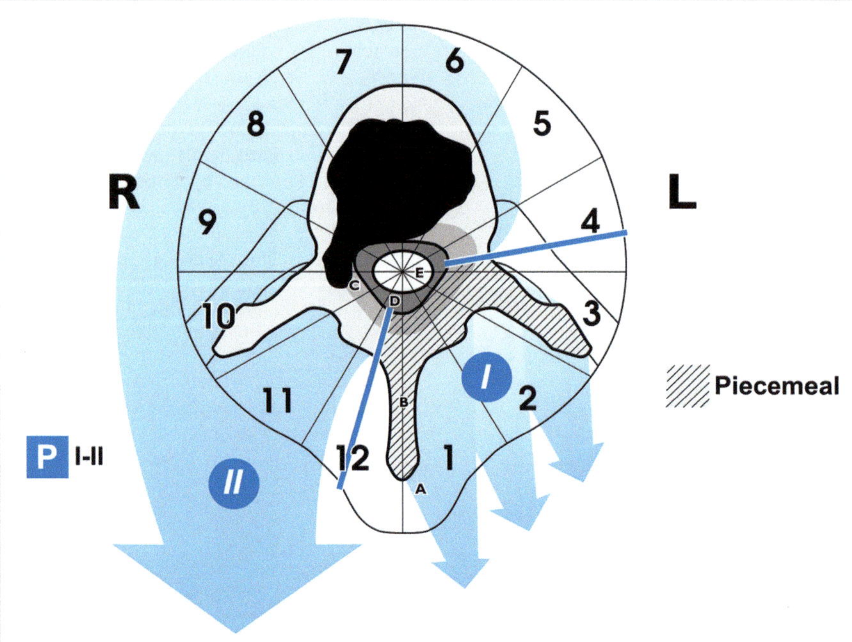

Fig. 17.4 Resection type 2B: Single posterior approach (P) for tumors arising from a vertebral body in the thoracic spine. To achieve appropriate margins, tumor must be completely removed from sector(s) 9 and/or 4. The lesion will be penetrated in cases where tumor extends into extraosseous tissues adjacent to the dura (compartment D) and during release from anterior structures when it extends anterior to the spinal column. Surgical steps I and II are shown. This resection type is difficult to apply in the lumbar spine.

tumor from sectors 9 and/or 4. There will be intralesional penetration during release from the dura in cases where the tumor grows in compartment D, and during release from anterior structures when it grows in compartment A.

Two Steps

First: Perform piecemeal excision of the posterior arch not involved by the tumor. At least four sectors are required, starting from sector 4 or from sector 9. The tumor is released from the dura, and the nerve root(s) involved by the tumor are sectioned. Second: Perform a blunt dissection of the anterior part of the vertebral body from the mediastinum, with osteotomy or diskectomy above and below the tumor. Then obtain a full release from the dura and finalize the resection.

The technique illustrated in ▶ Fig. 17.4 is difficult to apply to lumbar vertebrae. Digital blunt dissection of the anterior circumference is demanding or impossible due to the psoas muscle, the dimension of the vertebral body, and the major vessels that are closely connected to the spine by the transverse segmental vessels. In these cases, the approaches defined as type 3a and type 5 are safer and more appropriate.

Type 2C: Single Posterior Approach with Sagittal Osteotomy

A single posterior approach with sagittal osteotomy enables en bloc resection by a single posterior approach of a tumor growing eccentrically in the thoracic and lumbar spine (▶ Fig. 17.5), provided the body is not involved over sector 5 on the left or over sector 8 on the right. At least three posterior sectors must remain uninvolved by the tumor (4 to 1–2, or 9 to 11–12).

Four Steps

First: Provide the appropriate margin over the posterior aspect of the tumor by resecting inside the posterior muscles covering the tumor mass if it is expanding in compartment A (I). Release will then proceed laterally to the lateral side of the vertebral body. In the thoracic spine, the pleura can be left on the tumor; in the lumbar spine, the posterior part of the psoas must be dissected, but segmental vessels must be found and ligated. Second: Perform a piecemeal excision of the posterior arch not involved by the tumor (II). During the approach to the canal, release of the dura from the tumor, and section of the involved nerve root(s), dissection of the dura will result in intralesional penetration if the tumor grows in compartment D. Third: Carefully displace the dura and perform osteotomy from posterior to anterior in sector 8 or 5. Fourth: Remove the specimen.

Type 3A: Sequential Anterior and Posterior Approaches

A sequential approach to the tumor using two approaches, anterior first and posterior second, in the thoracic and lumbar spine, is proposed when a vertebral body tumor is growing anteriorly into compartment A (▶ Fig. 17.6).

Four Steps

First: Perform an anterior approach to provide a wide/marginal margin under visual control. In cases where the tumor grows from the vertebral body into anterior structures (compartment A), the anterior approach must be the first step to enable release of the tumor from the mediastinum in the thoracic spine, or from the retroperitoneum in the lumbar spine, eventually leaving involved structures as tumor margin. A sheet of Silastic or similar material can be left as protection. Second: Via a posterior approach, perform piecemeal excision of the posterior arch not involved by the tumor. At least three to four sectors are required, starting from sector 4 or sector 9. Third: Release the dura from the tumor, section the involved nerve root(s), and provide an appropriate margin over the tumor on its posterior aspect by resecting inside the posterior muscles

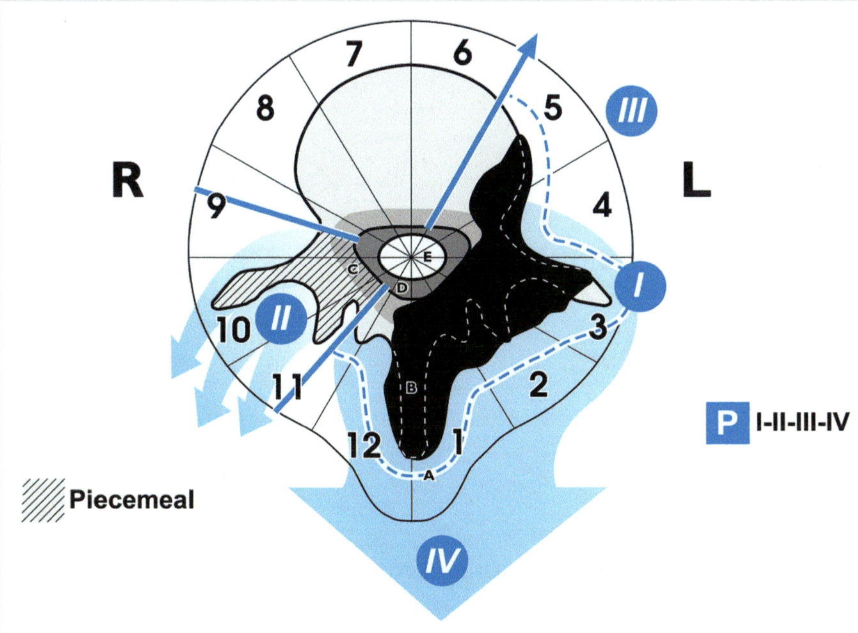

Fig. 17.5 Resection type 2C: Single posterior approach (P) with sagittal osteotomy for resection of a tumor growing eccentrically in the thoracic or lumber spine. For en bloc resection under full visual control with this approach, the tumor must be absent from sectors 6–7, and at least three posterior sectors must be free of tumor (sectors 4 to 1–2 or 9 to 11–12). Surgical steps I, II, III, IV are shown.

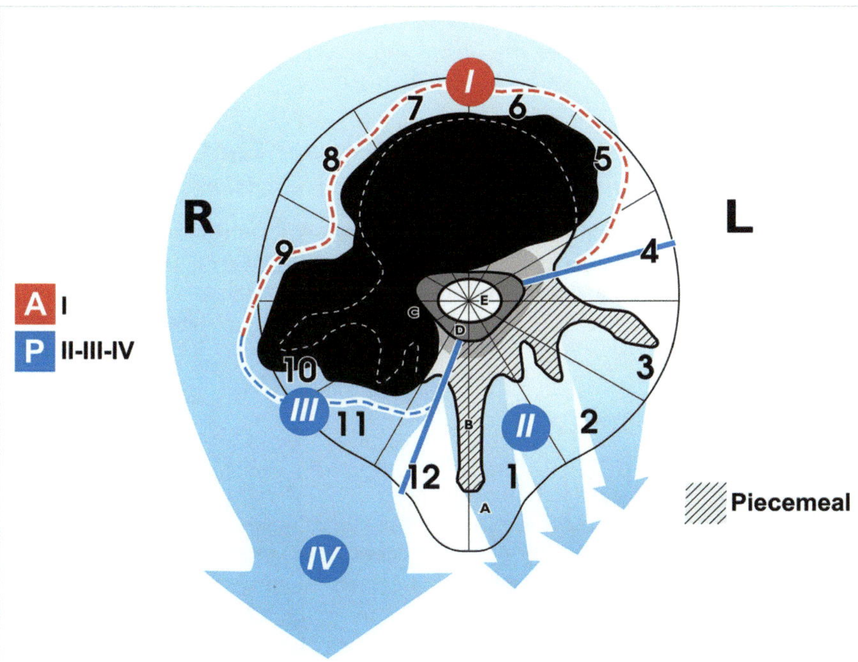

Fig. 17.6 Resection type 3A: Sequential anterior (A) and then posterior (P) approaches for tumors originating from a vertebra of thoracic or lumber spine and extending anteriorly into extraosseous tissues anterior to the spinal column (compartment A). Surgical steps I, II, III, IV are shown.

covering the tumor mass if it is expanding in compartment A. Fourth: Remove the specimen by rotating around the dural sac. This technique requires the section of at least one nerve root in order to rotate the specimen around the thecal sac when removing it via a posterior approach. If the nerve roots are not involved by the tumor and are functionally relevant, a type 5 resection may provide a safer approach.

Type 3B: Sequential Anterior and Posterior Approaches

An anterior approach first, followed by a posterior approach, should be considered in cervical spine tumors partially occupying the vertebral body and the posterior arch in cases where at least three sectors, including sectors 6 and 7, are not involved (▶ Fig. 17.7). When sectors 6 and/or 7 are involved, approach type 4 may provide a better approach.

Five Steps

First: Perform the anterior approach to leave healthy tissue over the lateral aspects of the tumor. Second: Create a sagittal groove reaching up to the epidural space in the vertebral body. Diskectomies are performed or transverse grooves are created in the vertebral bodies to define the upper and lower margins, including ligation of the vertebral artery (II). Third: Open a posterior

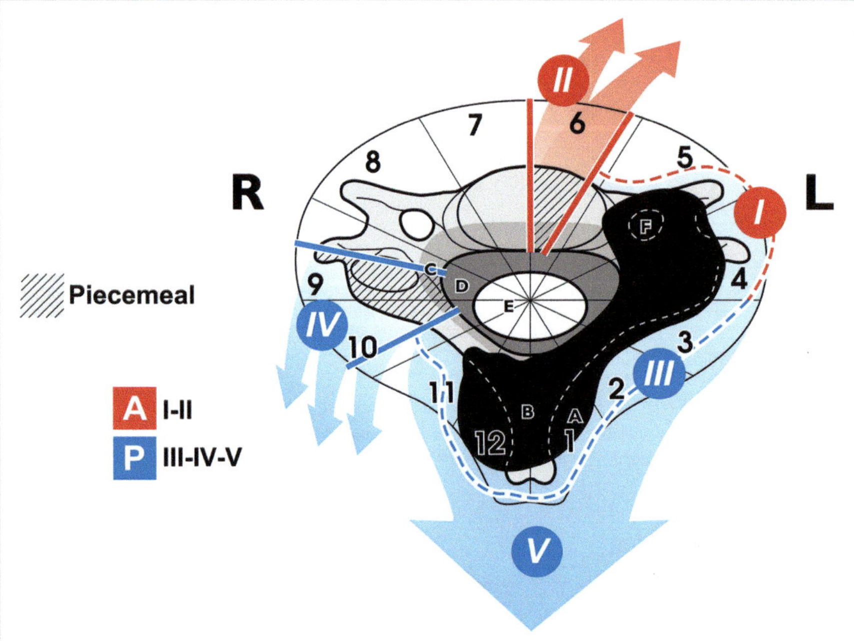

Fig. 17.7 Resection type 3B: Sequential anterior (A) and then posterior (P) approaches for tumors in the cervical spine that partially occupy the vertebral body and posterior arch. To achieve en bloc resection under full visual control, at least three sectors, including sectors 6 and 7, must be free of tumor involvement. Surgical steps I, II, III, IV, V are shown.

approach. Create an appropriate margin over the posterior aspect of the tumor by resecting inside the posterior muscles covering the tumor mass if it is expanding into compartment A. Fourth Use piecemeal excision to remove the posterior arch not involved by the tumor. At least three sectors are removed, starting from sector 4 or sector 9. This allows the release of the dura from the tumor and section the nerve root(s) involved by the tumor. Fifth: After the upper and lower extent of resection is finalized by diskectomy or osteotomy, remove the specimen by rotating it around the dural sac.

Type 3C: Sequential Anterior and Posterior Approaches for Eccentric Tumors

In cases where the tumor is growing eccentrically in the thoracic or lumbar spine, two approaches are recommended, anterior first and posterior second (▸ Fig. 17.8). Sagittal osteotomy is considered safe to obtain an appropriate margin.

Five Steps

First: Perform the anterior approach to provide a wide/marginal margin under visual control enabling release of the tumor from the mediastinum in the thoracic spine or from peritoneal structures in the lumbar spine, eventually leaving involved structures as margin (I). Diskectomies or transverse grooves in vertebral bodies are performed to define the upper and lower margins. A sheet of Silastic or any other tissue can be left as protection. Second: Perform a posterior approach with piecemeal excision of the posterior arch not involved by the tumor. At least three sectors are required, starting from sector 4 or sector 9. Third: Provide the appropriate margin over the posterior aspect of the tumor by resecting inside the posterior muscles covering the tumor mass if it is expanding in compartment A. Fourth: Release the dura from the tumor, section the nerve roots crossing the tumor, and perform an osteotomy posterior to anterior at some distance from the tumor in order to leave uninvolved bone as a margin. Fifth: Remove the resected specimen after the upper and lower extremities of the resection have been finalized with diskectomies or osteotomies.

Type 4: Posterior, Anterior Contralateral, and Anterior Ipsilateral Approaches

In some huge tumors of the cervical spine that extend over the midline, three approaches are required for a safe and oncologically appropriate surgery: first posterior, second anterior contralateral to the tumor, third anterior ipsilateral to the tumor (▸ Fig. 17.9).

Five Steps

First: With the patient in the prone position, perform piecemeal excision of the posterior arch not involved by the tumor. At least three sectors must be removed, starting from sector 4 or sector 9. Second: In cases where the tumor extends posteriorly and invades compartment A, an appropriate margin must be provided by resecting inside the posterior muscles covering the tumor mass. Then release the dura from the tumor and section the nerve root(s) crossing the tumor. If the tumor grows into compartment D, the margin will result in intralesional penetration. Patient is placed in the supine position. Third: Place the patient in a supine position. Using an anterior approach contralateral to the tumor, a sagittal groove is created in the vertebral body not occupied by the tumor up to the vertebral artery, which must be saved, as the contralateral artery is involved by the tumor and must be sacrificed. Fourth: The anterior margin is provided by leaving healthy soft tissue over the tumor mass. Perform diskectomies or create transverse grooves in vertebral bodies to define the upper and lower margins of the resection. Fifth: Via an anterior approach ipsilateral to the tumor, perform the upper and lower diskectomies or osteotomies, including ligation of the vertebral artery, and remove the mass.

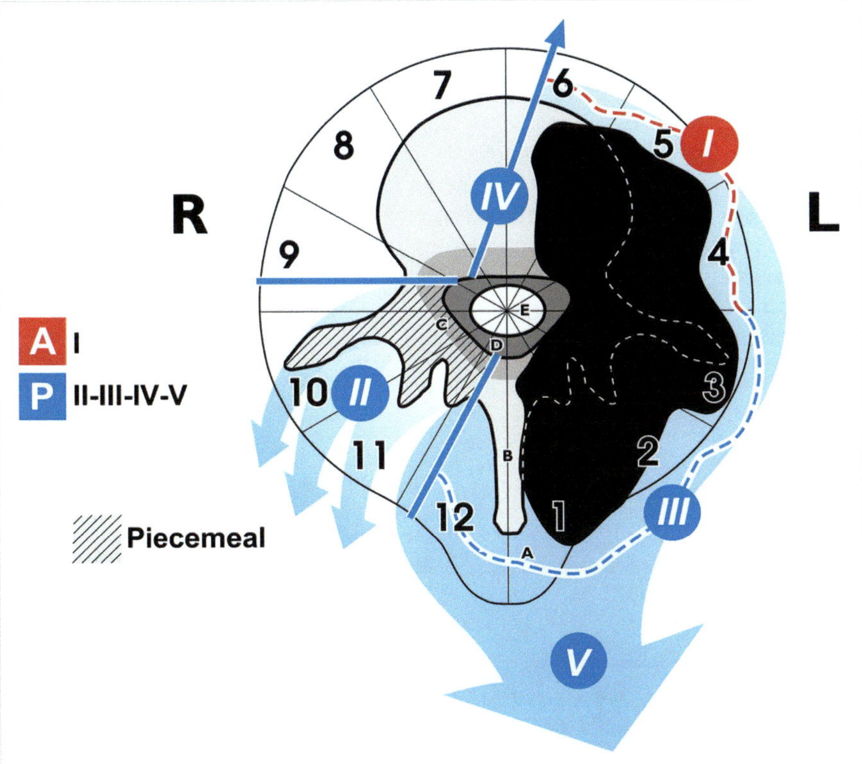

Fig. 17.8 Resection type 3C: Sequential anterior (A) and then posterior (P) approaches for tumors growing eccentrically in the thoracic or lumbar spine. Surgical steps I, II, III, IV, V are shown.

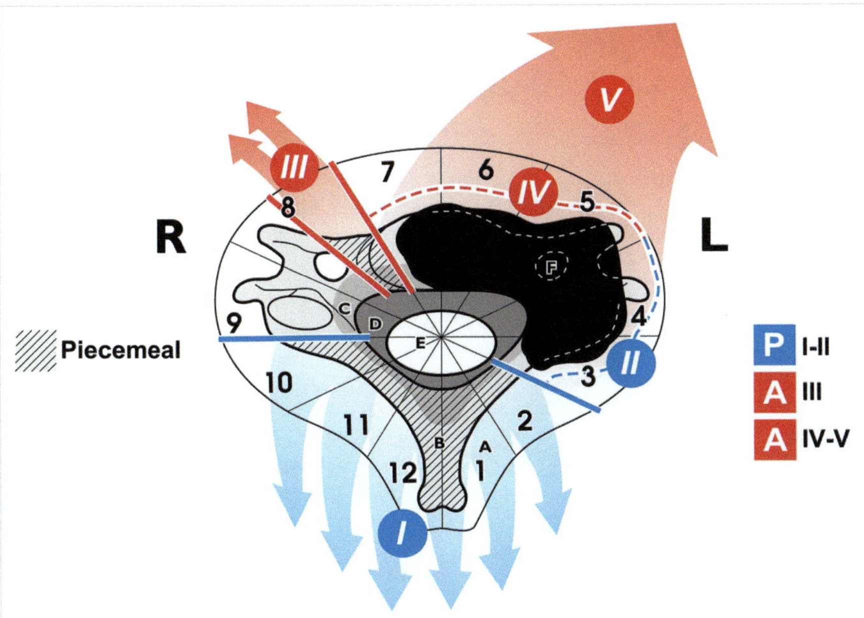

Fig. 17.9 Resection type 4: Three surgical approaches, posterior (P), anterior contralateral to the tumor (A III), and anterior ipsilateral to the tumor (A IV–V), are required for en bloc resection under full visual control of very large tumors in the cervical spine that extend over the midline. Surgical steps I, II, III, IV, V are shown.

Type 5: Posterior Followed by Simultaneous Anterior/Posterior Approaches

For lumbar tumors expanding anteriorly, surgery may best be performed in two stages. First a posterior approach is performed, and second resection is performed with simultaneous anterior and posterior approaches (▶ Fig. 17.10). This type of resection is associated with the highest rate of morbidity and complications[23]; however, this approach has an important advantage compared to type 3A (▶ Fig. 17.6) because no nerve roots are sacrificed if they are not directly involved by the tumor.

Four Steps

First: Via a posterior approach, with the patient placed in the prone position, perform piecemeal excision of the posterior arch not involved by the tumor. At least three sectors are required, starting from sector 4 or sector 9. Second: In cases where the tumor extends posteriorly and invades compartment

A, an appropriate margin must be provided by resecting inside the posterior muscles covering the tumor mass. Release the tumor from the dura, and resect the nerve roots crossing the tumor. If the tumor grows in compartment D, the margin will result in intralesional penetration. Third: The patient is placed in a lateral position. Diskectomies or transverse grooves in vertebral bodies are used to define the upper and lower margins of the resection. Resect the tumor from the surrounding soft tissue along with a layer of pleura or psoas to provide an appropriate margin. Use spiral wires to embolize the segmental arteries and thus simplify release of the aorta on the contralateral side. Fourth: Finalize the upper and lower diskectomies or osteotomies and remove the specimen by combined maneuvers.

Type 6: Anterior Contralateral, Posterior, and Simultaneous Anterior/Posterior Approaches

Three approaches should be planned to resect a tumor of L5: first an anterior approach on the contralateral side of the tumor, second a posterior approach, and third simultaneous anterior and posterior approaches (▶ Fig. 17.11). The double anterior approach is required to fully release the aorta/cava bifurcation.

Five Steps

First: With the patient in the supine position, release the aorta/cava bifurcation and perform partial diskectomies or osteotomies

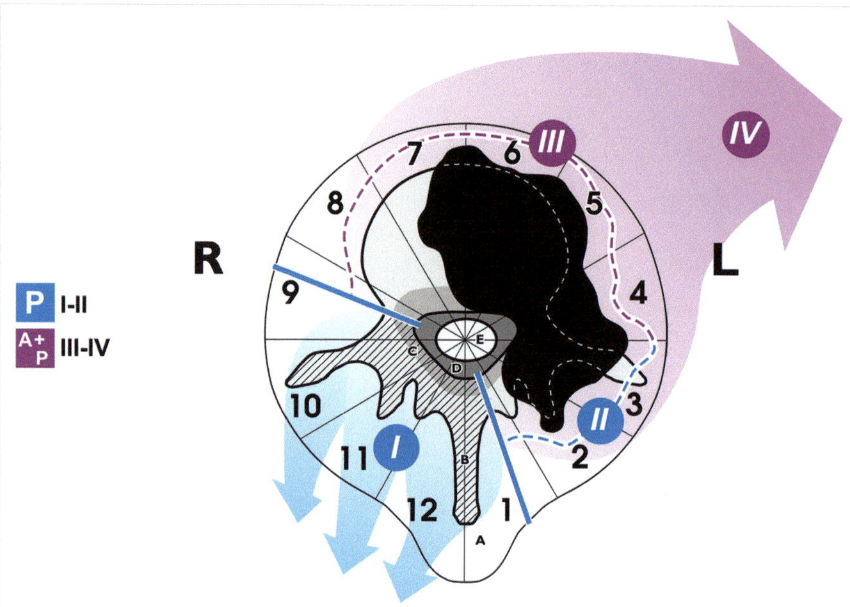

Fig. 17.10 Resection type 5: A posterior approach (P) followed by simultaneous anterior (A) and posterior approaches may be performed for large tumors of the lumbar spine extending anterior to the spinal column. It is associated with the highest rate of morbidity and complications; however, this technique may provide the option to preserve nerve roots that are not directly involved by the tumor. Surgical steps I, II, III, IV are shown.

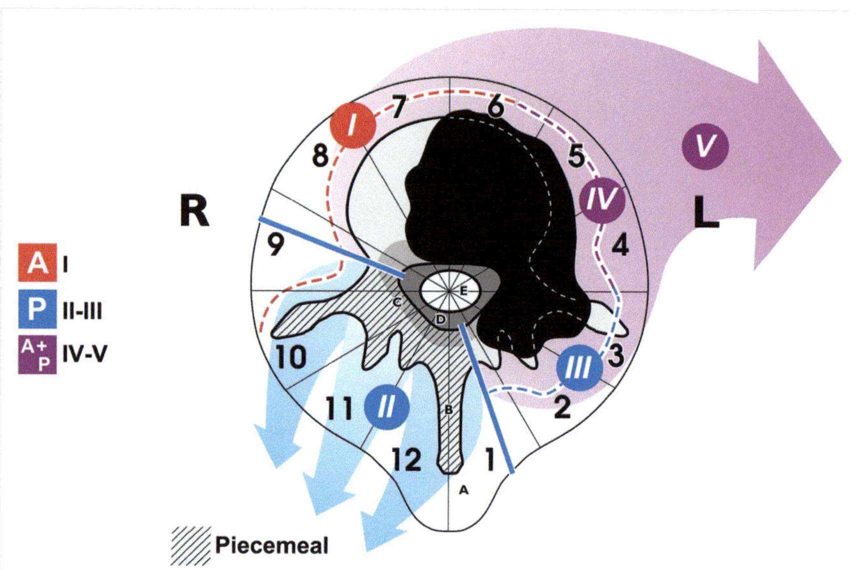

Fig. 17.11 Resection type 6: An anterior approach (A) contralateral to the tumor, then a posterior approach (P), and finally a simultaneous anterior (A) and posterior (P) approaches may be appropriate for removal of large tumors involving L5. Surgical steps I, II, III, IV, V are shown.

to define the upper and lower margins of the resection. Place the patient in the prone position. Second: Using a posterior approach, perform piecemeal excision of the posterior arch not involved by the tumor. At least three sectors must be removed, starting from sector 4 or sector 9. In cases where the tumor extends posteriorly and invades compartment A, an appropriate margin must be provided by resecting inside the posterior muscles covering the tumor mass. Then release the dura from the tumor and section the nerve root(s) crossing the tumor. If the tumor grows in compartment D, the margin will result in intralesional penetration. Perform diskectomies or create transverse grooves in vertebral bodies. Fourth: Place the patient in the lateral position. Perform a retroperitoneal approach and reopen the posterior approach. Provide an appropriate margin over the tumor by leaving it covered by psoas. Fifth: Finalize the diskectomies or transverse grooves in vertebral bodies and remove the specimen by the anterior approach.

17.2.5 Osteotomy of the Spine to Finalize the En Bloc Resection

In the original papers by Roy Camille et al,[34] the technique to perform the osteotomy began with an anterior-to-posterior cut using a Gigli saw to remove two-thirds of the vertebral body. Removal was then finalized with osteotomies to prevent inadvertent injury of the dural sac due to loss of control of the Gigli saw during the final steps. Tomita et al[32] later proposed use of a thinner saw and an original set of instruments to protect the dura from accidental injury while cutting anterior-to-posterior.

We propose an alternative technique[35] based on the need to protect the dura from injury during instrumentation. A malleable protector is inserted between the dura and the posterior vertebral wall and fixed to one of the rods (▶ Fig. 17.12). This system provides solid and sound protection from accidental injury, relieving the surgical assistant of this heavy responsibility.

17.3 Case Report

A 53-year-old woman presented with isolated metastases at T11 from colon carcinoma (▶ Fig. 17.13a). Her tumor was considered to have poor response to radiotherapy, and the primary lesion was fully controlled 3 years after surgery; thus en bloc resection was deemed the optimal approach to achieve local control. A type 3A en bloc resection was planned (▶ Fig. 17.6). To achieve en bloc resection with a wide/marginal margin, the pleura would be left over the tumor expansion on the right side of the vertebral body (compartment A, ▶ Fig. 17.13a). The anterior approach was performed via thoracoscopy. A video still (▶ Fig. 17.13b) shows the pleura resected over the right side of the vertebral body. The posterior approach was opened, and the dura was released from the tumor. At the last step, the Promid device (Novatek) was firmly fixed to the rod (▶ Fig. 17.13c) to guide the Gigli saw and protect the dural sac anteriorly. T11 osteotomy was performed. Note the perfectly flat surface of the osteotomy (▶ Fig. 17.13d, e) in comparison with the often oblique or irregular surface that is typically achieved with an osteoma. The smooth surface allows full contact between residual

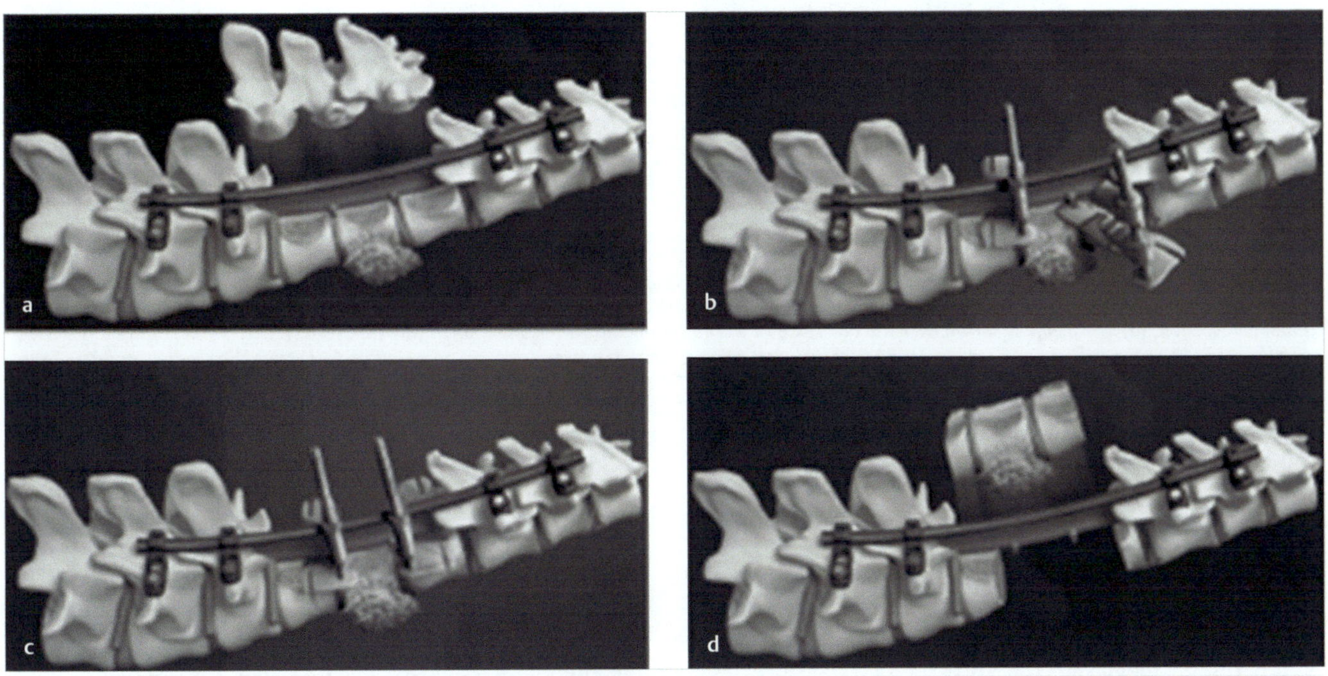

Fig. 17.12 **(a)** Operative schema of vertebrectomy and removal of the affected sections of vertebral body with the wire-cutting device. Resection of the posterior elements. **(b)** The device is positioned under the dural sac and unilateral bar connection. **(c)** Osteotomy with the thread wire saw through the vertebral body, proximally and distally from the tumor. **(d)** En bloc resection of the affected vertebra. **(e)** Intraoperative view of the Promid device (Novatek) connected to the stabilization rod where it provides guidance to the wire saw during complete section of the vertebral body or intervertebral disk. (Source: Gasbarrini A, Simoes CE, Amendola L, et al. Influence of a thread wire saw guide and spinal cord protector device in "en bloc" vertebrectomies. J Spinal Disord Tech 2012;25(2):E7–12.)

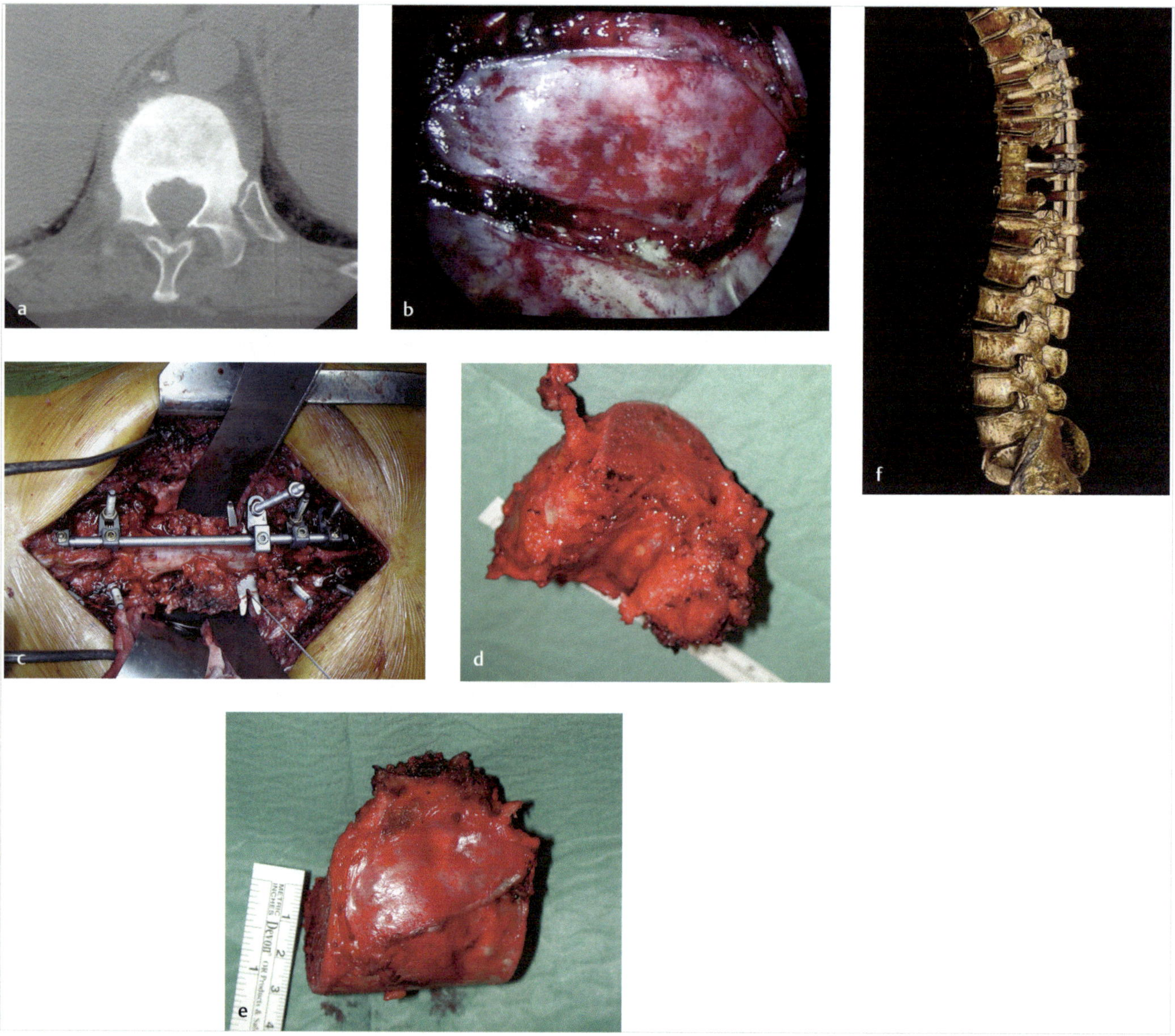

Fig. 17.13 **(a)** Axial noncontrast CT scan showing metastasis of a primary colon carcinoma at T 11 in a 53-year-old woman. Her primary tumor was well controlled, and the spine lesion was the sole systemic metastasis. Pleura on the right side of the vertebral body was removed to provide a margin for en bloc resection. **(b)** The pleura is shown over the right side of the vertebral body after resection in this video still. **(c)** The Promid device is shown firmly anchored to the rod, where it will guide the Gigli saw and protect the dura from accidental penetration. **(d,e)** Note the smooth surface of the osteotomy. **(f)**Three-dimensional reconstruction of the postoperative CT shows the implanted graft and cage.

bone and the implanted cage and graft, for a satisfying reconstruction and good sagittal balance (▶ Fig. 17.13f).

17.4 Discussion and Conclusions

En bloc resection in the spine is a very demanding surgical procedure. This operation can be safely performed and can achieve oncological effectiveness if some mandatory steps are followed.

1. *Diagnosis and staging must suggest en bloc resection as the procedure of choice.* The Enneking staging system has been adopted over the last 30 years in many tumor centers, and numerous reports have reviewed and confirmed its validity.[5,8] En bloc resection is proposed for aggressive benign (stage 3) and low-grade malignant tumors (stage 1). For high-grade malignant tumors, en bloc resection is a valid option in some circumstances, but must always be associated with chemotherapy or radiotherapy according to the sensitivity of the specific tumor.
2. *Tumor extension and surgical anatomy must meet criteria for performing a tumor-free margin en bloc resection safely and with acceptable functional loss.* The WBB system was proposed in 1997[24] for the surgical staging of primary spine tumors based on their extensions, using computer-based terminology that includes numeric descriptors for sections of the vertebra involved and letters to define intra-/extracompartmental extension. This system has been validated as

reliable and reproducible by a multidisciplinary group of experts in spine oncology.[8]

3. *Planning of the surgical procedure must consider the two previous points.* Selection of one surgical approach or a combination of approaches and their timing must be decided based on tumor extensions and regional anatomy, with consideration of the margins that must be achieved. If the tumor is expanding anteriorly or a nonexpendable anatomical structure is close to the anterior surface of the tumor, an anterior approach is mandatory to leave a layer of healthy tissue over the tumor. In the cervical and lower lumbar spine it is frequently necessary to combine multiple approaches due to the complexity of the anatomy.
4. *Osteotomies at the superior and inferior edges of the surgical field must be performed safely and achieve a regular and orthogonal cutting surface.* The final surgical step in resection types 2B, 3A, 5, and 6 is spinal osteotomy, which is performed only after anterior structures are protected and the dural sac has been dissected free, or, as rarely required, resected and left connected to the tumor mass. The choice of technique and device to perform osteotomy should be based on the personal experience of the surgeon. Roy-Camille et al[34] first proposed use of the Gigli saw and osteotome, Tomita et al[32] proposed a thinner saw for the complete cut with a system to protect the dura that relied, in part, on the handheld positioning by the surgical assistant. Today the ultrasound scalpel presents a new and interesting option, although its popularity is constrained by the limited availability of blades of appropriate length.

The Gigli or Tomita saws seem the best devices to achieve a regular and fully flat cutting surface. An original system, which is connected to the rods of the implanted device, has been proposed to protect the dura.[35] This system is sound and stable, and relieves the surgical assistant of the heavy responsibility of protecting the dura.

17.4.1 Conflicts of Interest

Dr. Itshayek is the recipient of research support from MFast, a distributor of a wide range of surgical devices in Israel. The other authors disclose no conflicts of interest.

17.4.2 Acknowledgments

The authors acknowledge the invaluable contribution of Carlo Piovani for data collection and original drawings.

References

[1] Falicov A, Fisher CG, Sparkes J, Boyd MC, Wing PC, Dvorak MF. Impact of surgical intervention on quality of life in patients with spinal metastases. Spine. 2006; 31(24):2849–2856

[2] Harel R, Angelov L. Spine metastases: current treatments and future directions. Eur J Cancer. 2010; 46(15):2696–2707

[3] Hayat MJ, Howlader N, Reichman ME, Edwards BK. Cancer statistics, trends, and multiple primary cancer analyses from the Surveillance, Epidemiology, and End Results (SEER) Program. Oncologist. 2007; 12(1):20–37

[4] Hsu W, Kosztowski TA, Zaidi HA, Dorsi M, Gokaslan ZL, Wolinsky JP. Multidisciplinary management of primary tumors of the vertebral column. Curr Treat Options Oncol. 2009; 10(1-2):107–125

[5] Fisher CG, Keynan O, Boyd MC, Dvorak MF. The surgical management of primary tumorsof the spine: initial results of an ongoing prospective cohort study. Spine. 2005; 30(16):1899–1908

[6] Fisher CG, Saravanja DD, Dvorak MF, et al. Surgical management of primary bone tumors of the spine: validation of an approach to enhance cure and reduce local recurrence. Spine. 2011; 36(10):830–836

[7] Chan P, Boriani S, Fourney DR, et al. An assessment of the reliability of the Enneking and Weinstein-Boriani-Biagini classifications for staging of primary spinal tumors by the Spine Oncology Study Group. Spine. 2009; 34(4):384–391

[8] Boriani S, Bandiera S, Casadei R, et al. Giant cell tumor of the mobile spine: a review of 49 cases. Spine. 2012; 37(1):E37–E45

[9] Harrop JS, Schmidt MH, Boriani S, Shaffrey CI. Aggressive "benign" primary spine neoplasms: osteoblastoma, aneurysmal bone cyst, and giant cell tumor. Spine. 2009; 34(22) Suppl:S39–S47

[10] Boriani S, Saravanja D, Yamada Y, Varga PP, Biagini R, Fisher CG. Challenges of local recurrence and cure in low grade malignant tumors of the spine. Spine. 2009; 34(22) Suppl:S48–S57

[11] Schwab J, Gasbarrini A, Bandiera S, et al. Osteosarcoma of the mobile spine. Spine. 2012; 37(6):E381–E386

[12] Sciubba DM, Okuno SH, Dekutoski MB, Gokaslan ZL. Ewing and osteogenic sarcoma: evidence for multidisciplinary management. Spine. 2009; 34(22) Suppl:S58–S68

[13] Boriani S, Amendola L, Corghi A, et al. Ewing's sarcoma of the mobile spine. Eur Rev Med Pharmacol Sci. 2011; 15(7):831–839

[14] Boriani S, Weinstein JN. The role of "tumor-free margins" in the resection of spinal tumors: who should be treating spinal tumors? Sem Spine Surg. 2009; 21(2):76–85

[15] Fisher CG, DiPaola CP, Ryken TC, et al. A novel classification system for spinal instability in neoplastic disease: an evidence-based approach and expert consensus from the Spine Oncology Study Group. Spine. 2010; 35(22):E1221–E1229

[16] Patchell RA, Tibbs PA, Regine WF, et al. Direct decompressive surgical resection in the treatment of spinal cord compression caused by metastatic cancer: a randomised trial. Lancet. 2005; 366(9 486):643–648

[17] Loblaw DA, Perry J, Chambers A, Laperriere NJ. Systematic review of the diagnosis and management of malignant extradural spinal cord compression: the Cancer Care Ontario Practice Guidelines Initiative's Neuro-Oncology Disease Site Group. J Clin Oncol. 2005; 23(9):2028–2037

[18] Li H, Gasbarrini A, Cappuccio M, et al. Outcome of excisional surgeries for the patients with spinal metastases. Eur Spine J. 2009; 18(10):1423–1430

[19] Yao KC, Boriani S, Gokaslan ZL, Sundaresan N. En bloc spondylectomy for spinal metastases: a review of techniques. Neurosurg Focus. 2003; 15(5):E6

[20] Tomita K, Kawahara N, Kobayashi T, Yoshida A, Murakami H, Akamaru T. Surgical strategy for spinal metastases. Spine. 2001; 26(3):298–306

[21] Gasbarrini A, Li H, Cappuccio M, et al. Efficacy evaluation of a new treatment algorithm for spinal metastases. Spine. 2010; 35(15):1466–1470

[22] Boriani S, Bandiera S, Donthineni R, et al. Morbidity of en bloc resections in the spine. Eur Spine J. 2010; 19(2):231–241

[23] Boriani S, Weinstein JN, Biagini R. Primary bone tumors of the spine. Terminology and surgical staging. Spine. 1997; 22(9):1036–1044

[24] Fisher CG, Andersson GB, Weinstein JN. Spine focus issue. Summary of management recommendations in spine oncology. Spine. 2009; 34(22) Suppl:S2–S6

[25] Biagini R, Casadei R, Boriani S, et al. En bloc vertebrectomy and dural resection for chordoma: a case report. Spine. 2003; 28(18):E368–E372

[26] Murakami H, Kawahara N, Tomita K, Demura S, Kato S, Yoshioka K. Does interruption of the artery of Adamkiewicz during total en bloc spondylectomy affect neurologic function? Spine. 2010; 35(22):E1187–E1192

[27] Fujimaki Y, Kawahara N, Tomita K, Murakami H, Ueda Y. How many ligations of bilateral segmental arteries cause ischemic spinal cord dysfunction? An experimental study using a dog model. Spine. 2006; 31(21):E781–E789

[28] Kato S, Kawahara N, Tomita K, Murakami H, Demura S, Fujimaki Y. Effects on spinal cord blood flow and neurologic function secondary to interruption of bilateral segmental arteries which supply the artery of Adamkiewicz: an experimental study using a dog model. Spine. 2008; 33(14):1533–1541

[29] Kawahara N, Tomita K, Baba H, et al. Cadaveric vascular anatomy for total en bloc spondylectomy in malignant vertebral tumors. Spine. 1996; 21 (12):1401–1407

[30] Ueda Y, Kawahara N, Tomita K, Kobayashi T, Murakami H, Nambu K. Influence on spinal cord blood flow and function by interruption of bilateral segmental arteries at up to three levels: experimental study in dogs. Spine. 2005; 30 (20):2239–2243

[31] Kawahara N, Tomita K, Kobayashi T, Abdel-Wanis ME, Murakami H, Akamaru T. Influence of acute shortening on the spinal cord: an experimental study. Spine. 2005; 30(6):613–620

[32] Tomita K, Kawahara N, Baba H, Tsuchiya H, Fujita T, Toribatake Y. Total en bloc spondylectomy. A new surgical technique for primary malignant vertebral tumors. Spine. 1997; 22(3):324–333

[33] Roy-Camille R, Mazel CH, Saillant G, Lapresle PH. Treatment of malignant tumors of the spine with posterior instrumentation. In: Sundaresan N, Schmidek HH, Schiller AL, Rosenthal DI, eds. Tumors of the Spine: Diagnosis and Clinical Management. Philadelphia: W.B. Saunders; 1990:473–492

[34] Roy-Camille R, Saillant G, Bisserié M, Hautefort E, Mamoudy P. Total excision of thoracic vertebrae (author's transl.) [in French]. Rev Chir Orthop Reparatrice Appar Mot. 1981; 67(3):421–430

[35] Gasbarrini A, Simoes CE, Amendola L, et al. Influence of a thread wire saw guide and spinal cord protector device in "en bloc" vertebrectomies. J Spinal Disord Tech. 2012; 25(2):E7–E12

18 Corrective Osteotomies in the Cervical Spine

Venu M. Nemani, Peter B. Derman, Han Jo Kim

Abstract

Deformities of the cervical spine are among the most disabling of all spinal pathologies. Patients can present with a myriad of symptoms including pain and difficulty with horizontal gaze, radiculopathy, myelopathy, and dysphagia. Malnutrition, soft tissue deficiency, and osteoporosis can also complicate the treatment of this patient population. Here we review the appropriate clinical and radiographic workup of the patient with a cervical spinal deformity. We also describe the various types of osteotomies available to treat patients with rigid deformities, including anterior osteotomies, posterior column osteotomies, and three-column resections, and we present some of the technical nuances of the various approaches. Selecting an appropriate osteotomy is based on many factors, including experience and comfort level with the various approaches. There continues to be many unanswered questions with regards to goals for cervical deformity correction, and further work is necessary to help standardize the decision-making process to achieve optimal radiographic and clinical results with the least amount of surgical risk.

Keywords: cervical deformity, cervical kyphosis, myelopathy, osteotomies

18.1 Introduction

Cervical deformities can cause significant functional disability and pain as a result of the deformity causing difficulty with forward gaze as well as dysphagia, both of which can have a significant impact on health-related quality of life. In addition, cervical deformities can also result in dynamic cervical spinal cord compression, further disabling patients due to gait ataxia, manual dexterity issues, and bowel and bladder dysfunction.

Cervical kyphosis is the most common cervical deformity encountered, although scoliosis can also be present. While flexible deformities can be treated with a variety of options, including anterior, posterior, or combined approaches, patients with rigid, ankylosed cervical spines will require an osteotomy for appropriate correction and neural decompression. The osteotomies that can be performed in the cervical spine are largely similar to those that are more commonly performed in the thoracolumbar spine; however, anatomical constraints (e. g., the vertebral artery) make these more challenging to perform and pose a higher risk for complications. Here we describe a systematic approach for evaluating patients with cervical spine deformities and provide a method to formulate a surgical treatment plan. In addition, we review the various types of cervical osteotomies that can aid in deformity correction and our surgical technique for performing them safely.

18.2 Clinical Symptoms and Natural History

Although multiplanar deformities can occur in the cervical spine, kyphosis predominates and may be attributable to a number of causes. These include iatrogenic factors (e. g., postlaminectomy), spondylosis, infection, inflammatory arthritides (e. g., ankylosing spondylitis), neuromuscular diseases, and metabolic diseases.[1,2,3,4,5] Kyphotic deformity tends to progress over time and may result in pain, myelopathy, radiculopathy, difficulty achieving horizontal gaze or upright posture, aspiration, swallowing dysfunction, social impairment, and even chest pressure sores in severe cases.[4,5] Neck pain in these cases is multifactorial and may be attributable to facet joint and intervertebral disk degeneration, compression of neural structures, and from cervical extensor muscular pain as they fatigue and struggle to maintain normal alignment.[4,5]

Although cervical myelopathy is most commonly attributable to spondylosis,[6] cervical kyphosis has also been associated with myelopathy.[7] As the cervical spine develops progressively increased kyphosis, the spinal cord is stretched and flattened against the posterior aspect of the vertebral bodies, leading to microvascular disruption, demyelination, and neuronal loss.[8,9] Patients may therefore experience symptoms typical of myelopathy, such as gait instability, neck pain, diminished manual dexterity, bladder and bowel dysfunction, paresthesias, and extremity weakness.[7,10,11,12,13,14]

Studies of nonoperative management of cervical myelopathy reveal that myelopathy symptoms tend to progress in the absence of surgical intervention.[15] While these studies were performed in patients suffering from myelopathy due to cervical spondylosis, not all of whom necessarily had any deformity, myelopathy secondary to cervical deformity may exhibit a similar natural history.

18.3 Physical Exam

Because the behavior of each spinal region is dependent on that of the others, physical examination of the patient with cervical deformity should begin with a careful assessment of global spinal alignment.[2,16,17] Normal alignment places the cranium over the pelvis with approximately 40 degrees of cervical lordosis, 50 degrees of thoracic kyphosis, 60 degrees of lumbar lordosis, and no deviation from midline in the coronal plane.[18] The patient should be observed while standing upright, sitting, prone, and in supine and/or hyperextension positions. This allows the clinician to identify spinal deformities and coexistent hip/knee pathology, and to determine if the deformities are rigid or flexible.[2,19]

In patients with ankylosing spondylitis, loss of lumbar or cervical lordosis or an increase in thoracic kyphosis may result in fixed global kyphosis due to a loss of compensatory mechanisms. This can result in an inability to achieve horizontal gaze, which may significantly impact a patient's ability to perform activities of daily living. The chin–brow vertical angle (CBVA) is a means to quantify horizontal gaze. While it can be estimated based on visual inspection of a patient standing with hips and knees extended, the CBVA can be more precisely measured on either a clinical photograph (▶ Fig. 18.1) or a standing radiograph. To measure CBVA, a line is first drawn between the tip of a patient's chin and the tip of the brow. The angle subtended by this line and the vertical plane represents the CBVA, with positive angles indicating a downward gaze.[20] Normal CBVA values have not been defined, but postoperative values of approximately −10 to +10 degrees have been associated with acceptable clinical outcomes.[20,21,22] Another clinical measure of overall sagittal imbalance is the occiput-to-wall measure, which is the horizontal distance from the wall to the occiput when the patient is standing against the wall with hips and knees extended (▶ Fig. 18.1). A value of 0 to 2 cm is considered normal.[2]

After assessing overall alignment, the cervical spine may be more closely examined for the presence of coronal, sagittal, and/or rotational deformity. Evaluate for neck tenderness, stiffness, and pain with motion. Pain with attempted neck extension may indicate spinal stenosis or nerve root compression.[10]

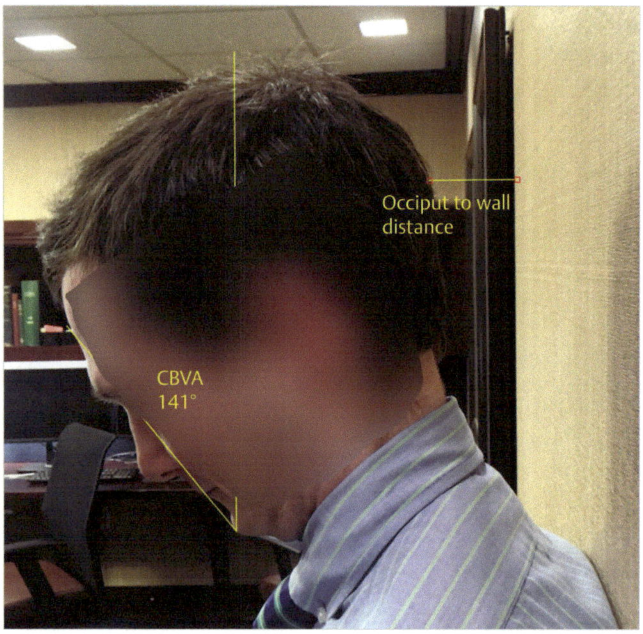

Fig. 18.1 Clinical photograph showing the measurement of chin–brow vertical angle and occiput to wall distance in a patient with cervical kyphosis.

A complete neurologic exam should be performed to detect weakness, motor abnormalities, and sensory changes. Signs of myelopathy include difficulty with heel-to-toe walking, Romberg's sign, wasting of the intrinsic hand musculature, the finger escape sign, dysdiadochokinesia, diminished sensation, hyperreflexia, clonus, Hoffmann's reflex, the Babinski sign, and the inverted radial reflex. Shoulder girdle muscle wasting may also be observed in patients with C 4–C 6 stenosis as a result of loss of function of anterior-horn cells.[10]

18.4 Radiographic Evaluation

Given the close relationship between the alignment of each spinal region, radiographic evaluation of patients with cervical deformities begins with standing full-length 3-foot anteroposterior and lateral radiographs.[17,23] Dedicated anteroposterior, lateral, and flexion/extension radiographs of the cervical spine are also indicated.[7,10] These studies may demonstrate pathology such as disk narrowing, osteophytes, canal stenosis, ossification of the posterior longitudinal ligament, dynamic instability, as well as coronal and sagittal plane deformity.[10]

There are several described techniques for quantifying sagittal plane curvature of the cervical spine (▶ Fig. 18.2). The Cobb angle method measures the lordosis from either C 1 or C 2 to C 7, using the angle subtended by a line either from the midpoints of the C 1 anterior and posterior tubercles or along the inferior end plate of C 2, to a line drawn along the inferior end plate of C 7.[24] Lordosis is typically indicated by a negative number. Because the majority of normal cervical lordosis comes from the C 1–C 2 level (− 32.2 degrees), cervical Cobb angles will differ based on whether C 1 or C 2 is selected as the proximal level. The mean C 1–C 7 lordosis is − 41.8 degrees, and the mean C 2–C 7 lordosis is − 9.6 degrees. Furthermore, younger individuals typically have less lordosis, whereas older people exhibit more.[18,25]

In the Jackson physiological stress line method of measuring cervical sagittal alignment, lines are drawn parallel to the

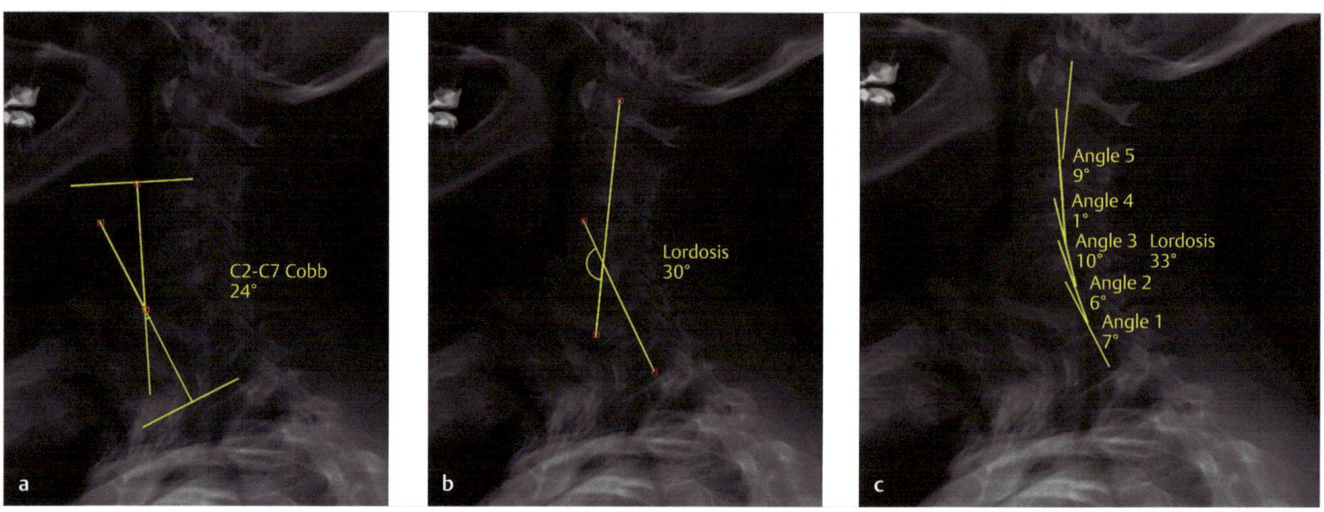

Fig. 18.2 **(a)** Lateral EOS images of the cervical spine showing the measurement of cervical lordosis using the Cobb method, **(b)** the Jackson physiological stress line method, and **(c)** the Harrison posterior tangent method.

posterior surface of the C2 and C7 vertebral bodies, and the angle subtended between them is measured.[26,27]

The Harrison posterior tangent method is similar to the Jackson method but involves projecting lines parallel to each vertebral body from C2 through C7 and then summing the segmental angles to obtain an overall measure of cervical lordosis or kyphosis.[24]

In a direct comparison of the Cobb and Harrison posterior tangent methods, investigators found that the C1–C7 Cobb angle tended to overestimate cervical curvature, while the C2–C7 Cobb angle underestimated it. They suggested that the Harrison method was a more reliable technique for quantifying cervical curvature.[24] However, use of the Cobb method remains widespread, likely as a result of its ease of use and good inter- and intraexaminer reliability.[28]

Cervical spinal alignment can be further described in terms of sagittal plane translation. The cervical sagittal vertical axis (SVA) is such a measure of translation and is defined as the horizontal distance between the posterior superior aspect of the C7 vertebral body and a plumb line dropped from the center of the C2 vertebral body (▶ Fig. 18.3). Positive values indicate that the center of the C2 body lies anterior to the posterior superior aspect of the C7 body. The normal cervical SVA in asymptomatic individuals has been quantified at 15.6 ± 11.2 mm, and increasing values (especially those ≥ 40 mm) have been shown to negatively impact health-related quality of life in patients who have undergone posterior cervical fusion surgery.[18,29] While lordosis may affect the cervical SVA, note that patients with identical cervical Cobb angles may have large differences in their cervical SVA depending on alignment at the cervicothoracic junction.

More recent efforts to evaluate cervical spinal alignment have focused on the interaction between the upper thoracic spine and the sagittal balance of the cervical spine and head (▶ Fig. 18.4). Lee et al defined three relevant parameters: (1) the thoracic inlet angle (TIA) is the angle subtended by a line extending perpendicularly from the center of the T1 upper end plate and a line from the center of the T1 upper end plate to the cephalad aspect of the sternum, (2) the T1 slope (T1S) is the angle between the T1 upper endplate and the horizontal plane, and (3) the neck tilt (NT) is the angle between a line extending from the upper end of the sternum to the center of the T1 upper end plate and the vertical plane.[30] Like pelvic incidence, the TIA is a constant anatomical parameter, which is uninfluenced by posture. Furthermore, similar to the relationship between pelvic incidence, sacral slope, and pelvic tilt, the following formula holds true: TIA = T1S + NT.

MRI is indicated for patients with cervical deformity and longstanding arm or neck pain, neurologic abnormalities, or worsening symptoms. This imaging modality is useful in evaluating soft tissue pathology, such as intervertebral disk herniation and

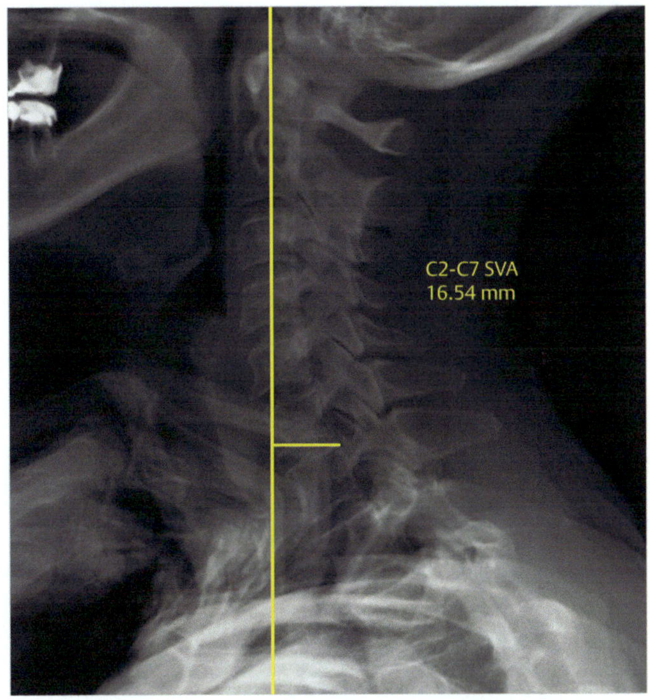

Fig. 18.3 Lateral EOS image of the cervical spine showing the measurement of C2–C7 sagittal vertical axis (C2–C7 SVA).

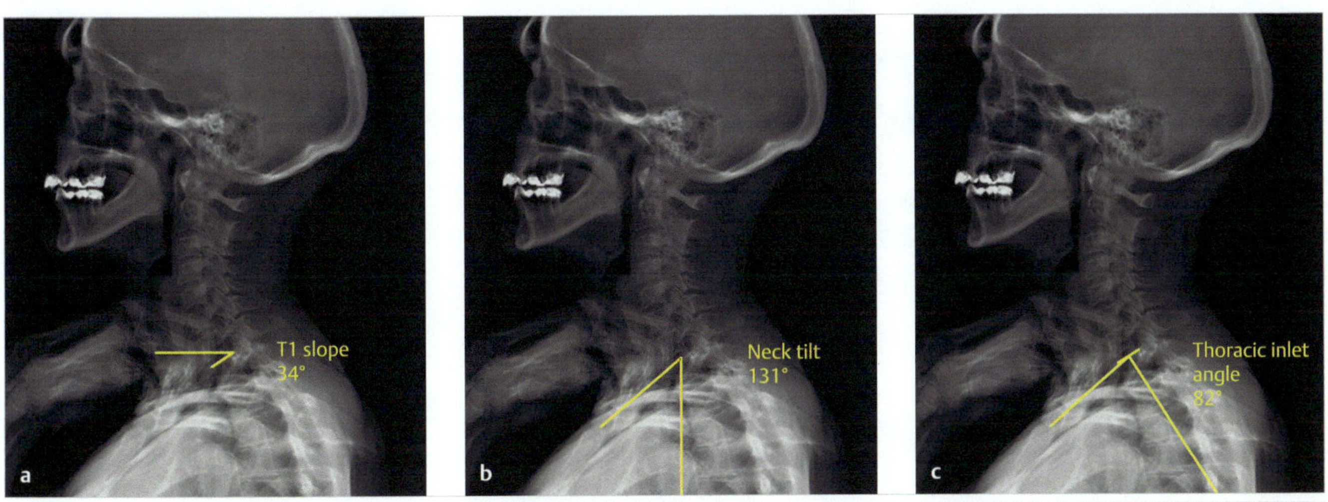

Fig. 18.4 Lateral EOS images of the cervical spine showing the measurement of the cervicothoracic junction parameters: **(a)** T1 slope, **(b)** neck tilt, and **(c)** thoracic inlet angle (TIA). The mathematical relationship between these parameters is TIA = T1 slope + neck tilt.

ligamentum flavum hypertrophy and buckling. Furthermore, it can be used to quantify the extent of cord compression, flattening, myelomalacia, and syrinx formation, as well as concomitant nerve root impingement, if present (▶ Fig. 18.5). Cord atrophy may be observed in long-standing cases.[7,10] These cord changes increase the risk of neurologic deficit with surgery.[7]

Finally, given its superior osseous resolution, CT may also be considered for preoperative planning purposes. To minimize the risk of intraoperative damage, the location and course of the vertebral artery should be closely scrutinized using CT angiography or magnetic resonance angiography prior to any cervical deformity surgery.[7]

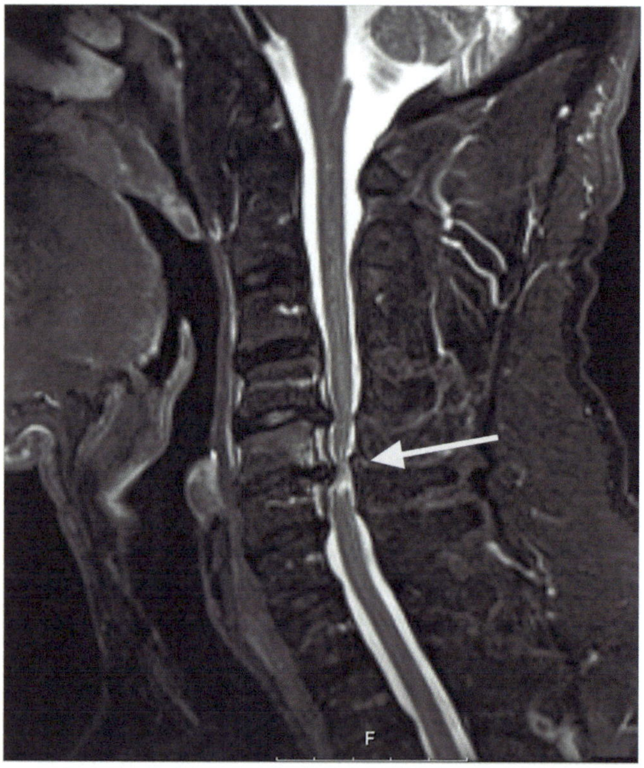

Fig. 18.5 Midsagittal fluid-sensitive MRI sequence showing severe spinal cord compression and myelomalacia (*arrow*) from central disk herniations, posterior longitudinal ligament hypertrophy, and ligamentum flavum buckling.

18.5 Assessment and Preoperative Planning

A full assessment of the patient's deformity and neurologic status requires a careful critique of the history, a physical exam, and radiological studies. Patients with progressive myelopathy should have spinal decompression as there is a very limited role for nonoperative treatment in this setting. Additionally, these patients should also have correction of their cervical deformity as kyphosis and increased C 2–C 7 SVA have both been shown to affect spinal cord pressure[31] and neurologic outcome in patients undergoing surgery for myelopathy.[29,32,33,34,35] In the absence of myelopathy, correction of cervical deformity is indicated in a patient who has loss of horizontal gaze, difficulty swallowing, and/or pain and who has failed conservative treatment. It is important that the patient has exhausted all potential forms of nonoperative treatment because the operations necessary to correct cervical deformity are generally extensive and can have serious complications.

Currently, no published classification system exists that encompasses all of these factors and guides treatment for patients with cervical deformity. However, there are several key criteria that play a critical role in the assessment of patients with cervical deformity and affect the choice of operation that is to be performed.

18.5.1 Location of the Deformity

First, one must determine the primary location of the patient's deformity. Because of the close relationship of both the global and the regional spinal sagittal alignment to the alignment of the cervical spine, it is important to assess the alignment of the spinal column in its entirety with the appropriate radiographs (▶ Fig. 18.6). Indeed, loss of sagittal balance from a primary

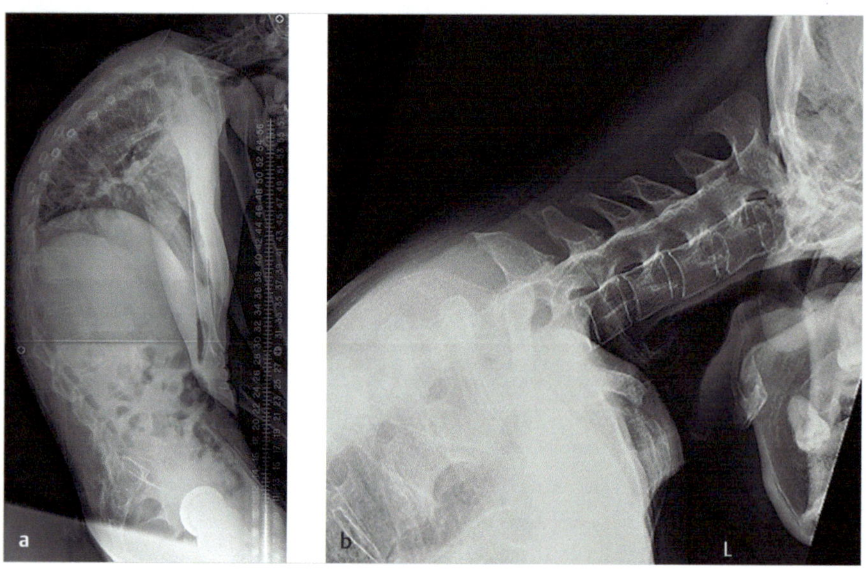

Fig. 18.6 (a) Lateral scoliosis and **(b)** lateral cervical spine X-rays showing global sagittal imbalance in a patient with fixed and ankylosed thoracolumbar kyphosis as well as fixed and ankylosed cervical kyphosis in the setting of ankylosing spondylitis.

thoracolumbar deformity has been shown to affect the alignment of the cervical spine.[25] In a similar fashion, deformities at the craniocervical junction or in the upper cervical spine can cause secondary deformities in the subaxial spine and vice versa. Further, the presence of deformities elsewhere in the spine may alter the desired deformity correction to maintain overall balance and function. For example, in patients with subaxial cervical spine kyphosis, fusion of the occipitocervical junction alone in a neutral position may leave them with difficulty in horizontal gaze and a markedly positive CBVA. Thus it is important to evaluate the entire spinal axis as well as the lower extremities when planning a surgical correction.

18.5.2 Previous Surgery

A large proportion, if not a majority, of patients presenting with cervical deformity will have had previous cervical spine operations. The details of what operation was performed, the approach used, and the success of that operation with respect to decompression and fusion are crucial to devising an operative plan. If patients have had a previous anterior approach, an evaluation by an otolaryngologist is important to determine the function of the recurrent laryngeal nerve (RLN). If a previous operation resulted in injury to the RLN, then any future anterior approaches should be performed ipsilateral to the injured nerve to avoid the potential for bilateral RLN injuries resulting in devastating vocal cord dysfunction. However, if there has not been an injury to the RLN, and an anterior approach is indicated, it may be advisable to approach from the contralateral side to the previous surgery, which can make the approach easier to perform by avoiding scarred tissue planes.

Additionally, if a patient has had previous surgery, it is important to consider infection or pseudarthrosis, especially with new-onset pain after a pain-free interval or in the setting of a newly worsening deformity. If infection is suspected, inflammatory markers should be evaluated with a further workup as necessary. CT scans with coronal and sagittal reconstructions and/or flexion-extension radiographs can be helpful to evaluate for pseudarthrosis.[36]

18.5.3 Curve Rigidity and Degree of Deformity

The rigidity of the curve is a crucial factor when one is formulating a preoperative plan. If the curve is flexible, then gaining the necessary amount of correction is trivial as the head can be positioned intraoperatively in the desired position and then fused using an anterior, posterior, or combined approach depending on the amount of immediate stability needed. If the curve is rigid but not ankylosed, then anterior releases through diskectomies followed by anterior, with or without posterior fusion, is often sufficient for achieving the desired result. If, however, the curve is rigid and ankylosed, then some type of osteotomy will be required to obtain the necessary curve correction. In the setting of a previous operation, a careful review of preoperative imaging studies will allow the surgeon to determine where the spine has been previously fused (anterior or posterior). In general, the spine will need to be approached from the side where a previous fusion has been performed (e.g., a posterior approach with a posterior-based osteotomy in the setting of a prior posterior fusion) to mobilize the spine followed by either same-sided fusion alone or a combined approach.

The amount of angular and translational deformity in rigid deformities will also affect the surgical plan. Different types of osteotomies can achieve differing amounts of correction (see the section "Osteotomy Types"). A thorough analysis of sites of previous fusion as well as the amount of correction needed will allow the surgeon to formulate an appropriate plan for location and type of osteotomy to be performed.

18.5.4 Neurologic Status

Lastly, the presence of myelopathy or radiculopathy in a patient with cervical deformity is important for at least two reasons. First, decompression of the neural elements becomes an important goal of the procedure, which could have implications for the bony surfaces available for fusion after deformity correction, or may necessitate both anterior and posterior fusion due to the iatrogenic instability caused by the decompression. Second, there may be a higher risk of neurologic complications after deformity correction in patients who already have a "sick cord."[37]

18.6 Osteotomy Types

Many types of cervical spine osteotomies are largely similar to ones performed more frequently in the thoracolumbar spine. However, osteotomies in the cervical spine are technically more challenging to perform because of the need to protect the vertebral artery. The various osteotomies can be categorized by approach (anterior vs. posterior vs. combined), or by the number of columns involved in the osteotomy (posterior column osteotomy vs. pedicle subtraction osteotomy or vertebral column resection). Ames and colleagues recently developed a standard nomenclature regarding cervical spine osteotomies that is anatomically based and graduated in terms of degree of resection and provides a useful framework for understanding the different types of osteotomies.[16] Here we describe the various osteotomies in an anatomically based fashion while highlighting the various degrees of destabilization associated with each osteotomy.

18.6.1 Anterior Osteotomies

Anterior-based osteotomies can range from partial uncovertebral joint resection as performed during an anterior cervical diskectomy and fusion, a partial or complete corpectomy, or an osteotomy that exits through the uncovertebral joints out laterally into the transverse foramina. These are classified by Ames et al as grade 1, 3, or 4 osteotomies.[16] These osteotomies depend on motion through the facets to gain correction and therefore cannot be performed in isolation in patients with fused posterior elements.

The technique for an anterior osteotomy (grade 4) has been described in detail by Kim et al.[38] Briefly, the patient is positioned supine with support under the head in the case of a fixed, kyphotic deformity. Gardner–Wells tongs are placed with 2.2 kg of traction to stabilize the head. A Smith–Robinson approach is used to approach the convexity of the deformity if there is a concomitant scoliosis in addition to kyphosis. Blunt dissection lateral to the uncinates is performed with a Penfield no. 4 and/or no. 2 and is used to identify the fused disk space, which is located just medial to the cranial border of the costal process. Caspar pins are placed in a divergent fashion (perpendicular to the anterior plane of the deformed cervical spine), which can help produce lordosis after completion of the osteotomy. The osteotomy is initiated using a 3-mm matchstick bur, with the carpentry being tailored to match the patient's unique deformity so that there is proper alignment when the osteotomy is closed down. The bony resection is taken all the way back to the posterior longitudinal ligament. When burring laterally it is imperative to protect the vertebral arteries using a Penfield no. 4 or 2, or a cottonoid patty. It is also advisable to perform a foraminotomy at the level of the osteotomy to prevent nerve root compression with closure of the osteotomy. With the osteotomy complete, the deformity reduction is performed by removing the supports under the head and pushing on the forehead through the sterile drapes. This can be done in conjunction with distraction along the Caspar pins or by using a laminar spreader in the osteotomy defect. The traction weight is increased from 9 to 11.3 kg to maintain the correction. A graft with a large surface area is shaped to fit the defect to reduce the risk of subsidence, and an anterior cervical plate is placed with fixed-angle screws. Adjunctive posterior fusion is performed as necessary for increased stability.

Kim et al showed that anterior osteotomies provide on average 23 degrees of angular correction and 1.3 cm of translational correction.[38] If performed in combination with posteriorly based Smith–Petersen osteotomies (SPOs), they obtained an average angular correction of 33 degrees and translational correction of 3.7 cm, although most of these were performed only for additional stabilization.

18.6.2 Posterior Osteotomies

Posterior-based osteotomies can range from partial facet joint resection to total facet resection (SPO or Ponte-type) to a closing-wedge pedicle subtraction osteotomy (PSO). These have been classified by Ames et al[16] as grades 1, 2, 5, or 6 depending on the degree of instability produced.

The SPO or Ponte-type osteotomy is performed by completely resecting both the superior and the inferior articulating facets at a given spinal segment. This may be performed in conjunction with resecting the ligamentum flavum, lamina, and spinous processes. These osteotomies depend on residual anterior column mobility to obtain the necessary correction and are typically performed at multiple levels to obtain increased correction (▶ Fig. 18.7). Importantly, these osteotomies do not involve any resection of the pedicles or the vertebral body. The foramen transversarium is left intact as the vertebral artery runs just anterior to the level of the resection anterior to the facets and exiting nerve roots.

An opening wedge osteotomy, or grade 5 resection, involves complete resection of the posterior elements, lamina, spinous process, and facets, followed by osteoclasis with subsequent lengthening of the anterior column. This was originally described by Mason and colleagues[39] and modified by several people, including Urist[40] and McMaster,[41] and is typically used in the treatment of patients with ankylosing spondylitis. Because it lengthens the anterior column, it is a relatively dangerous osteotomy with significant risks to the anterior soft tissue structures (trachea, esophagus).

A PSO grade 6, alternatively, is a spinal-shortening, closing wedge osteotomy that is inherently safer than the opening wedge osteotomy, in addition to being more stable upon osteotomy closure. Both of these resections are typically performed at the cervicothoracic junction at C 7 for several reasons: (1) the safe location of the vertebral artery in front of the transverse processes of C 7, (2) the size of the spinal canal at C 7–T 1, (3) the mobility of the spinal cord and eighth cervical nerve in this region, and (4) the limited impairment in hand function if a C 8 nerve root injury were to occur. Prior to performing a PSO at C 7, however, it is critical to evaluate the preoperative imaging studies carefully to make sure the vertebral artery does not take an aberrant course through the C 7 foramen transversarium, which occurs in 2 to 5% of patients.[42]

The technique for cervical PSO has been previously described in detail by Wollowick et al.[43] Briefly, the patient is positioned prone on a Jackson table on bolsters positioned to accommodate the deformity, with the table in maximum reverse Trendelenburg. The head is suspended in Gardner–Wells tongs with 7 kg traction, with a second traction rope positioned to provide an extension moment after completion of the osteotomy to hold the reduction. Posterior cervical and upper thoracic exposure is performed per routine. If motion is preserved at the craniocervical junction the fusion will stop proximally at C 2, but it is taken to the occiput in a completely ankylosed spine for improved fixation. Distal fixation is to T 3 or T 4. Instrumentation is placed segmentally with lateral mass screws and pedicles screws where appropriate, skipping C 6 or T 1. The osteotomy is begun with a complete laminectomy of C 7 as well as a partial laminectomy of the inferior half of C 6 and the superior half of T 1. The lateral masses of C 7 are then removed using a rongeur and a high-speed bur. Great care must be taken to remove any overhanging bone on osteotomy closure from the facets of C 6 and T 1 to prevent C 8 nerve root impingement. After identifying and protecting the thecal sac medially, the C 7 nerve root superiorly, and the C 8 nerve root inferiorly, a bur is used to decancellate the C 7 pedicle and vertebral body. Pituitary rongeurs and reverse-angle curets are used to remove the bony walls of the pedicle, along with further decancellation of the body. Finally, the dorsal cortex of the vertebral body is impacted into the previously created decancellation cavity to complete the osteotomy. The osteotomy is closed and the deformity corrected by fixing prebent rods to the thoracic pedicle screws, and then extending the neck by pulling up on the Gardner–Wells tongs and seating the rods into the cervical lateral mass and/or pedicle screws. The C 7 and C 8 nerve roots again must be meticulously checked to rule out any signs of impingement. The neuromonitoring should also be checked carefully to ensure no signs of spinal cord compromise. Once the deformity is corrected, adjunctive anterior plating with screws above and below the osteotomy can be performed for additional stability.

Kim et al showed that with isolated cervical PSOs, the mean angular correction achieved was 34.5 degrees with a mean translational correction of 2.5 cm.[44] Interestingly, they found that by combining an anterior osteotomy with posterior SPOs, they achieved a mean angular correction of 27.8 degrees with a

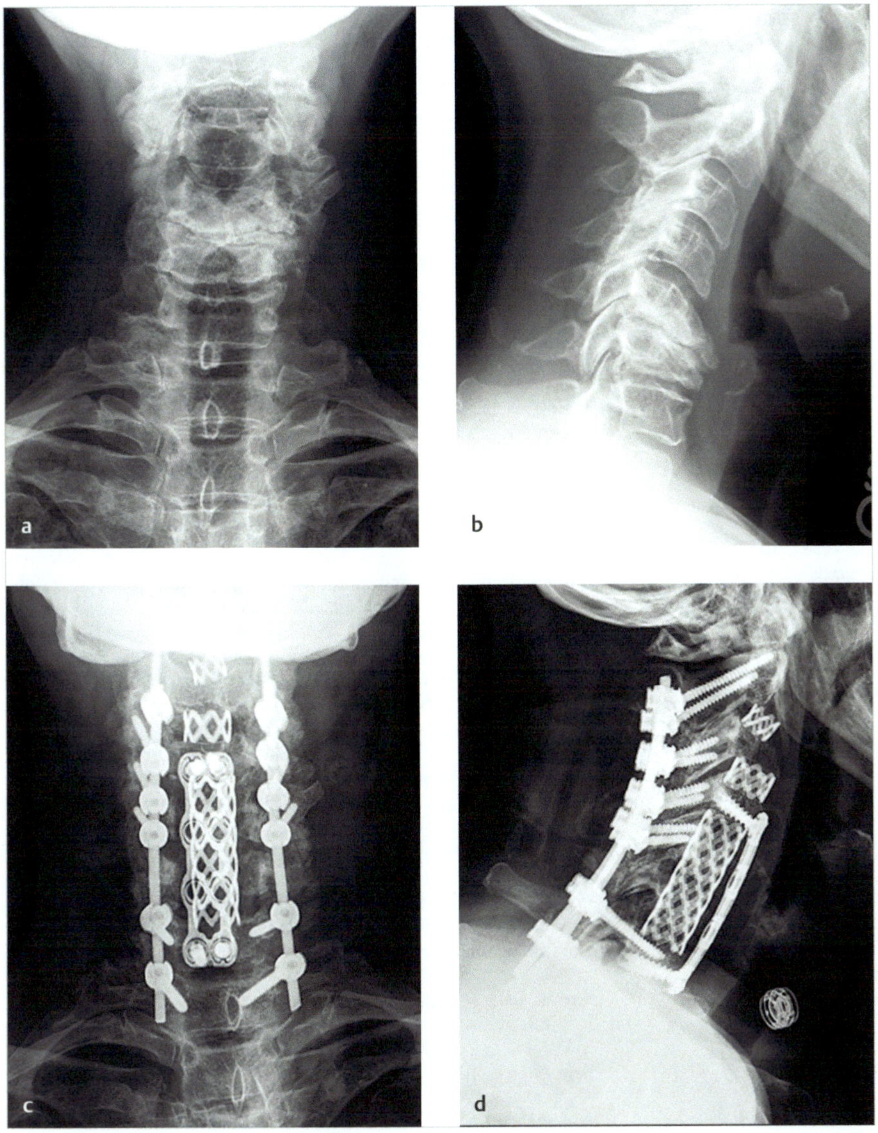

Fig. 18.7 (a) Preoperative anterior and (b) lateral radiographs of a patient with cervical kyphosis and myelopathy. (c, d) The patient underwent an anterior/posterior procedure with an anterior corpectomy, anterior cervical diskectomy and fusion, and posterior fusion with instrumentation with several Smith–Petersen osteotomies to aid in deformity correction.

mean translational correction of 2.6 cm, which were both statistically equivalent to those achieved with an isolated PSO, and with significantly less blood loss. Because of this, if technically feasible, they recommend combining anterior osteotomies with SPOs rather than an isolated PSO.

18.6.3 Combined Osteotomies

For severe deformities, both anterior and posterior osteotomies can be combined to achieve significant curve correction. As stated earlier, it has recently been shown that combining an anterior osteotomy with posterior SPOs can provide similar correction to an isolated PSO.[44] In certain, rare, situations a severe deformity may require removal of a complete vertebral segment (grade 7), consisting of the entire vertebral body, the adjacent disks, the complete uncovertebral joint, the lamina, and the facets. This type of osteotomy, called a vertebral column resection, is rarely performed in the cervical spine except for oncologic resections due to the need to protect the vertebral arteries. If necessary, it is performed via a combined approach.

18.7 Conclusion

There remain many unanswered questions regarding the pathophysiology of cervical deformity and the optimal treatment, including the role of spinal osteotomies to correct these deformities. Our understanding of global spinal sagittal balance has increased tremendously in recent years, especially in relation to pelvic morphometric parameters (e.g., pelvic incidence) and lumbar lordosis. Current research directed at increasing our understanding of the thoracic inlet angle and T 1 slope and how that affects cervical spine alignment and positioning of the skull in space will undoubtedly be critical. Indeed, these parameters may eventually be useful to guide the surgical approach or procedure as we develop a deeper understanding of their meaning. Additionally, more research is needed on the effects of deformity correction on myelopathic symptoms and axial neck pain. Finally, our goals for deformity correction are currently guided by normal values that may not pertain to the entire population across the age spectrum, because life is a "kyphosing event." More research is needed to determine what an appropriate cervical sagittal profile is for different age groups, and how to best maintain or achieve that alignment while minimizing the risks of treatment.

The treatment of cervical deformity is complex, but the principles are straightforward—obtaining a balanced correction with adequate neural decompression by performing an operation with the least amount of surgical risk. In cases of rigid deformities, cervical osteotomies, which present increased risk, are often necessary to obtain the desired correction. However, with a full understanding of the anatomical limitations of the various approaches and techniques, one can treat a variety of complex deformities effectively and safely.

References

[1] Cha TD, An HS. Cervical spine manifestations in patients with inflammatory arthritides. Nat Rev Rheumatol. 2013; 9(7):423–432

[2] Kubiak EN, Moskovich R, Errico TJ, Di Cesare PE. Orthopaedic management of ankylosing spondylitis. J Am Acad Orthop Surg. 2005; 13(4):267–278

[3] Nguyen HV, Ludwig SC, Silber J, et al. Rheumatoid arthritis of the cervical spine. Spine J. 2004; 4(3):329–334

[4] O'Shaughnessy BA, Liu JC, Hsieh PC, Koski TR, Ganju A, Ondra SL. Surgical treatment of fixed cervical kyphosis with myelopathy. Spine. 2008; 33 (7):771–778

[5] Scheer JK, Tang JA, Smith JS, et al. International Spine Study Group. Cervical spine alignment, sagittal deformity, and clinical implications: a review. J Neurosurg Spine. 2013; 19(2):141–159

[6] Karadimas SK, Erwin WM, Ely CG, Dettori JR, Fehlings MG. Pathophysiology and natural history of cervical spondylotic myelopathy. Spine. 2013; 38(22) Suppl 1:S21–S36

[7] Albert TJ, Vacarro A. Postlaminectomy kyphosis. Spine. 1998; 23(24):2738–2745

[8] Breig A, el-Nadi AF. Biomechanics of the cervical spinal cord. Relief of contact pressure on and overstretching of the spinal cord. Acta Radiol Diagn (Stockh). 1966; 4(6):602–624

[9] Shimizu K, Nakamura M, Nishikawa Y, Hijikata S, Chiba K, Toyama Y. Spinal kyphosis causes demyelination and neuronal loss in the spinal cord: a new model of kyphotic deformity using juvenile Japanese small game fowls. Spine. 2005; 30(21):2388–2392

[10] Emery SE. Cervical spondylotic myelopathy: diagnosis and treatment. J Am Acad Orthop Surg. 2001; 9(6):376–388

[11] Herman JM, Sonntag VK. Cervical corpectomy and plate fixation for postlaminectomy kyphosis. J Neurosurg. 1994; 80(6):963–970

[12] Nagano A, Miyamoto K, Fushimi K, Hosoe H, Shimizu K. Failure of reconstruction surgery using anterior fibular strut grafting to correct postlaminectomy kyphosis. J Clin Neurosci. 2007; 14(4):376–379

[13] Park Y, Riew KD, Cho W. The long-term results of anterior surgical reconstruction in patients with postlaminectomy cervical kyphosis. Spine J. 2010; 10(5):380–387

[14] Zdeblick TA, Bohlman HH. Cervical kyphosis and myelopathy. Treatment by anterior corpectomy and strut-grafting. J Bone Joint Surg Am. 1989; 71 (2):170–182

[15] Rhee JM, Shamji MF, Erwin WM, et al. Nonoperative management of cervical myelopathy: a systematic review. Spine. 2013; 38(22) Suppl 1:S55–S67

[16] Ames CP, Smith JS, Scheer JK, et al. International Spine Study Group. A standardized nomenclature for cervical spine soft-tissue release and osteotomy for deformity correction: clinical article. J Neurosurg Spine. 2013; 19(3):269–278

[17] Joseph SA, Jr, Moreno AP, Brandoff J, Casden AC, Kuflik P, Neuwirth MG. Sagittal plane deformity in the adult patient. J Am Acad Orthop Surg. 2009; 17 (6):378–388

[18] Hardacker JW, Shuford RF, Capicotto PN, Pryor PW. Radiographic standing cervical segmental alignment in adult volunteers without neck symptoms. Spine. 1997; 22(13):1472–1480, discussion 1480

[19] Bridwell KH, Lenke LG, Lewis SJ. Treatment of spinal stenosis and fixed sagittal imbalance. Clin Orthop Relat Res. 2001(384):35–44

[20] Suk KS, Kim KT, Lee SH, Kim JM. Significance of chin-brow vertical angle in correction of kyphotic deformity of ankylosing spondylitis patients. Spine. 2003; 28(17):2001–2005

[21] Deviren V, Scheer JK, Ames CP. Technique of cervicothoracic junction pedicle subtraction osteotomy for cervical sagittal imbalance: report of 11 cases. J Neurosurg Spine. 2011; 15(2):174–181

[22] Zheng GQ, Song K, Zhang YG, et al. Two-level spinal osteotomy for severe thoracolumbar kyphosis in ankylosing spondylitis. Experience with 48 patients. Spine. 2014; 39(13):1055–1058

[23] Ames CP, Blondel B, Scheer JK, et al. Cervical radiographical alignment: comprehensive assessment techniques and potential importance in cervical myelopathy. Spine. 2013; 38(22) Suppl 1:S149–S160

[24] Harrison DE, Harrison DD, Cailliet R, Troyanovich SJ, Janik TJ, Holland B. Cobb method or Harrison posterior tangent method: which to choose for lateral cervical radiographic analysis. Spine. 2000; 25(16):2072–2078

[25] Kim HJ, Lenke LG, Oshima Y, et al. Cervical Lordosis Actually Increases With Aging and Progressive Degeneration in Spinal Deformity Patients. Spine Deform. 2014; 2(5):410–414

[26] Gore DR. Roentgenographic findings in the cervical spine in asymptomatic persons: a ten-year follow-up. Spine. 2001; 26(22):2463–2466

[27] Jackson R. The Cervical Syndrome. 2nd ed. Springfield, IL: Charles C. Thomas; 1958

[28] Côté P, Cassidy JD, Yong-Hing K, Sibley J, Loewy J. Apophysial joint degeneration, disc degeneration, and sagittal curve of the cervical spine. Can they be measured reliably on radiographs? Spine. 1997; 22(8):859–864

[29] Tang JA, Scheer JK, Smith JS, et al. ISSG. The impact of standing regional cervical sagittal alignment on outcomes in posterior cervical fusion surgery. Neurosurgery. 2012; 71(3):662–669, discussion 669

[30] Lee SH, Kim KT, Seo EM, Suk KS, Kwack YH, Son ES. The influence of thoracic inlet alignment on the craniocervical sagittal balance in asymptomatic adults. J Spinal Disord Tech. 2012; 25(2):E41–E47

[31] Chavanne A, Pettigrew DB, Holtz JR, Dollin N, Kuntz C, IV. Spinal cord intramedullary pressure in cervical kyphotic deformity: a cadaveric study. Spine. 2011; 36(20):1619–1626

[32] Suda K, Abumi K, Ito M, Shono Y, Kaneda K, Fujiya M. Local kyphosis reduces surgical outcomes of expansive open-door laminoplasty for cervical spondylotic myelopathy. Spine. 2003; 28(12):1258–1262

[33] Baba H, Uchida K, Maezawa Y, Furusawa N, Azuchi M, Imura S. Lordotic alignment and posterior migration of the spinal cord following en bloc open-door laminoplasty for cervical myelopathy: a magnetic resonance imaging study. J Neurol. 1996; 243(9):626–632

[34] Ferch RD, Shad A, Cadoux-Hudson TA, Teddy PJ. Anterior correction of cervical kyphotic deformity: effects on myelopathy, neck pain, and sagittal alignment. J Neurosurg. 2004; 100(1) Suppl Spine:13–19

[35] Villavicencio AT, Babuska JM, Ashton A, et al. Prospective, randomized, double-blind clinical study evaluating the correlation of clinical outcomes and cervical sagittal alignment. Neurosurgery. 2011; 68(5):1309–1316, discussion 1316

[36] Song KS, Piyaskulkaew C, Chuntarapas T, et al. Dynamic radiographic criteria for detecting pseudarthrosis following anterior cervical arthrodesis. J Bone Joint Surg Am. 2014; 96(7):557–563

[37] Kim HJ, Nemani VM, Daniel Riew K. Cervical osteotomies for neurological deformities. Eur Spine J. 2015; 24 Suppl 1:S16–S22

[38] Kim HJ, Piyaskulkaew C, Riew KD. Anterior cervical osteotomy for fixed cervical deformities. Spine. 2014; 39(21):1751–1757

[39] Mason C, Cozen L, Adelstein L. Surgical correction of flexion deformity of the cervical spine. Calif Med. 1953; 79(3):244–246

[40] Urist MR. Osteotomy of the cervical spine; report of a case of ankylosing rheumatoid spondylitis. J Bone Joint Surg Am. 1958; 40-A(4):833–843

[41] McMaster MJ. Osteotomy of the cervical spine in ankylosing spondylitis. J Bone Joint Surg Br. 1997; 79(2):197–203

[42] Wakao N, Takeuchi M, Kamiya M, et al. Variance of cervical vertebral artery measured by CT angiography and its influence on C 7 pedicle anatomy. Spine. 2014; 39(3):228–232

[43] Wollowick AL, Kelly MP, Riew KD. Pedicle subtraction osteotomy in the cervical spine. Spine. 2012; 37(5):E342–E348

[44] Kim HJ, Piyaskulkaew C, Riew KD. Comparison of Smith-Petersen osteotomy versus pedicle subtraction osteotomy versus anterior-posterior osteotomy types for the correction of cervical spine deformities. Spine. 2015; 40 (3):143–146

19 Junctional Corrective Osteotomies (Cervicothoracic, Thoracolumbar, Lumbosacral)

Claudio Lamartina, Riccardo Cecchinato

Abstract

This chapter focuses on the vertebral osteotomies for the correction of spinal deformities, either degenerative or congenital, and the treatment of deformities resulting from conditions such as ankylosing spondylitis, infections such as tuberculosis, proximal or distal junctional kyphosis in patients with spinal fusion, or postsurgical flat back syndrome. The main objective of this chapter is to provide information regarding the application of these techniques in the junctional regions, namely, the cervicothoracic, thoracolumbar, and lumbosacral junctions. Surgical techniques of different type of osteotomies (Smith-Petersen, pedicle subtraction, corner, and vertebral column resection) are described, and their indications are explained. Each junctional area of the spine, the cervicothoracic, the thoracolumbar, and the lumbosacral regions, is deeply analyzed and each peculiarity of the application of these techniques in these different anatomies are explained. The steps of the different surgical techniques are described in detail and illustrative cases are shown to help the reader's understanding of the treatment of these complex spinal pathologies. A description of the requirements of preoperative patient preparation is also provided based on the personal experience of the authors and on literature findings.

Keywords: spinal osteotomy, pedicle subtraction osteotomy, Smith-Petersen osteotomy, posterior vertebral column resection, corner osteotomy

19.1 Introduction

A local kyphosis of the junctional transitional regions of the spine (cervicothoracic, thoracolumbar, and lumbosacral) can produce a painful state with a worsening in the patient's quality of life. The global sagittal balance of these patients can be altered, especially in cases of kyphotic deformity of the lower junctional segments (thoracolumbar and lumbosacral). When this happens, compensation mechanisms can arise to preserve a normal C 7 plumb line. These mechanisms, however, require a large amount of energy to be maintained and are themselves a source of pain. A local kyphosis can further lead to abnormal biomechanics, thus accelerating degenerative processes and increasing the pain.

The main causes of deformity of the junctional segments of the spine can be classified as follows:

- Degenerative process.
- Posttraumatic deformity.
- Congenital deformity.
- Ankylosing spondylitis.
- Proximal/distal junctional kyphosis in subjects with a previous instrumentation of the spine.
- Result of a tubercular/infective process of the spine.
- Postsurgical flat back syndrome.

Frequently, these kinds of deformities are rigid and require aggressive and complex osteotomies of the spine to restore a correct sagittal and coronal balance. If a coronal imbalance coexists with a sagittal kyphotic deformity, the surgery required to correct the problem on both planes is even more elaborate. Despite their difficulty, even in expert hands, asymmetrical osteotomies can provide excellent correction on sagittal and coronal planes, restoring a good balance of the spine and increasing the patient's quality of life.

19.2 Preoperative Evaluation

The preoperative evaluation of patients with a kyphotic deformity of the junctional regions of the spine is based on clinical and radiologic examination.

Clinically it is important to notice any coronal or sagittal deformity. In case of a coronal deformity, a lateral positioning of the head relative to the pelvis can be observed. Sagittal imbalance, however, implies more mechanisms that appear evident during a clinical examination. Thoracic hypokyphosis to compensate a lumbar deformity, pelvic retroversion, and knee flexion are the first compensational mechanisms observed during an office examination. Any thoracic or lumbar hump can further indicate a rotational deformity of the spine.

Regarding the radiologic exams, the following should be performed before considering any type of surgery for adult deformity, especially if an osteotomy is thought to be required:

- Full standing X-rays of the spine in double projection—anteroposterior (AP) and lateral.
- Bending X-rays magnetic resonance imaging (MRI).
- Computed tomography (CT) scan.

Full standing X-rays offer a complete view of the spine, allowing the evaluation of the patient's global balance. On this kind of exam we can calculate preoperative spinopelvic parameters (pelvic incidence, pelvic tilt, sacral slope, lumbar lordosis, thoracolumbar and thoracic kyphosis, cervical lordosis, spinosacral angle), and assess the sagittal balance with the calculation of the sagittal vertical axis (SVA, the distance between the C 7 plumb line and the posterosuperior corner of S 1). A comprehension of the coronal alignment on the AP view is also fundamental to plan an adequate surgery with a correction on both planes. All these considerations should be completed in order to perform an optimal corrective surgery.

Bending X-rays are useful to determine the flexibility of the curves. In case of a sagittal deformity, a supine lateral view can establish the flexibility of the kyphotic deformity. In some cases, when the deformity is prevalently in the thoracic or thoracolumbar area with an acute angle, the positioning of a support under the apex of the curve can allow the surgeon to determine the flexibility of this deformity. If a coronal deformity exists, the AP view of a degenerative deformity can help the surgeon to assess the changes of the spine between standing and lying positions. This is important when a rotation of the vertebra is present, as in degenerative worsening of an idiopathic scoliosis.

MRI can show any cord abnormality, disk herniation, or stenotic segments of the spine. This is important in considering decompression techniques to be associated with an osteotomy of the spine.

Finally, a preoperative CT scan of the junctional segment can provide information on any bony abnormalities, such as bony spurs, previous vertebral fractures resulting in vertebral body abnormalities, or pedicle abnormalities. The CT scan can be helpful in determining the length and diameter of the screws for each single level. In cases of cervicothoracic osteotomies, where cervical vertebrae need to be instrumented to give stability to the osteotomy, the CT scan can show any abnormality of the vertebral artery foramina.

19.3 Cervicothoracic Kyphotic Deformity and Corrective Osteotomies

Cervicothoracic kyphosis is a disabling pathology causing a chin-on-chest deformity in the majority of cases. The affected patients have a limitation in forward gaze, and they often present with difficulty in swallowing and jaw opening, episodes of choking, and problems with personal hygiene and self-image. Cervical and cervicothoracic kyphosis can be due to multiple etiologies. Usually, congenital deformities related to genetic syndromes affect the mid or the upper part of the cervical region. Midcervical kyphosis is observed in patients with Larsen syndrome and diastrophic dysplasia, whereas upper cervical spine instability and deformity can be found in Down syndrome, pseudoachondroplasia, Morquio syndrome, spondyloepiphyseal dysplasia congenita, and Kniest syndrome. More often, cervicothoracic deformities can be observed in ankylosing spondylitis, in degenerative processes, and in posttraumatic kyphosis, even if this last cause is less frequent, happening especially in patients with ankylosing spondylitis. More often in recent years, proximal junctional kyphosis after long thoracic or thoracolumbar instrumented fusions or distal junctional pathology after cervical fusions are the cause of cervicothoracic kyphotic deformity. A review by Lawrence et al in 2012 found a prevalence of distal segment pathology after cervical fusion ranged from 11 to 12% at 5 years, 16 to 38% at 10 years, and 33% at 17 years.[1] Proximal junctional kyphosis at the cervicothoracic region has an incidence that ranges from 26 to 39%, depending on the studies.[2,0,0] While the distal junctional kyphosis can often be treated with a selected fusion of the pathological level, proximal junctional kyphosis after long thoracic or thoracolumbar fusions can often present as a fixed deformity, severe in nature, needing complex osteotomies to restore the alignment of the spine.

19.3.1 Patient Preparation

All patients undergoing a corrective osteotomy for cervicothoracic kyphosis must have continuous neuromonitoring during all phases of the surgery. The neurophysiologist that will perform neuromonitoring throughout the procedure should place the needles before the patient is positioned on the operating table. Neuromonitoring is a crucial aspect of all the techniques of cervicothoracic osteotomies. A continuous examination during surgery is mandatory to detect any alteration in signal transmission during the correction maneuvers. Advances in neuromonitoring now make it possible to monitor the cord and nerves in real time using sensory and motor evoked potentials. The major risks of cord damage are during the corrective maneuvers, but the risk remains after surgery because failure of the implant and spine subluxation can produce irreversible damage. We can consider a three-step procedure when evoked potentials disappear or their amplitude falls below 20% of the reference value; this procedure can also be applied in thoracolumbar and lumbosacral osteotomies, or in major spinal surgeries in which large corrections are performed. Whenever there is a decrease in amplitude, the technical causes are found and eventually repaired. Second, optimization of hemodynamic changes and possible restoration of higher blood pressure are obtained by the anesthesiologist. Finally, as a third step if the signal amplitude remains low, the previous surgical corrective maneuvers are considered to be the cause of the alteration in neuromonitoring. Therefore, if possible, the corrective maneuvers are reversed. If doubts arise as to the reliability of neuromonitoring, a Stagnara wake-up test should be performed.

The positioning of a halo cast or a Mayfield ring is not always necessary and depends on the surgeon's preference. Both devices provide traction during surgery and a better manipulation during corrective maneuvers. A halo cast is also indicated when a brace supporting the ring is supposed to be worn after the surgery.

Patient positioning on the operating table is crucial to obtaining the best surgical outcomes. Some authors performing cervicothoracic osteotomies consider having the patient in a sitting position, but this leads to some technical difficulties in the osteotomy procedure. In the sitting position the stabilization of the obtained correction is technically difficult because the rods have to be contoured in an extreme lordosis shape. Second, when a halo cast has been implanted, the operating area is reduced, thereby limiting the distal fixation procedure. This is why we prefer the prone position for this kind of procedure, though there are some important factors to consider. When a cervicothoracic kyphotic deformity is present, prone placement causes the head to be in a very low position. This can produce two different kinds of problems. First, the edema and pressure around the eyes and the face can increase significantly in respect to nondeformity spinal procedures. Second, raised intraocular hydrostatic pressure can lead to central optic neuropathy and, consequently, to blindness. The facial edema can be reduced using a halo device, thereby avoiding the positioning of facial padding and the compression on the head.

19.3.2 Technical Considerations

The preferred site for cervicothoracic osteotomies is at C 7 or T 1 for the following reasons: first, the spinal canal is wider here than in the cervical region, and the cord, nerve roots, and vertebral artery are favorably placed. Second, the C 8 nerve roots are more mobile, and damage to these roots is less detrimental to hand function. Finally, the vertebral arteries pass anterior to the transverse process of C 7 before entering the foramen. Thus the risk of kinking on neck extension during the osteotomy and the correction is low.

We can basically consider two kinds of wedge osteotomies of the cervical spine: the anterior opening/posterior closing osteotomy, and the posterior closing-wedge osteotomies.

The first descriptions of cervical osteotomies were those of Urist in 1958 and of Law in 1959.[0,0] These authors proposed techniques similar to that of Smith-Petersen, with removal of the spinous process and lamina at the selected levels and an extension opening osteotomy of the cervical spine. In fact these techniques produced an anterior wedge with disruption of the intervertebral disk and the anterior longitudinal ligament, using the posterior longitudinal ligament as the hinge of the correction and leaving a bony gap in the anterior column. Simmons proposed variations to these techniques in 1972.[0] The author introduced a so-called controlled fracture of C 7 in patients with ankylosing spondylitis, with an opening wedge to restore normal alignment of the cervicothoracic junction. This technique has been the gold standard in sagittal balance reconstruction of the cervicothoracic junction for many years and is still widely used. However, the instability provided by an anterior opening osteotomy, together with serious vascular and neurologic complications due to the elongation of the anterior column, led to the introduction of the pedicle subtraction osteotomy (PSO) in the cervical spine. The cervicothoracic junction PSO can offer a more controlled closure of the wedge than the Simmons technique, showing greater biomechanical stability and avoiding the problem of the anterior open-wedge defect. In fact, as mentioned earlier, the Smith-Petersen osteotomy (SPO) in the cervical spine often produces a disruption of the intervertebral disk and a tear of the anterior longitudinal ligament, leaving an anterior gap and decreasing the stability in the treated region. This happens often in patients with ankylosing spondylitis, where the anterior components are fused and thus less mobile and flexible than in normal patients. Subsequently, PSO creates a large bone-on-bone contact, with a wide bearing surface, even when compared to an SPO that is fully closed posteriorly. Variations of the PSO technique have been proposed in recent years by various authors.[8,9] The one we usually apply is a traditional PSO performed with consecutive increasing tapping of the pedicles. This technique has also been described by Deviren, Scheer, and Ames in 2011.[0] These authors describe the results of 11 patients treated with this kind of cervical PSO, having no postoperative neurologic complications. A posterior incision from C 2 to T 3 or T 5 and a meticulous dissection of the paravertebral muscles is performed. The upper level of instrumentation can usually be C 2, in order to obtain a solid bicortical screw placement, with a stronger fixation than lateral mass screws in the lower levels. Distally, T 3 can be considered the lower instrumented vertebra if the upper thoracic region shows no hyperkyphosis, whereas in case of sagittal deformity of the upper thoracic region, the fusion should go caudally almost to T 5. The main rule is to give at least three levels of stability above and below the osteotomy level and to avoid stopping the instrumentation at the apex of the thoracic kyphosis. If the patient has bone of good quality, a two-level fusion above and below the osteotomy can provide enough stability. The osteotomy can begin after screw implantation. First, a complete laminectomy of C 7 is performed, with the removal of the spinous process, lamina, and articular facets. At this point a complete C 6–C 7 and C 7–T 1 bilateral foraminotomy is performed. The view of C 7 and C 8 bilateral roots is mandatory for the removal of any scar tissue in cases of previous posterior cervical surgery. After the isolation of the C 7 pedicles, apposite rongeurs are used to remove the pedicles, and taps of increasing size are used to create bilateral holes to the vertebral body, which finally connect in the midline. Osteotomes and downpushing curets are needed to create a wedge in the vertebral body. The lateral walls of the C 7 vertebra are then identified and dissected: when complete visualization is obtained, a rongeur or an osteotome can be used to remove a triangular part of the lateral walls, corresponding to the wedge in the vertebral body. This procedure is followed by the removal of the posterior wall to complete the osteotomy. The neck can then be extended to close the osteotomy using the anterior ligament as a hinge for the corrective procedure, and two rods are placed and locked to maintain the obtained correction. We suggest controlling the rotational alignment during this maneuver, checking the position of the nose, to avoid malalignments that can lead to a lateral rotation of the head and consequently of sight in relation to the rest of the body. Because this is a shortening procedure of the spine, this should not cause neurologic problems as long as the laminectomy provides adequate space to the neurologic elements posteriorly. Local bone graft and eventually iliac bone graft are then placed after decortication of the laminae and lateral masses to obtain a solid bony fusion. With this technique the theoretical correction can reach 30 degrees, even if in their work Deviren et al had an average correction of 19 degrees, with a mean overall cervical correction of 49.9 ± 7.2 degrees.[0] This technique can also be applied to T 1. In some cases, when previous surgery and eventual decompression have been performed at the cervicothoracic junction, a lower osteotomy (T 2 or T 3) can provide adequate correction without managing the epidural scarring tissue (▶ Fig. 19.1a–e). The amount of the needed correction must be calculated preoperatively. A slight undercorrection of the deformity is desirable as opposed to overcorrection, allowing for a good compromise between a horizontal gaze and looking at the floor during walking, or handling a pen or a keyboard on a desk during work activities.

There are many variations on this technique. Initially Shimizu[11] and McMaster[12] used sublaminar wires to correct the spine, but the frequent ankylosis of the posterior bony elements and the possibility of tearing the underlying adherent dura made this technique fall out of use. Chin and Ahn[13] suggested the use of high-speed burs and osteotomes to complete the osteotomy but, as also suggested by Deviren et al,[14] we consider that consecutive tapping creates a reproducible osteotomy and is a quick way to obtain the wedge with minimal risks.

Anterior support is at times mandatory, especially when a cervicothoracic kyphosis occurs after a vertebral fracture (this happens frequently in proximal junctional kyphosis after long thoracic or thoracolumbar instrumented fusions). Support can be provided with an anterior approach, a corpectomy of the fractured vertebra, and the implant of an expandable cage. We suggest performing the anterior part after the posterior one, because it is the latter that allows for the majority of the correction, being that the anterior cage (and eventual plating) provides support for only the anterior column.

The diameter and material of the rods still remain under open debate among spine surgeons. In the 56th Annual Meeting

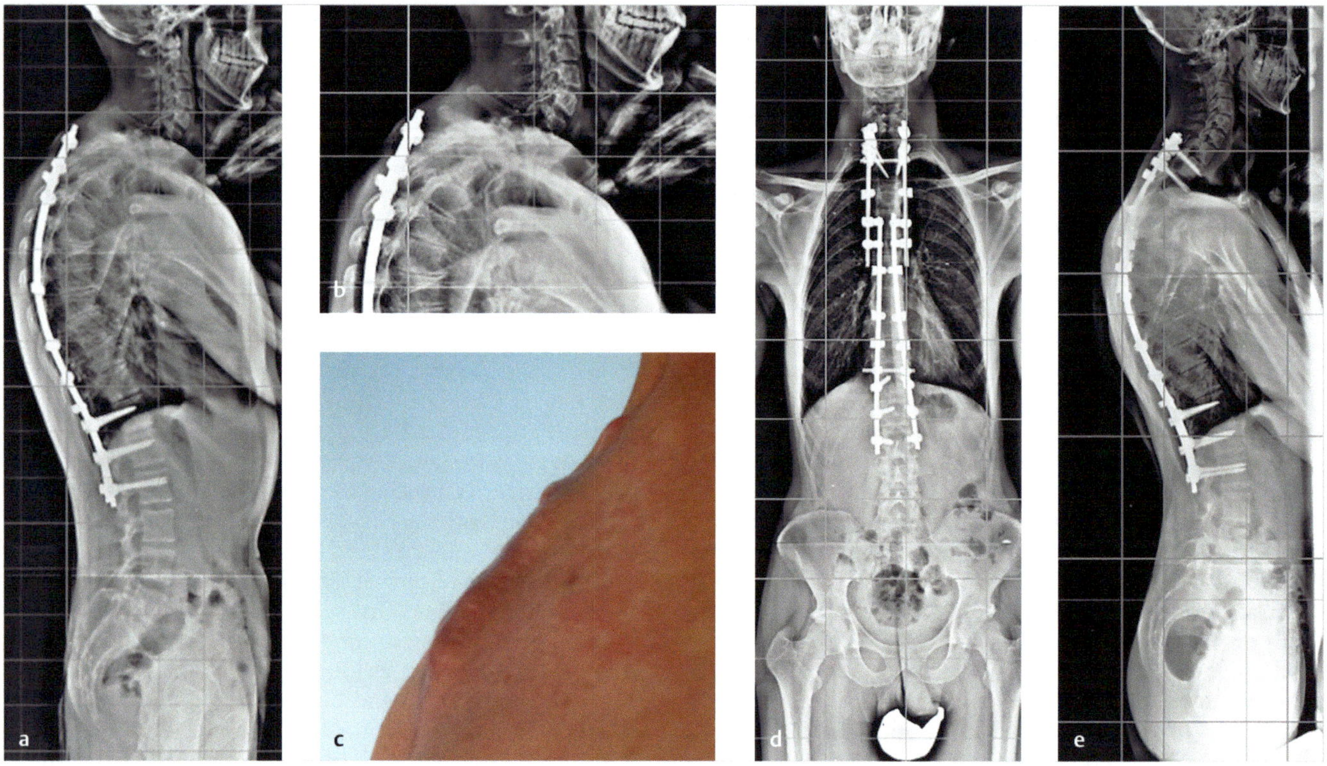

Fig. 19.1 (a) Proximal junctional kyphosis in a 36-year-old man treated for Scheuermann kyphosis with a T2–L2 fusion. **(b)** Detail of the proximal junctional kyphosis. **(c)** Clinical detail of the skin prominence due to hardware mobilization. **(d, e)** Postoperative result after a cervicothoracic pedicle subtraction osteotomy and cranial extension.

of the Orthopaedic Research Society, Scheer et al presented "Biomechanical Characterization of Fusion Constructs across the Cervicothoracic Junction."[15] The authors performed an extensive study on the biomechanics of opening- and closing-wedge osteotomies at the cervicothoracic junction. Eight fresh-frozen C3–T4 spinal sections were harvested from the original specimens and cleaned of paravertebral muscles, without disrupting ligaments. All the vertebrae were instrumented with posterior screw–rod hardware, with lateral mass screws in the cervical region and pedicle screws in the thoracic vertebrae. Half of the specimen had an opening-wedge osteotomy at C7, whereas those remaining had closing-wedge osteotomies. The study aimed to evaluate any difference in stress-loading capacity of two different rod diameters, 3.5 mm and 4.5 mm. The study achieved the following results: Regardless of the type of osteotomy, 4.5 mm rods increased rigidity in all bending directions (flexion/extension, lateral bending, axial rotation) compared to 3.5 mm rods. Considering closing-wedge osteotomies only, 4.5 mm rods increased flexion/extension and axial rotation rigidity, while there was no significant difference between rod sizes in any bending direction with the opening-wedge osteotomies. Scheer et al also published a paper in the *Journal of Neurosurgery: Spine* in 2011 on the biomechanics of cervicothoracic junction osteotomies in a cadaveric model of ankylosing spondylitis.[16] In this study the authors tested three different types of rods: 3.2 mm titanium, 3.5 mm titanium, and 3.5 mm cobalt–chrome (CoCr) rods. C7–T1 opening-wedge osteotomies were performed in 10 fresh-frozen human spine specimens stabilized from C3 to T4. The authors' findings were that the 3.5 mm CoCr rods yielded stiffer constructs than titanium rods of the same diameter, and both of them were stiffer than 3.2 mm titanium rods. In any case, the greater stiffness obtained when using larger or CoCr rods is not a clear indication to use these kinds of hardware. Adjacent segment problems, such as disk degeneration or vertebral fracture, can occur when a stiff construct is implanted in poor-quality bone after large corrections. Each case should be considered individually, and the hardware used must be customized based on the patient's characteristics. On the other hand, as discussed earlier, adjacent segment disease is more frequently becoming a cause of cervicothoracic hyperkyphosis after long thoracolumbar fusions and thus remain an unsolved problem in major spine surgery. A final consideration can be made on vertebral column resection (VCR) of the cervical spine. Although it is a difficult technique to be performed in the cervical spine, VCR can be performed at C7 or T1 levels. However, the inability to sacrifice the C8 or T1 nerve roots due to their motor contribution to the hand, combined with the more effective and relative ease of performing a posterior column osteotomy, makes VCR an infrequently used technique for cervicothoracic kyphosis correction.

19.4 Thoracolumbar Corrective Osteotomies

Thoracolumbar deformity can have various causes, the most common being degeneration of the intervertebral disks, a fracture of the thoracolumbar junction, and infective and tubercular localization with deformity of the vertebra–disk complex. Iatrogenic thoracolumbar kyphosis often occurs after a previous failed surgery for a thoracolumbar fracture. Rarely, genetic syndromes, such as achondroplasia, Stickler syndrome, and Marfan syndrome are associated with thoracolumbar deformity. The most common cause of thoracolumbar kyphotic deformity is, however, posttraumatic. A fracture of the thoracolumbar region with a local kyphosis of more than 20 degrees can hide an injury of the posterior elements, with the possibility of developing a posttraumatic kyphosis. This deformity can be subdivided into "acute" and "late" types, depending on the time elapsed between the fracture and the kyphotic deformation. Late deformities may be caused by the progression of the vertebral body collapse or may result from the surgical treatment of the fracture. The most common causes of late kyphotic deformities related to treatment are implant failure, deep infection, pseudarthrosis, short fusion, and aggressive laminectomy.

Patients with a sagittal imbalance related to the thoracolumbar kyphotic deformity usually show a hyperlordosis of the lumbar tract and a hypokyphosis of the upper thoracic region, with a pelvic retroversion in the worst scenarios. If there is hyperlordosis of the lumbar region, the overloading of the articular facets can generate pain in the lower region of the spine, even if the fracture and the correlated deformity are cranial.

The posttraumatic deformity is usually an abnormality referred only to the sagittal plane. If a degenerative pathology is the cause of thoracolumbar deformity, the curves are usually combined on the sagittal and coronal planes, requiring more complex surgeries to correct both the imbalances.

19.4.1 Patient Preparation

Preoperative evaluation of the patient should include a standing full spine frontal and lateral X-ray, including from the acoustic meatus down to the first part of the femoral shaft. After analyzing all the sagittal pelvic and spinal parameters and verifying the coronal alignment, the authors' preferred method for determining the indication for surgery is based on Farcy's sagittal index. This parameter is calculated by the difference between the kyphotic angle measured at the level of the deformity (between the intact end plate of the fractured vertebra and the same end plate—cranial or caudal—of the next vertebra across the fracture) and the normal alignment of the segment where the kyphosis occurs. In the case of the thoracolumbar junction, the normal alignment of the area is 0 degrees of kyphosis. Patients with a Farcy's sagittal index under 15 degrees usually compensate with few symptoms, while a Farcy's index higher than 20 degrees is generally a source of pain and hides the risk of progression, providing the indication for surgery. Between 15 and 20 degrees a decision should be made depending on the patient's symptoms.

Additionally, MRI is useful to rule out spinal cord or nerve root compression, whereas a CT scan can offer a better picture of anterior or lateral bony spurs or bridges. Both these exams are mandatory if an anterior approach for a corpectomy is planned.

The day before surgery, a complete intestinal preparation is performed. We usually dispense 140 mg of macrogol oral powder in 2 L of water. This frequently avoids any postoperative abdominal complication, such as fecal impaction.

The day of surgery, general anesthesia with tracheal intubation is performed and neuromonitoring needles are placed. The patient is placed prone on a Jackson table, with appropriate foam supports on the thorax and on the anterosuperior iliac spines. If a Jackson table is not available, a Risser frame should be preferred to a foam cushion to support the patient. The Risser frame offers greater space for the abdomen, resulting in lower vascular compression and decreased blood loss during surgery.

If a lateral access is performed, as for an anterior corpectomy or a cage implant, the patient is placed in a lateral decubitus position. Foam cushions are placed under the head, the lower arm, and between the legs. A support is used to hold the arm opposite to the bed in a forward extension position. A first tape is used to fix the thorax to the bed, and a second is fixed at the level of the patient's hips. A third tape starts from the hip down along the leg (with care to avoid compression of the peroneal head, where the external sciatic-peroneal nerve lies), turns around the table, and joins the tape around the hips on the front side (▶ Fig. 19.2). Once the patient is firmly affixed to the

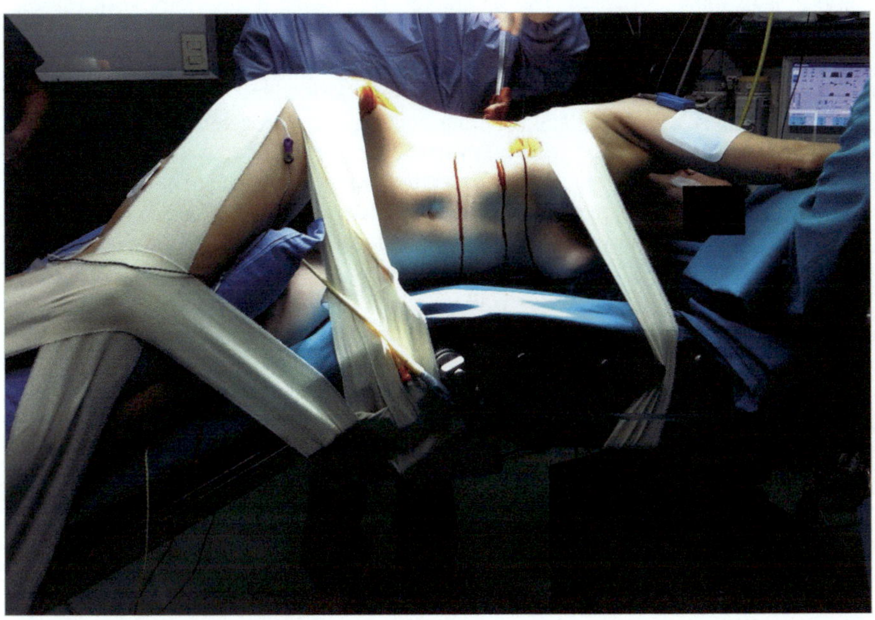

Fig. 19.2 Taping the patient for firm positioning on the operating table to provide access for an extreme lateral interbody fusion.

table, lateral and anteroposterior fluoroscopy will show the orientation of the spine. The Jackson bed is then turned to the left or right side, and the head of the bed is bent up or down to obtain a perfect lateral and AP projection of the target vertebra. If a Jackson table is not available, the fluoroscopy and correction of the patient's position must be performed before the tapes are definitively affixed. This allows the surgeon to work in a straight position, without the use of angled instruments.

19.4.2 Technical Considerations

The surgical techniques applied in the thoracolumbar kyphotic deformity can be subdivided into posterior osteotomies and anterior lengthening procedures.

Posterior osteotomies include posterior column–shortening osteotomies, such as the Ponte osteotomy or the SPO, and PSO. The first two techniques are less able to correct an angular kyphotic deformity, since they restore few grades of lordosis per level and are more adequate in treating a multilevel global deformity, as in Scheuermann disease in the thoracic spine. Additionally, the Ponte osteotomy and the SPO require a flexible intervertebral disk at the treated level; considering post-traumatic angular kyphosis, an anterior bony bridge frequently fuses the spine at the affected level, thus limiting the efficacy of these techniques. PSOs are widely used in the treatment of angular thoracolumbar kyphotic deformity because they permit a large correction (up to 30 degrees) at a single level and, due to their tricolumnar resection, are able to restore spine alignment in fixed deformities. Moreover, PSOs allow treatment of the pathological segment from a single approach, which is more familiar to most spinal surgeons and allows simultaneous implant revision in cases with previous surgery or nerve root/ cord decompression. Difficulties related to epidural scarring, frequent in cases of revision surgery on a previous decompression and fusion for a vertebral fracture, can limit the efficacy of PSO or extend the surgical time, with greater blood loss and complications related to anesthesia and positioning. Further on, in cases with a severe collapsed vertebral body, PSO efficacy is limited in restoring a sufficient amount of lordosis. In our experience, a PSO of the thoracolumbar region requires at least four fixation points cranial and caudal to the level of the osteotomy, usually fixing with pedicle screws two levels above and below the treated level. One alternative configuration in cases with low-grade corrections and with a good restoration of the sagittal alignment is to implant sublaminar bands in combination with pedicle screws just one level above and below the PSO to save as many motion segments as possible. The sublaminar bands improve the screws' resistance to pull-out stresses anchoring to the lamina, one of the toughest structures of the whole vertebra. A variation of PSO we often use in this kind of surgery is the corner PSO, a slightly different technique proposed by the senior author (CL) that provides wider bone-to-bone contact and higher rates of fusion. Both PSO and corner PSO techniques will be described in the subsequent section on lumbosacral osteotomies. However, it is important to emphasize how both of these techniques create instability of the anterior column. We always suggest the implant of intersomatic cages in the mobile levels (both the upper and lower in a traditional PSO, only the caudal in a corner PSO) to stabilize the anterior column and improve the chances of fusion. The ideal level for PSO in thoracolumbar kyphosis is the apex of the kyphotic deformity. The presence of implants, solid mass fusion, or scar tissue can make it convenient to perform the osteotomy at a more cranial or caudal level (the second to be preferred because of greater efficacy in translating the C7 plumb line and reducing compensating mechanisms).

When anterior lengthening procedures are considered, a mobile posterior column is required to obtain the maximal correction. The advantages of this approach include blood loss reduction during anterior column reconstruction compared with posterior osteotomies of the anterior column, the avoidance of dealing with epidural adherent scar tissue in revision surgery with a previous laminectomy, the ability to reconstruct the anterior column and, in selected cases, the possibility to obtain a perfect reduction with a two-stage procedure. Disadvantages of the anterior techniques are the need for an anterior approach, which can be unfamiliar to some spinal surgeons; the frequent need for a thoracotomy with handling of the diaphragm; and the risk of a range of complications that are unique to the anterior approach, such as pleural effusion, pneumothorax, hemothorax, atelectasis, vascular injuries, thoracic duct lesions, and lumbar plexus lesions.

We prefer to use lateral access for an anterior column corpectomy and cage implant in the thoracolumbar region, conventional open thoracotomy, or laparotomic transdiaphragmatic access, but these techniques are accompanied by significant approach-related and postoperative complications that decrease their value. Usually, the minimally invasive approach to T12 is performed on the left side. An oblique incision is performed after the identification of the level, and the ribs are exposed. At the T11 and T12 levels the rib heads are located inferiorly to the disk space and are resected with a portion of the rib itself in order to obtain enough working space. The diaphragm provides the limit between the thoracic cavity and the peritoneum. This muscle has lateral costal and posterior lumbar attachments. These can be mobilized around the thoracolumbar junction without the need for a dissection and then a transdiaphragmatic approach. Sometimes an angled approach can be used to avoid the diaphragm, but we don't suggest this option, even in the hands of an expert surgeon. The pleura can be mobilized anteriorly with the diaphragm in a smooth manner to expose the T12 vertebral body and the cranial and caudal disks. Once these structures are isolated, diskectomies can be performed in a traditional lateral way, cutting any eventual bony bridge. Corpectomy can now be performed with two vertical cuts, the first anterior and the second posterior. We are used to leaving a thin shell of bone corresponding to the anterior wall in order to protect the great vessels. We perform the same technique for the posterior cut if a decompression of the canal is not necessary. Otherwise, a careful removal of the posterior wall with curets and rongeurs allows the surgeon to enter the spinal canal to decompress the cord. Once the vertebral body has been removed, an adequate expandable cage filled with autologous bone graft is implanted and gradually spread. If necessary, lateral access can be used to perform even a double corpectomy (▶ Fig. 19.3).

A successful anterior correction depends on the observance of some key factors. First of all, flexibility of the deformity is needed; when a fixed kyphosis is present, a circumferential release of the anterior annulus fibrosus or the osteotomy of any bony bridge should be performed. After the release, a

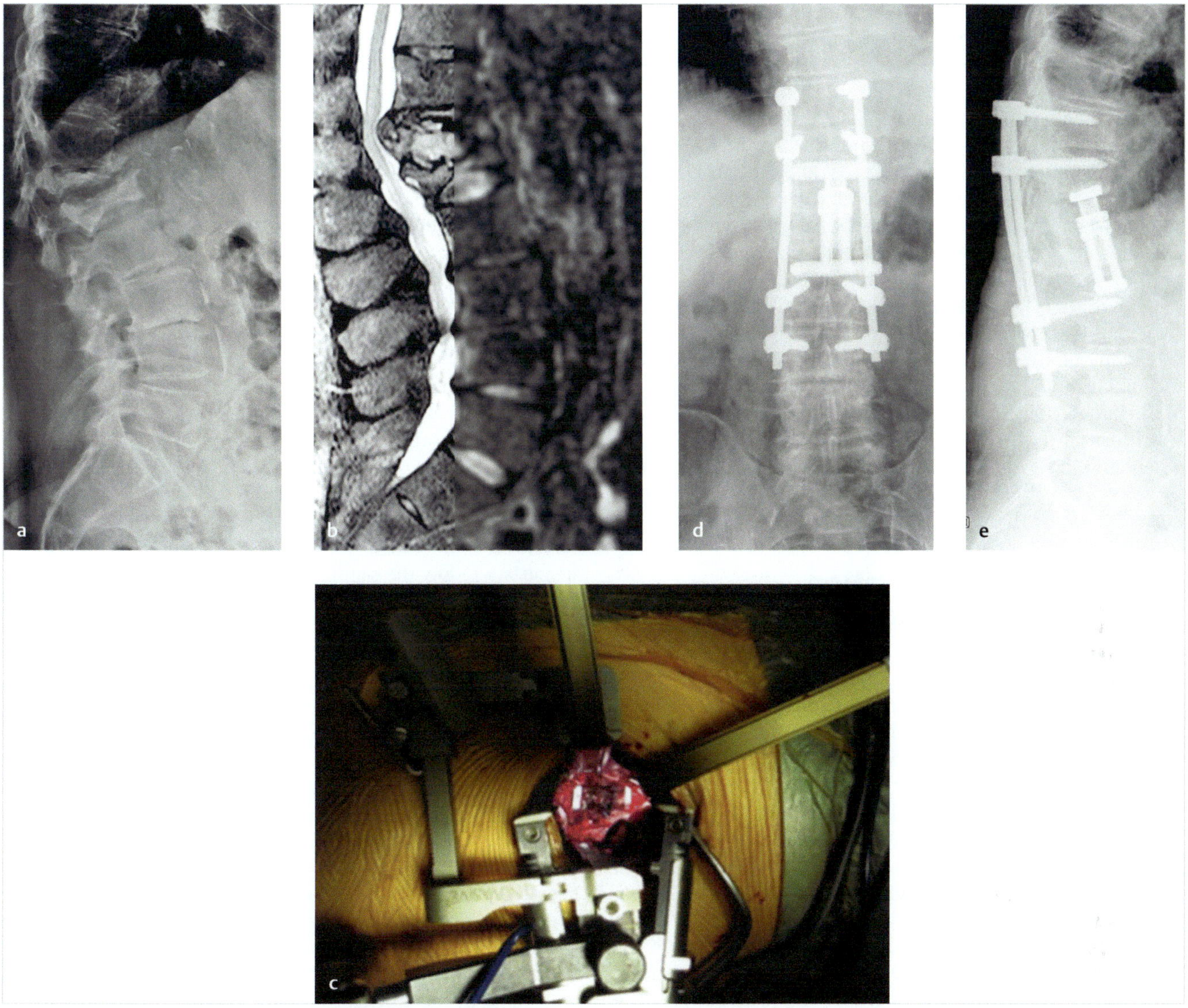

Fig. 19.3 **(a)** Lateral X-ray and **(b)** MRI sagittal scan details a burst fracture of T 12 and L 1 in a 67-year-old man, associated with local thoracolumbar kyphosis of 32 degrees. **(c)** Intraoperative detail of the lateral access for T 12 and L 1 corpectomy and cage implant. **(d)** Postoperative X-rays of a T 12–L 1 corpectomy and cage implant and posterior percutaneous T 10–L 3 fixation. **(e)** The local deformity was restored to 10 degrees of thoracolumbar kyphosis.

three-point stress (directed from posterior to anterior at the level of corpectomy, and from anterior to posterior above and below this level, generally at the sternum and at the iliac spine) is useful to verify the reducibility of the deformity. The second consideration regards the integrity of the end plates. Obviously, the cartilage layer has to be removed to promote bony fusion, but no violation of the subchondral bone should be performed. The resistance of this layer to compression stresses is useful to reduce the risk of subsidence of the cage. Third, we suggest the use of a cage with wide plates to distribute the weight across a larger surface, and contacting the periphery of the end plate, where the bone is more resistant. Finally, the quality of the bone graft should be adequate to promote a fusion of the anterior column.

After the suture of the diaphragm and of the superficial layers of the access, the patient is carefully turned in a prone position. A posterior stabilization is required at least one level cranial and caudal to the implanted cage. When needed, the SPO or Ponte osteotomy of the posterior bony elements can be performed to gain more degrees of lordosis and restore the balance of the thoracolumbar junction.

19.5 Lumbosacral Corrective Osteotomies

The causes of sagittal imbalance are many, but most commonly these include lumbar disk degeneration, posttraumatic or postlaminectomy kyphosis, iatrogenic flat back syndrome, and ankylosing spondylitis.

Lumbosacral corrective osteotomies are frequently performed in patients affected by sagittal unbalance. This kind of surgery is used to restore a correct SVA, as determined by a vertical line starting from the center of the C7 body. In sagittally balanced subjects, this line is found less than 5 cm ahead of or behind the posterosuperior corner of S1. When a sagittal imbalance occurs, the forward bending of the spine brings this line in front of the femoral heads, thus making the SVA greater than 5 cm. This is why most of the osteotomies performed to correct a sagittal imbalance involve L4 or L5: the lower the osteotomy, the greater the effect on the backward translation of C7. A second consideration is that the distribution of the lordosis in the lumbar spine is not homogeneous. It is well known that one-third of the lordosis lies between L1 and L3, while the remaining two-thirds are enclosed between L4 and S1. An osteotomy of the upper lumbar spine will hypercorrect this region, creating a nonphysiological distribution of the lordosis of the lumbar spine. The third and last consideration, but not of less importance, is that the spinal cord generally reaches L2, whereas in the lower lumbar spine only the cauda is present. In the lower lumbar region the dura can then be manipulated easily, with less risk of neurologic complications.

19.5.1 Patient Preparation

As in the thoracolumbar kyphotic deformities, the patient needs complete intestinal preparation before surgery to avoid abdominal complications after surgery. This should be done the day before surgery. The day of surgery, the patient is intubated and neuromonitoring needles are inserted. The patient is then placed in a prone position on a Jackson table, with foam pillows under the legs to hyperextend the hips. The positioning of the patient is a critical part of the surgery, because it will determine a better result of the operation. The Jackson table we use has the possibility to be bent at the midline, allowing a correction in kyphosis or lordosis of the spine. This is useful when the osteotomy is completed: bending the table in a lordosis fashion permits the closure of the osteotomy without pushing on the bony elements or on the screws. In the absence of a Jackson table, a Risser frame should be preferred to a foam cushion. The hyperextension of the hips is useful to create as much lordosis as possible in the lumbar spine to gain correction and reduce the stress on the hardware during corrective maneuvers.

The correct preoperative planning is mandatory for a good surgical outcome. The type of deformity is classified following the rules described by the senior author (CL) and Berjano.[17,18] We also measure the spinopelvic parameters to consider the lack of lordosis of the patient. Once we have all the needed parameters and the appropriate classification of the deformity, we can plan the area of fusion and, considering the difference between actual and needed lordosis, the adequate osteotomy to treat the deformity and achieve the appropriate spinopelvic balance for the patient can be chosen. The coronal profile of the spine indicates if asymmetric osteotomies should be performed to correct the alignment on both sagittal and coronal planes.

19.5.2 Technical Considerations

We can consider the osteotomies performed at L4 and L5 as lumbosacral osteotomies because they are performed in the lower part of the lumbar spine. There are three main types of osteotomies usually performed at this level: the SPO, the PSO, and the VCR. The use of one of these osteotomies depends on many factors. First, in the sagittal plane, the lack of lordosis guides the surgeon in the choice of one type of osteotomy over another: whereas an SPO can restore up to 10 degrees of lordosis per level, a PSO can reach a value of 30 degrees and a VCR of 45 degrees. The second aspect that has to be considered is the mobility of the spine at the lower lumbar levels. SPOs work on the flexibility of the intervertebral disk, using the posterior longitudinal ligament as a hinge for the posterior closure of the osteotomy. If the anterior structures are fused, as in ankylosing spondylitis, an SPO won't be effective in correcting the lordosis at the desired level. Third, the coronal plane must be observed. A rigid coronal deformity cannot be well corrected by an SPO alone, whereas an asymmetric PSO or a VCR performed at the apex of the curve can better correct the deformity on both planes.

The SPO was first described in 1945 to treat rheumatoid arthritis kyphotic deformities.[19] This technique is less invasive than the other two, and the invasion of the canal is minimal. After a longitudinal incision and exposure of the spine, pedicle screws are implanted. To choose the appropriate levels of fusion, we follow the sagittal deformity classification of Lamartina and Berjano, as explained earlier. Once the pedicle screws are implanted, the osteotomy procedure can begin. After the identification of the level, the interspinous ligament and the adjoining spinous processes are resected. A V-shaped osteotomy of the lamina is then performed, with the removal of the underlying ligamentum flavum. Typically, the width of the osteotomy should be about 7 to 10 mm. An intuitive rule to follow is that for each millimeter of removed bone, 1 degree of correction is obtained. Another rule that should be followed is to direct the osteotomy line laterocranially, with an angle of about 30 to 40 degrees in respect to the midline. Once the osteotomy reaches the isthmus bilaterally, a progressive compression of the posterior elements or the bending in lordosis of the table (if a Jackson table is used) allows the osteotomy to be closed. If a mild coronal deformity has to be corrected, the osteotomy of the convex side must be wider than the one on the concave side. However, as stated earlier, we don't consider SPO to be the best osteotomy for treating a complex sagittal and coronal deformity.

PSO is a more powerful option for restoring lordosis. It was first described by Thomasen as a transpedicular cortical decancellation osteotomy, in which the posterior column is shortened without lengthening the anterior one. The advantage of PSO is its capacity to restore lumbar lordosis, with the potential to obtain up to 30 degrees of lordosis from a single-level osteotomy. On the other hand PSO greatly destabilizes the anterior column and leads to a large amount of blood loss during the procedure. After the spine is exposed and the pedicle screws have been implanted, the PSO starts with a wide laminectomy. The whole spinous process, the lamina, and the ligamentum flavum are removed to allow reveal both the upper and the lower roots on both sides. The pedicle is then removed with a rongeur, and a tap is used to open a hole in the remaining part of the pedicle. Bigger convergent taps are sequentially introduced into the vertebral body to create two cavities that are connected in the midline of the vertebra. Downpushing curets and rongeurs are then used to create a wedge in the vertebral body. Once the cavity is completed, the thin posterior wall is broken with an apposite flat instrument that is placed between the dura and the bone and then carefully hammered.

After careful isolation of the lateral walls and bilateral removal of the transverse processes, the lateral walls are cut with apposite rongeurs in a triangular shape. At this point the osteotomy is complete and can be closed by bending the Jackson table or compressing the adjoining pedicle screws. This procedure should be performed carefully in order to verify any entrapment of the dura or the four roots. If compression of the screws is performed, the surgeon must be careful to verify any screw pullout, especially in osteoporotic bone.

Continuous neuromonitoring must be performed throughout the entire procedure to control nerve function during the corrective maneuvers; kinking of the dura cannot be avoided in the correction of lordosis, but excessive flexion can cause neurologic damage. When the osteotomy closure is complete and the correction has been obtained, two precontoured rods are connected to the screws and fixed with appropriate caps. PSO is an effective technique for correcting combined sagittal and coronal deformities. If a rigid coronal curve is present, the removal of a wider section of the lateral wall on the convex side can correct the deformity on both planes.

Though it is a powerful technique for correcting spinal deformities, PSO has some disadvantages that can compromise the surgical outcome. The massive bleeding that usually happens during the osteotomy derives from the vertebral body, and the closure of the osteotomy is an effective way to stop this blood loss. Thus the osteotomy should be performed as quickly as possible to reduce the amount of blood loss. Moreover, the removal of both pedicles makes it impossible to place screws or any kind of hardware to stabilize the osteotomized vertebra. This is an obvious cause of instability at the level of the osteotomy. Furthermore, the posterior wide decompression usually leaves a discontinuity of the posterior column that cannot be bridged by the bone grafts, and the bilateral removal of the transverse processes impedes a good intertransversary fusion. These factors increase the risk of pseudarthrosis and subsequent implant failure. This is why some modifications to the original PSO technique have been proposed.

The transdiskal wedge osteotomy is an example of an original PSO variation. In this technique, the resection wedge crosses the disk between two vertebrae. In this way, a triangle of the upper part of the caudal vertebra and a triangle of the lower part of the cranial vertebra are removed together with the intervertebral disk. The closure of the osteotomy allows a large area of contact between two trabecular bony surfaces, reducing the instability at the level of the osteotomy and promoting fusion. However, this is a complex technique, with prolonged surgery time and requiring the removal of portions of two different vertebrae. For these reasons the PSO variation we prefer is the so-called corner PSO, a variation we have conceived (▶ Fig. 19.4).

In the corner PSO the wedge removed from the vertebral body includes only a part of the cranial intervertebral disk. After the decompression and removal of the pedicles, as previously described for the normal PSO technique, the sequential tapping of the vertebral body and the wedge creation includes the trabecular bone underlying the upper end plate of the vertebra. After the wedge is created, the subchondral bone and the corresponding part of the upper end plate are removed. From the wide laminar decompression a partial diskectomy is performed, and the corresponding lower end plate of the upper vertebra is prepared as for an intersomatic fusion. After removal of the cartilage, the closure of the osteotomy allows a large area of contact between two trabecular bone surfaces, with a higher possibility for fusion.

In traditional PSO, but also in any modified technique presented in the literature, the vertebra that undergoes the osteotomy cannot be instrumented. This, as emphasized earlier, is a cause of instability and consequently increases the risk of pseudarthrosis. This is why we always perform an interbody fusion of the adjacent levels. If an L4 traditional PSO is performed, we suggest implanting cages at L3–L4 and L4–L5 levels. If a corner PSO is used to correct a fixed kyphosis of the lumbar region, an L4–L5 interbody fusion is mandatory. This increases the stability of the anterior column and promotes its fusion, diminishing the rates of pseudarthrosis and hardware failure. We prefer to use lateral access (also known as extreme lateral interbody fusion) for implanting the intersomatic cages in lumbar osteotomies. This kind of access does not require widening of the posterior decompression; thus it increases the posterior bony surface for placement of the bone graft.

Revision rates in adult deformity surgery reach values of 30% in the literature. This is partly due to pseudarthrosis at the level of the osteotomy and to the consequent implant failure. As mentioned earlier, it is important to consider the small surface left for fusion after the PSO procedure and the discontinuity of the posterior column. However, other factors intervene in implant failure after a PSO, as described by Berjano et al: the insufficient correction is a key factor in determining the failure of surgery, thus underlining the importance of adequate preoperative planning.[20] The rods also play a fundamental role in this kind of surgery. The aggressive bending of CoCr or titanium rods creates a series of notches on the surface of the rod itself; these marks act as stress risers, lowering the resistance of the material to fatigue stresses. Finally, an insufficient distal foundation of the hardware can be a cause of failure. This is why we suggest, when performing an L4 or L5 osteotomy, enhancing spinal stabilization with iliac screws. The different orientation in the axial plane of the divergent pelvic screws in respect to the S1 convergent screws is the key for increasing the construct's resistance to pullout.

The last option for correcting a kyphotic deformity of the lumbar spine is a VCR. This technique was first proposed by Bradford[21] in the late 1980s, and can be performed with a single posterior approach, the so-called posterior vertebral column resection (PVCR), or with a combined anterior/posterior approach. PVCR provides a trapezoidal space after the removal of the lamina and the underlying ligamentum flavum, the pedicles, and the entire vertebral body. After a complete bony removal, an expandable cage or a mesh cage is placed in the anterior column replacing the vertebral body, and a posterior compression approaches the residual spinous processes, creating lordosis. However, we prefer using PVCR in corrective surgery of the thoracic area, performing a double anterior/posterior approach in the surgery of the lower lumbar spine.

We perform L4 corpectomy in cases of posttraumatic lower lumbar kyphosis or, rarely, in cases of pseudarthrosis resulting from a previous PSO that has led to the vertebral body's collapse. In these cases, we prefer a double approach to perform the column resection, position the cage, and then implant the

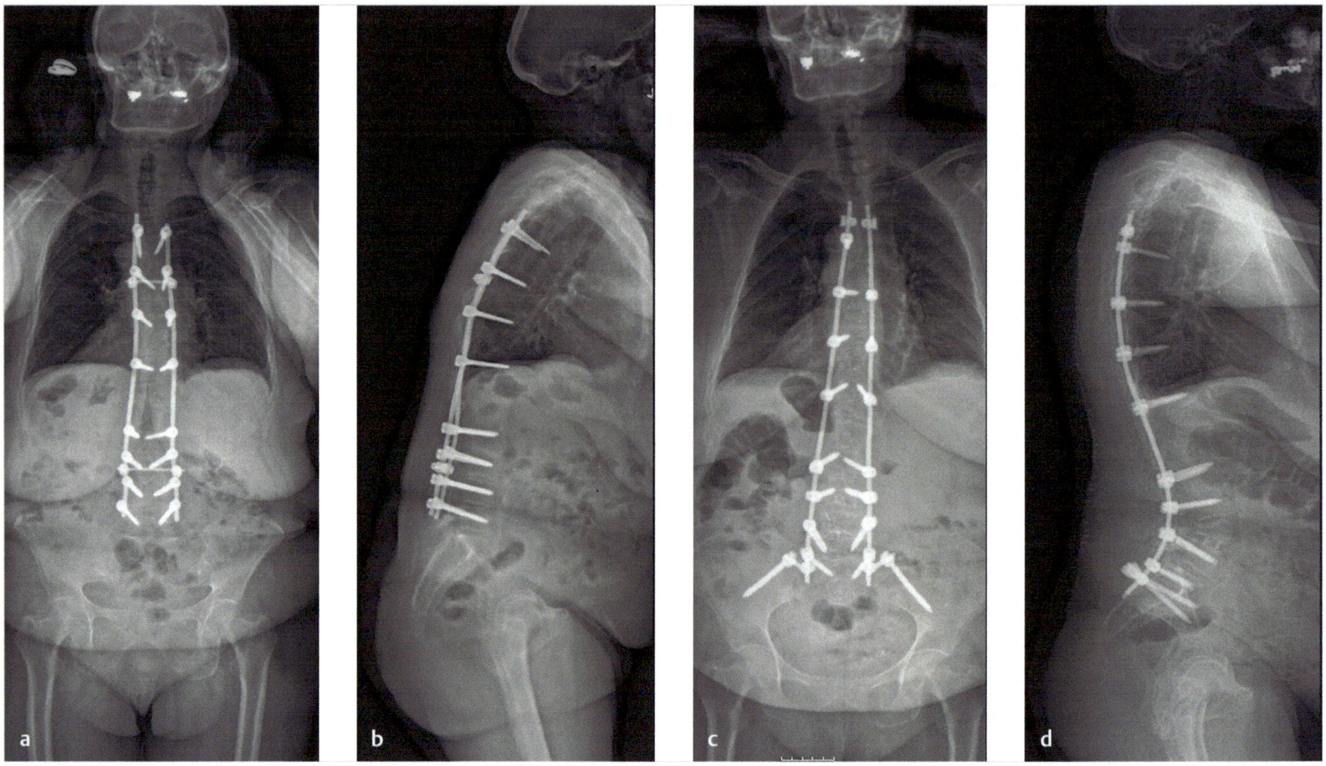

Fig. 19.4 **(a)** Preoperative anteroposterior and **(b)** lateral X-rays of a 66-year-old woman showing sagittal imbalance after a previous T5–L5 fusion. **(c)** Postoperative anteroposterior and **(d)** lateral control X-rays showing revision of the hardware, with a caudal extension to the pelvis, L4 corner pedicle subtraction osteotomy, and L4–L5 intersomatic cage implant through an extreme lateral interbody fusion access.

pedicle screws. The first part of the surgery is performed through lateral access to the spine, which exposes the entire vertebral body and the cranial and caudal intervertebral disks. A complete diskectomy of the two disks is performed, and the osteotomy of the vertebral body begins. We usually perform a vertical cut with a large osteotome in the anterior part of the body, leaving a thin shell of bone attached to the anterior longitudinal ligament. A second vertical cut is then performed posteriorly, removing as much bone as possible to create the space in which to implant the expandable cage. Aggressive curets and rongeurs are used to remove the cancellous bone and to enlarge the osteotomy. The posterior vertebral wall is taken out if a decompression of the canal is needed. When enough space has been created for the cage, the end plates of the upper and lower vertebrae are prepared, and an adequate expandable cage, filled with autologous bone, is placed. After closure of the lateral access, the patient is carefully turned in a prone position and a revision of the posterior hardware or new pedicle screws are implanted. Compression of the posterior elements is needed to close the osteotomy and improve local lordosis, and precontoured rods are positioned to stabilize the spine and correct the deformity.

References

[1] Lawrence BD, Hilibrand AS, Brodt ED, Dettori JR, Brodke DS. Predicting the risk of adjacent segment pathology in the cervical spine: a systematic review. Spine 2012; 37(22, Suppl)S52–S64

[2] Hollenbeck SM, Glattes RC, Asher MA, Lai SM, Burton DC. The prevalence of increased proximal junctional flexion following posterior instrumentation and arthrodesis for adolescent idiopathic scoliosis. Spine 2008;33(15):1675–1681

[3] Watanabe K, Lenke LG, Bridwell KH, Kim YJ, Koester L, Hensley M. Proximal junctional vertebral fracture in adults after spinal deformity surgery using pedicle screw constructs: analysis of morphological features. Spine 2010;35 (2):138–145

[4] Kim YJ, Bridwell KH, Lenke LG, Glattes CR, Rhim S, Cheh G. Proximal junctional kyphosis in adult spinal deformity after segmental posterior spinal instrumentation and fusion: minimum five-year follow-up. Spine 2008;33 (20):2179–2184

[5] Urist MR. Osteotomy of the cervical spine; report of a case of ankylosing rheumatoid spondylitis. J Bone Joint Surg Am 1958;40-A(4):833–843

[6] Law WA. Osteotomy of the cervical spine. J Bone Joint Surg Br 1959;41-B:640–641

[7] Simmons EH. The surgical correction of flexion deformity of the cervical spine in ankylosing spondylitis. Clin Orthop Relat Res 1972;86(86):132–143

[8] Berjano P, Pejrona M, Damilano M, Cecchinato R, Aguirre MF, Lamartina C. Corner osteotomy: a modified pedicle subtraction osteotomy for increased sagittal correction in the lumbar spine. Eur Spine J 2015;24(Suppl 1):58–65

[9] Wang Y, Li C, Liu L, Qi L. One-level mini-open pedicle subtraction osteotomy for treating spinal kyphosis in patients with ankylosing spondylitis. BMC Musculoskelet Disord 2021;22(1):101

[10] Deviren V, Scheer JK, Ames CP. Technique of cervicothoracic junction pedicle subtraction osteotomy for cervical sagittal imbalance: report of 11 cases. J Neurosurg Spine 2011;15(2):174–181

[11] Shimizu K, Matsushita M, Fujibayashi S, Toguchida J, Ido K, Nakamura T. Correction of kyphotic deformity of the cervical spine in ankylosing spondylitis using general anesthesia and internal fixation. J Spinal Disord 1996;9 (6):540–543

[12] McMaster MJ. Osteotomy of the cervical spine in ankylosing spondylitis. J Bone Joint Surg Br 1997;79(2):197–203

[13] Chin KR, Ahn J. Controlled cervical extension osteotomy for ankylosing spondylitis utilizing the Jackson operating table: technical note. Spine 2007;32 (17):1926–1929

[14] Deviren V, Scheer JK, Ames CP. Technique of cervicothoracic junction pedicle subtraction osteotomy for cervical sagittal imbalance: report of 11 cases. J Neurosurg Spine 2011;15(2):174–181

[15] Scheer JK, Tang JA, Deviren V, et al. (2010, March). Biomechanical Characterization of Fusion Constructs Across the Cervicothoracic Junction. [Poster]. 56th Annual Meeting of the Orthopaedic Research Society. New Orleans, LA.

[16] Scheer JK, Tang JA, Deviren V, et al. Biomechanical analysis of cervicothoracic junction osteotomy in cadaveric model of ankylosing spondylitis: effect of rod material and diameter. J Neurosurg Spine 2011;14(3):330–335

[17] Lamartina C, Berjano P. Classification of sagittal imbalance based on spinal alignment and compensatory mechanisms. Eur Spine J 2014;23(6):1177–1189

[18] Berjano P, Lamartina C. Classification of degenerative segment disease in adults with deformity of the lumbar or thoracolumbar spine. Eur Spine J 2014;23(9):1815–1824

[19] Smith-Petersen MN, Larson CB, Aufranc Otto E. Osteotomy of The Spine for Correction of Flexion Deformity in Rheumatoid Arthritis. The Journal of Bone & Joint Surgery 1945;27(1):1–11

[20] Berjano P, Bassani R, Casero G, Sinigaglia A, Cecchinato R, Lamartina C. Failures and revisions in surgery for sagittal imbalance: analysis of factors influencing failure. Eur Spine J 2013;22(Suppl 6):S853–S858

[21] Bradford DS. Vertebral column resection: orthopedic transaction. J Bone Joint Surg Am 1985;9:130

Further Reading

Berjano P, Damilano M, Lamartina C. Sagittal alignment correction and reconstruction of lumbar post-traumatic kyphosis via MIS lateral approach. Eur Spine J. 2012; 21(12):2718–2720

Cecchinato R, Berjano P, Damilano M, Lamartina C. Spinal osteotomies to treat post-traumatic thoracolumbar deformity. Eur J Orthop Surg Traumatol. 2014; 24 Suppl 1:S31–S37

Kim HJ, Bridwell KH, Lenke LG, et al. Proximal junctional kyphosis results in inferior SRS pain subscores in adult deformity patients. Spine. 2013; 38(11):896–901

Kim YC, Lenke LG, Hyun SJ, Lee JH, Koester LA, Blanke KM. Results of Revision Surgery after Pedicle Subtraction Osteotomy for Fixed Sagittal Imbalance With Pseudarthrosis at the Prior Osteotomy Site or Elsewhere: Minimum 5 years post-revision. Spine. 2014; 39(21):1817–1828

Lamartina C, Berjano P, Petruzzi M, et al. Criteria to restore the sagittal balance in deformity and degenerative spondylolisthesis. Eur Spine J. 2012; 21 Suppl 1:S27–S31

Munting E. Surgical treatment of post-traumatic kyphosis in the thoracolumbar spine: indications and technical aspects. Eur Spine J. 2010; 19 Suppl 1:S69–S73

20 Corrective Strategies and Management of Rigid Sacropelvic Pathologies

Yechiel N. Gellman, Josh Schroeder, Meir Liebergall

Abstract

In this chapter, we discuss the rare condition of rigid sacroiliac pathologies, which are usually of post-traumatic nature. We discuss the clinical presentation and radiographic evaluation of these complex disorders. Afterwards, we discuss the management of these pathologies, including nonsurgical treatment, but mainly the surgical reconstruction of the pelvic girdle and other salvage procedures to address specific, usually neurological, pathologies caused by the disfigured pelvic ring. Lastly, we describe use of a modern approach using computer-assisted surgery in order to plan and execute it to the fullest.

Keywords: sacro-pelvic fractures, post-traumatic deformity, sacral osteotomies, pelvic osteotomies, computer-assisted surgery

20.1 Introduction

Rigid pathologies involving the sacrum and pelvis are rare. Congenital and acquired conditions might cause such deformities, leading to significant morbidities. The most common condition requiring corrective surgery is posttraumatic pelvic deformity. This deformity is generally due to high-energy trauma and is associated with concomitant injuries, although in recent years there have been many reports on osteoporotic insufficiency fractures leading to major disability.[1] Better management of such severely injured individuals, which has prolonged their survival, has increased the number of post-traumatic deformities.

Tile et al estimated that there are 5% residual severe deformities following major disruptions of the pelvic ring.[2] Higher rates of deformities are found in different patterns of fracture (i. e., vertically unstable fractures raise the rate of deformities to 55–75% of all cases).[3]

Malunion and nonunion fractures of the pelvic ring are associated with many factors, including posterior disruption of the pelvis, failure of reduction, failure of fixation, and delayed treatment prior to bone healing.[4] Location and type of the malunion and nonunion fractures are crucial in understanding the presenting symptoms and require different corrective treatment. Rigid sacropelvic pathologies include internal and external malalignment, posterior and anterior displacement, and cranial and caudal displacement of the hemipelvis. Cephalad displacement of 1 cm and rotation of up to 20 degrees are considered acceptable; however, any larger deviation causes increased morbidity. Some cases may include a combination of these pathologies. Corrective treatment is difficult to attain in these rigid sacropelvic pathologies and usually requires excellent technique and equipment.

In a significant number of patients (10–40%) there are associated internal organ problems, such as gynecourological, neurologic, and others. The treatment and the clinical meaning of these pathologies will not be addressed in this chapter.

20.2 Presenting Symptoms

Symptoms of rigid sacropelvic pathologies vary based on location and type. These symptoms include pain, gait abnormalities, pelvic instability, pelvic obliquity with or without limb length discrepancy (LLD), and the aforementioned gynecourinary malfunction, nerve damage, and altered conduction.

Pain is usually the most common symptom (97%) that necessitates orthopaedic referral. This symptom can be exacerbated by movement or posture. Pain while bearing weight is usually posterior to the sacroiliac region.[5] Posterior pain is hypothesized to be due to axial forces that are transmitted mainly through the posterior region rather than the anterior pelvis (around 90% of the axial load) and is therefore increased with weight bearing. Traditionally it was thought that mainly injuries of the posterior pelvic elements would result in symptoms. Nonetheless, pain could also occur in the anterior, or both the anterior and posterior regions. Although malunion sites are often associated with pain, location of the malunion is important because posterior malunion or sacroiliac instability is more prone to pain than anterior malunion, which can be pain free. Pain while sitting or lying down is caused by anatomical deformities. Ischial imbalance (which is seen especially in cranial malunions) causes pain while sitting, whereas displacement of the posterior superior iliac spine (PSIS) (which occurs especially in sagittal malrotation malunions) causes pain during lying down.

The second most common orthopaedic complaint is gait abnormalities (67.4%), which include antalgic gait, Trendelenburg gait, and the use of walking aids. These abnormalities are attributed to both LLDs and pelvic deformities or instability. Furthermore, internal and external malformation of the pelvis might lead to intoed gait, which may lead to unphysiological gait, in turn leading to referred back pain.

A substantial number of patients will report pelvic instability (60.3%), which can be either clinical instability or radiographical instability (as shown by stress views, which will be discussed later in this chapter). Patients can suffer from LLDs (24.8%), which are usually due to cranial displacement of the ipsilateral leg. Research has shown that unstable vertical fractures of the pelvis will lead to an average LLD of 3 to 6 cm.[6]

Since the pelvic girdle encompasses many organs, associated injuries, such as gynecourinary malfunction might persist. A large cohort of 298 patients, collected by Wright et al, showed sexual and excretory dysfunction of 21% and 8%, respectively.[7] Rotational malunions, especially internal-rotation hemipelvic malunions and superior rami malunions, might cause impingement or herniation of the bladder. Other organs that are in danger include the vagina, causing dyspareunia, with a sporadic case of clitoral stimulation following weight bearing secondary to an unstable pubic symphysis. Other complications include herniation of the bowel and bladder through malunited fracture regions.[8]

Pelvic misalignment may cause compression and altered nerve conduction, leading to neurologic pain and damage. Vertically unstable fracture may lead to neurologic damage in 24 to 60% of the cases at the time of the fracture, leading to chronic damage in a malreduced fracture or a fracture that was treated nonsurgically.

20.3 Radiographic Evaluation

After a careful and complete physical exam is performed, radiographs of the pelvis must be obtained. Whereas most deformities will require a complete set of radiographs that includes anteroposterior (AP), inlet and outlet pelvic views, and the Judet series if acetabular involvement is suspected (depending on the underlying pathology), other deformities will require additional stress views to fully assess the deformity. Radiographs of both the original injury and the subsequent malformation should be obtained to fully assess the deformity and the deforming forces affecting the deformity.

Stress views and standing views are important for further assessing pelvic stability, which is defined by Dickson as "the ability of the pelvis to withstand physiological forces without abnormal deformation."[9] The common tests include the anterior superior iliac spine compression test and the iliac wing compression test, in which sacroiliac displacement of more than 5 mm in any plane shows instability of the pelvic girdle. Siegel et al described other radiographs in a study that reviewed 38 patients with pelvic instability and pain, in which single-leg-stance radiographs were more indicative of instability than standard radiographs, and showed that up to 5 cm of symphyseal translation can be present with these injuries.[10] Because this test can cause significant pain for some patients, this test should be done under local anesthesia or prior to fixation of the deformity. Other tests include traction of the affected side with internal rotation of the pelvis, for which either anesthesia or heavy sedation is sometimes recommended. Widespread use of CT scans, especially three-dimensional reconstructions, has eliminated the need for most radiographs, besides stress views.

Any radiographs, especially when used with CT, enable the surgical team to better define the deformation, which might be on the x, y, or z-axis (▶ Fig. 20.1). X-axis deformation causes either impaction or diastasis malformation, whereas y-axis deformation causes cephalad or caudad malformation, and z-axis deformation can cause anterior or posterior malformations. Newer software enables virtual surgical correction, including using a mirror image of the healthy side (if present) as a template.

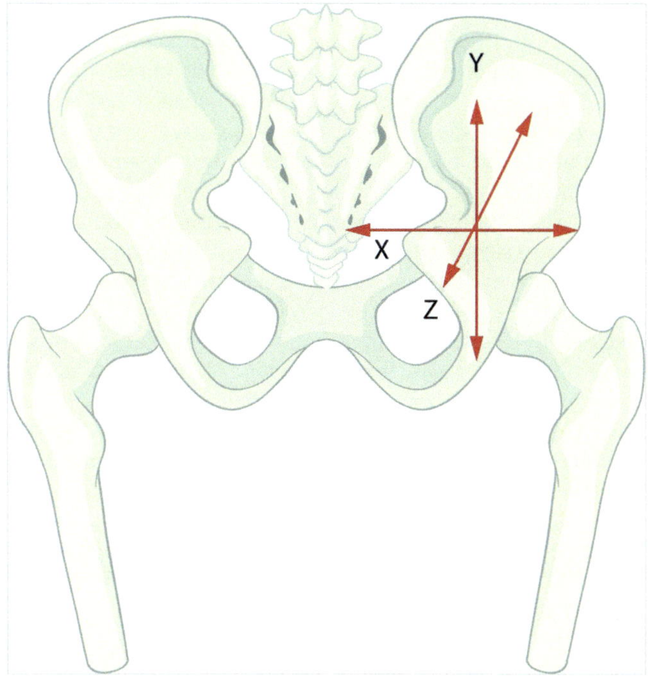

Fig. 20.1 A pelvis diagram with three different axes. Each axis can have either a translational deformity or a rotational deformity. X-axis: translation impaction/diastasis; rotation flexion/extension. Y-axis: translation cephalad/caudad; rotation internal/external. Z-axis: translation anterior/posterior; rotation abduction/adduction.

20.4 Management

Patients involved in major traumas are often deferred from surgery due to the extreme comorbidities they sustain that require extensive nonsurgical care. Remedies including analgesics, heel lift, or other shoe inserts for LLDs and local steroid injection to sites of specific pain might provide transient relief. We feel that these patients require close follow-up to determine when surgical treatment is needed. If surgical intervention is needed for fracture reduction it is logical to intervene early, prior to bone healing, rather than dealing with malunion that demands osteotomy and further fixation. However, the clinical outcome is not predictable.

Surgical treatment might be necessary in some indications, as listed earlier, including debilitating pain, gait abnormalities, associated deformities of the limbs or spine, and associated injuries involving the genitourinary system and neurologic compromise.

Surgical treatment can be divided in two major groups: (1) Reconstruction of the original pelvis, which usually includes reduction of the original fracture, either due to nonunited fractures or by recreating the original fracture line, and fixation of the fracture. At times, surgical corrective osteotomies and bone grafting might be necessary in order to achieve union and physiological pelvic alignment. (2) Other salvage procedures addressing specific, usually neurologic, problems.

20.4.1 Reconstruction of the Pelvic Girdle

Letournel and Matta were the first to describe the multistaged procedure, usually a three-stage reconstruction of the pelvis, which can be performed either with the anterior-posterior-anterior approach, or the posterior-anterior-posterior approach.[6,11] These stages require extensive soft tissue releases and mobilization of the fracture zone on both hemipelvises, and reduction and fixation in the final stage of the surgery. Matta et al described these procedures in 37 patients, with good results in 32 patients, who were satisfied with their outcome. Nonetheless, 19% of patients suffered complications.[6] For example, Matta and Yerasimides described a three-stage reconstruction for a 39-year-old man with sacral nonunion.[12] This involved placing the patient supine and reopening his lower abdominal incision, removing the plates, and mobilizing the symphysis. Then a distal femur traction pin was placed and the patient was turned prone. A pelvic frame was applied on the uninjured hemipelvis, and a longitudinal incision was made lateral to the PSIS, with removal of the old sacroiliac screws, and the nonunion site was mobilized and debrided. The traction pin and pelvic frame provided adequate fixation, and greater fixation was achieved using trans-sacral screws and a posterior tension band plate. Then traction was removed and the symphysis was fixated using an eight-hole plate. Oransky and Tortora described adequate methods for reduction and fixation using a single- or two-stage approach using more modern clamps, external fixation, and skeletal traction.[13] The largest series to date was reported on by Mears and Velyvis, who operated on 204 patients with pelvic nonunions and malunions using the staged reconstruction method.[14] They introduced a new classification system, with type I being underformed nonunions; type II stable (true) malalignments; type III unstable, ununited malalignments; and type IV partially stable malalignments with incomplete stabilization by callus and heterotopic bone. Almost all the patients achieved union (96%), and disabling pain reduced from 36% preoperatively to 0% postoperatively. No patients reported postoperative instability. All patients with nonunions were satisfied on follow-up (79% were extremely satisfied and 21% satisfied), whereas patient with malunion were satisfied in 89% of the cases (57% extremely satisfied, 32% satisfied).

It should be noted that because these malunion pathologies are usually rigid, it is sometimes hard to find the original fracture line, which requires osteotomies of those anatomical regions in order to achieve the original three-dimensional structure of the pelvis.

20.4.2 Sacral Osteotomies

Sacral osteotomies are rare and are mainly used in the setting of sacral fractures with either unstable configurations[15] or associated neurologic deficit.[16] Since the main objective of such procedures is either to release the injured nerve roots or to prevent further deterioration of the neurologic condition, the natural history of such fractures has been pursued. It had been shown that most will either be recovery without need of surgery, therefore advocating non-surgical treatment[17] or that original injuries were so substantial that operative treatment might not help. The second option was reinforced by intraoperative findings of highly injured nerves in such conditions.[18] The largest study, performed by Schildhauer et al, showed that of 18 patients with irreducible Roy-Camille type 2–4 sacral fractures with instability and cauda equina deficits, 15 patients had full or partial recovery of bowel and bladder function through the use of open reduction, sacral decompression, and lumbopelvic fixation.[19]

The classic sacral osteotomy using a posterior approach to the sacrum through a midline incision, then local skeletonization of the posterior sacrum, is performed up to the iliac crests, lifting the muscle bed in a thick, single layer. Pedicle screws are placed in the L4 and L5 vertebrae and in the S2 and pelvic girdle via S1 and S2 iliac bolts. Laminectomy of S1 is done until the first sacral foramina are reached, then pedicle subtraction osteotomy (PSO) of the S1 pedicles and separation of the superior end plate of S1 is performed. Two additional vertical osteotomies are performed on the lateral wings of the sacrum, creating a fracture similar to an H-type fracture of the sacrum, leaving only the anterior sacral cortex intact and allowing a closing-wedge effect. Then closure is possible using compression between the pedicular lumbar screws and the iliac screws. The major limitations with such an approach are the limited access, especially to the sacroiliac joint, unless an extensive incision is done from the L4 level to S3–S4, and the risk of secondary infection of an incision as distal as this one is.

20.4.3 Pelvic Osteotomies

Pelvic osteotomies can be divided into two groups, osteotomies that will affect alignment and osteotomies to correct preexisting deformities, which were mentioned earlier. There are currently two described methods for iliac osteotomy that effect alignment between the spine and pelvis: the posterior iliac osteotomy and the bilateral modified Salter osteotomy. The main objection of these osteotomies is to increase pelvic tilt and decrease the sacral slope, by extending the distal pelvis compared to the proximal pelvis. Although no biomechanical studies have been performed, the expected overall effect should be increased pelvic incidence and decreased lumber lordosis.

Lindseth was the first to use the posterior iliac osteotomy to correct pelvic obliquity, in nine children with myelomeningocele and fixed pelvic obliquity due to uncorrectable lumbosacral scoliosis.[20] This was done using an Opening-wedge osteotomy and local bone graft (▶ Fig. 20.2). The exposure of the posterior aspect of the ilium needed in this osteotomy is from the sciatic notch to the proximal posterior ilium, allowing vertical osteotomies starting at the sciatic notch to the proximal posterior ilium. This is usually achieved with two L-shaped incisions, which are parallel and slightly lateral to the iliac crest and parallel to the sacrum, ranging from the PSIS to the posterior inferior iliac spine (PIIS).

Bilateral modified Salter osteotomies were originally used for treatment of developmental dysplasia of the hip (▶ Fig. 20.3). Wilson and Levine were the first to use this osteotomy for a patient with ankylosing spondylitis.[21] The exposure of the anterior two-thirds of the ilium needed in this osteotomy is from the sciatic notch to the anterior ilium, allowing osteotomies from the sciatic notch to the anterior iliac, between the anterior superior iliac spine and the anterior inferior iliac spine (AIIS). This is usually achieved with two incisions along the iliac crest and extending laterally on both sides.

Bodin and Roussouly have shown on cadaveric models that, although a Slater osteotomy is simpler to perform and is efficient in restoring sagittal balance of the spine, the posterior sacral approach is more powerful.[22]

20.4.4 Other Salvage Procedures

The aforementioned surgical options require extensive surgeries; thus, a more limited approach has been pursued. Alexander et al addressed this problem by performing decompression of the L5 nerve root alone in four patients with residual root injury due to pelvic fractures. All these cases ended with resolution of their neurological pain and no pelvic nor L5-S1 instability was noted on repeat radiographs.[23]

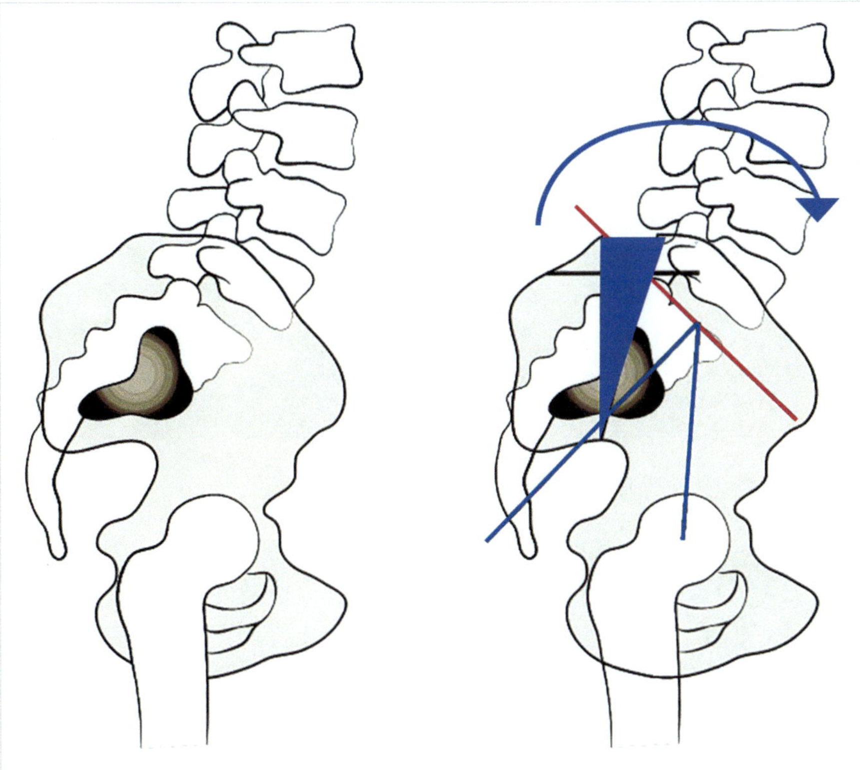

Fig. 20.2 Pelvic incidence can be changed by posterior iliac osteotomy. Here, an opening-wedge osteotomy is utilized (*blue triangle*) through the posterior iliac wing rotating the native sacroiliac join and increasing the pelvic incidence (the angle formed by the *blue lines*). Alternatively, a closing-wedge osteotomy through the sacroiliac joints will decrease pelvic incidence.

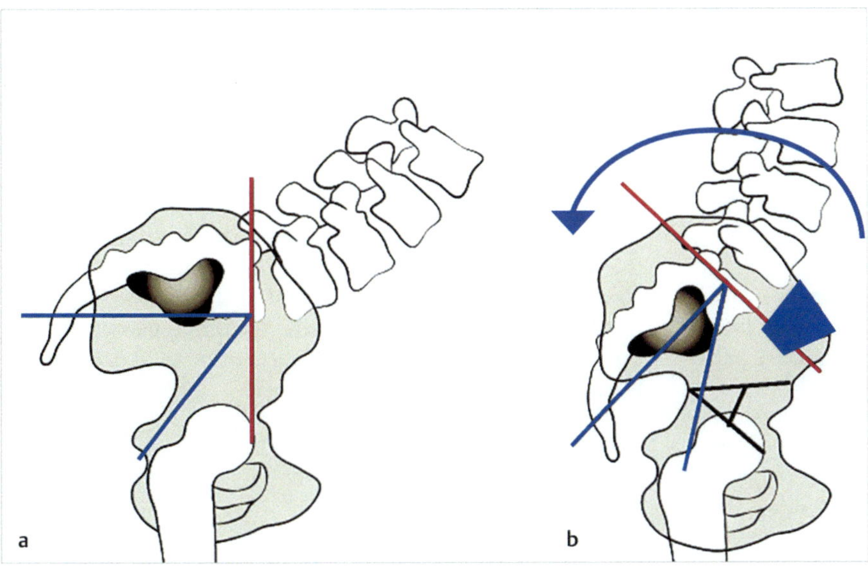

Fig. 20.3 Pelvic incidence can be changed by a Salter pelvic osteotomy. **(a)** Normal lumbar lordosis with a high pelvic incidence (the angle formed by the *blue lines*) will lead to a highly positive sagittal balance. **(b)** Bilateral Salter osteotomies (trapezoid blue, filled will tricortical bone graft) will reduce pelvic incidence by rotating the cephalad half of the pelvis posteriorly.

20.4.5 Computer-Assisted Surgery

Computer-assisted surgery seems attractive for pelvic and spinal surgery and includes navigation and robotics.[2,24,25] However, although it has been available for almost two decades it is not yet the standard of care. The merging of preoperative CT images with the real environment of the operating room may be beneficial, especially for pelvic osteotomy and fixation. CT-guided navigation in fracture nonunion was first described by Huegli et al, who treated a delayed union site percutaneously in a single-step procedure using a CT navigation system for drilling the delayed union, autologous bone grafting, and screw fixation.[26] Lee et al later described treating a single case of nonunion of the sacrum and ramus pubis using bone grafting through a posterior approach and CT-guided percutaneous guided iliosacral screw fixation combined with anterior external fixation.[27]

Emerging computer-assisted surgery has assisted surgeons in decreasing the amount of radiographs needed intraoperatively,

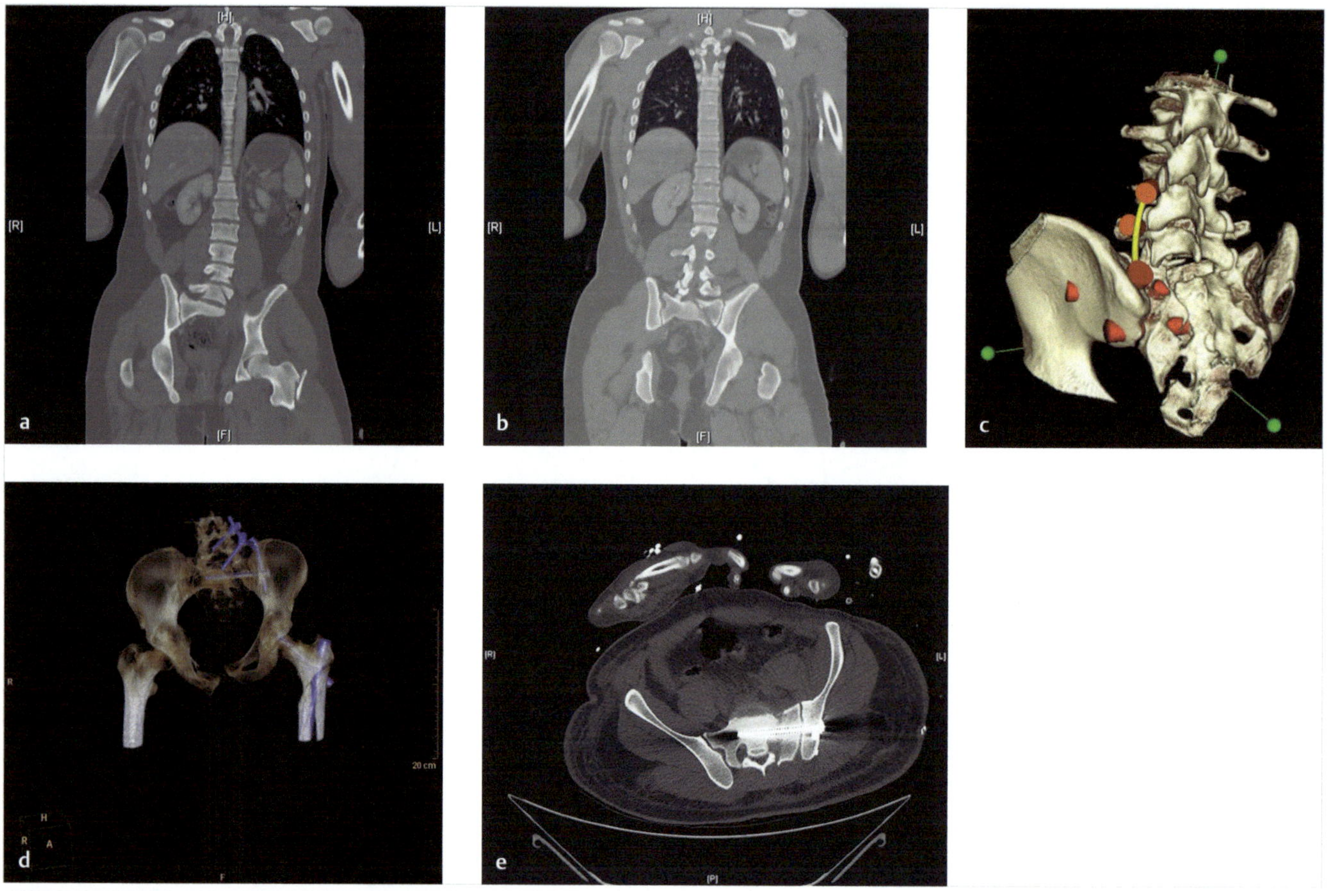

Fig. 20.4 (a, b) A CT scan showing a left subtrochanteric femoral fracture, L5 vertebral and Denis type II sacral injury in a 17-year-old patient who fell from height. **(c)** Preoperative planning and execution was done using the Renaissance robotic system. **(d, e)** Final CT scan and CT reconstructions showed excellent placement of the pedicular and iliosacral screws, not involving the foramen.

and allowed surgeons to fully understand the three-dimensional anatomy, thereby enabling them to place fixation devices in the appropriate anatomical sites and achieve a lower complication rate. Delécrin used a computer to superimpose a virtual image of the instruments on the CT images, thereby allowing precise insertion of the two transiliosacral screws into S 1 and S 2 percutaneously with minimal neurologic risk.[28]

Advances in robotic technology have allowed surgeons to place screws even more accurately. The authors have successfully repaired an L 5 fracture with an associated Denis type II sacral fracture acutely using the Renaissance robotic system (▶ Fig. 20.4). A 17-year-old patient presented to our emergency room after falling from a height, resulting in a subtrochanteric fracture of his left femur and the fractures already mentioned. The subtrochanteric fracture was repaired immediately using the proximal femoral nail antirotation (PFNA) system, and the sacrospinal fracture waited until preoperative planning was performed. A preoperative CT scan was obtained, the femoral fracture was done immediately and the pelvic spinal fracture was deferred until adequate planning was done. The patient was then taken to the operating room and placed prone on a radiolucent table with a bed-mounted robotic platform. A Kirschner wire was then placed in the level of the L 2 spinous process in order to fully mount the robotic system. Then the robotic bridge was connected and registration was performed using an X-ray machine followed by further verification using the robotic system. The robotic system was then moved to the correct position to enable placement of the screws. Postoperative CT scans showed that the screw position was as planned preoperatively. Follow-up images showed proper healing of the fractures.

20.5 Summary

Pelvic and sacral malunions can cause extreme morbidity leading to the need for corrective surgery. Because the surgical care is major, with a high risk of complications, patients should be informed of the procedure and the risks involved; however, with the use of newer techniques, these risks may be reduced.

References

[1] Tsiridis E, Upadhyay N, Giannoudis PV. Sacral insufficiency fractures: current concepts of management. Osteoporos Int. 2006; 17(12):1716–1725

[2] Tile M, Helfet DL, Kellam JF, Vrahas M. Fractures of the Pelvis and Acetabulum: Principles and Methods of Management. 4th ed. New York: Thieme/AO; 2015

[3] Matta JM, Saucedo T. Internal fixation of pelvic ring fractures. Clin Orthop Relat Res. 1989(242):83–97

[4] Dickson, K. F. (2012). Malalignment, 157–164. Chapter 16. http://www.acetabulumdoco.com/doc/2/pelvic%20malalignment.pdf

[5] Semba RT, Yasukawa K, Gustilo RB. Critical analysis of results of 53 Malgaigne fractures of the pelvis. J Trauma. 1983; 23(6):535–537

[6] Matta JM, Dickson KF, Markovich GD. Surgical treatment of pelvic nonunions and malunions. Clin Orthop Relat Res. 1996(329):199–206

[7] Wright JL, Nathens AB, Rivara FP, MacKenzie EJ, Wessells H. Specific fracture configurations predict sexual and excretory dysfunction in men and women 1 year after pelvic fracture. J Urol. 2006; 176(4 Pt 1):1540–1545, discussion 1545

[8] Tile M, Helfet DL, Kellam JF, eds. Fractures of the Pelvis and Acetabulum. 3 rd ed. Philadelphia, PA: Lippincott Williams and Wilkins; 2003

[9] Acetabulum & Pelvic | Acetabular Pelvic Injuries | Dr. Kyle Dickson. (n.d.). Retrieved April 14, 2015, from http://www.acetabulumdoc.com/injuries/2/acetabulum-pelvic.html

[10] Siegel J, Templeman DC, Tornetta P, III. Single-leg-stance radiographs in the diagnosis of pelvic instability. J Bone Joint Surg Am. 2008; 90(10):2119–2125

[11] Letournel E. (1993). No Title. In Fractures of the acetabulum and pelvis. Paris: Ninth AFOR Course and Workshop

[12] Matta JM, Yerasimides JG. Table-skeletal fixation as an adjunct to pelvic ring reduction. J Orthop Trauma. 2007; 21(9):647–656

[13] Oransky M, Tortora M. Nonunions and malunions after pelvic fractures: why they occur and what can be done? Injury. 2007; 38(4):489–496

[14] Mears DC, Velyvis J. Surgical reconstruction of late pelvic post-traumatic nonunion and malalignment. J Bone Joint Surg Br. 2003; 85(1):21–30

[15] Kim MY, Reidy DP, Nolan PC, Finkelstein JA. Transverse sacral fractures: case series and literature review. Can J Surg. 2001; 44(5):359–363

[16] Ebraheim NA, Biyani A, Wong F. Nonunion of pelvic fractures. J Trauma. 1998; 44(1):202–204

[17] Sabiston CP, Wing PC. Sacral fractures: classification and neurologic implications. J Trauma. 1986; 26(12):1113–1115

[18] Phelan ST, Jones DA, Bishay M. Conservative management of transverse fractures of the sacrum with neurological features. A report of four cases. J Bone Joint Surg Br. 1991; 73(6):969–971

[19] Schildhauer TA, Bellabarba C, Nork SE, Barei DP, Routt MLC, Jr, Chapman JR. Decompression and lumbopelvic fixation for sacral fracture-dislocations with spino-pelvic dissociation. J Orthop Trauma. 2006; 20(7):447–457

[20] Lindseth RE. Posterior iliac osteotomy for fixed pelvic obliquity. J Bone Joint Surg Am. 1978; 60(1):17–22

[21] Wilson PD, Jr, Levine DB. Compensatory pelvic osteotomy for ankylosing spondylitis. A case report. J Bone Joint Surg Am. 1969; 51(1):142–148

[22] Bodin A, Roussouly P. Sacral and pelvic osteotomies for correction of spinal deformities. Eur Spine J. 2015; 24 Suppl 1:S72–S82

[23] Alexander JJ, Brennan M, Rahm MD. L5 nerve root decompression after malunion of surgically managed vertically unstable pelvic ring injuries. Am J Orthop. 2013; 42(4):E23–E25

[24] Liebergall M, Ben-David D, Weil Y, Peyser A, Mosheiff R. Computerized navigation for the internal fixation of femoral neck fractures. J Bone Joint Surg Am. 2006; 88(8):1748–1754

[25] Tornetta P, Court-Brown C, Heckman JD, McKee M, McQueen MM, Ricci W. Rockwood and Green's Fractures in Adults. 8th ed. Philadelphia, PA: Lippincott Williams & Wilkins; 2014

[26] Huegli RW, Messmer P, Jacob AL, Regazzoni P, Styger S, Gross T. Delayed union of a sacral fracture: percutaneous navigated autologous cancellous bone grafting and screw fixation. Cardiovasc Intervent Radiol. 2003; 26(5):502–505

[27] Lee SY, Niikura T, Sakai Y, et al. Sacral Fracture Nonunion Treated by Bone Grafting through a Posterior Approach. Case Rep Orthop. 2013; 2013:932521

[28] Delécrin J, Gouin F, Passuti N. Computer-assisted insertion of polyaxial screws for sacroiliac fixation in patients with sacral nonunion. J Bone Joint Surg Br. 2005; 87-B SUPP II117

21 Ankylosing Spinal Disorders

Roongrath Chitragran, Rune Hedlund

Abstract

Ankylosing spondylitis (AS) and diffuse idiopathic skeletal hyperostosis (DISH) lead to ankylosis of the spinal column, which makes it susceptible to unstable fracture, even from minor trauma, and to rigid kyphotic deformity in AS.

The chapter outlines the specific nature of hyperextension spine fractures in AS and DISH, and the problem of kyphotic deformity in AS. In fractures the difficulties in diagnosis, the high incidence of neurologic complications, and the frequent necessity of surgical fixation are underlined, as well as the risk of displacement of the fracture during routine care. In DISH, the awareness is lower about potentially unstable hyperextension fracture than in AS, and delayed diagnosis is frequent. Although the posterior column in DISH, as opposed to AS, is intact, the risk of neurological compromise is similarly increased, and the indication for surgical stabilization is strong. For both AS and DISH, posterior surgical fixation is recommended, including two to three levels above and below the injury.

AS is associated with kyphotic deformity with a forward-leaning posture, resulting in substantial functional disability and problems with horizontal gaze. Surgical correction demands osteotomy of the ankylosed spine, most often with a pedicle subtraction osteotomy (PSO). A PSO is a high-risk procedure but can result in dramatic improvements in AS patients' quality of life. The higher risk of complications in cervical (C7) PSO as compared to lumbar PSO is underlined. However, swallowing or breathing problems can only be addressed by a cervical or T1 osteotomy.

Keywords: spinal deformity, kyphosis, ankylosing spondylitis, diffuse idiopathic skeleton hyperostosis, ankylosed spine fracture

21.1 Introduction

Despite their different etiologies, the three primary ankylosing spinal disorders—ankylosing spondylitis (AS), diffuse idiopathic skeletal hyperostosis (DISH), and ossification of the posterior longitudinal ligament (OPLL)—have several similarities. They all lead to ankylosis of the spinal column, which results in a variety of problems caused by altered biomechanical properties. The spine becomes more susceptible to unstable fracture, even after minor trauma, and also to rigid kyphotic deformity in the advanced stage of AS (▶ Fig. 21.1, ▶ Fig. 21.2). This chapter discusses only AS and DISH; OPLL presents quite differently.

The etiology of AS is not clearly understood, but several theories have been proposed. AS is strongly associated with the human leukocyte antigen B27 (HLA-B27) gene, which can be demonstrated in 90 to 95% of patients. The diagnosis is based on the clinical picture as well as on a positive HLA-B27 test. AS occurs globally; the prevalence has been estimated to be between 0.1 and 1.4% in different populations, and it has been reported to be more common and aggressive in men.

AS is a chronic inflammatory rheumatic disease. Its most pronounced effects are on the axial skeleton, initially causing sarcoiliitis, with inflammation gradually spreading cranially up the spine, ultimately involving the upper cervical spine in advanced cases.[1] Low back pain is a typical symptom in the early phase of the disorder. The pain is frequently worse in the morning and will improve with activity.

The pathogenesis involves the formation of bony syndesmophytes across the disk spaces, which appear to flow from one vertebra to the next, resulting in a characteristic radiographic appearance of a "bamboo spine," with calcifications of the disk spaces, the facet joints, and the supraspinous ligament. Once the articulations are anchylotic, patients become pain free. Severe kyphosis in the thoracolumbar and cervicothoracic regions may occur in the later stages (▶ Fig. 21.3).

21.2 Ankylosing Spondylitis with Fracture

The brittleness of the spine renders the spine susceptible to fracture, which is four times more common than in the general population.[2] Furthermore, after spine fracture the incidence of neurogenic complication is more than 10 times higher than in the normal population, and the mortality rates are between 18 and 32%.[3] Spinal fractures frequently result from low-energy trauma.

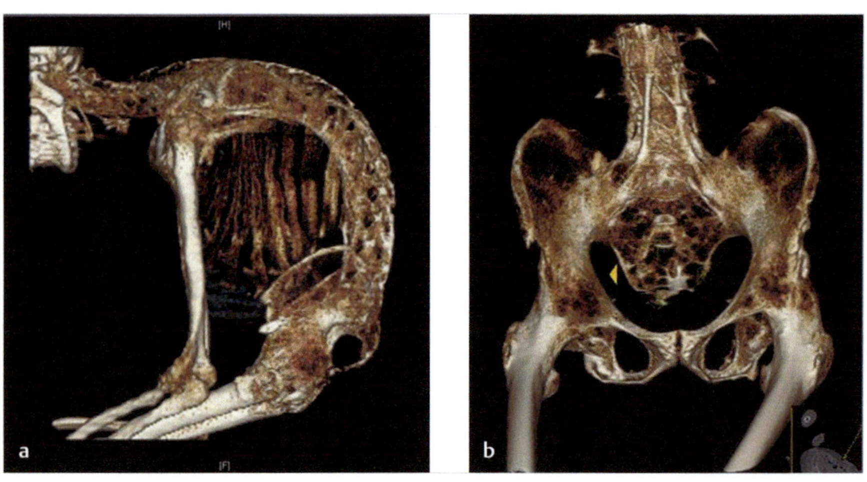

Fig. 21.1 (a, b) Three-dimensional CT reconstruction of a 37-year-old man with severe juvenile ankylosing spondylitis. Ankylosed spine, sacroiliac joints, hip joints.

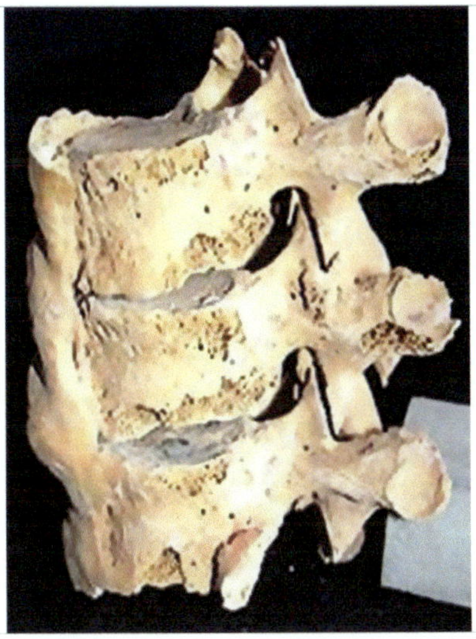

Fig. 21.2 Specimen showing morphological changes typical of diffuse idiopathic skeletal hyperostosis, with a calcified anterior longitudinal ligament, most pronounced on the right side.

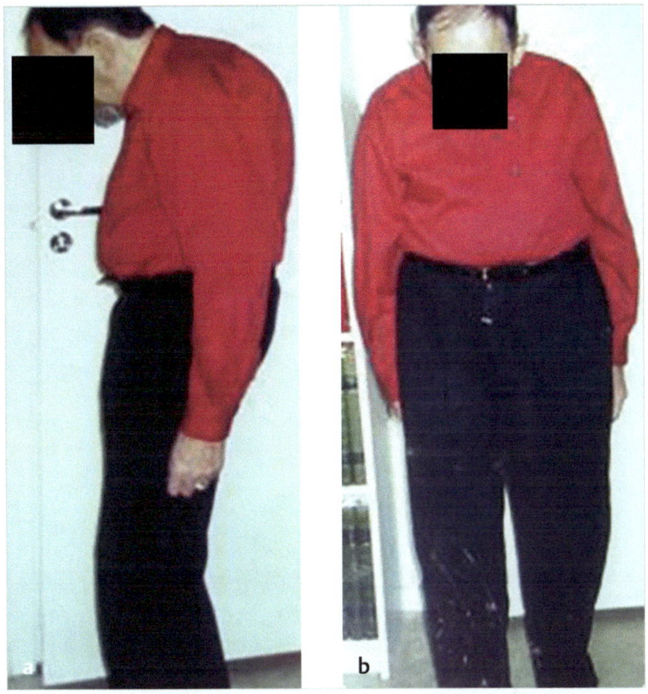

Fig. 21.3 (a, b) A 60-year-old man with severe kyphosis, limiting the horizontal gaze.

There are many factors contributing to fracture, including the long lever arms resulting from the ankylosis as well as the accompanying osteoporosis, gait disturbance, and sagittal imbalance.

Most fracture occurs in the cervical region (81.2%, most commonly C5–C6, C6–C7).[3] The most common injury mechanism is a simple fall and hyperextension, either backward or forward. Because of the decreased elasticity of the intervertebral disk, many fractures pass through the entire disk. Cervical fractures in AS are highly unstable, with an increased risk for neurologic deficits (29–91%),[4] and are associated with a doubled mortality rate compare to the general population. Unfortunately, the diagnosis is frequently delayed or missed; patients with AS often present late because they can't distinguish acute fracture pain from chronic inflammatory pain. Fracture may also be missed in plain radiographs due to preexisting kyphotic deformity with distorted anatomy and high-riding shoulders. In Anwar et al's retrospective review of AS with cervical spine injuries, 60% of fractures were missed in the initial radiographs.[5] This is now generally recognized, and a CT scan is necessary in AS patients with cervical spine trauma (▶ Fig. 21.4). To visualize the spinal cord an MRI scan should be performed in any case with a neurologic deficit. It should also be noted that AS patients with spine fracture have an increased risk of epidural hematoma, which may need to be evacuated.

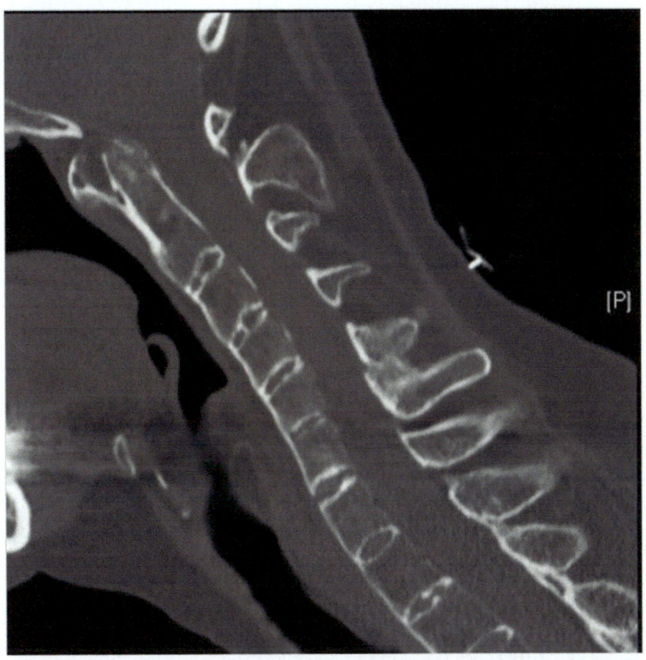

Fig. 21.4 A 70-year-old woman with ankylosing spondylitis and fracture at C6–C7 after a fall. The observations on this CT scan revealed that the vertebrae were anchored from C2 to the thoracic vertebrae.

Thoracolumbar fractures in AS are less common than cervical fractures. As in the cervical spine, the most common mechanism in the thoracolumbar spine is extension injury, and, also as in the cervical spine, the fracture is highly unstable, with disruption of both the anterior and posterior columns[6] (▶ Fig. 21.5a). Associated heart conduction abnormalities and pulmonary disease are common, and vessel injury may occur.[7]

Treatment is determined by fracture severity and the patient's general medical condition. Treatment options include orthoses, halo vest, or operative treatment. In general, fractures in AS are unstable, and the indication for surgery is strong. In more minor fractures one may try conservative treatment, such as immobilization in a rigid cervical collar or a thoracolumbosacral orthosis. However, in conservative treatment the patient has to be followed closely because of the risk of displacement and catastrophic neurologic compromise. There is increasing evidence of a higher complication rate in conservative treatment

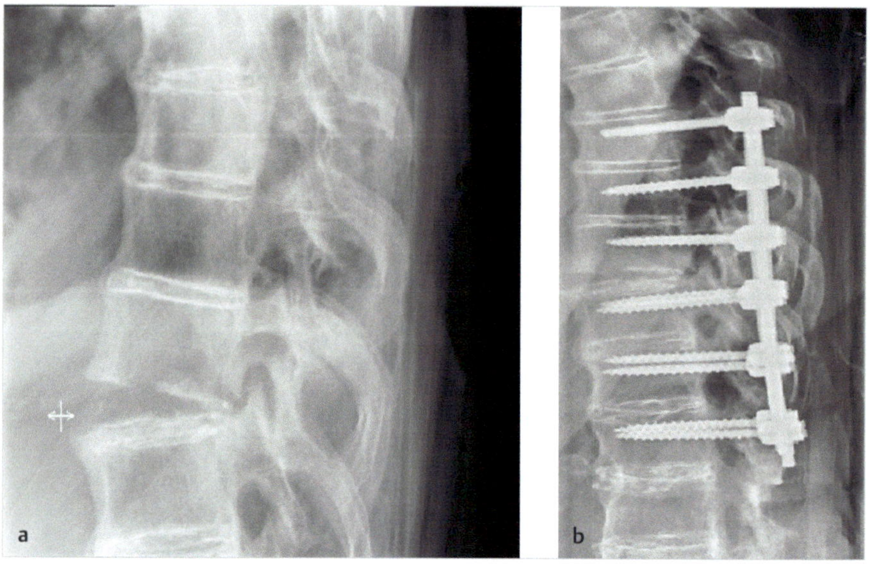

Fig. 21.5 (a) Typical highly unstable hyperextension fracture of the thoracic spine in a patient with ankylosing spondylitis. (b) Extension fracture using a posterior approach, three levels above and below the fracture. Slight extension remains at the fracture site, of possible advantage to the patient.

compared to surgical treatment (51% vs. 23%).[3] In a Swedish national registry cohort study by Robinson et al, 990 patients with AS spine fractures were identified, with about 70% being operated on. They reported a 3-month mortality rate of 17%, and that comorbidities and spinal cord injury increased the mortality rate, whereas surgical treatment decreased it.[8] It is of great importance to avoid aggravating the injury by extending the trunk while the patient is in the bed or during radiographic examinations.

Of equally great importance is to avoid displacement while turning the patient prone onto the operating table. The surgery is performed using a posterior approach, mainly because a solid fixation in osteopenic bone is easier to realize from the back (▶ Fig. 21.5b). Decompression is performed if indicated[9] (i. e., if there is neurologic compromise and a compressive mechanism, bony, soft tissue, or epidural hematoma). Posterior instrumentation should extend two to three levels above and below the injury in the thoracolumbar spine, and three levels above and below in the cervical spine. In surgical treatment one may use the occurrence of the fracture to the patients' advantage and correct some of the kyphotic deformity. The general recommendation, however, is to fix the spine in the preexisting kyphotic position. In patients without neurologic symptoms, closed reduction and percutaneous instrumentation constitute an attractive treatment model, minimizing surgical trauma. Fusion is not necessary in the already ankylosed AS spine.

21.3 Ankylosing Spondylitis with Kyphotic Deformity

The primary goals of operative treatment in AS with progressive kyphotic deformity include restoration of sagittal balance and horizontal gaze. The forward-leaning posture, which is sometimes severe, creates substantial functional disability. If the hips are involved, the patient may have great difficulties walking and may need a wheelchair (▶ Fig. 21.6a). In the extreme forms, patients cannot see forward and may choose to walk backward, while looking backward between the legs. A primary complaint by these patients is the inability to use a horizontal gaze, which has profound negative impacts on the ability to move around and on social life, given the difficulties of interacting.

If symptomatic kyphotic deformity has developed, there are no conservative treatment options, other than supporting compensatory functions by physiotherapy. Modern operative treatment today means a pedicle subtraction osteotomy (PSO). Historically a so-called open wedge osteotomy described by Smith–Petersen was used, but it was abandoned because of the risk of aortic rupture. Similarly, extensive front and back surgeries with multiple osteotomies have been proposed, but they have also been abandoned since the advent of the PSO. The PSO results in a major correction of the deformity at one single level (30 degrees per level), and also leads to a quick consolidation on the osteotomy secondary to bone–bone contact.

A lumbar osteotomy is usually performed even if the deformity is in the thoracic or cervicothoracic region. Doing so minimizes the risk of spinal cord injury and also achieves greater restoration of sagittal balance correction by the long lever arm. Also, a larger wedge can be removed in the lumbar spine than in the thoracic spine. Spinal deformity must be assessed both clinically and radiographically as part of the preoperative planning (▶ Fig. 21.6b). Hip joints should always be assessed, since they may contribute to the sagittal imbalance and the functional disability. The severity of spinal deformity versus hip involvement will aid in determining whether total hip replacement should be performed, and if so when. If hip arthritis significantly contributes to the disability most surgeons recommend that total hip replacement should be performed before spinal osteotomy.

In the radiological analysis, the sagittal balance is assessed in a standardized fashion. Normal individuals are able to compensate for kyphotic deformity through changes in, for example, pelvic version, hip extension, and knee flexion. In patients with AS, however, these normal compensatory changes are ameliorated by loss of motion in these joints, as well as in the spine.

The PSO is typically performed at the L3 or L4 level. At least two levels above and below should be fixated; most surgeons recommend three levels above and below. The rate of

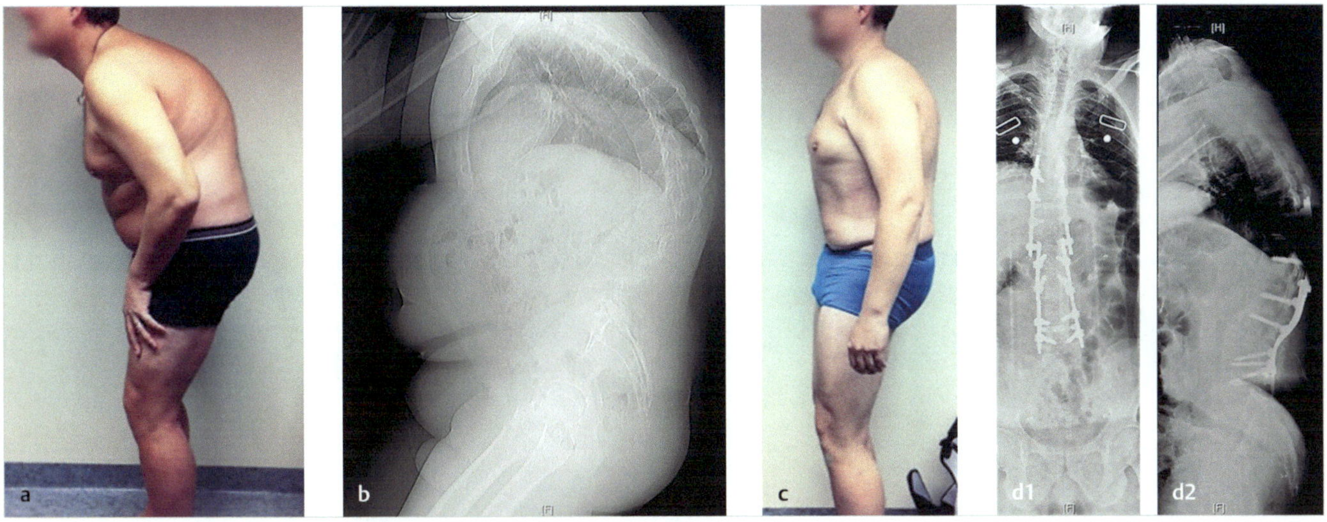

Fig. 21.6 **(a)** A patient with severe ankylosing spondylitis, leaning forward, barely managing a horizontal gaze. He uses walking supports indoors and a wheelchair outdoors. **(b)** Overview CT scan showing an ankylosed spine and 92-degree kyphosis. **(c)** The patient postoperatively, after double pedicle subtraction osteotomies at T12 and L3. **(d1, d2)** Standing postoperative radiographs.

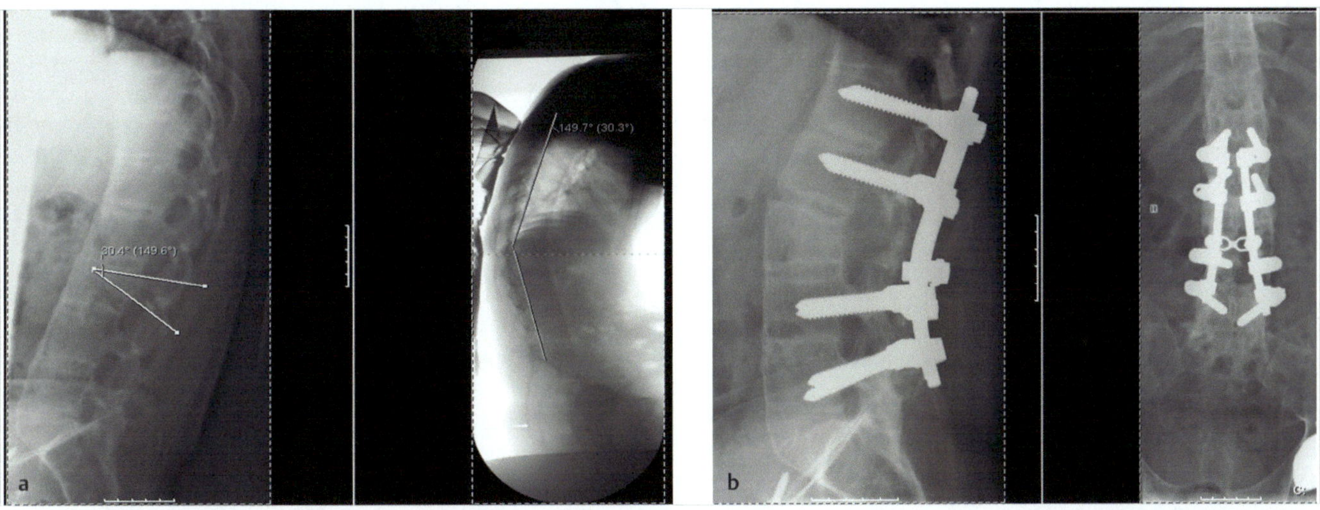

Fig. 21.7 **(a)** A 41-year-old man with ankylosing spondylitis, with no pain but a severe horizontal gaze problem. Previous total hip replacement. Severe sagittal imbalance. **(b)** Postoperatively (L3 pedicle subtraction osteotomy with a 30-degree wedge taken out), the patient has normalized gaze and cosmesis and improved functional level.

complications with the PSO is substantial; in the literature, up to 45% has been reported.[10] The PSO is a technically demanding procedure with a significant risk of complications, such as blood loss, deep vein thrombosis, wound infection, pseudarthrosis, proximal junctional kyphosis (PJK), and neurologic deficit.[11] The neurologic complication rate has been reported to be around 11% in the lumbar spine, most of which are temporary, with only 2.8% being permanent.[11] Technical details on surgery are beyond the scope of this chapter.

Cervicothoracic kyphosis in AS can be extremely disabling and can significantly interfere with activities of daily living. Patients may develop difficulty with forward gaze, eating, swallowing, hygiene, and breathing. Independent ambulation becomes increasingly difficult because of a combination of factors, including sagittal imbalance, stiffness and/or pain in the hips and knees, as well as the inability to look forward.

Patients often have kyphosis of the cervical as well as the thoracolumbar spine. The symptoms decide the level of the osteotomy. If the problem is the forward-leaning posture or lack of horizontal gaze, the PSO should be performed in the lumbar spine (▶ Fig. 21.7a, b). In some patients two PSOs may be necessary to sufficiently correct the deformity (▶ Fig. 21.6c, d). Positioning on the operating table is often difficult in cases of severe kyphosis, a stiff spine prone to fracture (particularly the cervical spine), and stiff shoulders and hips. The author has found halo traction to be helpful in protecting the eyes as well as to control the cervical spine, particularly during the correction maneuver (▶ Fig. 21.8a, b).

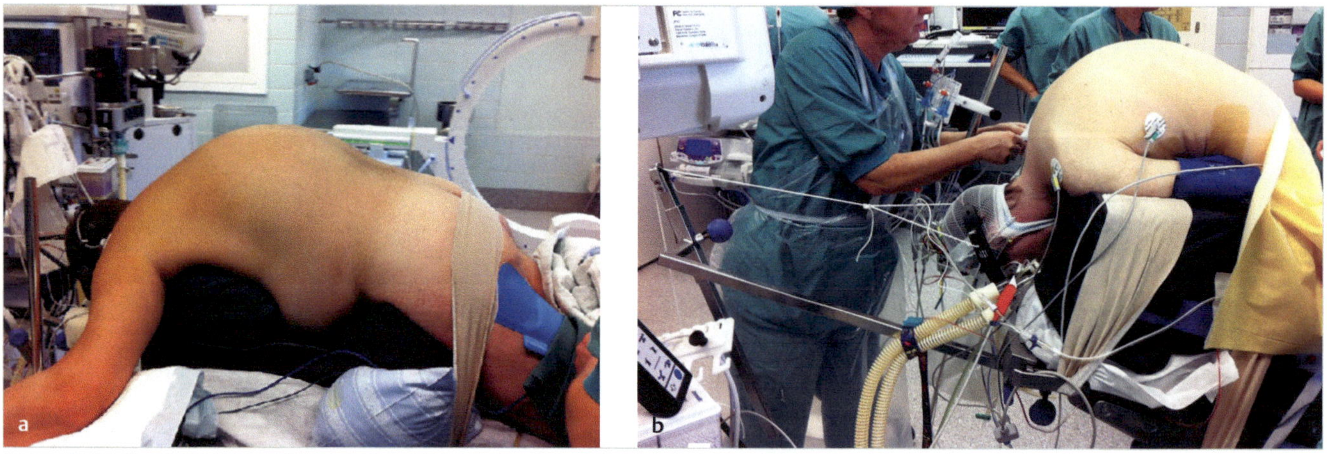

Fig. 21.8 (a) Operating table view before a planned double pedicle subtraction osteotomy (PSO) in a patient with ankylosing spondylitis (AS). Note halo traction to relieve pressure on the face and eyes and to facilitate the correction maneuver. The table may be tilted to additionally facilitate correction, but this is not always needed. **(b)** Patient with extreme AS (see ▶ Fig. 21.1 for CT reconstruction) placed on the operating table before planned triple PSOs. Placement was planned the day before surgery with the patient awake. Note the use of halo traction.

If the problem is dysphagia or dyspnea, one must consider a cervical osteotomy, usually performed at the C7 level. The PSO of the cervical spine can improve cervical spine alignment and that patient's ability to swallow and to maintain horizontal gaze to perform activities of daily living.[12] Before performing a C7 osteotomy one must exclude the possibility of the vertebral artery entering at the C7 level,[13] which is usually at C6 (> 85% of cases).[13] A halo vest is recommended for postoperative immobilization, especially in osteoporotic patients, but it is not obligatory if fixation can be considered solid.

Only highly experienced surgeons should perform a C7 osteotomy[14] (▶ Fig. 21.9a, b, c). The risk of catastrophic neurologic complications must not be underestimated with this procedure. The PSO at the cervical spine is much more hazardous than at the lumbar level. The overall rate of neurologic complications has been reported to be approximately 23%.[15] Often, but not always, the neurologic deficits, most commonly C8 palsy, are transient. Other complications include pseudarthrosis, wound infection, and dysphagia.

21.4 Diffuse Idiopathic Skeletal Hyperostosis with Fracture

The clinical appearance of senile vertebral ankylosing hyperostosis was first described by Forestier and Rotes-Querol in 1950.[16] It was considered a noninflammatory disorder in which spinal longitudinal ligaments and their insertions slowly become ossified, leading to decreased mobility and ultimately to complete ankylosis. Similar to the situation in AS the etiology of DISH is not clearly understood. As a reflection of the complex background, genetic, metabolic, endocrinologic, environmental, as well as toxic factors have been suggested to play a role in the pathogenesis. DISH has been associated with obesity, hyperlipidemia, and type 2 diabetes mellitus.

Verlaan et al found DISH-like changes in human remains excavated from an abbey court in the Netherlands, speculating it was a reflection of "a monastic way of life" (i. e., too much food and too little activity)[17] (▶ Fig. 21.10). The prevalence ranges from 2.9 to 25% in different populations. DISH is more common in males than females; an 8% prevalence has been reported in Finnish males.[18] An increasing amount of evidence suggests this disease is less rare than previously thought. The associations with advanced age have been demonstrated by several authors; therefore the incidence is likely to increase in the future as a result of global demographic changes, with an aging population. Furthermore, the increase in body weight observed in many countries may add to this problem.

On physical examination patients with DISH have reduction in neck rotation and in thoracic and lumbar mobility. In advanced stages, spinal ossifications may lead to complete ankylosis of the spine and postural changes similar to those in long-standing cases of AS, including forward stooping of the neck, high thoracic kyphosis, and loss of normal lumbar lordosis. According to Resnick, DISH is characterized by (1) new bone formation along the anterolateral aspect of the thoracic spine at four or more contiguous vertebral bodies, (2) preservation of the intervertebral disk space, and (3) absence of apophyseal joints or sacroiliac inflammatory changes.[19]

Most of the symptoms are mild with gradually developing stiffness. Major cervical spondylophytes may result in dysphagia and make endotracheal intubation difficult. Spondylophytes may also result in cervical spinal canal stenosis and myelopathy. Although some authors have speculated that DISH patients are at a higher risk for spinal fractures after minor trauma, generally the risk of fracture is not increased in DISH, as opposed to AS.

Individuals with DISH sustain fractures of similar nature to those with AS (i. e., hyperextension fractures that may result in severe neurologic compromise). The fracture morphology is slightly different between the two disorders. Fractures in AS tend to occur more often at the level of the disk, whereas DISH fractures tend to occur at the level of the vertebral body, most likely reflecting the fact that the ossification in DISH is concentrated at the disk level, protecting it from fracture. Also, fractures in DISH typically involve only the anterior column since the posterior column is not ankylosed. Importantly, as a result of this, the instability in DISH fractures is less pronounced than in AS fractures.

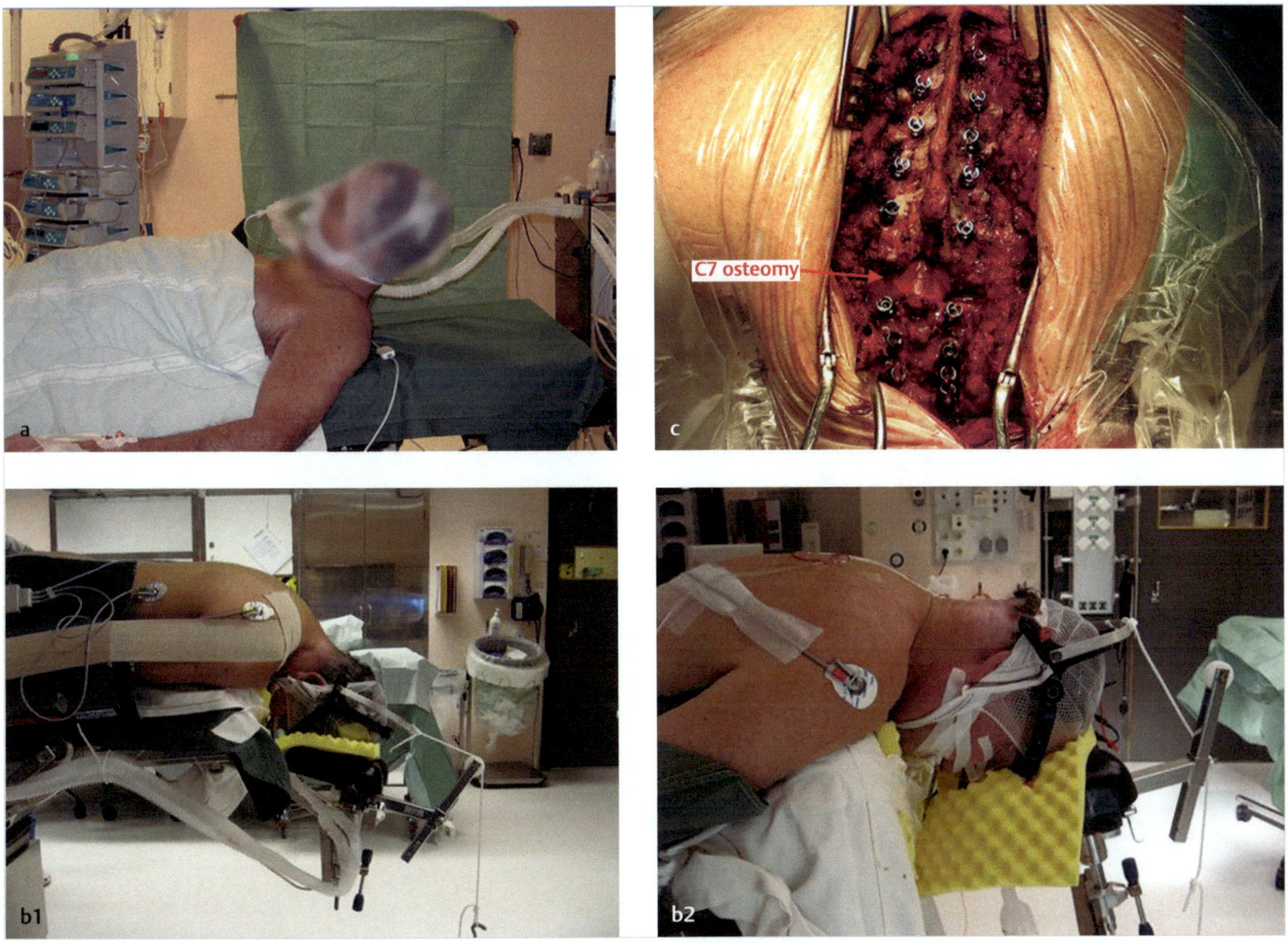

Fig. 21.9 (a) A patient with malunited fractures of C 2 as well as C 6, with chin-on-chest deformity and problems with horizontal gaze and swallowing. Note the complete stiffness of the cervicothoracic deformity. **(b1, b2)** Patient on the operating table before and after a C 7 osteotomy and fixation of C 4 to T 5. Note also the mandatory neuromonitoring. **(c)** Lateral mass screws have been implanted at C 3–C 6, pedicle screws at T 1–T 4, and hooks at T 5. Note the wide osteotomy at C 7 before closure.

As in AS, diagnosis of acute fracture is often delayed in DISH patients because patients have underlying spinal complaints that may not be easily distinguished from acute fracture pain. Also, a fracture may not be considered in patients with DISH given that these fractures, as in AS, often result from minor trauma. Furthermore, awareness among physicians is lower about potentially unstable hyperextension fractures in DISH than in AS, leading to underdiagnosis. Finally, the spinal radiographs may be difficult to interpret due to preexisting pathological changes, which may mask acute fractures (▶ Fig. 21.11, ▶ Fig. 21.12). Thus, as in AS, there is a low threshold for fracture in DISH patients, and a CT scan should be performed in every patient with a clinically suspected fracture. An MRI scan should be added in most patients to exclude posterior ligamentous injury and also to demonstrate compressive mechanisms on the spinal cord.[20] Most fractures are localized in the cervical spine (60%), some in the thoracic spine (33%), and very few in the lumbar spine. Neurologic deficit has been reported to occur in up to 40%. Worsening of neurologic deficit due to inadequate immobilization and inconsiderate transfers has been reported by several authors.[20,21,22]

Westerveld et al reported that hyperextension injury is the most common mechanism, occurring in about half of patients. Compression fractures are less common, and there have been no reports of flexion injury. Surgical treatment is preferred in hyperextension fractures because this treatment option is associated with lower complication and mortality rates and more predictably leads to neurologic improvement.[21] As for AS pedicle screw fixation, the recommendation is for at least two levels above and below. Posterior fusion with local bone graft can be considered sufficient. For compression fractures conservative or surgical treatment is chosen, depending on the severity of the fracture and the integrity of the posterior ligamentous complex. In conservative treatment, however, close follow-up is mandatory.

Although the evidence-based medicine (EBM) situation on how to treat DISH fractures is weak, the Spine Trauma Study Group, composed of international experts in spinal trauma care, strongly recommends surgical treatment in hyperextension DISH fractures of the spine, in accordance with the recommendation for those in AS.[22]

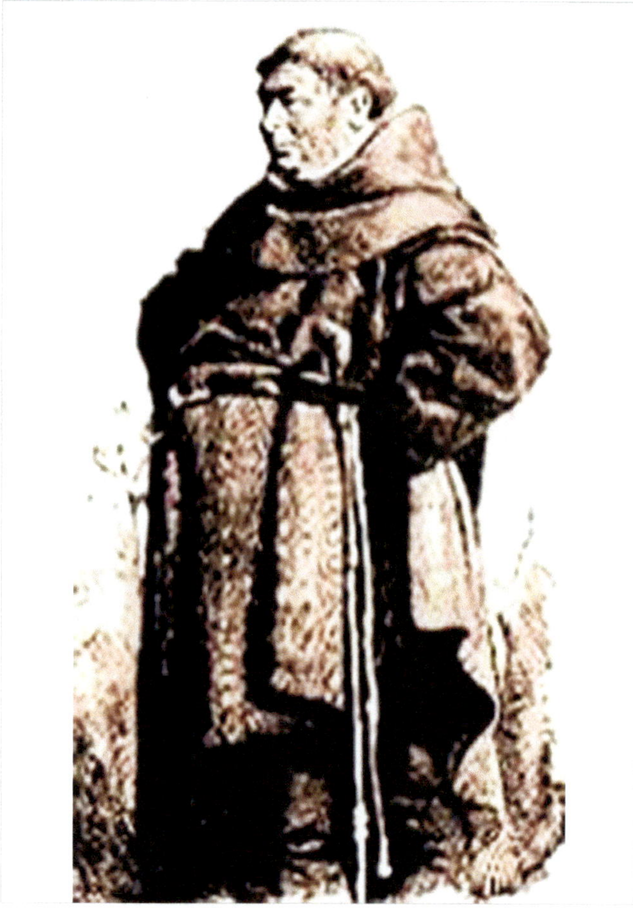

Fig. 21.10 Diffuse idiopathic skeletal hyperostosis has been suggested to be caused by a monastic way of life.

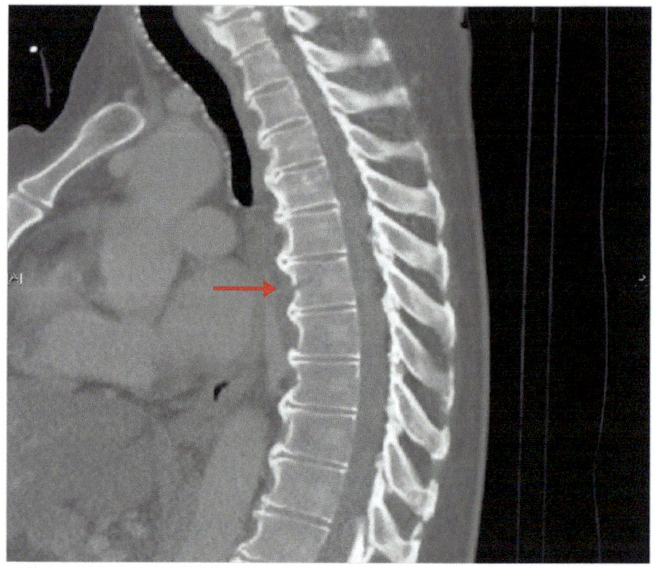

Fig. 21.12 A 52-year-old man with a psychiatric background and drug abuse. Simple fall. Initially suspected cardiac or neurologic cause. CT showed diffuse idiopathic skeletal hyperostosis with fracture at T 6 (*red arrow*), probably of an extension type. Treated successfully with brace for 3 months.

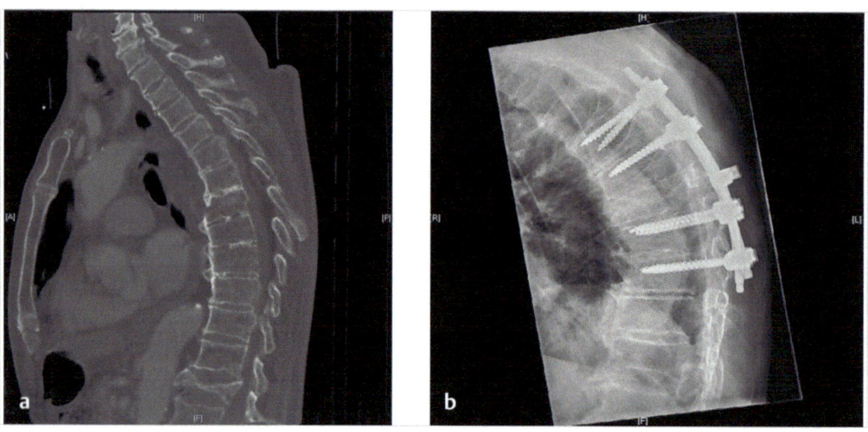

Fig. 21.11 **(a)** An 84-year-old man. Motor vehicle accident. Previous stroke with right-sided weakness. No new neurology. Preoperative CT shows T 7 fracture with slight translation. Also an acetabular fracture. **(b)** Postoperative radiograph shows fixation at T 5–T 9. No complications.

References

[1] Braun J, Bollow M, Remlinger G, et al. Prevalence of spondylarthropathies in HLA-B27 positive and negative blood donors. Arthritis Rheum. 1998; 41 (1):58–67

[2] Braun J, Sieper J. Ankylosing spondylitis. Lancet. 2007; 369(9570):1379–1390

[3] Caron T, Bransford R, Nguyen Q, Agel J, Chapman J, Bellabarba C. Spine fractures in patients with ankylosing spinal disorders. Spine. 2010; 35(11):E458–E464

[4] Fox MW, Onofrio BM, Kilgore JE. Neurological complications of ankylosing spondylitis. J Neurosurg. 1993; 78(6):871–878

[5] Anwar F, Al-Khayer A, Joseph G, Fraser MH, Jigajinni MV, Allan DB. Delayed presentation and diagnosis of cervical spine injuries in long-standing ankylosing spondylitis. Eur Spine J. 2011; 20(3):403–407

[6] Hitchon PW, From AM, Brenton MD, Glaser JA, Torner JC. Fractures of the thoracolumbar spine complicating ankylosing spondylitis. J Neurosurg. 2002; 97(2) Suppl:218–222

[7] Taggard DA, Traynelis VC. Management of cervical spinal fractures in ankylosing spondylitis with posterior fixation. Spine. 2000; 25(16):2035–2039

[8] Robinson Y, Willander J, Olerud C. Surgical stabilization improves survival of spinal fractures related to ankylosing spondylitis. Spine. 2015; 40(21):1697–1702

[9] Kanter AS, Wang MY, Mummaneni PV. A treatment algorithm for the management of cervical spine fractures and deformity in patients with ankylosing spondylitis. Neurosurg Focus. 2008; 24(1):E11

[10] Bridwell KH, Lewis SJ, Edwards C, et al. Complications and outcomes of pedicle subtraction osteotomies for fixed sagittal imbalance. Spine. 2003; 28 (18):2093–2101

[11] Buchowski JM, Bridwell KH, Lenke LG, et al. Neurologic complications of lumbar pedicle subtraction osteotomy: a 10-year assessment. Spine. 2007; 32 (20):2245–2252

[12] Kim HJ, Piyaskulkaew C, Riew KD. Comparison of Smith-Petersen osteotomy versus pedicle subtraction osteotomy versus anterior-posterior osteotomy types for the correction of cervical spine deformities. Spine. 2015; 40 (3):143–146

[13] Argenson Cl, Francke JP, Sylla S, et al. Les artères vertébrales (segments V1 et V2). Anatomia Clinica 2 2005:29–41

[14] Wollowick AL, Kelly MP, Riew KD. Pedicle subtraction osteotomy in the cervical spine. Spine. 2012; 37(5):E342–E348

[15] Etame AB, Than KD, Wang AC, La Marca F, Park P. Surgical management of symptomatic cervical or cervicothoracic kyphosis due to ankylosing spondylitis. Spine. 2008; 33(16):E559–E564

[16] Forestier J, Rotes-Querol J. Senile ankylosing hyperostosis of the spine. Ann Rheum Dis. 1950; 9(4):321–330

[17] Verlaan JJ, Oner FC, Maat GJR. Diffuse idiopathic skeletal hyperostosis in ancient clergymen. Eur Spine J. 2007; 16(8):1129–1135

[18] Julkunen H, Heinonen OP, Knekt P, Maatela J. The epidemiology of hyperostosis of the spine together with its symptoms and related mortality in a general population. Scand J Rheumatol. 1975; 4(1):23–27

[19] Resnick D, Niwayama G. Radiographic and pathologic features of spinal involvement in diffuse idiopathic skeletal hyperostosis (DISH). Radiology. 1976; 119(3):559–568

[20] Finkelstein JA, Chapman JR, Mirza S. Occult vertebral fractures in ankylosing spondylitis. Spinal Cord. 1999; 37(6):444–447

[21] Verlaan JJ, Diekerhof CH, Buskens E, et al. Surgical treatment of traumatic fractures of the thoracic and lumbar spine: a systematic review of the literature on techniques, complications, and outcome. Spine. 2004; 29(7):803–814

[22] Hedlund R, Verlaan JJ. Thoracolumbar hyperextension injuries in the stiff spine. In: Vaccaro AR, Fehlings MG, Dvorak MF, eds. Spine and Spinal Cord Trauma: Evidence Based Management. New York, NY: Thieme; 2011:391–399

22 Osteotomies in Revision Surgery

Ahmet Alanay, Çağlar Yılgör

Abstract

In a revision case, vertebral osteotomies are indicated when the deformity is too rigid to be corrected either with instrumentation alone or with the addition of posterior ligament and simple facet joint releases. Osteotomies in revision surgery can be performed via anterior-only, posterior-only, or combined anterior-posterior approaches, and can be classified into different grades based on the extent of anatomical resection. The main aims are to correct the multiplanar deformity, relieve compression of the spinal cord, and allow functional improvement. Yet, the deformities in children, adolescents, and adults have different characteristics in regards to growth, rigidity, and bone quality. Although osteotomies offer adequate correction and yield satisfactory outcomes, they are also associated with an increased risk of intraoperative and follow-up complications. Plus, all the osteotomy types are technically demanding and should be performed under intraoperative neurophysiologic monitoring. During preoperative planning, the decision-making on selection of osteotomies should not be solely based on the deformity, but the patient's age, neurologic status, bone quality, and medical comorbidities should also be considered, as well as the surgeon's experience and comfort level.

Keywords: spinal deformity, vertebral osteotomies, pedicle subtraction osteotomy, vertebral column resection, preoperative planning

22.1 Introduction

Rapid improvements and advances in spinal deformity surgery have resulted in an increased number of children, adolescents, and adults undergoing surgery worldwide. The number of revision cases has increased accordingly.

In general, vertebral osteotomies are indicated when the deformity is too rigid to be corrected either with instrumentation alone or with the addition of posterior ligament and simple facet joint releases. The main aims of an osteotomy in a revision are to correct the multiplanar deformity, thus the appearance, and to restore sagittal balance, enable a more erect posture, and relieve compression of the spinal cord and visceral organs and allow functional improvement.

It must be kept in mind that the decision to perform an osteotomy cannot be based solely on the deformity. The patient's age and chief complaint as well as the natural history of the deformity and/or the underlying disease, neurologic status, bone quality, and medical comorbidities should also be considered.

The deformities in children, adolescents, and adults have different characteristics. In children, because growth is an ongoing process, a deformed spinal section influences the growth of the remaining spine, chest wall, lungs, and extremities. Respecting the remaining spinal growth is of the utmost importance when planning a revision osteotomy in a child. Therefore, osteotomies and fusion should be performed for short segments to correct the deformity and cease progression while allowing further growth and improving pulmonary function. In general, adult curves tend to be more rigid than adolescent curves. Cosmetic concerns are more important in the pediatric and adolescent population, whereas adult patients frequently present with pain, alterations in gait, and neurologic symptoms. Bone quality can be a major concern in the elderly population

Osteotomies in revision surgery can be performed via an anterior-only, a posterior-only, or an anterior and posterior combined (circumferential) approach. Our experience, and that cited in the recent literature, suggests that the posterior-only approach is safe and efficient to adequately address very rigid or fixed deformities.[1,2] Revision spinal osteotomies have satisfactory results, and they can be life-saving procedures in cases where standard approaches are incapable of offering adequate treatment. Yet they have an increased risk of intraoperative and follow-up complications. Therefore, surgeons should choose the most appropriate type of osteotomy and surgical approach based on the type of deformity, curve magnitude, stiffness, bone density, and operative goals, as well as the surgeon's experience and comfort level.[3,4]

22.2 General Indications

In general, an osteotomy is necessary if the deformity cannot be corrected by diskectomy and/or facetectomy and soft tissue releases. In revision osteotomy, the index fusion is revised with osteotomy with or without extension of posterior fusion. In the thoracic region, thoracoplasty can be additionally performed to reduce the rib hump appearance.[5] In children, crankshaft phenomenon, junctional deformity, and progression may require revision osteotomy. Crankshaft phenomenon is the progression of rotational and angular deformity due to continued anterior growth in the setting of a previous posterior fusion. In adult spinal deformity, revision osteotomies are commonly used for loss of lumbar lordosis and fixed kyphosis and more rarely for coronal plane deformity and imbalance.

Appropriate preoperative clinical and radiographic evaluations are mandatory. A thorough history and evaluation of the patient's general health status and the whole locomotor system should be performed. Evaluation of the hip joints is important owing to their contribution to the sagittal plane. A careful neurologic examination is essential. In children, the ability to sit, stand, and walk is evaluated.

Radiologic evaluation starts with standing whole-spine radiographs in anteroposterior and lateral views (sitting radiographs may be obtained in nonambulatory patients). Supine bending, lateral fulcrum, and lateral flexion and extension radiographs demonstrate the flexibility of the deformity. Axial traction X-rays under general anesthesia provide greater detail as to flexibility.[6,7]

Revision osteotomies should be performed under intraoperative neurophysiologic monitoring. Somatosensory evoked potential, motor evoked potential, and real-time electromyography as well as pedicle screw stimulation may be used. The neurologic status of the patient at the beginning of the operation after positioning, during the osteotomy, and during the correction of the deformity should be carefully recorded. A wake-up test can occasionally be necessary.

22.3 Osteotomies

Osteotomy options in revision spinal surgery are the Ponte osteotomy, Smith-Petersen osteotomy (SPO), pedicle subtraction osteotomy (PSO), bone-disk-bone osteotomy (BDBO), and vertebral column resection (VCR). Recently, Schwab et al[8] classified these osteotomies into six categories based on anatomical grades of resection.

Grade 1 osteotomies involve the resection of the joint capsule and inferior facet. Grade 2 osteotomies involve removal of all posterior ligaments (supraspinous, intraspinous, and ligamentum flavum) and facet joints. Grade 3 osteotomies involve the removal of the pedicles and partial body. Grade 4 osteotomies involve the removal of the pedicles, partial body, and disk. Grade 5 osteotomies involve the removal of a complete vertebra and disks. Grade 6 osteotomies involve the removal of several adjacent vertebrae, at least one complete vertebral body, and a partial or complete second vertebra.

All the osteotomy types are technically demanding and have potentially high rates of complications. The appropriate selection of the osteotomy grade depends on the surgeon's experience, the type of deformity, and the magnitude of the curve. In general, varied clinical and radiologic scenarios may necessitate different grades/types of osteotomies.[3]

- If the surgeon is less experienced with osteotomies or the patient is in poor medical condition, intraoperative halo-femoral traction and grade 1 osteotomies may be performed.
- If the kyphosis is gradual or sweeping, the degree of sagittal imbalance is moderate, and the disk space is mobile, then grade 2 osteotomies should be sufficient.
- Fixed disk space and severe sagittal imbalance generally necessitate grade 3 or 4 osteotomies.
- Sharp and focal kyphotic deformities in the lumbar region are also addressed with grade 3 and 4 osteotomies.
- Thoracic sharp and focal kyphosis may be corrected with grade 5 and 6 osteotomies.

Lafage et al[9] reported on the fundamental role of the pelvis in sagittal plane evaluation. Therefore, spinopelvic parameters such as the sagittal vertical axis, the pelvic tilt, and the relationship between pelvic incidence and lumbar lordosis should be an indispensable part of the surgical planning. These parameters were shown to correlate with pain and disability.

22.3.1 Grade 1 Osteotomies

Grade 1 osteotomies are opening-wedge osteotomies that involve the resection of the joint capsule and inferior facet. Hence, they are partial facet joint resections. Anterior column mobility is a prerequisite for this procedure, which has limited deformity correction ability. SPO and chevron osteotomies are examples of grade 1 resections.

The chevron osteotomy was described through unfused facets.[10] SPO is performed through previously fused facet joints, and 5 to 7 degrees of correction can be obtained per level.[11]

In a study comparing SPO and PSO, single-level PSO caused nearly twice as much bleeding as three levels of SPO.[12] SPO had a greater tendency toward coronal decompensation.[12] In our clinical experience, SPOs are technically easier and safer to perform when compared to other spinal osteotomy types. SPOs cause less blood loss, have a decreased risk of neurologic injury, and require a shorter operative duration.

22.3.2 Grade 2 Osteotomies

Grade 2 osteotomies involve removal of all posterior ligaments (supraspinous, intraspinous, and ligamentum flavum) and facet joints. Hence, they are complete facet joint resections. The Ponte osteotomy may be an example of grade 2 resections. It can be performed at several levels and can provide up to 10 to 15 degrees of correction per level based on the amount of bone resected. Compression of the osteotomy sites provides correction of kyphosis. During the correction, strong segmental fixation is mandatory to prevent loss of the reduction achieved. Additionally, compression leads to narrowing of the neural foramina, which necessitates a preceding wide facetectomy to prevent nerve root impingement.[3]

Ponte osteotomies can be performed asymmetrically to correct the coronal imbalance as well as the sagittal imbalance. It is important that the anterior disk be mobile. If the disk is severely degenerated or collapsed, placement of a structural interbody graft anteriorly would allow for greater correction through a posterior osteotomy closure.

22.3.3 Grade 3 Osteotomies

Grade 3 osteotomies involve the removal of the pedicles and partial body. PSO[13] and closing-opening wedge osteotomy[14] may be examples of grade 3 resections. They can provide up to 15 to 20 degrees and 30 to 40 degrees of focal sagittal correction at each segment in the thoracic and lumbar spine, respectively. Closing-opening wedge osteotomy may provide more sagittal alignment correction than PSO.[8] In grade 3 osteotomies, the anterior column does not lengthen, and an anterior bone defect is not created, while the posterior and middle columns shorten. Thus they provide a more stable correction. PSO can also be performed asymmetrically to achieve coronal correction in combination with sagittal correction. According to the definition, a PSO that extends into adjacent disk spaces would be a grade 4 resection.[8]

Placing a temporary rod on the contralateral side while working on one side will help avoid any translocation during the osteotomy. The hips and knees may be hyperextended when the osteotomy site is compressed to facilitate closure of the osteotomy. After closing the osteotomy site, any dural buckling or nerve impingement should be controlled to avoid neurologic injury.

PSO was reported to result in 29% of pseudarthroses[15] and 11.1% of neurologic deficits,[16] of which only 2.8% were permanent over a 10-year follow-up. Although complication rates were high, patients reported improved Oswestry disability index (ODI) and Scoliosis Research Society scores at 2-year follow-up.[17] Similarly, closing-opening wedge osteotomy was reported to yield an 86% satisfaction rate.[14] Pseudarthrosis is more common in the segments where the disk height and thus

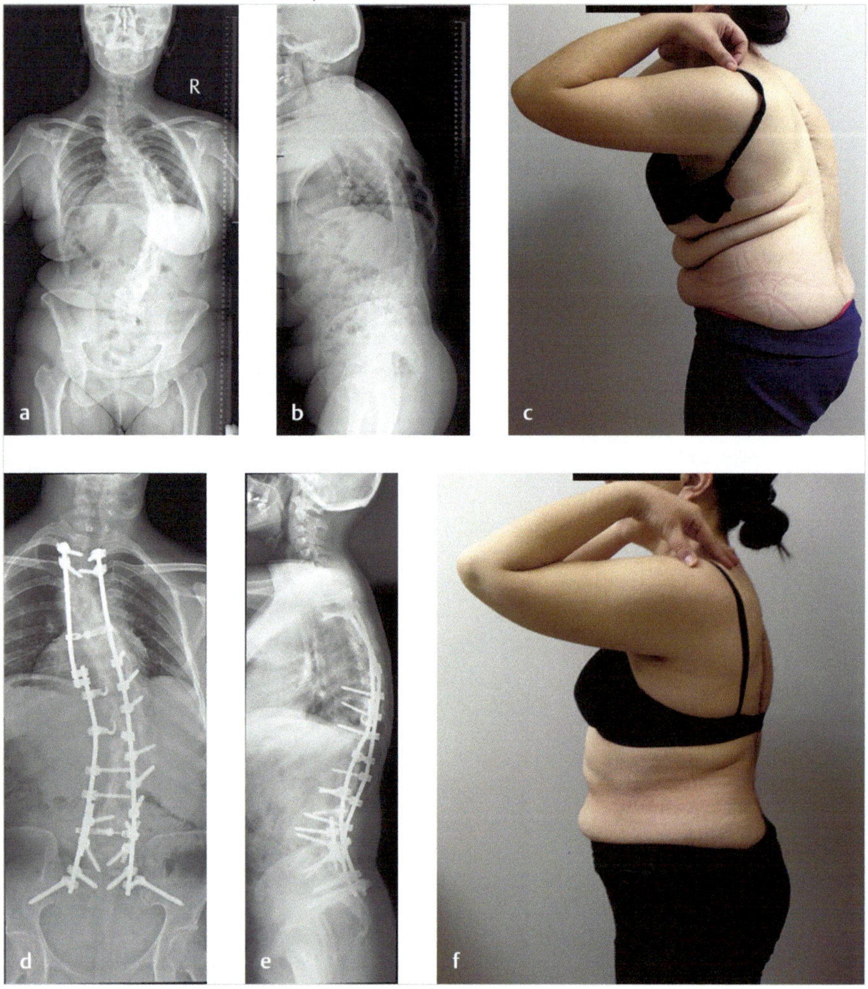

Fig. 22.1 (a, b) Preoperative coronal and sagittal X-rays of a 41-year-old woman. The patient had had three previous operations. A Harrington rod was applied when she was 12, and it was revised with sublaminar wiring when she was 23 years old. Subsequently implant removal was applied. **(c)** Sagittal profile of the patient when she first applied to our clinic. She had right leg pain and claudication with the ability to walk less than 100 meters. T2 to iliac posterior instrumented fusion was performed with an L4 pedicle subtraction osteotomy (PSO) and T7–T8, T8–T9, T9–T10, T10–T11, and T11–T12 Ponte osteotomies at our institution. A double-rod technique was used at the PSO site. **(d, e)** Postoperative radiographic and **(f)** clinical status of the patient. Her symptoms of back and leg pain as well as claudication were resolved.

the mobility are preserved. In such cases, posterior or anterior interbody arthrodesis above and below the PSO level can be carried out. Another method to decrease the rates of nonunion is to increase the number of rods that cross the osteotomy site. In the so-called double-rod technique the osteotomy site can be closed via two rods, one on each side that is connected to the screws one level above and below the osteotomy. Two other rods are used to connect the whole construct. The rods on each side can be connected by a domino connector or left independent. Similarly, the use of a central hook–rod construct is a quick and safe method that can be used to decrease the undue stress across the osteotomy site, which can lead to pseudarthrosis and fixation failure.[18] Pseudarthrosis after grade 3 osteotomies in the pediatric population is reported less frequently in comparison to adults.

A demonstrative patient for grade 3 osteotomy in a revision case is shown in ▸ Fig. 22.1.

22.3.4 Grade 4 Osteotomies

Grade 4 osteotomies can be performed in different ways to provide different amounts of correction rates ranging from 35 to 60 degrees. They involve the removal of the pedicles, partial body, and disk. BDBO may be an example of grade 4 resections. Grade 4 osteotomies may be an alternative to grade 5 osteotomies in patients with severe and rigid thoracolumbar and lumbar deformities, particularly when the apex or the center of rotational axis (CORA) of the deformity is at a disk level.

The advantages of BDBO when compared to PSO include correction of the deformity at its apex, higher correction rates, and a potential decrease in pseudarthrosis rates due to disk removal. The major advantage compared to VCR is its applicability at the lumbar spine without sacrificing the nerve roots while providing correction rates closer to those of VCR. Ozturk et al[19] reported an average 38 degrees of correction in the sagittal plane without any neurologic injury or pseudarthrosis during a 2-year follow-up after BDBO.

22.3.5 Grade 5 and 6 Osteotomies

Grade 5 osteotomies involve the removal of a complete vertebra and disks. They provide the greatest amount of correction and play an important role in the treatment of severe deformities that cannot be effectively corrected by less aggressive methods. Single-level VCR may be an example of grade 5 resections. Removal of several adjacent vertebrae, at least one complete vertebral body, and a partial or complete second vertebra is classified as a grade 6 resection. The decision as to the number of vertebral bodies to be resected is based on the rigidity and characteristics of the spinal deformity. Grade 5 and 6 resections can be performed as a combined anterior and posterior procedure. Deformity correction is performed gradually by

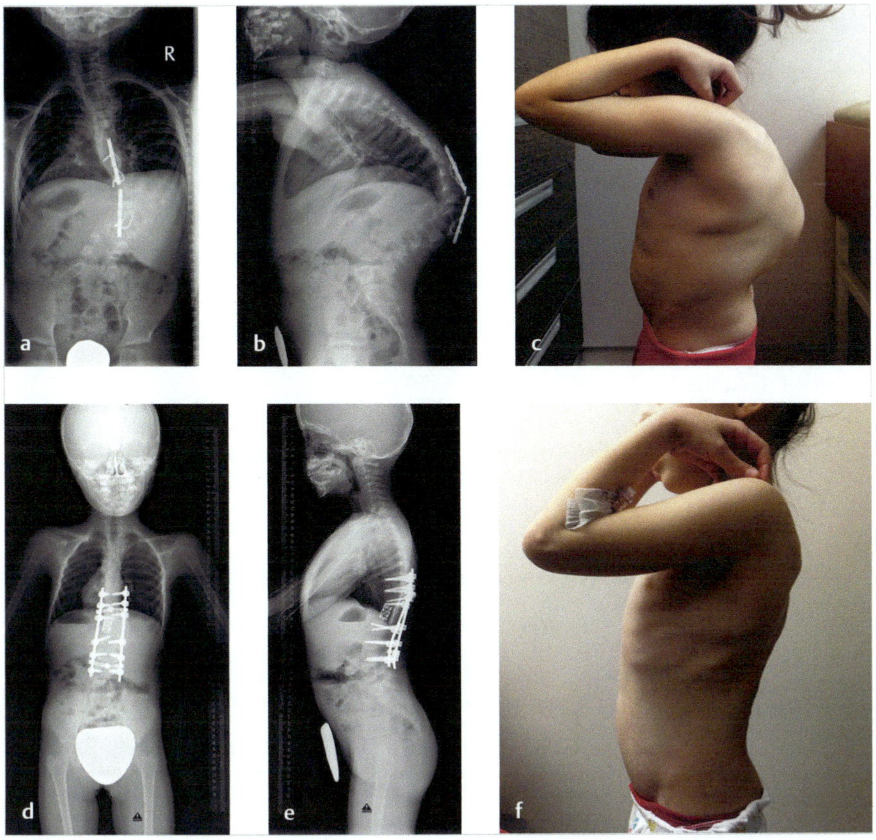

Fig. 22.2 (a, b) Preoperative coronal and sagittal X-rays of a 6-year-old girl diagnosed with congenital kyphoscoliosis with T 12 and L 1 hemivertebrae and implant failure. She had six previous operations with a partially fused thoracolumbar spine. Although the exact details were not available due to missing records, as far as the family reported, three of these surgeries were major deformity correction attempts, and three were minor revision/debridements. **(c)** Sagittal profile of the patient when she first applied to our clinic. T 9 to L 4 posterior instrumented fusion was applied with T 12–L 1 PVCR at our institute. **(d, e)** Postoperative coronal and sagittal radiographs and **(f)** clinical status of the patient.

compression, in situ contouring, and replacing the kyphotic rods with rods precontoured to the physiological contours. In contrast to other osteotomy grades, grade 5 and 6 resections are usually not bone-to-bone contact osteotomies and require structural allografts, autografts, or a cage to reconstruct the vertebral column after resection.

Posterior vertebral column resection (PVCR) was first introduced by Suk et al[20], and was popularized by Lenke et al[21] for severe deformities of the spinal column. It enables translational and rotational correction of the spinal column and provides a controlled manipulation of both the anterior and posterior columns simultaneously through a single approach. PVCR is a technically demanding procedure with a high rate of neurologic injury and should be performed by experienced spine surgeons and spine teams under neurologic monitoring. Furthermore, in revision cases spinal angiography may be required. In their series of 102 severe adult spinal deformity patients, Hamzaoglu et al[22] reported an average correction rate of 62% and 72% in coronal and sagittal planes, respectively. Suk et al[20] reported a correction of 59% in the coronal plane with significant improvement of the sagittal imbalance. In a series of 35 children, Lenke et al[21] noted major curve improvement that varied between 51 and 60% for idiopathic and congenital scoliosis, kyphosis, and kyphoscoliosis cases with PVCR.

The relative complexity of the procedure causes high rates of neurologic and overall complications. Neurologic injury can be caused by a direct insult, subluxation of the spinal column, dural buckling, and/or compression of the spinal cord by residual bone or soft tissues during or after correction. Reported overall complication rates range from 7.84% up to 40%, with neurologic complications ranging from 1.96% to 17.1%.[20,21,22]

A demonstrative patient for grade 5 osteotomy in a revision case is shown in ▶ Fig. 22.2.

22.4 Difficulties in Performing Osteotomies in Revision Cases

Revision cases are the perfect candidates for osteotomies as most of them are fixed—stuck in a less than perfect position—and do not have enough mobility to benefit from simple soft tissue releases. However, revision surgeries carry certain disadvantages for performing osteotomies. The exposure carries the risk of dural injury, particularly in the setting of previous laminectomy. Dural adhesions caused by a previous surgery may make it difficult to mobilize the spinal cord to resect the bone, and injury to dural tissue can easily happen. Working in collaboration with neurosurgeons may help to release the dura and prevent dural tears.

Another important difficulty is the placement of pedicle screws due to the landmarks obscured by fusion. Fully or partially intact transverse processes in the thoracic and lumbar spine may be helpful to find the entry points but should definitely be checked under fluoroscopy. Navigation, if available, would be very useful to find the pedicle paths and to place screws safely. It is important to be able to place pedicle screws bilaterally to have better control of the osteotomy sites and to manipulate the spinal column effectively and safely. Performing laminotomies to find the pedicles may also help for secure placement. Power drills are very helpful in breaking fusion at the osteotomy site. Diamond tips should be preferred when working close to the dura.

Preoperative planning and adhering to the plan are more important than in primary cases, particularly when the osteotomy is to be performed in a patient with a long fusion and very few mobile segments. In this case, one should provide a perfect alignment by the osteotomy because there will be no or very few mobile segments to compensate for any miscalculation or a less than perfect correction in alignment.

22.5 Conclusions

Osteotomies in revision surgery are proven to be highly efficient in pediatric and adult patients. They are powerful techniques enabling the spine surgeon to balance the spinal column. Achieving a well-balanced and aligned spinal column is the main goal of spine surgery. Advances in anesthetic and surgical techniques and the use of intraoperative neurophysiologic monitoring allow correction of rigid deformities that were previously thought to be inoperable. Furthermore, these challenging bony resections can safely be done via a posterior-only approach.

All the osteotomy types are technically demanding. Preoperative planning is very important as well as the operative procedure itself for obtaining satisfactory results. Neurophysiologic monitoring should be an indispensable part of the procedure. The patient's general health status and the surgeon's experience also significantly influence successful outcomes. Working in collaboration with a rehabilitation team is also essential.

In conclusion, we consider revision spinal osteotomies to be effective procedures for the treatment of severe deformities if an experienced surgical team performs them.

References

[1] Lenke LG, Sides BA, Koester LA, Hensley M, Blanke KM. Vertebral column resection for the treatment of severe spinal deformity. Clin Orthop Relat Res. 2010 Mar; 468(3):687–699

[2] Suk SI, Chung ER, Lee SM, Lee JH, Kim SS, Kim JH. Posterior vertebral column resection in fixed lumbosacral deformity. Spine. 2005; 30(23):E703–E710

[3] Dorward IG, Lenke LG. Osteotomies in the posterior-only treatment of complex adult spinal deformity: a comparative review. Neurosurg Focus. 2010; 28(3):E4

[4] Enercan M, Ozturk C, Kahraman S, Sarıer M, Hamzaoglu A, Alanay A. Osteotomies/spinal column resections in adult deformity. Eur Spine J. 2013; 22 Suppl 2:S254–S264

[5] Kim HJ, Cunningham ME, Boachie-Adjei O. Revision spine surgery to manage pediatric deformity. J Am Acad Orthop Surg. 2010; 18(12):739–748

[6] Davis BJ, Gadgil A, Trivedi J, Ahmed NB. Traction radiography performed under general anesthetic: a new technique for assessing idiopathic scoliosis curves. Spine. 2004; 29(21):2466–2470

[7] Liu RW, Teng AL, Armstrong DG, Poe-Kochert C, Son-Hing JP, Thompson GH. Comparison of supine bending, push-prone, and traction under general anesthesia radiographs in predicting curve flexibility and postoperative correction in adolescent idiopathic scoliosis. Spine. 2010; 35(4):416–422

[8] Schwab F, Blondel B, Chay E, et al. The comprehensive anatomical spinal osteotomy classification. Neurosurgery. 2015; 76 Suppl 1:S33–S41, discussion S41

[9] Lafage V, Schwab F, Patel A, Hawkinson N, Farcy JP. Pelvic tilt and truncal inclination: two key radiographic parameters in the setting of adults with spinal deformity. Spine. 2009; 34(17):E599–E606

[10] Bridwell KH. Decision making regarding Smith-Petersen vs. pedicle subtraction osteotomy vs. vertebral column resection for spinal deformity. Spine. 2006; 31(19) Suppl:S171–S178

[11] Bridwell KH, Lenke LG, Lewis SJ. Treatment of spinal stenosis and fixed sagittal imbalance. Clin Orthop Relat Res. 2001(384):35–44

[12] Cho KJ, Bridwell KH, Lenke LG, Berra A, Baldus C. Comparison of Smith-Petersen versus pedicle subtraction osteotomy for the correction of fixed sagittal imbalance. Spine. 2005; 30(18):2030–2037, discussion 2038

[13] Bridwell KH, Lewis SJ, Rinella A, Lenke LG, Baldus C, Blanke K. Pedicle subtraction osteotomy for the treatment of fixed sagittal imbalance. Surgical technique. J Bone Joint Surg Am. 2004; 86-A Suppl 1:44–50

[14] Chang KW, Cheng CW, Chen HC, Chang KI, Chen TC. Closing-opening wedge osteotomy for the treatment of sagittal imbalance. Spine. 2008; 33(13):1470–1477

[15] Kim YJ, Bridwell KH, Lenke LG, Cheh G, Baldus C. Results of lumbar pedicle subtraction osteotomies for fixed sagittal imbalance: a minimum 5-year follow-up study. Spine. 2007; 32(20):2189–2197

[16] Buchowski JM, Bridwell KH, Lenke LG, et al. Neurologic complications of lumbar pedicle subtraction osteotomy: a 10-year assessment. Spine. 2007; 32 (20):2245–2252

[17] Rose PS, Bridwell KH, Lenke LG, et al. Role of pelvic incidence, thoracic kyphosis, and patient factors on sagittal plane correction following pedicle subtraction osteotomy. Spine. 2009; 34(8):785–791

[18] Hyun SJ, Lenke LG, Kim YC, Koester LA, Blanke KM. Long-term radiographic outcomes of a central hook-rod construct for osteotomy closure: minimum 5-year follow-up. Spine. 2015; 40(7):E428–E432

[19] Ozturk C, Aydogan M, Karadereler S, Tezer M, Alanay A, Hamzaoglu A. Inter-radicular Bone-Disc-Bone Osteotomy (BDBO): An Alternative to Other Osteotomy Types for the Correction of Thoracolumbar and Lumbar Spine Deformities. Spine: Affiliated Society Meeting Abstracts 2010:77

[20] Suk SI, Chung ER, Kim JH, Kim SS, Lee JS, Choi WK. Posterior vertebral column resection for severe rigid scoliosis. Spine. 2005; 30(14):1682–1687

[21] Lenke LG, O'Leary PT, Bridwell KH, Sides BA, Koester LA, Blanke KM. Posterior vertebral column resection for severe pediatric deformity: minimum two-year follow-up of thirty-five consecutive patients. Spine. 2009; 34(20):2213–2221

[22] Hamzaoglu A, Alanay A, Ozturk C, Sarier M, Karadereler S, Ganiyusufoglu K. Posterior vertebral column resection in severe spinal deformities: a total of 102 cases. Spine. 2011; 36(5):E340–E344

23 Classification and Definition of Rigid Spine Deformity

Josh Schroeder, Janina Kueper, Leon Kaplan

Abstract

Rigid spine deformity represents a variation from the normal spinal alignment in the child and the adult. Variance from the alignment in the coronal plane is termed scoliosis, whereas variance from the alignment in the sagittal plane is termed kyphosis or lordosis, depending on the orientation of the curve's convexity. The deformity itself may be caused by a variety of underlying diseases, such as congenital and developmental disorders; skeletal dysplasia; and infectious, traumatic, surgical, or neoplastic sequelae. The etiology of the most frequently diagnosed spinal deformity, idiopathic scoliosis, has, as the name suggests, not been established to date. The classification of the deformities in the pediatric and the adult patient population enable a structured approach to the patient and allow physicians to compare and determine treatment options most suitable to the severity of the deformity. Spinal deformities in the pediatric patient present an additional challenge, as the effect of vertebral growth must be considered when possible conservative, or in some severe cases surgical, treatments are being debated.

Keywords: hemivertebrae, failure of formation, failure of segmentation, congenital scoliosis

23.1 Introduction

Hippocrates of Cos (4th–5th century BC), the philosopher and physician from the Age of Pericles in ancient Greece, was the first to describe the curvatures and diseases of the spine.[1] His treatise "On Fractures and On Joints" discussed both the physiological anatomy and the pathology of the human spine. He provided a precise description of the structure of the vertebrae, the motion segments, and the normal shapes of the curves of the spine. In addition, he discussed a variety of diseases that altered the spine's shape, including posttraumatic kyphosis and scoliosis, outlining treatment strategies that would become the cornerstone of surgical management of spinal deformity.[2]

Rigid spine deformity is the most frequently diagnosed form of congenital orthopaedic anomaly.[3] Spinal deformities encompass a broad spectrum of physical manifestations of aberrations in the magnitude and orientation of the vertebral curves. Patients may present with deformity at differing stages of life depending on the etiology of the underlying disease. In addition to the average age at the development of the deformity, each disease has characteristic concomitant symptoms and features that allow a physician to capture the underlying condition.

The organization of the vertebrae and intervertebral disks in successive curvatures is vital for maintaining an erect position, which allows mobility. The definition of normal spinal alignment differs with respect to age and sex. The spine is divided into the following curves: cervical lordosis (C 1–C 7), thoracic (dorsal) kyphosis (T 1–T 12), lumbar lordosis (L 1–L 5), and sacral kyphosis (S 1–S 4/S 5). Any reversals or significant increases in the spinal curvatures as well as deviations in the coronal or sagittal plane are considered pathological. Generally, females as well as both men and women of older age, may present with curvatures of a greater magnitude.

Any deviation that differs from the physiological alignment may, depending on its magnitude, lead to faults in the balance of the vertebral column. Scoliosis describes a curve in the coronal plane that is often associated with an element of rotation and causes loss of balance. Hyperkyphosis and hyperlordosis are deviations in the sagittal plane that may cause forward or backward imbalance. All curvatures may be defined as either primary, or major, and secondary, or minor. Primary curves are mostly rigid and result from structural changes to the vertebrae. Secondary curves are the body's compensatory response to primary curves and will generally be smaller and have some flexible elements. The secondary curve may aid the body in maintaining balance and mobility through the redistribution of weight, leading to more efficient energy consumption.

The scope of treatment options for rigid spine deformities has expanded significantly in the past few decades. As the etiologies of pediatric and adult spinal deformities have become better understood, patient-centered conservative and surgical treatment strategies have been advanced. Harrington rods, which were originally developed for the correction and stabilization of scoliosis in patients with poliomyelitis, introduced the concept of spinal instrumentation to the orthopaedic community, and it has since rapidly evolved.[4]

23.2 Definition

In the next paragraphs we will define the disorders that create a rigid spine deformity.

23.2.1 Pediatric Rigid Spinal Deformity

In skeletally immature patients, spinal deformity can result from a variety of causes, including but not limited to congenital anomalies, syndromatic disorders, neuromuscular deformities, and skeletal dysplasia.[5,6] The diagnosis of idiopathic scoliosis, which is found in 70% of all structural deformities of the pediatric population, is made once generalized syndromes and inflammatory causes have been excluded.[7] Syndromatic causes, such as Marfan's syndrome, VATER/VACTERL (V, vertebrae; A, imperforate anus or anal atresia; C, cardiac anomalies; TE, tracheoesophageal fistula; R, renal anomalies; and L, limb anomalies) association, Poland syndrome, osteogenesis imperfecta, and neurofibromatosis should be evaluated carefully by an interdisciplinary team of physicians and geneticists because the deformity of the spine will possibly overshadow other issues the patient may be experiencing. Spinal deformities are associated with renal, cardiofacial, tracheoesophageal, anorectal, and cardiac malformations.

The most important consideration in the classification and treatment of pediatric spinal deformity are the effects that skeletal growth will have on the deformity. Anticipating the extent of vertebral growth allows for a more precise treatment strategy resulting in a more successful control of curve progression.

The two main growth spurts occur between birth and 5 years of age and during puberty. Skeletal growth slows down significantly approximately 18 months after menarche in girls, and at age 18 in boys. During the growth spurt occurring at puberty the thoracic spine grows 1.2 cm per year, while the lumbar spine grows 0.6 cm per year.[8] Based on these calculations made by Dimeglio and Bonnel, physicians may roughly approximate how skeletal development may alter the deformity or the decision of surgical corrections made before or during periods of growth.

23.2.2 Idiopathic Scoliosis

Idiopathic scoliosis is the most frequent diagnosis in spinal deformities of the child and the adolescent and is made once generalized syndromes and inflammatory causes have been excluded.[7] Little insight into the cause of idiopathic scoliosis has been established, though the deformity has been found to have a familial tendency and a bimodal frequency distribution.[9] Bunnell found that approximately 10% of adolescents have minor degrees of curvature (<10 degrees), but of these individuals only 2% warrant medical attention due to curve progression.[11] The prevalence of scoliosis >20 degrees is 0.3 to 0.5%, and the prevalence of curves with a magnitude of >40 degrees is 0.1%.[6] The deformity is generally categorized based on the age when it first becomes apparent, being broadly divided into infantile scoliosis (<3 years of age), juvenile scoliosis (3–9 years of age), and adolescent scoliosis (>10 years of age).[11,12,13] A younger age of onset correlates with severe curve progression due to the growth of the spine, which may result in curves >100 degrees restricting the adequate development of the lungs.[6] Adolescent idiopathic scoliosis is 10 times more prevalent in girls, whereas infantile idiopathic scoliosis is more common in boys.[14,15] The typical deformity pattern in adolescent idiopathic scoliosis in girls is a primary right thoracic curve with a secondary compensatory left lumbar curve.[16] The curves in infantile idiopathic scoliosis are, in contrast to adolescent idiopathic scoliosis, most commonly left thoracic curves with minor compensatory curves.[15]

23.2.3 Congenital Deformity

Anomalies in the formation of vertebral elements during the embryological period result in congenital deformities that will continue to develop and grow unevenly in the child. These vertebral anomalies develop during the first 6 weeks of pregnancy, when other organ systems, such as the genitourinary tract and the heart, are being formed as well, which result in a high rate of multiple associated anomalies the physician should attempt to identify through a thorough patient evaluation.[17] The vertebral anomalies are broadly categorized as follows:

- Formation failures, such as hemivertebrae and wedged vertebrae.
- Segmentation failures, such as block vertebrae or segmented or unsegmented bars.
- Mixed deformities.[18]

Approximately 75 to 90% of congenital vertebral anomalies resulting in a rigid spine deformity will progress as the child develops, with thoracic or thoracolumbar deformities with an unsegmented bar and a convex hemivertebra having the poorest prognosis.[17,19]

23.2.4 Neuromuscular and Paralytic Scoliosis

Neuromuscular scoliosis or paralytic scoliosis includes deformities resulting from progressive muscular dystrophies, cerebral palsy, and other neurologic disorders. Despite the wide variety of neuromuscular disorders, 25 to 100% of them cause some type of spinal deformity because of the spine's dependence on secondary stabilization from well-innervated skeletal muscle.[20] Due to erroneous or disrupted neural signaling to or from the neuromuscular junction, the central nervous system loses command and is no longer able to control muscular activity.[21] The severity of the disease and therefore the degree of paralysis or muscular atrophy correlate directly with the magnitude and the progression of the deformity. Patients presenting with neuromuscular scoliosis frequently have additional comorbidities, such as additional neurologic problems, joint contractures and dislocations, and poor bone quality. They present with a variety of curves of different magnitudes, which are characterized by an early-onset and unhalted progression, even once skeletal maturity has been reached.[20]

23.2.5 Scheuermann's Kyphosis

Scheuermann's kyphosis is defined as a structural thoracic or thoracolumbar hyperkyphosis that can be radiographically identified by at least three adjacent wedged vertebrae angled at a minimum of 5 degrees. The reported incidence ranges from 0.4 to 8%.[22] The etiology of the deformity is unknown, though defective asymmetrical endochondral ossification, increased mechanical stress, and juvenile osteoporosis have been postulated to play roles in the development of the disease.[23,24] The disease is usually identified during early adolescence, though patients with mild cases of Scheuermann's kyphosis may not present until adulthood.[25] Though the natural history of the disease remains debated, the deformity is generally accepted to have a benign course and not progress significantly once skeletal maturity has been reached.[26]

23.2.6 Adult Spinal Deformity

In skeletally mature adults, a preexisting deformity stemming from childhood, degenerative changes to the vertebrae, systemic disease, trauma, or surgical intervention may cause rigid spinal deformity. Spinal deformity has been demonstrated to have a significantly negative impact on the health-related quality of life.[10,27] Degenerative spinal deformity is becoming increasingly common due to the aging population. The asymmetry of the vertebrae or adjacent disk degeneration causing the deformity leads to an unequal distribution of stress on the structural elements over time in the adult, resulting in the disproportionally accelerated degeneration of disks and facet joints.

Adults who had been diagnosed with spinal deformity in childhood, or with endocrinological issues resulting in osteoporosis or osteopenia are at an increased risk for curve progression. The weakened vertebrae result in a decrease of the stability of the motion segments and therefore increased susceptibility to forces acting on the spine. If the loss of bone quality is advanced, it may result in compression fractures of the vertebrae combined with pain associated with the fractures and inactivity that may drive the progression of the deformity. The secondary dynamic support of the aging spine provided by the ligaments as well as the paraspinal muscles may weaken and atrophy in age, further destabilizing the deformity.[28] Compression of neural structures due to foraminal or central canal stenosis resulting from degenerative changes or fractures may occur.

23.3 Classification

A range of classification systems exist for both pediatric and adult rigid spinal deformities. The parameters considered differ depending on the population and the primary diagnosis the classification was designed for. Classifications are created to allow a structured approach to a disease and to allow physicians to perform treatment options using an evidence-based approach according to the disease state. A classification system should allow the physician to identify a pattern in the patient and attribute it to a disease state (frequently in a hierarchical manner correlating to the severity of the disease), ease communication among health care professionals, allow a more comprehensive study of various treatment options in comparison with the identical disease state, and allow the creation of standardized treatment recommendations for the individual disease states identified.[29]

The parameters assessed for the classification should be directly related to the severity of the disease to allow for high construct validity. The classification system should have high intrarater and interrater reliability and therefore be easily reproducible.

23.3.1 Pediatric Spinal Deformity Classifications

Pediatric classification systems for spinal deformity are generally based on the identification of a morphological type of curve, to allow for a prognosis as to the potential for progression of the deformity. This approach ultimately allows the physician to determine a treatment strategy most suitable for the patient's deformity.

Idiopathic Scoliosis Classifications

Idiopathic scoliosis can occur at any age of the growing child. It is categorized based on the age when it first develops, being broadly divided into infantile scoliosis (<3 years of age), juvenile scoliosis (3–9 years of age), and adolescent scoliosis (>10 years of age).[11,12,13]

King Classification

The King classification was developed in the early 1980 s for the treatment of spinal deformities with Harrington rods. It is based on the examinations of anteroposterior radiographs obtained from 149 patients. A line was drawn on the radiographs through the center of the sacrum and another line perpendicular to the iliac crests. The vertebrae centered closest to the line were designated as stable. King et al established five curve patterns based on the number and location of the curves (primary or secondary curve; thoracic and/or lumbar curve), the flexibility of the deformity, and the magnitude of the curves.[30] The classification does not take the three-dimensional characteristics of deformity into account. Intra- and interreporter reliability have been reported as poor to fair, specifically when compared to the Lenke classification.[31,32]

Lenke Classification

Lenke et al's classification was developed toward the end of the 20th century as a classification to address the shortcoming of the widely used King classification. The classification system was devised to be more comprehensive, to consider sagittal alignment, and to have a good intra- and interobserver reliability.[32] During the design of the system, anteroposterior, lateral, and right- and left-side-bending radiographs were evaluated. The scoliosis is classified according to the location of the deformity and the number of curves (1–6), which is combined with a lumbar spine modifier grading the severity of the lumbar curve (A, B, or C) and a sagittal thoracic modifier that describes the degree of thoracic kyphosis (–, N, or +) .

Congenital Scoliosis Classification

Congenital scoliosis classifications are more descriptive according to the bony anomalies in the spine. MacEwen[33] in 1968 divided the congenital spinal anomalies into three types: failure of formation, failure of segmentation, and mixed-type deformity. McMaster et al[19] in 1982 expanded the classification into defects in segmentation and defects in formation with multiple subtypes of each defect. If kyphosis is present as well, it is generally classified into three types according to the Winter[34] classification: type I develops through a failure of anterior vertebral body formation (posterior hemivertebra), type II is characterized by an anterior unsegmented bar, and type III represents mixed defects. Upper thoracic type I deformities have the worst prognosis in terms of progression during the growth period of the child.[17]

In 2009 Kawakami et al[35] developed a new classification and algorithm of care for congenital spinal deformities, based on three-dimensional understanding of the pathology. They state that using only two-dimensional images underestimates the pathology and a full three-dimensional estimation is needed. The pathologies are divided into solitary and multiple pathologies. There are four subtypes of pathologies: type I—simple solitary anomaly, type II—multiple solitary anomalies, type III—complex type deformity, and type IV—no formation anomaly present, only a segmentation failure.

Adult Spinal Deformity Classifications

Aebi Classification

The Aebi classification,[36] divided deformities into three subtypes. Type 1, primary degenerative scoliosis (de novo form), is usually located in the thoracolumbar or lumbar spine. The primary degenerative curve develops mostly on the grounds of primarily limited disk degeneration in one or more motion segments. These curves could also be referred to as diskogenic curves and are the result of an asymmetric degenerative change of the disk with the consecutive development of a frontal deviation and concomitant rotation with the facet joints on one side as a pivot leading to facet subluxation. The apex of these curves is usually between L2 and L3, and L3 and L4. These curves tend to accompany a significant rotational translation of the apical vertebra. The sagittal malalignment with concomitant instability is usually responsible for the severe postural back pain of these patients. The disk degeneration leads to spondylosis, disk bulging, osteophyte formation, hypertrophic facet joint osteoarthritis with hypertrophic ligamentum flavum, and calcification of these structures with osteophytes, all at the cost of the space in the spinal canal and foramina, thus contributing to the formation of lumbar spinal stenosis.

Type 2, progressive idiopathic scoliosis of the thoracic, thoracolumbar, and/or lumbar spine. These curves present themselves in a variety of forms, depending on whether they have been treated in childhood. The deformity can present in both the sagittal and coronal planes. The sagittal deformity almost always results in a flat back syndrome in the lumbar spine, corresponding with mechanical back pain and limitation of mobility. In cases in which a fusion was performed prior to degeneration a stenotic level may be present adjacent to a previously fused spine.

Type 3, secondary degenerative scoliosis, is divided into two subtypes. The first is scoliosis following idiopathic or other forms of scoliosis or occurring in the context of a pelvic obliquity due to a leg-length discrepancy, hip pathology, or a lumbosacral transitional anomaly, usually located in the thoracolumbar, lumbar, or lumbosacral spine. These secondary curves, with the causes being primarily external to the spine, do not have a relevant rotation; however, they are basically deviations in the frontal plain.

The second type of secondary degenerative scoliosis is scoliosis secondary to metabolic bone disease (mostly osteoporosis) combined with asymmetric arthritic changes or erosive (inflammatory) diskitis or vertebral fractures. Owing to bone weakness, there may be fractures, which create an asymmetric configuration with expression of either kyphosis or scoliosis or both.

Schwab–Scoliosis Research Society Classification

The Schwab–Scoliosis Research Society classification[37] is aimed at describing the relevant coronal aspects of the deformity. The sagittal components of the deformity are characterized through the three modifiers. The curve type is determined on the basis of maximal coronal angle measured according to the standard Cobb technique.

Curve type T: Patients with a thoracic major curve of >30 degrees (apical level of T9 or higher) are classified with curve type T.

Curve type L: Patients with a lumbar or thoracolumbar major curve of >30 degrees (apical level of T10 or lower) are classified with curve type L.

Curve type D: Patients with a double major curve, with each curve >30 degrees are classified with curve type D.

Curve type N: Patients with no coronal curve >30 degrees (i. e., no major coronal deformity) are classified with curve type N (normal).

The first sagittal modifier takes into account two radiographical parameters: pelvic incidence (PI) and lumbar lordosis (LL). The PI-LL modifier represents the difference between the angle measure of the PI and the angle measure of the LL. Patients with a PI-LL value of less than 10 degrees are classified with a PI-LL modifier of zero (0). Patients with a PI-LL value between 10 and 20 degrees are classified with a PI-LL plus modifier (+). Patients with a PI-LL value of greater than 20 degrees are classified with a double-plus PI-LL modifier (++).

The second modifier is in regard to the amount of pelvic tilt (PT) the patients have, indicating the amount of pelvic retroversion. Patients with a PT of less than 20 degrees are classified with a PT modifier of zero (0). Patients with a PT between 20 and 30 degrees are classified with a plus PT modifier (+). Patients with a PT greater than 30 degrees are classified with a double-plus PT modifier (++).

The global alignment modifier is the third modifier of the classification. It is based on the sacral vertical axis (SVA). The SVA is defined as the offset between the sagittal C7 plumb line and the posterior, superior corner of the sacrum. Patients with an SVA of less than 40 mm are classified with an SVA modifier of zero (0). Patients with an SVA between 40 and 95 mm are classified with a plus SVA modifier (+). Patients with an SVA greater than 95 mm are classified with a double-plus SVA modifier (++).

23.4 Conclusions

Over the years the classifications for scoliosis have evolved concordant with newer imaging modalities and newer instrumentation in order to provide caregivers a better understanding of the underlying pathology, the risks of progression, and the means needed to correct the deformity. Knowledge of the older classifications allows us to fully understand the pathology and develop new and more comprehensive classifications allowing better patient care.

References

[1] Marketos SG, Skiadas P. Hippocrates. The father of spine surgery. Spine. 1999; 24(13):1381–1387

[2] Hippocrates. On joints. In: Capps E, Page TE, Rouse WHD, Withington ET, eds., trans. Hippocrates: The Loeb Classical Library, vol III. London: W. Heinemann; 1927:200–397

[3] Dayer R, Haumont T, Belaieff W, Lascombes P. Idiopathic scoliosis: etiological concepts and hypotheses. J Child Orthop. 2013; 7(1):11–16

[4] Harrington PR. Treatment of scoliosis. Correction and internal fixation by spine instrumentation. J Bone Joint Surg Am. 1962; 44-A:591–610

[5] Abel MF, Shaffrey CI, Menezes AH. Pediatric spinal deformities. In: Benzel EC, ed. Spine Surgery: Techniques, Complication Avoidance, and Management. Philadelphia, PA: Churchill-Livingstone; 1999:565–612

[6] Weinstein SL. The Pediatric Spine: Principles and Practice. Vol. 1. New York, NY: Raven Press; 1994

[7] Lonstein JE, Winter RB, Bradford DS, et al. Moe's Textbook of Scoliosis and other Spinal Deformities. 3 rd ed. Philadelphia, PA: W.B. Saunders; 1995

[8] Dimeglio A, Bonnel F. Growth of the spine. In: Raimondi AJ, Choux M, Di Rocco C, eds. The Pediatric Spine. New York, NY: Springer-Verlag, 1989:39–83

[9] Wynne-Davies R. Familial (idiopathic) scoliosis. A family survey. J Bone Joint Surg Br. 1968; 50(1):24–30

[10] Bunnell WP. The natural history of idiopathic scoliosis. Clin Orthop Relat Res 1988(229):20–25

[11] Dobbs MB, Weinstein SL. Infantile and juvenile scoliosis. Orthop Clin North Am. 1999; 30(3):331–341, vii

[12] James JI. Idiopathic scoliosis; the prognosis, diagnosis, and operative indications related to curve patterns and the age at onset. J Bone Joint Surg Br. 1954; 36-B(1):36–49

[13] Gillingham BL, Fan RA, Akbarnia BA. Early onset idiopathic scoliosis. J Am Acad Orthop Surg. 2006; 14(2):101–112

[14] Miller NH. Cause and natural history of adolescent idiopathic scoliosis. Orthop Clin North Am. 1999; 30(3):343–352, vii

[15] James JIP, Lloyd-Roberts GC, Pilcher MF. Infantile structural scoliosis. J Bone Joint Surg Br. 1959; 41-B:719–735

[16] Goldstein LA, Waugh TR. Classification and terminology of scoliosis. Clin Orthop Relat Res. 1973(93):10–22

[17] Hedequist D, Emans J. Congenital scoliosis. J Am Acad Orthop Surg. 2004; 12 (4):266–275

[18] McMaster MJ. Congenital scoliosis. In: Weinstein SL, ed. The Pediatric Spine: Principles and Practice. 2nd ed. New York, NY: Lippincott Williams & Wilkins; 2001:161–177

[19] McMaster MJ, Ohtsuka K. The natural history of congenital scoliosis. A study of two hundred and fifty-one patients. J Bone Joint Surg Am. 1982; 64 (8):1128–1147

[20] Lonstein JE. Neuromuscular spinal deformities. In: Weinstein SL, ed. The Pediatric Spine: Principles and Practice. 2nd ed. New York, NY: Lippincott Williams & Wilkins; 2001:789–796

[21] McCarthy RE. Management of neuromuscular scoliosis. Orthop Clin North Am. 1999; 30(3):435–449, viii

[22] Sorensen KH. Scheuermann's Juvenile Kyphosis: Clinical Appearances, Radiography, Aetiology, and Prognosis. Copenhagen, Denmark: Blackwell Munkgaard; 1964

[23] Tribus CB. Scheuermann's kyphosis in adolescents and adults: diagnosis and management. J Am Acad Orthop Surg. 1998; 6(1):36–43

[24] Gordon GR. The Etiology of Scheuermann's Disease. The Textbook of Spinal Surgery. 2nd ed. Philadelphia, PA: Lippincott-Raven; 1997

[25] Wood KB, Melikian R, Villamil F. Adult Scheuermann kyphosis: evaluation, management, and new developments. J Am Acad Orthop Surg. 2012; 20 (2):113–121

[26] Murray PM, Weinstein SL, Spratt KF. The natural history and long-term follow-up of Scheuermann kyphosis. J Bone Joint Surg Am. 1993; 75(2):236–248

[27] Berven S, Deviren V, Demir-Deviren S, Hu SS, Bradford DS. Studies in the modified Scoliosis Research Society Outcomes Instrument in adults: validation, reliability, and discriminatory capacity. Spine. 2003; 28(18):2164–2169, discussion 2169

[28] Schwab FJ, Smith VA, Biserni M, Gamez L, Farcy JP, Pagala M. Adult scoliosis: a quantitative radiographic and clinical analysis. Spine. 2002; 27(4):387–392

[29] Bess S, Schwab F, Lafage V, Shaffrey CI, Ames CP. Classifications for adult spinal deformity and use of the Scoliosis Research Society-Schwab Adult Spinal Deformity Classification. Neurosurg Clin N Am. 2013; 24(2):185–193

[30] King HA, Moe JH, Bradford DS, Winter RB. The selection of fusion levels in thoracic idiopathic scoliosis. J Bone Joint Surg Am. 1983; 65(9):1302–1313

[31] Cummings RJ, Loveless EA, Campbell J, Samelson S, Mazur JM. Interobserver reliability and intraobserver reproducibility of the system of King et al. for the classification of adolescent idiopathic scoliosis. J Bone Joint Surg Am. 1998; 80(8):1107–1111

[32] Lenke LG, Betz RR, Harms J, et al. Adolescent idiopathic scoliosis: a new classification to determine extent of spinal arthrodesis. J Bone Joint Surg Am. 2001; 83-A(8):1169–1181

[33] MacEwen GD, Conway JJ, Miller WT. Congenital scoliosis with a unilateral bar. Radiology. 1968; 90(4):711–715

[34] Winter RB, Moe JH. Lonstein: Posterior spinal arthrodesis for congenital scoliosis: Analysis of cases of two-hundred ninety patients, five to nineteen years old. JBJS. 1984; 66A:1188–1197

[35] Kawakami N, Tsuji T, Imagama S, Lenke LG, Puno RM, Kuklo TR, Spinal Deformity Study Group. Classification of congenital scoliosis and kyphosis: a new approach to the three-dimensional classification for progressive vertebral anomalies requiring operative treatment. Spine. 2009; 34(17):1756–1765

[36] Aebi M. The adult scoliosis. Eur Spine J. 2005; 14(10):925–948

[37] Schwab F, Ungar B, Blondel B, et al. Scoliosis Research Society-Schwab adult spinal deformity classification: a validation study. Spine. 2012; 37(12):1077–1082

24 Strategies in the Correction of Rigid Spinal Deformities—Controversies between Anterior and Posterior Approach

Sebastien Charosky

Abstract

The author describes the surgical strategies and different treatment possibilities for surgical treatment of rigid spinal deformities. Anterior or posterior approach, rationale for the selection of either approach, and the correction strategy according to the location of the deformity, its shape and severity, the degree of flexibility or stiffness, and the global balance of the trunk in both coronal and sagittal planes, are all detailed in this chapter.

Keywords: rigid spinal deformity, anterior approach, PSO, vertebral column resection, VCR

24.1 Introduction

Combined anterior/posterior fusion procedures have traditionally been used to treat severe deformities. These procedures may include an anterior release with multiple disk excisions and grafting or even partial or total corpectomies performed, usually through a thoracotomy or thoracoabdominal approach followed in a staged or single session by a posterior spinal instrumentation and fusion. This combined approach has been promoted to provide increased deformity correction and fusion rates.[1,2,3,4,5] However, because the anterior approach has been shown to cause significant morbidity and complications,[5,6,7,8,9,10,11,12] a trend toward posterior-only surgery developed over the years. The development of more aggressive posterior approaches, including pedicle subtraction osteotomies and vertebral column resections, has shown the capability of very powerful deformity correction.[13,14,15,16,17] Nevertheless, the dramatic increase in neurologic and mechanical complications associated with these complex and challenging surgeries is a subject of increasing concern among the surgical community.[18,19,20,21,22,23] In response to this, there has been a resurgence of the anterior approach in recent years, with the development of minimally invasive techniques that address not the thoracic and thoracolumbar regions but the lumbar and lumbosacral regions.[24,25,26,27,28,29,30,31] These new minimally invasive anterior approaches provide an alternative to the deformity correction obtained by posterior-only surgery while lowering the complication rate. This chapter describes the advantages and disadvantages of these techniques and presents the author's view on the surgical options and strategies used to treat rigid deformities.

24.2 Patient Assessment and Surgical Strategy

The assessment of the spinal deformity patient is of capital importance and will determine the surgical strategy or strategies suitable to treat the problem. Several points need to be evaluated:

- The location of the deformity (thoracic, thoracolumbar, lumbar, lumbosacral).
- The shape and severity of the deformity (angular, short segment, or regular long segment).
- The degree of flexibility or rigidity of the deformity.
- Assessment of the global balance of the trunk (single plane or three-dimensional deformity; sagittal only or associated with a scoliosis).

24.2.1 Location of the Deformity

The area of the spine where the deformity is located is an essential point used to determine the surgical strategy. Every part of the spine is easily accessible from the back, but according to the level of the spine the morbidity associated with the anterior approach may differ. Thoracic and thoracolumbar deformities, when approached from the front, need a thoracotomy or even a thoracoabdominal approach, increasing the morbidity of the procedure and not always well tolerated in patients with a challenging respiratory situation.[6,7,9,10] Kim et al showed a fivefold increased risk of pulmonary embolism in patients undergoing a combined approach compared with a single posterior surgery.[7] These findings were confirmed by Piasecki et al[9] in their prospective study of 66 consecutive patients undergoing anterior/posterior spinal reconstructions for spinal deformity. They reported a high rate of thromboembolic disease for which a right-sided thoracoabdominal approach was an independent risk factor. Lee et al[6], in their recent literature review and meta-analysis, concluded that anterior fusion for adolescent idiopathic scoliosis leads to moderate to large declines in pulmonary function tests at 3 months postop, which later normalize at 2 years but do not increase beyond the preoperative levels. Furthermore, they report the same effect is seen with the less invasive video-assisted anterior approach. Burkett et al[32] showed a greater operative time and blood loss in the comparative analysis of fixed imbalance treated by posterior only or combined anterior/posterior approaches.

The situation is different in the lumbar or lumbosacral spine. In this region the anterior approach doesn't require the violation of the chest wall or the diaphragm and is hence much more easily tolerated, even by older patients. Newer techniques, with less invasive approaches of the lumbar and lumbosacral regions are available today and aim to minimize the risk of complications while allowing an efficient stabilization that may decrease the rate of mechanical failures associated with fusions of these segments. Mayer[27] described an anterior retroperitoneal approach to access the disks from L2 to L5. Molinares et al[24] showed that the oblique corridor to access L2 to L5 disks was found in 90% of the 133 MRI scans of their study and that the L5–S1 disk could be accessed by the same approach in 69% of the cases. The open lumbar interbody fusion technique, as described by Silvestre et al[26] in their series of 179 patients, was performed as a staged procedure after a posterior correction with instrumentation and fusion. They report an overall 11% complication rate. These results were confirmed by

Ohtori et al[25] in their series of 35 patients operated for lumbar degenerative disk disease. Another minimally invasive anterior approach to the lumbar spine is the extreme lateral approach. This technique includes a minimally invasive transpsoas retroperitoneal approach to access the lumbar disks from L 1 to L 5 and has gained popularity, especially in the United States. Although the reports from the literature[28,29,30,31] show a low complication rate between 6 and 12%, concern has been raised regarding the spinal nerve and psoas injuries following these procedures.[11,25]

In conclusion, regarding the location of the deformity, it could be advised that a posterior-based strategy is preferable when dealing with thoracic or thoracolumbar pathology, thereby avoiding violating the thorax or diaphragm. Regarding the lumbar and lumbosacral areas, an anterior approach represents a valid option as a first or second stage to achieve correction or to maximize the fusion rates. With the current available techniques these surgeries can provide good results in the correct indications with low complication rates. The decision as to whether a posterior only or a combined approach is indicated depends on the surgeon's experience and the patient's characteristics.

24.2.2 Shape and Severity of the Deformity

The shape and severity of the deformity will determine not only the degree of correction needed but also the extent of the fusion. Although short, angular deformities need a great degree of correction at the deformity site, thus implying a very aggressive release or even more frequently an osteotomy of some kind at the apex of the deformity, the extension of the fusion can usually be limited to the segments included in the deformed spine, and excluding the compensating areas above and below. On the other hand, when dealing with long, regular deformities the correction can be achieved by small amounts of correction distributed among several levels and thus including a longer fusion segment. While the first reports of vertebral column resection to treat severe spinal deformities included a double anterior and posterior approach like that described by Boachi-Adjei and Bradford,[33] most of the recently described techniques concern exclusively the posterior approach.[13,14,15,17,34]

A typical example of a short, angular deformity found frequently in today's practice is posttraumatic kyphosis. Although some authors, such as Steib et al,[35] still recommend a two-stage procedure, with first an anterior approach with release and strut awaiting graft followed by a second posterior instrumentation for correction and stabilization, most of the recent publications favor the single posterior approach.[21,36,37] A single posterior approach usually implies an osteotomy at the apex with either a pedicle subtraction or a vertebral column resection performed. These techniques are very powerful and efficient for correcting the deformity, but they are also associated with a high rate (30–68%) of complications. Despite this high rate of complications the clinical outcomes at 2 years do not seem affected.[21,36]

The author's preferred approach is a single-staged posterior surgery with a three-column osteotomy at the apex and placement of an expandable cage in the front that allows for partial lengthening of the anterior column. The careful lengthening of the anterior column enhances the possibility of correction by increasing the size of the hinge on which the correction is performed. This is followed by posterior closure of the osteotomy over the previously instrumented spine. This technique is useful to avoid overshortening of the spinal cord posteriorly and allows a very powerful correction of the kyphotic deformity (► Fig. 24.1).

In cases of severe, regular thoracic or thoracolumbar deformities, the situation is different. If the problem is the stiffness of the deformity, some kind of release of the spine is necessary. This can either be achieved through the disks or through the bone. If the surgeon wants to perform the release through the disks prior to the posterior correction a first anterior approach is necessary for disk excision and grafting. This poses a twofold

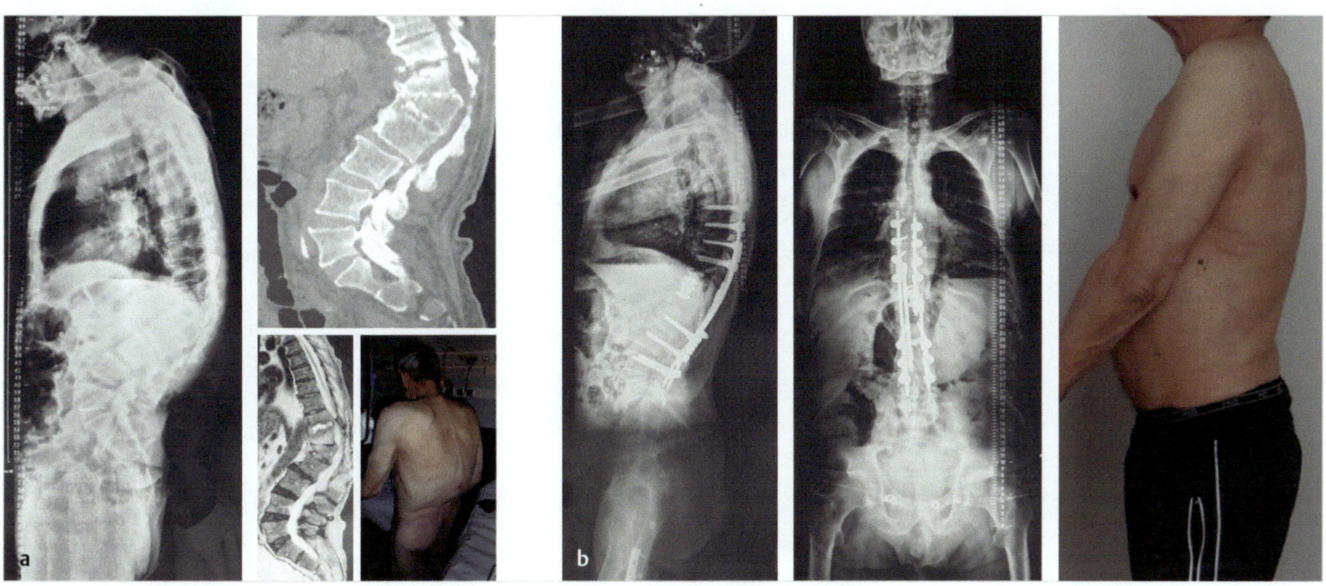

Fig. 24.1 **(a)** Preoperative severe posttraumatic kyphosis previously operated. Note the complete fusion of the vertebral bodies at the apex. **(b)** Two years postop: vertebral column resection at the apex of the deformity with expandable cage.

problem: the morbidity of the anterior thoracotomy or thoracoabdominal approach and the fact that the patient has to be bedridden until the posterior surgery is performed. This second concern can of course be avoided if both surgeries are performed in the same stage, which would on the other hand lengthen the procedure with the concomitant complications. The other option is to perform a more aggressive posterior approach that includes some kind of three-column osteotomy to correct the spine through the bone. Two examples are provided here. The first is a severe neglected thoracic idiopathic scoliosis. In this patient, a vertebral column decancellation was performed around the apex at the two adjacent levels to allow simultaneous correction of the frontal and sagittal planes. The resection according to this technique is a progressive removal of the cancellous bone inside the vertebral body so it will collapse under pressure during the reduction. To take into account the three-dimensional deformity and the correction needed, the amount of bone removed is more important on the convex side of the curve (▶ Fig. 24.2).

The second example is a severe neglected thoracolumbar kyphoscoliosis. In this case, even after multiple-level posterior column osteotomies the stiffness of the curve prevented satisfactory reduction. An asymmetrical pedicle subtraction osteotomy at the apex of the curve allowed excellent curve correction in the frontal plane while also correcting the thoracolumbar rotational kyphosis (▶ Fig. 24.3). Care must be taken when

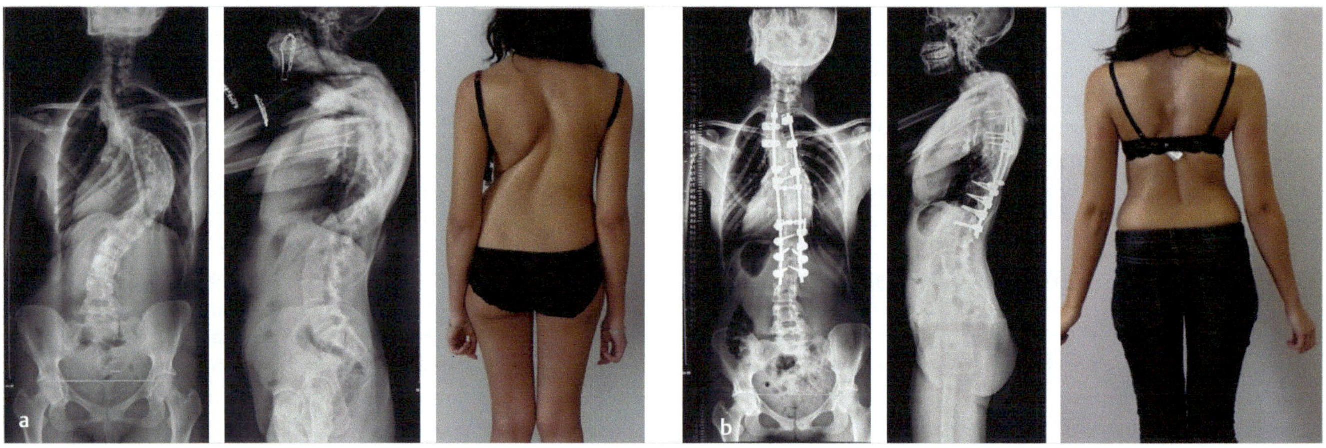

Fig. 24.2 (a) A 22-year-old patient with neglected thoracic idiopathic scoliosis. The main thoracic curve measures 98 degrees preoperatively. **(b)** At 5 years postoperative after T 2–L 2 correction and fusion with vertebral column decancellation D 8 and D 9.

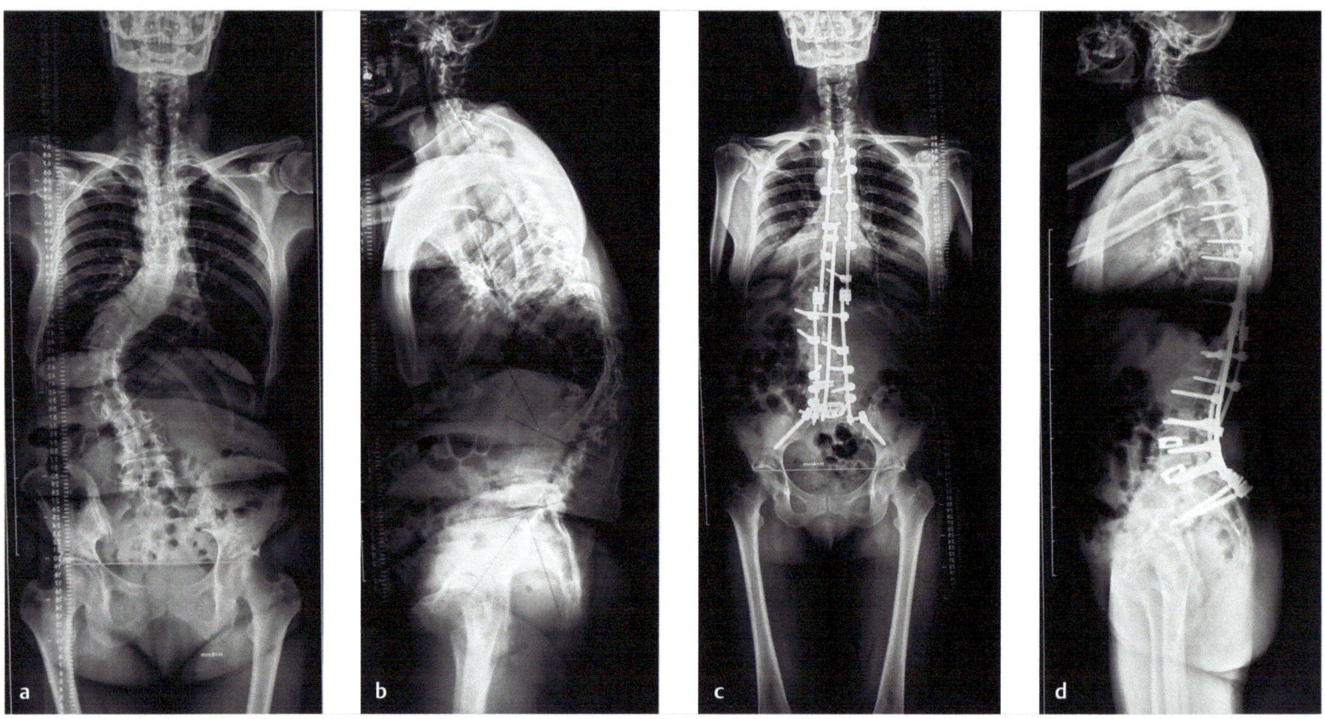

Fig. 24.3 (a–d) Pre- and postoperative X-rays of a 60-year-old patient with neglected idiopathic scoliosis. Surgery from T 2 to the pelvis, multiple posterior column osteotomies, and asymmetric posterior vertebral column resection at T 12.

performing osteotomies at the apex of these thoracolumbar curves because there is a high risk of residual frontal imbalance that may be due to overcorrection (imbalance toward the opposite convex side) or to undercorrection (imbalance to the same concave side). An intraoperative X-ray control with visualization of the pelvis is mandatory to avoid this complication.

24.2.3 Flexibility of the Deformity and Balance of the Trunk

Regarding flexibility, the spinal deformity can be described in terms of two extremes, with the majority of cases falling between those extremes, especially in cases of adult deformity. On one end there is the totally stiff spine in which every level is ankylosed and the disks are fused (ankylosing spondylitis or iatrogenic deformities after spinal fusion), and on the other end the flexible spine of juvenile idiopathic scoliosis. While the strategies are somewhat clear for the extreme cases, the debate persists concerning the vast majority of those that fall between them. We will concentrate here on the pathology of the lumbar segments, since the thoracic and thoracolumbar segments were already discussed.

The typical situation would be the patient with lumbar degenerative scoliosis and severe trunk imbalance in both the frontal and the sagittal planes, as shown in ▶ Fig. 24.4. Careful assessment shows disk spaces completely collapsed in several levels with vacuum phenomena and concave synostosic osteophytes. Despite the rigid aspect of the deformity and the severity of the imbalance the vacuum phenomena in the disks are a sign of potential mobility. The stiffness of this curve is largely the result of the locking osteoarthritic facets. After appropriate wide facet resection and eventually multiple posterior column osteotomies, the correction can be achieved without the need for pedicle subtraction osteotomy or other three-column procedures. This is a typical adult deformity case. The stiffness of the degenerative scoliosis patient is a combination of disk collapse, anterior and usually concave side synostosis, and facet osteoarthritis that may in reality be ankylosis.

Care must be taken to adequately restore the sagittal plane according to the pelvic parameters and respecting not only the value but also the distribution, shape, and length of the lumbar lordosis.[38,39] As always, after posterior column osteotomies the anterior opening of the concerned disks needs to be filled with structural graft. The anterior approach plays an important role here. Although interbody fusion is possible from the posterior approach, it demands entering the canal at multiple levels where it might not be necessary otherwise. Procedures such as transforaminal lumbar interbody fusion also increase the operative time, bleeding, and overall morbidity of this already complex surgery. Besides, it is our current opinion that restoration of lordosis is not as efficient, especially in the lumbosacral area where it is most needed. The preferred strategy in this kind of situation is to perform a staged anterior retroperitoneal paramedian approach that allows the surgeon to easily perform a fusion from the L3 to S1 disks with a single incision (▶ Fig. 24.5). This surgery can be delayed for 4 or 5 weeks, allowing the patient to recover conveniently from the first procedure and even to be discharged from the hospital before readmission for the anterior surgery.

Of course other strategies exist to treat the same problem. Supporters of the extreme lateral approach would probably start with a multilevel minimally invasive anterior approach followed by posterior instrumentation. Although this may be a suitable strategy, a word of caution is required regarding the first anterior approach, especially with long and wide rectangular cages. Restoration of disk height does not necessarily mean restoration of lordosis. This mistake is often seen and may have catastrophic consequences. Inability to restore the lumbar lordosis with the appropriate shape and distribution (around 70% at the L4–S1 segments) will lead to mechanical failure and proximal junctional kyphosis (▶ Fig. 24.6, ▶ Fig. 24.7). Another strategy that also carries potential complications is the all-posterior pedicle subtraction osteotomy in the context of mobile disks. Pedicle subtraction osteotomies are associated with an extremely high rate of mechanical failures.[21,22,23,36] It has been well demonstrated that the instability at the pedicle subtraction

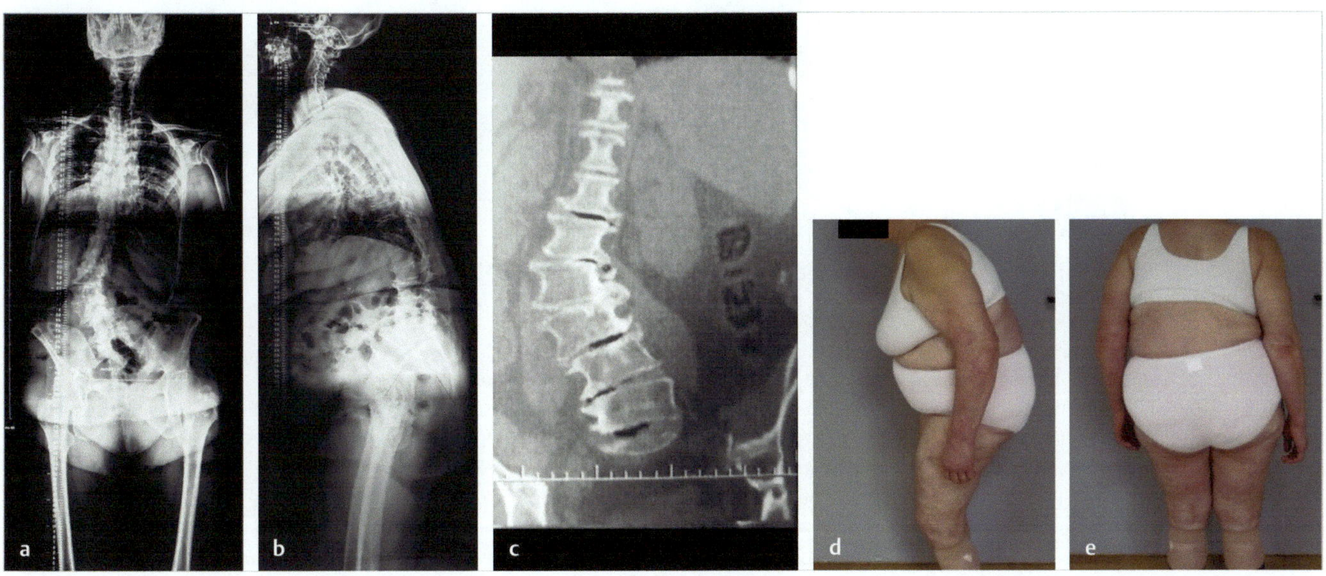

Fig. 24.4 (a–e) A 60-year-old patient with degenerative scoliosis. Frontal and sagittal imbalance with pelvic retroversion and loss of lumbar lordosis. Note vacuum phenomena in the lumbar disks and concave synostosis at the apex.

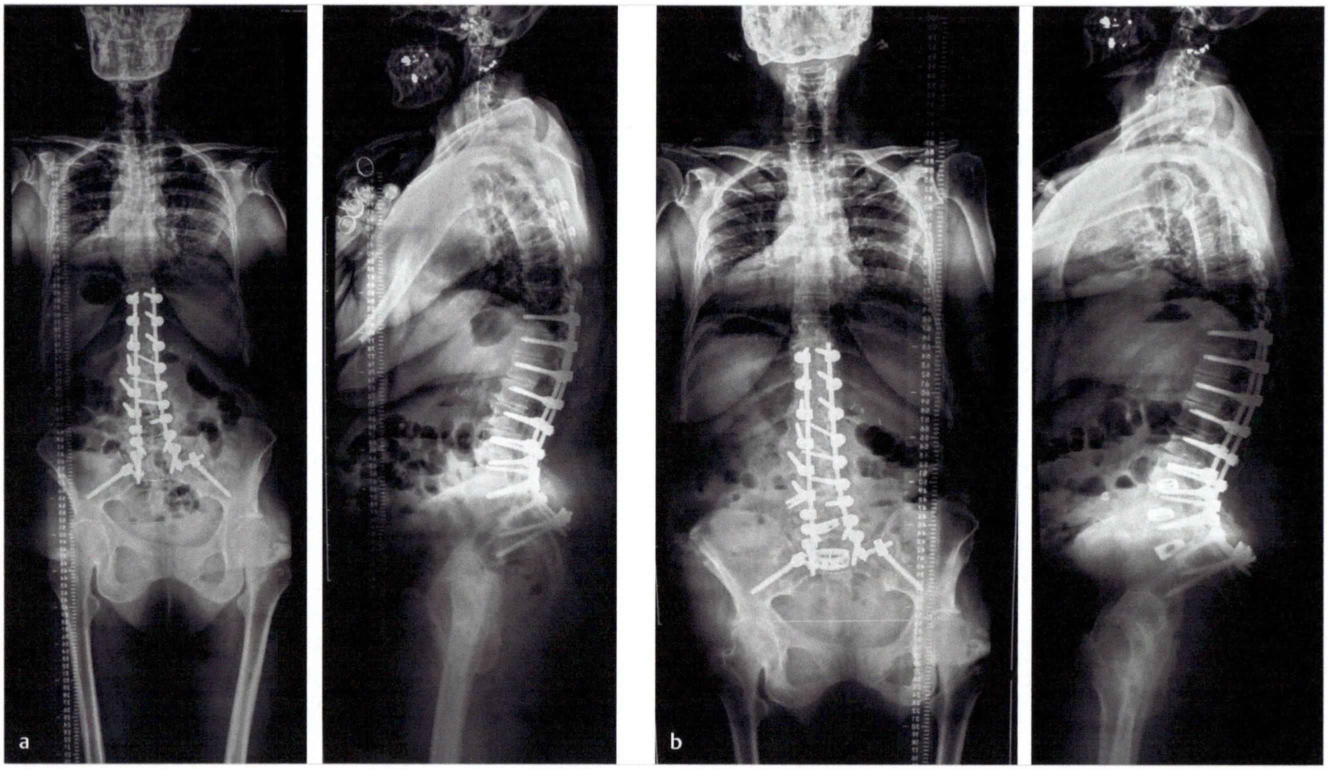

Fig. 24.5 **(a)** Postoperative after the first stage of posterior correction T 10–pelvis with multiple posterior column osteotomies. **(b)** Postoperative after second-stage anterior retroperitoneal paramedian approach from L 3 to S 1 performed 1 month later.

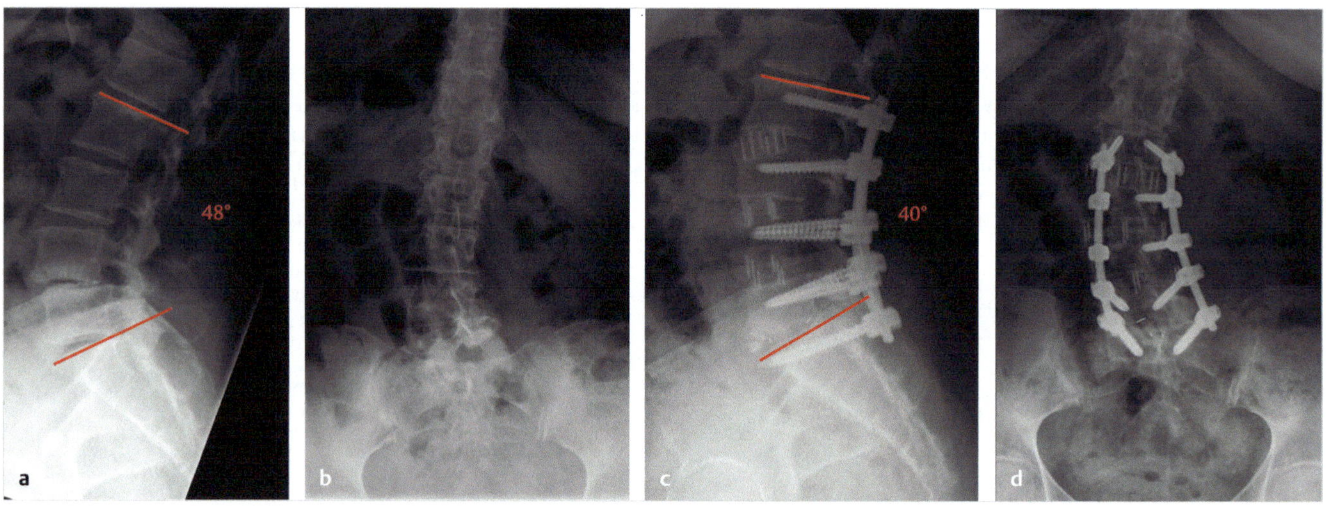

Fig. 24.6 **(a–d)** Pre- and postop X-rays of a patient who underwent first-stage anterior minimally invasive extreme lateral interbody fusion followed by posterior instrumentation. Note the decreased lordosis in the postoperative X-ray despite multilevel cages.

osteotomy is rotational in nature and increases with disk degeneration.[23] The only way to decrease this instability is to restore a solid anterior column that needs in most cases a staged anterior approach. The pedicle subtraction osteotomy loses in this context; one of the main reasons for performing it in the first place was the ability to solve the problem in a single posterior surgery and to avoid the anterior approach.

Another important issue that warrants discussion is the frontal balance of the trunk. In cases of scoliosis the imbalance on the frontal plane can either be toward the concavity or toward the convexity of the main lumbar or thoracolumbar curve. These situations and their treatment strategies are essentially different (▶ Fig. 24.8).

When the imbalance of the trunk is toward the concavity of the main lumbar or thoracolumbar curve, the correction of this curve will restore the appropriate balance. Furthermore, the correction of the thoracolumbar rotational kyphosis associated with the main curve goes in the same direction as the correction of

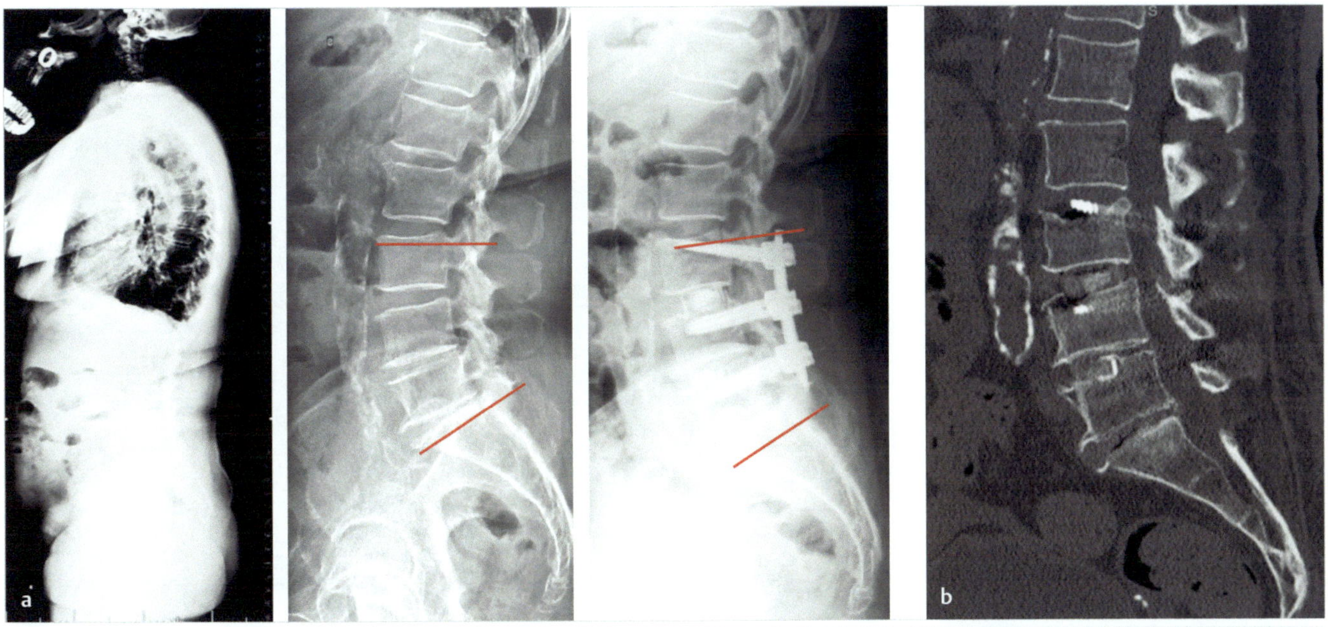

Fig. 24.7 **(a)** A 73-year-old patient who underwent first-stage extreme lateral interbody fusion followed by minimally invasive posterior instrumentation L 3–L 5. Preoperative L 3–S 1 lordosis is 35 degrees (*red line*). Postoperative L 3–S 1 lordosis is 25 degrees (*red line*). **(b)** Proximal junctional kyphosis of upper instrumented vertebra at 2 weeks postop.

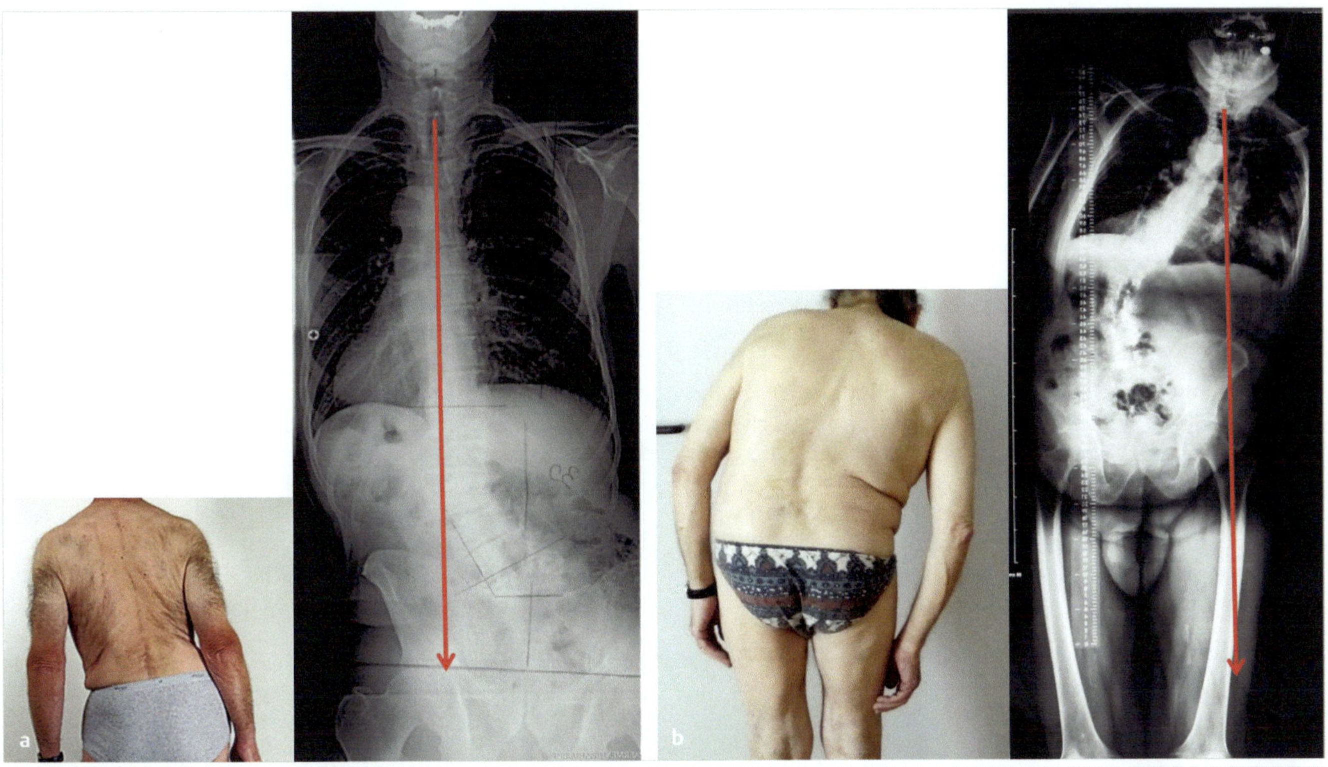

Fig. 24.8 Frontal Imbalance. **(a)** Imbalance toward the convex side of the main lumbar curve (*red arrow*). The origin of the imbalance is at L 5 (*gray line*). **(b)** Imbalance toward the concave side of the main thoracolumbar curve (*red arrow*).

the frontal imbalance. The correction strategy can then include every technique aimed at correcting the main curve: combined anterior/posterior surgery with disk excisions and grafting followed by posterior instrumentation with multiple wide facet resections or posterior column osteotomies; posterior approach with three-column osteotomy at the apex of the curve; or any other variation of these techniques. Special care must be given to the intraoperative assessment of the correction; X-ray control is mandatory to avoid overcorrection, especially when fusing to the pelvis (▶ Fig. 24.9).

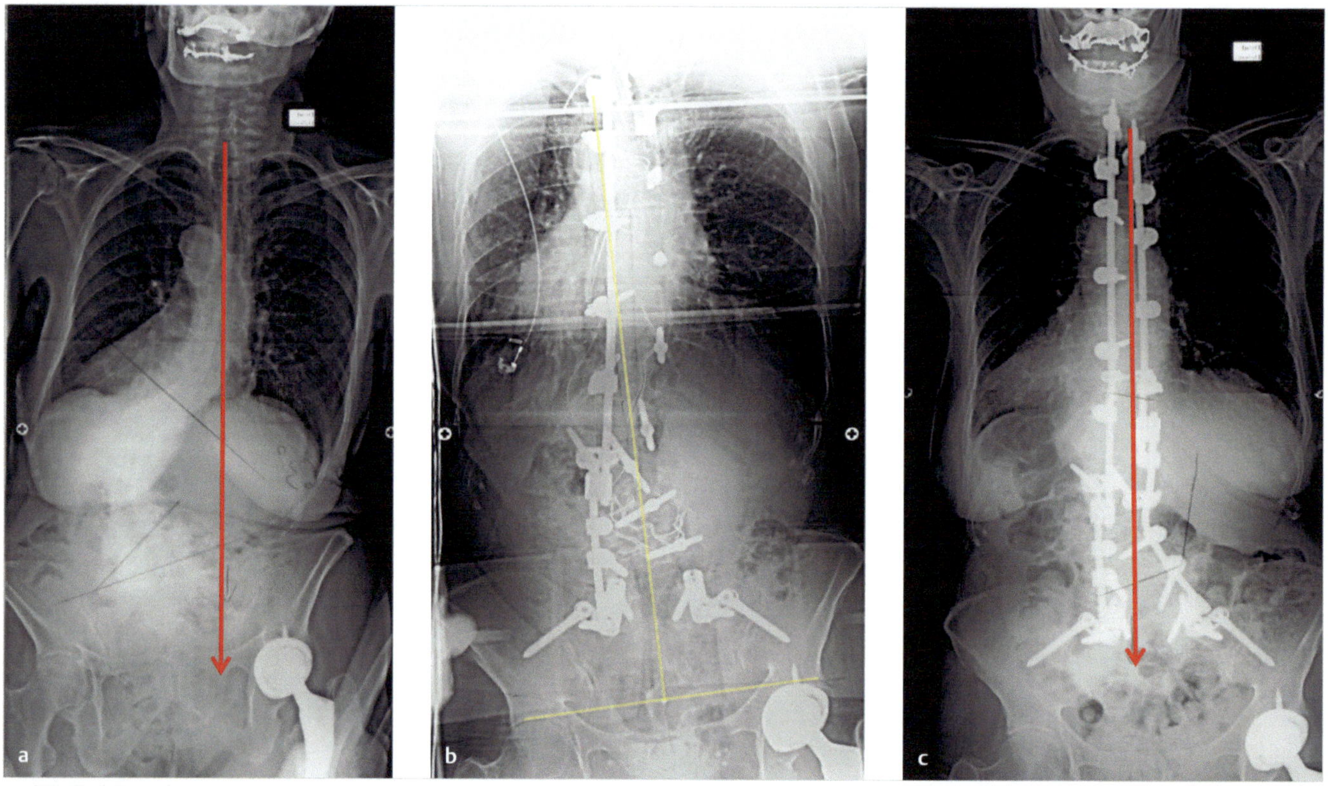

Fig. 24.9 **(a)** Patient with frontal imbalance toward the concavity of the main thoracolumbar curve (*red arrow*). **(b)** Intraoperative control with anteroposterior X-ray to evaluate frontal plane correction. Slight distraction was applied on the concave side rod. **(c)** Postoperative standing X-ray.

The other situation, when the trunk imbalance is toward the convexity of the main curve, is entirely different. The origin of the imbalance lies in the fractional lumbosacral curve. Three situations can give this same result as described by Chopin[40]:

1. Asymmetric lumbosacral disk degeneration, which results in the obliquity of L 4. This obliquity is at the beginning flexible but usually becomes fixed with evolution of the curve.
2. Malformative-like congenital or degenerative wedging of the L 5 vertebral body. An oblique takeoff of S 1 may also give rise to this situation with a degenerative curve that develops above.
3. Branch of candelabrum, typically over the age of 60. This presents with a short lumbosacral curve and a long curve above with major frontal imbalance and lumbosacral kyphosis with anterior imbalance of the trunk (▶ Fig. 24.10).

In these situations the maximum efforts of correction must be directed toward the lumbosacral region. Correction of the main and flexible lumbar curve above this fractional lumbosacral curve will result in increased frontal imbalance. The strategy has to be directed to the horizontalization of L 4. In some instances this can be achieved with posterior column osteotomies only, but very often a three-column osteotomy of either L 4 or L 5 is needed. Undercorrection of the main lumbar curve is advised to retrieve balance in the frontal plane.

24.3 Conclusion

Spine surgeons today have multiple techniques available for managing spinal deformities. Rather than always using the same technique to treat every patient, the surgeon should master several different techniques and apply each one of them in the right scenario. There is no such thing as the best technique for every deformity case; only the appropriate surgery applied to the right indication will provide a good outcome. On the other hand, there is not one single way to reach that objective. Different surgeons with different training and experiences may approach the same problem in different ways.

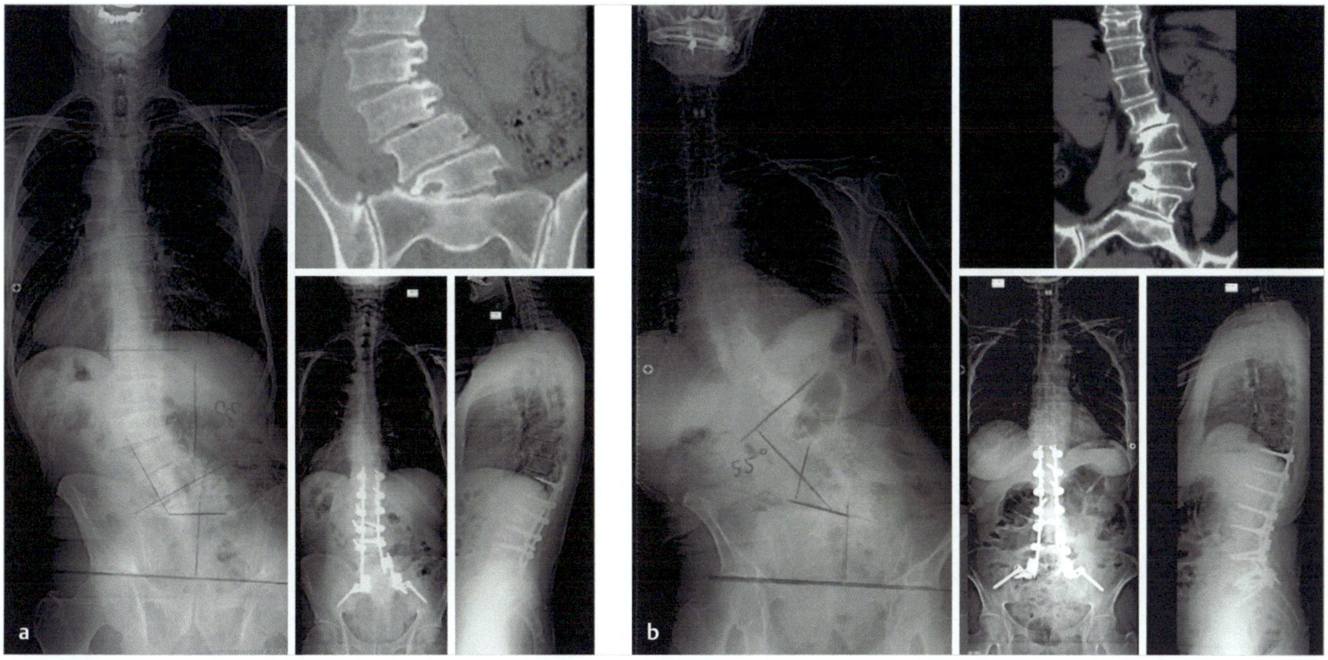

Fig. 24.10 (a) Malformative-like degenerative scoliosis with wedging of L 5. Correction with pedicle subtraction osteotomy (PSO) of L 5. **(b)** Asymmetric disk degeneration type. Correction with PSO of L 4.

References

[1] Bradford DS, Schumacher WL, Lonstein JE, Winter RB. Ankylosing spondylitis: experience in surgical management of 21 patients. Spine. 1987; 12(3):238–243

[2] Byrd JA, III, Scoles PV, Winter RB, Bradford DS, Lonstein JE, Moe JH. Adult idiopathic scoliosis treated by anterior and posterior spinal fusion. J Bone Joint Surg Am. 1987; 69(6):843–850

[3] DeWald RL, Faut MM. Anterior and posterior spinal fusion for paralytic scoliosis. Spine. 1979; 4(5):401–409

[4] Kaneda K, Matsuno S, Fujiya M, et al. Combined anterior and posterior procedure for severe spinal deformities. Orthop Trans. 1978; 2:280

[5] Berven SH, Deviren V, Smith JA, Hu SH, Bradford DS. Management of fixed sagittal plane deformity: outcome of combined anterior and posterior surgery. Spine. 2003; 28(15):1710–1715, discussion 1716

[6] Lee ACH, Feger MA, Singla A, et al. Effect of surgical approach on pulmonary function in adolescent idiopathic scoliosis patients. Spine. 2016; 22(41): E1343–E1355

[7] Kim HJ, Kepler C, Cunningham M, Rawlins B, Boachie-Adjei O. Pulmonary embolism in spine surgery: a comparison of combined anterior/posterior approach versus posterior approach surgery. Spine. 2011; 36(2):177–179

[8] Yagi M, Patel R, Boachie-Adjei O. Complications and unfavorable clinical outcomes in obese and overweight patients treated for adult lumbar or thoracolumbar scoliosis with combined anterior/posterior surgery. J Spinal Disord Tech. 2015; 28(6):E368–E376

[9] Piasecki DP, Poyton A, Mintz D, et al. Thromboembolic disease after combined anterior/posterior reconstruction for adult spinal deformity. Spine. 2008; 33 (6):668–672

[10] Pateder DB, Kebaish KM, Cascio BM, Neubaeur P, Matusz DM, Kostuik JP. Posterior only versus combined anterior and posterior approaches to lumbar scoliosis in adults: a radiographic analysis. Spine. 2007; 32(14):1551–1554

[11] Kim YB, Lenke LG, Kim YJ, et al. The morbidity of an anterior thoracolumbar approach: adult spinal deformity patients with greater than five-year followup. Spine. 2009; 34(8):822–826

[12] Good CR, Lenke LG, Bridwell KH, et al. Can posterior-only surgery provide similar radiographic and clinical results as combined anterior (thoracotomy/ thoracoabdominal)/posterior approaches for adult scoliosis? Spine. 2010; 35 (2):210–218

[13] Gertzbein SD, Harris MB. Wedge osteotomy for the correction of posttraumatic kyphosis. A new technique and a report of three cases. Spine. 1992; 17(3):374–379

[14] Suk SI, Kim JH, Kim WJ, Lee SM, Chung ER, Nah KH. Posterior vertebral column resection for severe spinal deformities. Spine. 2002; 27(21):2374–2382

[15] Charosky S, Harding IJ, Vialle R, et al. Transpedicular osteotomy in revision scoliosis surgery. J Bone Joint Surg. 2008; 90:450

[16] Dorward IG, Lenke LG, Stoker GE, Cho W, Koester LA, Sides BA. Radiographical and clinical outcomes of posterior column osteotomies in spinal deformity correction. Spine. 2014; 39(11):870–880

[17] Lenke LG, Sides BA, Koester LA, Hensley M, Blanke KM. Vertebral column resection for the treatment of severe spinal deformity. Clin Orthop Relat Res. 2010; 468(3):687–699

[18] Maier SP, Smith JS, Schwab FJ, et al. International Spine Study Group. Revision surgery after 3-Column osteotomy in 335 patients with adult spinal deformity. Spine. 2014; 39(11):881–885

[19] Xie JM, Zhang Y, Wang YS, et al. The risk factors of neurologic deficits of onestage posterior vertebral column resection for patients with severe and rigid spinal deformities. Eur Spine J. 2014; 23(1):149–156

[20] Pellisé F, Vila-Casademunt A, European Spine Study Group (ESSG). Posterior thoracic osteotomies. Eur J Orthop Surg Traumatol. 2014; 24 Suppl 1:S39–S48

[21] Auerbach JD, Lenke LG, Bridwell KH, et al. Major complications and comparison between 3-column osteotomy techniques in 105 consecutive spinal deformity procedures. Spine. 2012; 37(14):1198–1210

[22] Charosky S, Guigui P, Blamoutier A, Roussouly P, Chopin D, Study Group on Scoliosis. Complications and risk factors of primary adult scoliosis surgery: a multicenter study of 306 patients. Spine. 2012; 37(8):693–700

[23] Charosky S, Moreno P, Maxy P. Instability and instrumentation failures after a PSO: a finite element analysis. Eur Spine J. 2014; 23(11):2340–2349

[24] Molinares DM, Davis TT, Fung D. Retroperitoneal oblique corridor to the L2–S1 intervertebral discs: an MRI study. J Neurosurg Spine. 2016; 24(2):248–255

[25] Ohtori S, Orita S, Yamauchi K, et al. Mini-open anterior retroperitoneal lumbar interbody fusion: oblique lateral interbody fusion for lumbar spinal degeneration disease. Yonsei Med J. 2015; 56(4):1051–1059

[26] Silvestre C, Mac-Thiong JM, Hilmi R, et al. Complications and morbidities of mini-open lumbar interbody fusion: oblique lumbar interbody fusion in 179 patients. Asian Spine J. 2012; 6(2):89–97

[27] Mayer HM. A new microsurgical technique for minimally invasive anterior lumbar interbody fusion. Spine. 1997; 22(6):691–699, discussion 700

[28] Youssef JA, McAfee PC, Patty CA, et al. Minimally invasive surgery: lateral approach interbody fusion: results and review. Spine. 2010; 35(26) Suppl: S302–S311

[29] Rodgers WB, Gerber EJ, Patterson J. Intraoperative and early postoperative complications in extreme lateral interbody fusion: an analysis of 600 cases. Spine. 2011; 36(1):26–32

[30] Isaacs RE, Hyde J, Goodrich JA, et al. A prospective nonrandomized multicenter evaluation of extreme lateral interbody fusion for the treatment of adult degenerative scoliosis. Spine. 2010; 35 26S:S322–S330

[31] Phillips FM, Isaacs RE, Rodgers WB, et al. Adult degenerative scoliosis treated with XLIF: clinical and radiographical results of a prospective multicenter study with 24-month follow-up. Spine. 2013; 38(21):1853–1861

[32] Burkett B, Ricart-Hoffiz PA, Schwab F, et al. Comparative analysis of surgical approaches and osteotomies for the correction of sagittal plane spinal deformity in adults. Spine. 2013; 38(2):188–194

[33] Boachie-Adjei O, Bradford DS. Vertebral column resection and arthrodesis for complex spinal deformities. J Spinal Disord. 1991; 4(2):193–202

[34] Obeid I, Bourghli A, Boissière L, Vital JM, Barrey C. Complex osteotomies vertebral column resection and decancellation. Eur J Orthop Surg Traumatol. 2014; 24 Suppl 1:S49–S57

[35] Steib JP, Mezghani S, Charles YP, Mitulescu A. Double approach in thoracolumbar malunions. Eur Spine J. 2010; 19 Suppl 1:S48–S51

[36] Smith JS, Sansur CA, Donaldson WF, III, et al. Short-term morbidity and mortality associated with correction of thoracolumbar fixed sagittal plane deformity: a report from the Scoliosis Research Society Morbidity and Mortality Committee. Spine. 2011; 36(12):958–964

[37] El-Sharkawi MM, Koptan WM, El-Miligui YH, Said GZ. Comparison between pedicle subtraction osteotomy and anterior corpectomy and plating for correcting post-traumatic kyphosis: a multicenter study. Eur Spine J. 2011; 20 (9):1434–1440

[38] Roussouly P, Gollogly S, Berthonnaud E, Dimnet J. Classification of the normal variation in the sagittal alignment of the human lumbar spine and pelvis in the standing position. Spine. 2005; 30(3):346–353

[39] Mac-Thiong JM, Roussouly P, Berthonnaud E, Guigui P. Sagittal parameters of global spinal balance: normative values from a prospective cohort of seven hundred nine Caucasian asymptomatic adults. Spine. 2010; 35(22):E1193–E1198

[40] Chopin D. Spinal Stenosis and Degenerative Scoliosis. Cahiers d'ensignement de la SOFCOT. Paris: Elsevier; 2003:110–121

Further Reading

Bridwell KH. Decision making regarding Smith-Petersen vs. pedicle subtraction osteotomy vs. vertebral column resection for spinal deformity. Spine. 2006; 31(19) Suppl:S171–S178

MacLennan A. Scoliosis. BMJ. 1922; 2:864–866

O'Neill KR, Lenke LG, Bridwell KH, et al. Clinical and radiographic outcomes after 3-column osteotomies with 5-year follow-up. Spine. 2014; 39(5):424–432

25 Anesthesia for Spinal Surgery

Ruth Shaylor, Benjamin Drenger

Abstract

Anesthesia for spinal surgery can be challenging. The spinal cord has a complex blood supply that is susceptible to decreases in blood pressure. Patients presenting for spinal surgery may have multiple comorbidities or may have sustained trauma with other injuries present. A thorough preoperative assessment is essential in these cases. Airway management may be challenging and use of video laryngoscopy and, in some cases, fiberoptic intubation should be considered. These operations are long in duration and are often performed in the prone position. Meticulous care should be taken when positioning these patients to avoid pressure injuries. Neurophysiological monitoring limits the choice of anesthetic agents and techniques available. Use of a total intravenous anesthetic technique is almost ubiquitous. The specific drugs and doses used requires a thorough understanding of the effect of these agents on the type of monitoring used. Spinal surgery has traditionally been associated with large amounts of blood loss. Use of intraoperative cell salvage as well as other blood conservation techniques can limit the amount of blood transfusion required. In addition, pharmacological agents such as antifibrinolytics are also used to reduce blood loss. Pain should be aggressively managed with multimodal analgesia to minimize the risk of postoperative respiratory complications.

Keywords: anesthesia, preoperative assessment, transfusion, pain management

25.1 Introduction

Anesthesia for spinal surgery presents a challenge, not only because of the nature of the surgery itself but due to recent advances that have required a change in anesthetic technique. Surgeries are often long with a large anticipated blood loss. With the advent of neurophysiological monitoring (evoked potentials [EPs]), anesthesiologists are now required to convert from traditional inhalational anesthesia to a total intravenous anesthesia (TIVA) technique.

25.2 Spinal Cord

The spinal cord runs from the foramen magnum to the border of L1–L2 in the spinal canal formed by the cervical, thoracic, and lumbar vertebrae and is covered by three membranes. Attached to the spinal cord is the pia mater. The next layer of dura to surround the spinal cord is the arachnoid mater. Between the pia and arachnoid is the subarachnoid space that contains the cerebrospinal fluid (CSF). The CSF surrounds the spinal cord, supplying it with nutrients and removing waste products. The outermost layer of dura is the thick dura mater. Between the dura mater and the arachnoid is the subdural space, and between the dura and the bone is a potential space, the epidural space, that contains adipose tissue and the venous plexus.

Nerve transmission is arranged in different pathways depending on the type of information carried. These are referred to as tracts and named according to the different regions they travel to. Pain, proprioception, and vibration are carried in the dorsal column, whereas pain and temperature are carried in the anterolateral pathways. These are referred to as the ascending pathways. Nerve fibers enter at the level of the spinal cord and ascend on the ipsilateral side. At the level of the medulla they decussate and cross over to the contralateral side and continue to ascend to the sensory cortex.

The motor system is carried in the anterior descending pathway known as the corticospinal tract. It originates in the motor cortex, then descends on the ipsilateral side to the medulla where it decussates and continues to descend on the contralateral side. Ten percent of axons do not decussate, and instead, continue to descend on the ipsilateral side as the ventral corticospinal tracts.

Understanding the different spinal pathways can help predict the pattern of injury when different areas of the spinal cord are damaged.

25.3 Blood Supply

Traditionally blood supply to the spinal cord was thought to arise primarily from three main inputs: cephalic, caudal, and intermediate. The cephalic supply arises from the vertebral arteries; the intermediate input is via the intercostal arteries, including the large radicular artery, the artery of Adamkiewicz, originating between T8 and L1. The diameter of this artery is large at the caudal end, while the lower region of the anterior spinal artery has a small diameter and high resistance to flow; thus blood contribution to the central cord is marginal. The arterial blood flow in the major thoracic and lumbar spinal arteries is supported by a complex and intertwined spinal collateral arterial network (SCAN), which is nourished from the major aortic collaterals along the spinal cord. The caudal supply to the cord is from the internal iliac arteries.

Perfusion pressure in the SCAN = mean arterial pressure (MAP)—CSF pressure. The higher the MAP, the higher the perfusion pressure. The SCAN is a dynamic system able to undergo postoperative remodeling. Adaptations in response to decreased perfusion pressure include increasing the diameter of the anterior spinal artery and dilatation of the epidural veins. Later modifications include realignment of arterioles parallel to the spinal cord allowing for increased perfusion. These changes can be enhanced by increasing MAP and may reverse neurologic deficit if present.[1]

25.4 Preoperative Assessment

In the next paragraphs we will define the disorders that create a rigid spine deformity.

25.4.1 Preexisting Conditions

In patients with spinal deformities a detailed medical history should be taken. Patients with neurodegenerative disorders are at an increased risk for spinal deformities, as well as pulmonary and cardiovascular complications. In addition, succinylcholine is absolutely contraindicated in these patients.[2] Other neurologic diseases associated with spinal deformities include poliomyelitis, cerebral palsy, congenital myotonia, and neurofibromatosis.[3] Multiminicore disease is associated with scoliosis and malignant hyperthermia. Prevalence is unknown but inheritance is mainly autosomal recessive. Often it is asymptomatic and the scoliosis mild. As such, all patients with a scoliosis should also be questioned about a family history of muscle disease and of anesthetic complications, and there should be a high index of suspicion for malignant hyperthermia.[4] These days, increasingly large spinal operations are being performed on an aging population who may have other chronic health problems in addition to the spinal deformity itself.

25.4.2 Airway

All patients should have a thorough airway assessment prior to anesthesia. Patients with rheumatoid arthritis may have limited neck and jaw movements. Those with cervical spine disorder, should be assessed for a full range of neck movements. In addition, lateral cervical spine X-rays are mandatory in these patients prior to anesthesia. Patients presenting for cervical spine surgery may be in traction or a halo frame, making conventional intubation impossible, and awake fiberoptic intubation should be considered.

25.4.3 Respiratory System

Patients presenting for spinal surgery are at increased risk of preoperative respiratory problems, particularly those with scoliosis or neurodegenerative disorders. Scoliosis causes a restrictive lung defect, with chronic hypoventilation. The severity of pulmonary problems associated with scoliosis is related to the angle of the curvature, the cephalad location, and the number of vertebrae involved. All patients with thoracic scoliosis should undergo pulmonary function tests. A forced vital capacity of less than 30% predicted indicates an increased likelihood of needing postoperative ventilatory support. In addition to pulmonary function tests, arterial blood gas analysis should be carried out to assess the level of hypoventilation and ventilation perfusion mismatch. Arterial blood gas analysis may not be practical in the pediatric population. Those with a thoracic scoliosis curvature greater than 100 degrees are generally considered to be at risk of pulmonary complications, whereas those with a curvature less than 60 degrees are considered to be at low risk; however, severity of lung problems cannot be determined on angulature alone.[5] Patients who require continuous positive airway pressure (CPAP) at night are also considered high-risk patients and should have their CPAP machine available to them for immediate postoperative use. In addition to pulmonary function tests and arterial blood gas analysis, a chest radiograph should be taken and analyzed for signs of pulmonary and cardiac displacement or compression as well as signs of chronic infection.

25.4.4 Cardiovascular System

Patients presenting for spinal surgery may have a variety of cardiac problems either due to preexisting neuromuscular conditions or due to the spinal deformity itself. Scoliosis can cause right-sided heart failure from chronic hypoxemia leading to pulmonary hypertension secondary to distortion of the mediastinum and chest cavity. Patients with Duchenne muscular dystrophy have an increased risk of carodiomyopathy, which can lead to perioperative heart failure, and are susceptible to intraoperative fluid overload. In addition, changes in cardiac position intraoperatively during distraction and manipulation of the thoracic spine may cause unexpected life-threatening cardiac complications.

25.4.5 Neurologic System

A thorough neurologic exam should be performed and any preexisting neurologic deficits documented. Speech and swallowing should be assessed for any signs of bulbar palsy that may indicate a need for postoperative ventilation. In patients undergoing operations on the cervical spine it is vital that a full neurologic examination is recorded preoperatively to help determine if any postoperative deficit is the result of intubation, positioning, or the operation itself. In addition, patients with high spinal lesions may be at risk of autonomic hyperreflexia, which can cause problems with cardiovascular stability under anesthesia.

25.4.6 Trauma

In patients who suffer trauma to the spinal cord, neurogenic shock starts almost immediately after the injury and continues for around 3 weeks. These patients have a sympathectomy below the level of the lesion with associated vasodilatation, decreased systemic vascular resistance, and hypotension. If the lesion is above T6 there may be severe hypotension due to vasodilatation in the splanchnic vascular beds. Sympathetic supply to the heart is from T2–T6 and lesions above this may cause bradycardia as the parasympathetic stimulation is still preserved. Administration of large volumes of intravenous fluids in this situation is unlikely to treat the associated hypotension and may cause pulmonary edema. Vasopressors are the treatment of choice.[6]

Diaphragmatic innervation is from C3 to C5. Generally in lesions below C4 the diaphragm is preserved, but there is paralysis of the intercostal muscles with impaired cough and paroxysmal rib movement.[5] There is a reduction in respiratory reserve with a decrease in forced vital capacity and functional residual capacity, and an increase in expiratory reserve volume. Active expiration is also impaired.[7] Other complications associated with long-term spinal trauma include delayed gastric emptying, increased risk of venous thromboembolism, and impairment of thermoregulation.

Above the level of the lesion there may be vasoconstriction and tachycardia, an attempt to compensate for the vasodilatation and decreased systemic vascular resistance below the lesion. Autonomic dysreflexia presents 3 to 6 weeks post–spinal cord injury and is characterized by a heightened sympathetic response (tachycardia, hypertension), when the patient is stimulated below the level of the lesion. It tends to be more pronounced with more serious cardiac complications in lesions above T7.[8]

25.5 Induction and Maintenance

Anesthesia induction is determined by anatomical factors, muscular factors, and the need for neurophysiologic monitoring.

In those patients who do not need special airway management, induction may be achieved by intravenous agents or inhalational agents following adequate preoxygenation, depending on the patient's age and preexisting intravenous access. The use of muscle relaxants to assist intubation depends on the patient's preexisting conditions and whether or not neurologic monitoring is to be used. Succinylcholine is absolutely contraindicated in those with muscular dystrophies. In patients who have spinal trauma resulting in denervation there is an increased risk for succinylcholine-related electrolyte complications due to prejunctional nicotinic receptors that may lead to hyperkalemia and cardiac arrest when succinylcholine is used on induction. If a patient requires neuromonitoring then muscle relaxation interferes with these. A single reduced dose of an intermediate-acting nondepolarizing muscle relaxant (atracurium 0.4 mg/kg, or rocuronium 0.6 mg/kg) may be administered, as most of its effect has vanished by the time EPs are closely monitored.

Sedative premedication is generally avoided, especially in those with chronic hypoxia because this can exacerbate the hypoxia. Awake fiberoptic intubation should be considered for those with an unstable cervical spine or potentially difficult airway. If the patient is being considered for awake fiberoptic intubation then an antisialagogue, such as glycopyrrolate (200–400 µg IV or IM) may be considered. In addition, adequate anesthetization of the airway is essential. How this is carried out varies from physician to physician, but the patient's weight and maximum local anesthetic doses should be taken into account to avoid local anesthetic toxicity. Direct videolaryngoscopy is used frequently for difficult or nonconventional intubation. Whereas this minimizes cervical spine movement, it does not eliminate it; thus, awake fiberoptic intubation remains the gold standard when extension of the neck may illicit neurologic symptoms due to subluxation of C 1–C 2.[9]

Often, particularly in extensive corrective surgery, the surgeon may request a hypotensive technique to minimize blood loss. Generally, the anesthetic agents used during TIVA (i. e., propofol and remifentanil) are sufficient to achieve the desired MAP of 50–60 mm Hg. Rarely direct vasodilators are used, this is achieved either by an infusion of sodium nitroprusside or nitroglycerin because these are the easiest to titrate to effect. Sodium nitroprusside is metabolized to cyanide, and if this is used regular arterial blood gas analysis should be performed to monitor for increased arterial oxygen tension and acidosis, both of which are a sign of potential cyanide toxicity. If a hypotensive technique is being used then MAP should be kept above 60 mm Hg and tachycardia avoided.

In patients where neurophysiologic monitoring is not being used then anesthesia can be maintained with inhalational agents, muscle relaxants, and opioid boluses provided there are no other contraindications. The use of volatile anesthetics is contraindicated in patients where EPs are to be used, and a TIVA approach should be used. Most neurophysiologists will allow the use of nitrous oxide up to 50% before they start to see an effect on the quality of the EPs.

25.5.1 Neurophysiologic Monitoring

For surgeries where there is a potential for neurologic injury, monitoring of EPs is indicated. Nerve injury may be primary due to distractive forces or direct instrumental injury, or secondary due to ischemia caused by prolonged traction. The injury may be reversible if it is detected before the elastic limit of the nerve fiber is reached.

Monitoring EPs in spinal surgery usually consists of somatosensory evoked potentials (SSEPs) and transcranial motor evoked potentials (MEPs). SSEPs consist of a stimulus applied over a peripheral nerve and detected in the somatosensory cortex via scalp electrodes. It assesses the integrity of the posterior spinal tracts. A change in SSEP is thought to be significant if there is a 50% reduction in amplitude and a 10% increase in latency. MEPs consist of a stimulus applied to the motor cortex or directly to the spinal cord and detected over a peripheral nerve or muscle. MEPs are thus used to assess the integrity of the descending pathways. If MEPs are to be used it is essential to insert a bite block after induction to protect the patient's teeth and tongue. Hypotension increases the sensitivity of the spinal cord to injury, and there may be ischemic changes to the EPs without the presence of neurologic injury, or with small extraction forces applied.

Inhalational anesthetic agents greater than a minimum alveolar concentration (MAC) of 0.6 can interfere with interpretation of SSEPs via a dose-dependent reduction in amplitude and an increase in latency. Bolus administration of opioids produces a small but predictable reduction in amplitude and increase in latency in SSEPs, and muscle relaxants have no effect.

MEPs are exquisitely sensitive to both IV and inhalational anesthetics and a MAC of more than 0.6 should be avoided.[10] Even a bolus of 2 mg/kg of propofol will obliterate transcranial MEPs. MEPs can be made more reliable in the presence of anesthesia by using multiple pulse transcranial stimulation.

In operations where SSEPs and transcranial MEPs are being used, anesthesia maintenance is generally achieved by IV propofol 3–5 mg/kg/h plus remifentanil 0.03–0.05 µg/kg/min infusion with 50% nitrous oxide. In patients where the use of muscle relaxants is unavoidable (complex ventilation requirements), we recommend an infusion of rocuronium 2 µg/kg/min titrated to keep neuromuscular monitoring train-of-four twitch within 80% of baseline. In addition to monitoring physiologic parameters, close contact should be kept with the neurophysiologists to ensure that the dose of anesthetic (particularly propofol) does not interfere with adequate interpretation of EPs, and to ensure the depth of anesthesia is adequate in the electroencephalographic (EEG) monitoring.

25.5.2 Bispectral Index (BIS) Monitoring

In some surgeries, TIVA may be used without EP monitoring. In this situation, BIS monitoring is very useful. BIS is a monitor (Medtronic) that takes a modified EEG and by using Fourier analysis converts the EEG data into a single number between 0 and 100. A BIS result between 40 and 60 is considered to indicate an adequate plane of anesthesia. Below 40 and the patient is in deep anesthesia and above 60 there is a risk of awareness. BIS monitoring and its usefulness as a tool to reduce awareness during anesthesia remains controversial; however, a 2007 Cochrane Review concluded that BIS monitoring is a very useful method for managing adequate depth of anesthesia without muscle relaxants and could improve anesthesia delivery, particularly time to extubation, and decrease the risk of awareness in operations where end-tidal monitoring is not relevant or available.[11]

During TIVA use of BIS monitoring is essential to track the depth of anesthesia and adjust the rate of anesthetic infusions accordingly. If BIS is not available, the raw EEG tracing from the intraoperative EP monitoring may be used, but it is not continually controlled by the anesthesiologist, and its interpretation is more cumbersome.

25.5.3 Other Monitoring

Spinal surgeries tend to require long periods of anesthesia in positions that may cause physiological compromise. In addition to standard American Society of Anesthesiologists monitoring we also use invasive blood pressure monitoring usually via a radial arterial line. It allows beat-to-beat blood pressure monitoring, particularly critical when a hypotensive technique is required, as well as immediate identification of hemodynamic changes that may occur in the prone position or during spinal manipulation. Although transesophageal echocardiography may be tempting to use, the practicalities of inserting and using it in the prone position mean its use is not routine. This is particularly true when the probe has to be protected from biting during the use of MEPs.

Central venous pressure may be falsely elevated in the prone position due to increased intra-abdominal and thoracic pressures. In our institution we find that two large-bore peripheral cannulae provide adequate IV access; thus a central venous line is inserted only if the patient is expected to be hemodynamically unstable or there is an indication that potent ionotropic support may be required.

Temperature loss is almost inevitable during long operations with a large area of exposure. A forced air blanket and warming of IV fluids to 40 °C is used as a standard to minimize heat loss.

Finally a urinary catheter with urometer is inserted to monitor urine output, which can give an indication of prerenal fluid status and renal function.

25.6 Positioning

Patient positioning depends on the level of the spinal column that is to be operated on. Before induction, attention should be paid to contractures or any preexisting limitations to movement, and these should be considered prior to positioning the patient.

Operations on the lumbar spine are generally performed in the prone position. This requires the use of a special table that allows the abdomen to hang freely, reducing the increase in intra-abdominal pressure, aortocaval compression, and, more importantly, epidural venous pressure that causes an increase in blood loss and poor hemostasis of the surgical field. In the prone position it is essential that the head be at the same level as the shoulders with the neck in the neutral position. The face should be checked to make sure that there is no pressure on the nose and eyes, and this should be repeated at regular intervals throughout the operation. A special foam pillow can be used that has a hole cut out for the nose and eyes as well as a separate hole cut out for the endotracheal tube.

Ophthalmic complications have been described following spinal surgery, the most common of these being ischemic optic neuropathy. Initially this was thought to be due to direct pressure on the eyes when the patient is in the prone position. Recently, however, it has been shown that this is more likely due to hypotension during the procedure. One review of nine cases of postoperative visual loss found that risk factors for postoperative visual loss included repeat procedure, long procedure time, and large procedural blood loss. Perhaps more importantly, the authors also reported that in three of these cases the postoperative visual loss was reversed with prompt treatment of hypotension with fluid resuscitation. They do not recommend the use of vasopressors to treat hypotension as vasoconstriction may make the situation worse.[12]

The arms are generally bent and placed at the patient's sides, with padding at the elbows to protect the ulna nerve. Care should be taken to ensure the shoulders are not extended beyond 90 degrees to protect the brachial plexus. Depending on the operation the legs will either be level with or below the spine. Elasticated stockings (compression stockings) or Flowtron boots should be used to increase venous return and decrease the possibility of venous thromboembolism. Knees and ankles should be padded to prevent nerve injury.[13] During positioning from supine to prone and vice versa there is increased potential to accidentally remove indwelling catheters, or worse, accidentally extubate the patient, particularly if the patient is not paralyzed. Prior to moving the patient it is essential to ensure that he or she is sufficiently anesthetized to prevent coughing on transfer.

Thoracic surgery may be performed posteriorly in the prone position or anteriorly using a lateral approach. Patients placed in the lateral position may be supported via either a beanbag or a central chest support. It is essential to pad the knees and elevate the axilla slightly to avoid compression to the brachial plexus. This is usually done by placing a silicon roll under the chest. If lung deflation is required to increase access then a double-lumen endotracheal tube should be considered.

Cervical spine surgery may be performed via an anterior or a posterior approach. Posterior approach surgery is usually done with the head supported by a skull clamp so the position of the spine can be easily adjusted. Insertion of the pins is exquisitely painful but short-lived. A bolus of a short-acting opioid (e.g., alfentanil) provides adequate analgesia for this. If the head is instead placed on a horseshoe headrest then the orbits and maxilla are at risk of injury and should be checked regularly for pressure. Cervical spine surgery may carry increased risk for air embolism if the level of surgery is above the level of the heart. This risk is increased if the reverse Trendelenburg position is used to decrease venous bleeding. Anterior cervical surgery may require the use of an armored tube if there is a risk of edema or compression of the airway.

25.7 Blood Conservation Techniques

Blood loss during spinal surgery depends on the type of surgery and the number of levels exposed. In posterior spine surgery, veins adherent to bone are particularly prone to bleeding due to their poor ability to collapse. Due to the large surface area of decorticated bone that is exposed, blood loss is dependent on MAP, particularly if intra-abdominal pressure is also raised. Blood loss can be minimized by hypotensive techniques and special frames that allow the abdomen to hang free, thus reducing intra-abdominal pressure and epidural venous pressure. Even minor changes in position on the Wilson frame can reduce blood loss by 50% per spinal level.[14] Other techniques include hemodilution, autologous blood donation, cell saver, and pharmacological agents. Blood loss may be associated with poor wound healing and a higher incidence of wound infection.[15] Blood transfusion is not without its risks, including, hypothermia, infection, acute lung injury, and transfusion reactions from incompatible units.

Hemodilution involves removing blood from the patient after induction and replacing it with the same volume of crystalloid fluid. This is usually done on the basis of preoperative blood volume, and hematocrit. Usually patients are bled down to a hematocrit of 30%.

Volume removed = estimated blood volume × (initial hematocrit – target hematocrit) / mean hematocrit

At the end of the operation the blood is returned to the patient.[16]

In autologous blood donation, the patient donates units of blood 3 weeks before the operation. This may reduce blood loss by up to 75% in lumbar surgery. This technique is only suitable for patients over 30 kg, but it has the disadvantage of being expensive with potential for waste if the blood is not used.

Intraoperative cell salvage involves collecting intraoperative blood via special suction catheters, following which the red blood cells are separated from the rest of the fluid, washed, and returned to the patient. The returned blood does not contain any clotting factors, and these will need to be replaced using fresh frozen plasma. A consensus statement by the Royal College of Physicians concluded that despite initial costs cell salvage may well lead to an overall cost saving to the hospital.[17]

Pharmacological agents include antifibrinolytics and recombinant factor VII. Recombinant factor VII has not been found to significantly decrease blood loss in spinal surgery in randomized controlled trials. Unlike antifibrinolytic agents it is associated with an increase in thromboembolic events, and its use is not recommended.[5] Antifibrinolytic agents such as tranexamic acid, which is a lysine analogue, prevent clot breakdown by fibrinolysis. There have been several studies looking at the effectiveness of these agents given both systemically and topically via irrigation. Tranexamic acid has been shown to be effective in reducing blood loss and transfusion requirements when given both systemically and in surgical irrigation.[18]

25.8 Wake-Up Test

First described by Stangara in 1973, the wake-up test was considered for many years the gold standard in assessing neurologic function during spinal surgery. During the critical stage of the operation, after spine instrumentation, the patient is briefly woken up and asked to perform a range of commands (usually moving all four limbs) before being reanesthetized. It is essential that the procedure is fully explained to the patient prior to induction and that the surgeon gives enough prior warning to enable the anesthesiologist to prepare the anesthesia plan accordingly and adequately titrate the anesthesia. A variety of anesthetic techniques have been described, but they usually involve a remifentanil infusion plus either propofol or volatile anesthetic. At the surgeon's request either the propofol or the volatile anesthetic is stopped and the remifentanil infusion decreased to 0.05 µg/kg/min. The wake-up test is not without its risks, particularly that of extubation of a patient in the prone position. It also misses the exact onset or cause of injury. Today it is mainly used in centers where neurophysiologic monitoring is not available or where there is concern over the results of this monitoring.

25.9 Postoperative Considerations and Complications

Ideally the surgeon wants all patients to be woken and extubated as soon as possible after surgery to allow a full neurologic assessment. With the use of short-acting anesthetic agents such as propofol and remifentanil infusions, it relatively easy to wake patients enough to carry out a neurologic assessment and subsequently reanesthetize them if postoperative ventilation is required. The decision to extubate a patient postoperatively is multifactorial. In patients where preoperative pulmonary function tests indicate a need for postoperative ventilation, such as forced vital capacity <30%, it would be prudent not to attempt extubation in the operating room. Patients who use CPAP or other forms of noninvasive ventilation may be extubated directly to their noninvasive ventilation machine.[2]

Spinal surgery tends to involve long operations with the patient in the prone position. This leaves all patients liable to develop airway edema. Prior to any extubation it is essential to check for a leak around the cuff of the endotracheal tube. Patients who have suffered large blood loss (30 mL/kg) and who have received multiple blood transfusions are prone to postoperative respiratory complications, including transfusion-related lung injury.[19] In our center all spine surgery patients are observed in a high-dependency setting for 12 to 24 hours postoperatively and where a patient is transferred ventilated, extubation will be planned as early as possible.

Multimodal analgesia is essential following spinal surgery. In a recent survey of anesthetic practice, the use of epidural analgesia postoperatively was common in Australia and the United Kingdom.[20] Epidural catheters are inserted by the surgeon at the end of the procedure and connected to a patient-controlled anesthesia pump. The authors showed that epidural analgesia has been effective in decreasing hospital stay, and it has fewer systemic side effects.[21] Intrathecal analgesia has also been reported. Again, this is injected by the surgeon at the end of the operation; however it runs the risk of increased respiratory depression. The main option for postoperative analgesia following spine surgery is intravenous opioids administered via patient-controlled anesthesia. Other options include intrapleural analgesia if a thoracotomy has been performed. In all cases nonopioid adjuncts, such as paracetamol, should be added. Although these have not been shown to reduce opioid requirements they do reduce overall pain scores.[22] There has been some controversy surrounding the use of nonsteroidal anti-inflammatory drugs due to a reported delay in bone union, but this has subsequently been proven not to be the case.[23]

Respiratory complications occur in around 7% of patients undergoing spinal surgery. Patients are at increased risk of thromboembolic events postoperatively and precautions should be taken, including starting prophylactic low molecular weight heparin as soon as possible.[24]

25.10 Conclusions

Anesthesia for spinal surgery continues to be a challenging subspecialty. The advent of neuromonitoring, while making the surgery safer for the patient, has required a change in anesthetic technique. Postoperative morbidity remains a problem, and postoperative analgesia is important in preventing complications. It is a surgical specialty that continues to grow and become more challenging, and it is essential that the anesthetist adapts to the challenges this presents.

References

[1] Augoustides JG, Stone ME, Drenger B. Novel approaches to spinal cord protection during thoracoabdominal aortic interventions. Curr Opin Anaesthesiol. 2014; 27(1):98–105

[2] Birnkrant DJ, Panitch HB, Benditt JO, et al. American College of Chest Physicians consensus statement on the respiratory and related management of patients with Duchenne muscular dystrophy undergoing anesthesia or sedation. Chest. 2007; 132(6):1977–1986

[3] Gambrall MA. Anesthetic implications for surgical correction of scoliosis. AANA J. 2007; 75(4):277–285

[4] Jungbluth H. Multi-minicore disease. Orphanet J Rare Dis. 2007; 2:31

[5] Raw DA, Beattie JK, Hunter JM. Anaesthesia for spinal surgery in adults. Br J Anaesth. 2003; 91(6):886–904

[6] Fraser A, Edmonds-Seal J. Spinal cord injuries. A review of the problems facing the anaesthetist. Anaesthesia. 1982; 37(11):1084–1098

[7] Mansel JK, Norman JR. Respiratory complications and management of spinal cord injuries. Chest. 1990; 97(6):1446–1452

[8] Amzallag M. Autonomic hyperreflexia. Int Anesthesiol Clin. 1993; 31(1):87–102

[9] Sahin A, Salman MA, Erden IA, Aypar U. Upper cervical vertebrae movement during intubating laryngeal mask, fibreoptic and direct laryngoscopy: a video-fluoroscopic study. Eur J Anaesthesiol. 2004; 21(10):819–823

[10] Sloan T. Evoked responses. In: Albin MS, ed. A Textbook of Neuroanesthesia with Neurosurgical and Neuroscience Perspectives. New York NY: McGraw-Hill, 1996:221–276

[11] Punjasawadwong Y, Boonjeungmonkol N, Phongchiewboon A. Bispectral index for improving anaesthetic delivery and postoperative recovery. Cochrane Database Syst Rev. 2007(4):CD003843

[12] Stevens WR, Glazer PA, Kelley SD, Lietman TM, Bradford DS. Ophthalmic complications after spinal surgery. Spine. 1997; 22(12):1319–1324

[13] Schonauer C, Bocchetti A, Barbagallo G, Albanese V, Moraci A. Positioning on surgical table. Eur Spine J. 2004; 13 Suppl 1:S50–S55

[14] Park CK. The effect of patient positioning on intraabdominal pressure and blood loss in spinal surgery. Anesth Analg. 2000; 91(3):552–557

[15] Wimmer C, Gluch H, Franzreb M, Ogon M. Predisposing factors for infection in spine surgery: a survey of 850 spinal procedures. J Spinal Disord. 1998; 11 (2):124–128

[16] Copley LA, Richards BS, Safavi FZ, Newton PO. Hemodilution as a method to reduce transfusion requirements in adolescent spine fusion surgery. Spine. 1999; 24(3):219–222, discussion 223–224

[17] Allain J, Akehurst RL, Hunter JM. Autologous transfusion, 3 yr on-what is new? What has happened? Second Consensus Conference on Autologous Transfusion, held at the Royal College of Physicians, Edinburgh, November 11, 1998. Br J Anaesth. 1999; 82(5):783–784

[18] Elgafy H, Bransford RJ, McGuire RA, Dettori JR, Fischer D. Blood loss in major spine surgery: are there effective measures to decrease massive hemorrhage in major spine fusion surgery? Spine. 2010; 35(9) Suppl:S47–S56

[19] Vedantam R, Lenke LG, Bridwell KH, Haas J, Linville DA. A prospective evaluation of pulmonary function in patients with adolescent idiopathic scoliosis relative to the surgical approach used for spinal arthrodesis. Spine. 2000; 25 (1):82–90

[20] Palmer GM, Pirakalathanan P, Skinner AV. A multi-centre multi-national survey of anaesthetists regarding the range of anaesthetic and surgical practices for paediatric scoliosis surgery. Anaesth Intensive Care. 2010; 38(6):1077–1084

[21] Van Boerum DH, Smith JT, Curtin MJ. A comparison of the effects of patient-controlled analgesia with intravenous opioids versus Epidural analgesia on recovery after surgery for idiopathic scoliosis. Spine. 2000; 25(18):2355–2357

[22] Hiller A, Helenius I, Nurmi E, et al. Acetaminophen improves analgesia but does not reduce opioid requirement after major spine surgery in children and adolescents. Spine. 2012; 37(20):E1225–E1231

[23] Dodwell ER, Latorre JG, Parisini E, et al. NSAID exposure and risk of nonunion: a meta-analysis of case-control and cohort studies. Calcif Tissue Int. 2010; 87 (3):193–202

[24] Faciszewski T, Winter RB, Lonstein JE, Denis F, Johnson L. The surgical and medical perioperative complications of anterior spinal fusion surgery in the thoracic and lumbar spine in adults. A review of 1223 procedures. Spine. 1995; 20(14):1592–1599

26 Neuromonitoring in Rigid Spine Deformity Correction

Akiva Korn, Joseph Danto

Abstract

The application of intraoperative neurophysiologic monitoring has become a standard of care in the context of many spine surgeries, most prominently complex scoliosis correction. A multimodality monitoring approach includes the application of transcranial motor evoked potentials (tcMEP), somatosensory evoked potentials (SSEP), and free-running and triggered electromyography (EMG). These modalities are complementary and represent the functional integrity of different and respective neuroanatomical pathways in the spinal cord and surrounding neuroanatomical structures. Interpretation of the neurophysiological signals across these modalities differs based upon global physiological factors, neurophysiological principles, signal-to-noise ratios, time delays, and contexts such as surgical maneuvers. When taken together, the sensitivity and specificity values for detecting early stages of intraoperative neurological compromise are high, allowing for cessation or even reversal of surgical maneuvers that would otherwise result in significant permanent deficits.

Keywords: intraoperative neurophysiological monitoring, evoked potentials, SSEP, MEP, EMG

26.1 Introduction

Neurophysiologic intraoperative monitoring (NIOM) is the application of quantitative neurophysiologic methodologies designed to assess a patient's neurophysiologic status during a surgical procedure. The methodologies are focused on neurologic structures that are at risk during specific types of surgery. Electrophysiologic changes, such as attenuation or prolongation of evoked signals, are presumed to reflect dynamic clinical deterioration and can alert the surgical team to impending neural injury and thereby provide the opportunity, while the neurologic process is still reversible, to modify the operative technique and thus avoid or mitigate any permanent change in clinical function.

Dawson et al published a seminal paper paving the way for routine NIOM in deformity surgery by documenting and describing the efficacy of monitoring in a large series.[1] This survey of the Scoliosis Research Society reflected a 1.6% incidence of neurologic complication in scoliosis surgery, and is the basis for the almost universal definition of thresholds of 10% latency change and 50% amplitude change in somatosensory evoked potential (SSEP) monitoring data as portending neurologic compromise. With the subsequent introduction of multipulse transcranial motor evoked potential (tcMEP) monitoring, a multimodality approach combining both sensory and motor pathway central conduction assessment was established and remains the standard monitoring protocol in many international institutions to this day. These methods, together with electromyographic (EMG) recordings to reveal surgically evoked irritation to peripheral nerves and spinal nerve roots, have reached sensitivity and specificity values as high as 100%, and thus play a continued role in the modern-day comprehensive NIOM approach to complex spinal surgery, including treatment for rigid spine deformities.

NIOM, while originating in the spinal deformity context, has evolved over the past several decades to become a routinely applied adjunct in a plethora of other orthopaedic spine and neurosurgical procedures, including facial and peripheral nerve,[2,3] cervical spine,[4] intramedullary,[5,6,7] and extramedullary[8] spinal cord tumors and supratentorial brain surgery.[9,10,11,12]

26.2 NIOM Tools

Modalities included in modern intraoperative monitoring.

26.2.1 Somatosensory Evoked Potentials

SSEPs for intraoperative monitoring were described as early as the 1970 s by Nash et al.[13] They are responses to peripheral stimulation of afferent fibers of mixed nerves and reflect white matter conduction through the posterior columns to the appropriate sensory cortex. The stimulation typically consists of square wave electrical pulses applied to the wrists for median or ulnar nerve innervations and/or at the ankle, dorsal to the medial malleolus for posterior tibial nerve stimulation. Less commonly, they can also be undertaken at the popliteal fossae or at the lateral fibular head at the knee for peroneal nerve stimulation. Following stimulation, a traveling potential is generated, and these peripheral volleys may be recorded at the popliteal fossae (in case of posterior tibial nerve stimulation at the ankle) and along the lumbar spine. Similarly, stationary potentials can be recorded from generators, including the entry point into the spinal cord at the conus medullaris at the lower thoracic spine level, at the level of the upper cervical spine (P31), and at the brainstem level reflecting dorsal column and thalamic nuclei. Ultimately, a cortical response (P37) is recorded from scalp electrodes placed over the respective contralateral sensory cortex approximately 1 cm posterior to the C3 or C4 international 10–20 scalp position (▶ Fig. 26.1). The resultant data, measured in latency in milliseconds and amplitude in microvolts, are noted as a baseline measurement at the beginning of surgery, and then compared against constantly refreshed data collected repeatedly throughout the surgical procedure (▶ Fig. 26.2, ▶ Fig. 26.3). Special attention is given at surgical stages posing a higher risk of neurologic injury, for example, spinal osteotomy, placement of pedicle screws, and spinal corrective maneuvers.

The neurologic pathway of the SSEP is from the stimulated peripheral nerve to the primary sensory cortex by way of the lemniscal system situated in the posterior columns of the spinal cord. Among other insults, stretching, distraction, or compression of the spinal column, and thus indirectly (or directly), the spinal cord, can cause attenuation or abolishment of SSEP data. Compromise of the spinal cord blood flow along the posterior spinal arteries or their perforators will also disrupt normal

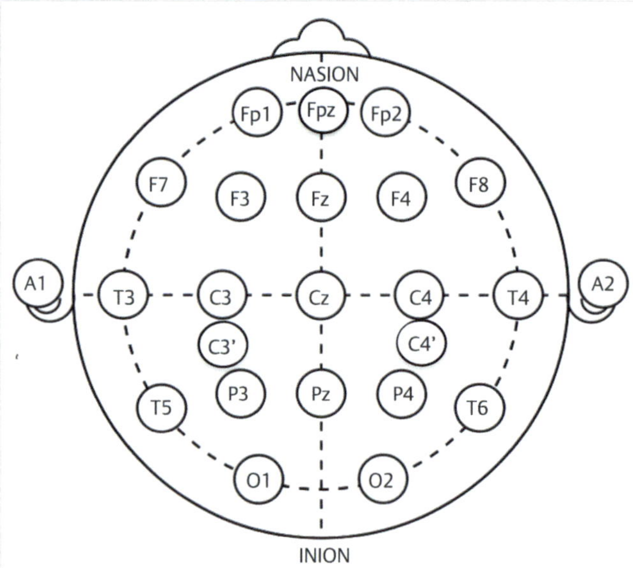

Fig. 26.1 Visual representation of the international 10–20 scalp electroencephalographic positioning system. The scalp surface is mapped into landmarks based on 10 and 20 % distances based on head circumference and inion–nasion distances. Common electrode positions for somatosensory evoked potential monitoring are C 3', C 4', and Fpz. Common positions for transcranial motor evoked potential stimulation are C 3, C 4, and Fpz.

lemniscal system transmission. If these adverse conditions are not identified and addressed in a timely manner, there is a high likelihood of permanent cord damage. The typical data (▶ Fig. 26.3) for lower-extremity data are biphasic waveforms with a positive peak at approximately 37 msec for the lower extremity SSEP (P37).

26.2.2 Transcranial Electric Motor Evoked Potentials

Marsden et al were early reporters of the ability to elicit motor responses from a transcranial stimulation.[14] The ability to more reliably collect the data under anesthesia was enhanced by the use of multipulse stimulation.[15] These data are generated by applying multipulse trains of electric stimuli transcranially and activating the pyramidal fibers in a nonselective manner. Compound muscle action potentials (CMAPs) are evoked from peripheral muscles following transcranial stimulation. The muscles typically chosen for tcMEP monitoring in long deformity rigid spine surgery include tibialis anterior or abductor hallucis brevis, with upper extremity muscles, such as abductor pollicis brevis, used as a positive control. The recording of upper extremity tcMEP data also has the added benefit of monitoring for upper extremity positioning complications, which are reported in lengthy surgery in the prone position.[16,17] Common stimulation sites are C 3 and C 4 of the international 10–20

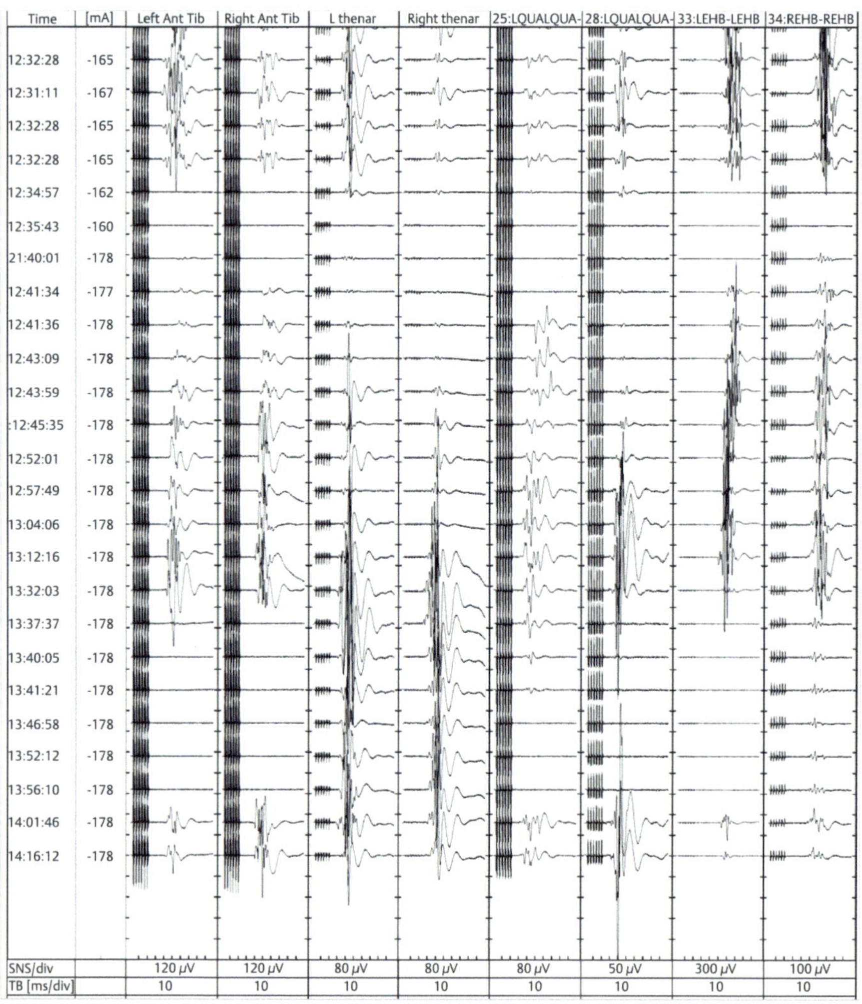

Fig. 26.2 Representative transcranial motor evoked potential (tcMEP) data during rigid spine surgery. Recording waterfalls from left to right are left tibialis anterior, right tibialis anterior, left abductor pollicis brevis, right abductor pollicis brevis, left quadriceps, right quadriceps, left abductor hallucis brevis, right abductor hallucis brevis. Baseline recordings at the top of the stack show availability of tcMEP data on all channels. At approximately 12:34 all data are abolished, including upper extremity, concomitant with a hemodynamic event and severe hypotension. All data are recovered with normotension at approximately 12:43. At 13:37, at spinal correction, lower-extremity tcMEP data were abolished with retained upper extremity data as control. These data returned approximately 23 minutes later, following a pause in the procedure, raising of the blood pressure, and initiation of a wakeup test. With the return of the affected data, the wakeup test was aborted. The patient emerged intact.

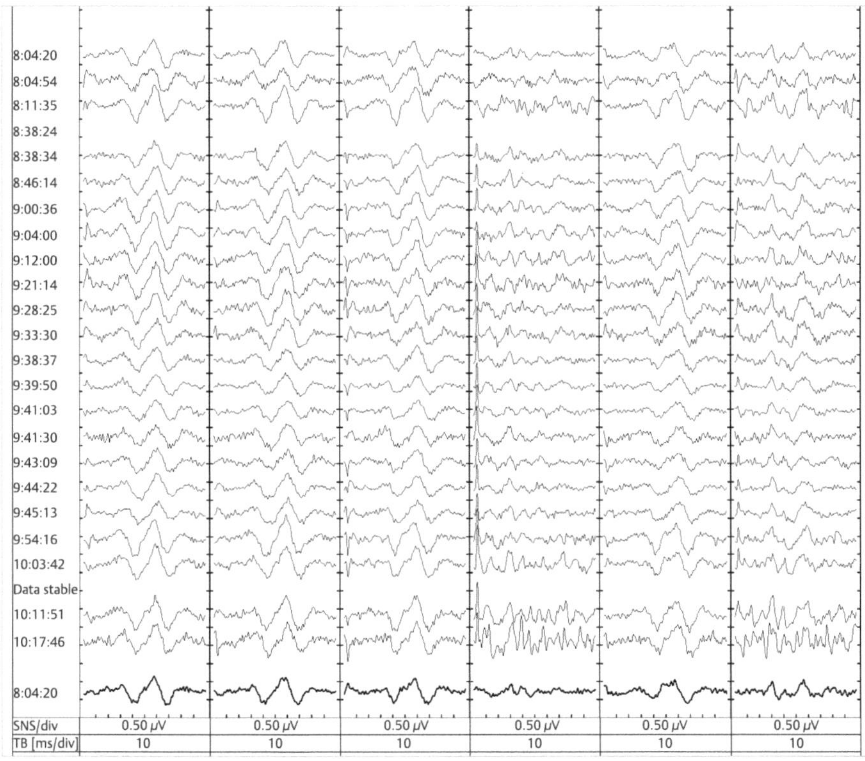

Fig. 26.3 Representative posterior tibial nerve somatosensory evoked potential (SSEP) data collected during adult scoliosis surgery. Recording waterfalls from left to right: left C 3/C 4, right C 3/C 4, left Cz/Fpz, left mastoid/Fpz, right Cz/Fpz, right mastoid/Fpz. Both cortically generated C 3, C 4, and Cz and subcortically generated SSEP data were collected in this procedure. The robust P37 waveform seen in the channels representing cortical activity can be appreciated. These data remained stable during the procedure despite aggressive spinal manipulation.

system (also termed M3 and M4). To close the electrical circuit, these electrodes can be referenced against each other or to a common Fpz site.[18]

Baseline tcMEP recordings are typically established either prior to or just following positioning, and as in SSEP, constantly refreshed data are collected throughout the procedure, with special attention given to "risky" stages. Unlike SSEP, the criteria for change and interpretation of tcMEP data is not linearly quantitative. Due to the natural fluctuations in upper to lower motor neuron excitability, and with the added complication of anesthetic effects, a large variability in tcMEP data exists regardless of surgical events. Therefore, the 50% amplitude attenuation criterion that has been described in SSEP is not applicable. Instead, an all-or-nothing approach is taken by most monitoring teams when interpreting tcMEP data to reflect long tract injury, although some semiquantitative models have been proposed, including changes in stimulation threshold necessary to provide a steady CMAP[19] or changes in the complexity of the tcMEP waveform.[20] It is our experience, however, that while the all-or-nothing approach is most applicable for predicting postoperative deficits involving the spinal cord pyramidal tracts, it is worthwhile to take note when sudden attenuation in tcMEP data occurs because it may signal the beginning of a more serious process. Likewise, if a given stage of surgery puts the peripheral nervous system at risk, including individual spinal nerve roots, significant attenuation of the tcMEP signal can be a criterion for alarm and should be addressed accordingly.

A corollary technique involves using a single-pulse stimulation from the same location but recording from an epidural electrode placed over the spinal cord through a flavotomy. These data are termed D wave volleys as they originate from direct stimulation of the pyramidal fibers at the cranial level.[5,21] Because they exclude the transmission from the upper to the lower motor neuron pathway, and they are not muscle responses, D waves are less susceptible to anesthetic agents and are not precluded by the use of muscle relaxants. Three caveats apply to D wave monitoring, however: (1) D wave data can only be recorded above T 10 and therefore only represent conduction above this level (e. g., the data would not be sensitive to specific injury to the conus medullaris).[5] (2) As spinal manipulation occurs typical to rigid deformity surgery, the orientation and positioning of the catheter electrode vis-à-vis the spinal cord can be altered resulting in false-positive changes.[22] (3) Since the electrode can only be placed in an invasive manner after flavotomy, and is removed prior to closure, a large part of the procedure would remain unmonitored. For these reasons, D waves are not used to monitor rigid spine surgery in our practice.

The tcMEP pathway is generated from the intracranial pyramidal tract at or through the internal capsule and is conducted through the brainstem and along the spinal cord via the anterior and anterolateral columns, through the anterior horn cell and lower motor neuron to the motor end plate. Compression or stretching of these fibers, or compromising blood supply to the anterior columns via the anterior spinal artery, would affect the tcMEP signal and raise alarm addressing significant concern for permanent motor impairment. Papers have shown tcMEP as a measure separate from SSEP and, when common damage has occurred, earlier changes were noted in the tcMEP compared with SSEP data.[17] TcMEP recording demands minimization of muscle relaxants and is precluded by the use of halogenated anesthetic agents, which must be balanced with surgical concerns.[23] The presence of a tcMEP signal at the conclusion of surgery is a good prognostic indicator of the avoidance of permanent neurologic damage.

26.2.3 Electromyography

The EMG is recorded as CMAP from monitored muscles innervated by root levels related to the focus of the surgical procedure. These are displayed on a screen and often delivered to a loudspeaker for immediate feedback. The EMG is usually recorded as an ongoing display of spontaneous muscle firing, but it can also be evoked from direct electrical stimulation of neural structures or surrounding ambiguous anatomy in the surgical field. For example, it has been shown that EMG can be useful in placement of pedicle screws by stimulation and EMG threshold testing.[24,25,26,27] In this method, when stimulating pedicle screws in situ, low thresholds of electrically evoked CMAPs in the lower extremities indicate a breach through the cortical wall of the corresponding pedicle. It is suggested that for lumbar-level pedicle screws the threshold of 11 mA or higher correlated with intact cortical bone surrounding the pedicle screw, whereas lower thresholds indicate a possible breach. The clinical caveats of EMG include the following: no muscle relaxant can be used or the alerting irritated muscle responses will be obliterated, and not all pedicle screw metals and constructs conduct the electrical stimulation in a universal manner. Recording of free-running EMG and spontaneous CMAP neuronic discharges from muscles innervated by the nerve roots at risk during a specific maneuver can alert the surgeon of irritation of the roots, for example, during screw placement, aggressive spinal manipulation, or introduction of spinal dissectors and other instruments in proximity to the lateral aspects of the spinal column.

26.2.4 Multimodality Approach

As monitoring progressed, investigators realized the value of simultaneously monitoring the multiple systems at risk during these procedures and hence used combined SSEP, tcMEP D wave, and free-running and triggered EMG.[28] The application of these measures allowed not just an overview as to whether a system is intact or not but introduced the ability to be more specific in the monitoring and mapping. For example, comparing results of corticobulbar MEP to spontaneous EMG can help differentiate subtle injuries that may affect roots versus peripheral nerves. In addition, the redundancy of multimodality data can provide "backup" systems, such as D waves when a muscle relaxant might obscure CMAP data.

Using a combined, multimodality approach to monitoring spinal surgery, the surgeon can obtain good feedback as to sensory and motor cord function and related spinal root integrity.

26.3 Clinical Applications

Positioning involves a potential risk for patients with compromised spinal canals. In patients with rigid spine diseases, these risks are exacerbated, particularly since the nature of the deformity often forces tortuous positioning postures to provide appropriate surgical and anesthesia management. Pedicle trajectories are often distorted, and the cord may be injured during column correction and shortening. The identification and progress of pedicle screw instrumentation become more of a challenge, with serious consequences. Correction of column deformities involves corrective forces that may impinge on the cord and may compromise blood flow. More direct handling of the cord, thecal sac, and nerve roots confronts the surgeon faced with the rigid spine deformity affecting these already vulnerable neural structures. And, as with any bone-sacrificing procedure, occult bone fragments add to the potential risks to the spinal cord. Vertebral column resection creates a threat of precipitous blood loss, and osteotomies are riskier with rigid spine deformities because of a restricted mobility of the disk, and the nature of the vertebral column resection further confronts the cord by shortening the column and possible additional torque on the cord.[29]

26.4 Conclusion

NIOM has been correctly established as a standard adjunct to rigid spinal deformity surgery. Given the inherent dangers of neurologic compromise in these procedures, NIOM can be a powerful tool used to mitigate unnecessary postoperative deficit. To use these tools most effectively, surgeons should be made aware of the variety of NIOM methodologies as well as their limitations and benefits.

References

[1] Dawson EG, Sherman JE, Kanim LE, Nuwer MR. Spinal cord monitoring. Results of the Scoliosis Research Society and the European Spinal Deformity Society survey. Spine. 1991; 16(8) Suppl:S361–S364

[2] Kline DG, Hackett ER, Happel LH. Surgery for lesions of the brachial plexus. Arch Neurol. 1986; 43(2):170–181

[3] Romstöck J, Strauss C, Fahlbusch R. Continuous electromyography monitoring of motor cranial nerves during cerebellopontine angle surgery. J Neurosurg. 2000; 93(4):586–593

[4] Epstein NE, Danto J, Nardi D. Evaluation of intraoperative somatosensory-evoked potential monitoring during 100 cervical operations. Spine. 1993; 18 (6):737–747

[5] Morota N, Deletis V, Constantini S, Kofler M, Cohen H, Epstein FJ. The role of motor evoked potentials during surgery for intramedullary spinal cord tumors. Neurosurgery. 1997; 41(6):1327–1336

[6] Sala F, Bricolo A, Faccioli F, Lanteri P, Gerosa M. Surgery for intramedullary spinal cord tumors: the role of intraoperative (neurophysiological) monitoring. Eur Spine J. 2007; 16 Suppl 2:S130–S139

[7] Sala F, Palandri G, Basso E, et al. Motor evoked potential monitoring improves outcome after surgery for intramedullary spinal cord tumors: a historical control study. Neurosurgery. 2006; 58(6):1129–1143, discussion 1129–1143

[8] Korn A, Halevi D, Lidar Z, Biron T, Ekstein P, Constantini S. Intraoperative neurophysiological monitoring during resection of intradural extramedullary spinal cord tumors: experience with 100 cases. Acta Neurochir (Wien). 2015; 157(5):819–830

[9] Neuloh G, Pechstein U, Cedzich C, Schramm J. Motor evoked potential monitoring with supratentorial surgery. Neurosurgery. 2004; 54(5):1061–1070, discussion 1070–1072

[10] Nossek E, Korn A, Shahar T, et al. Intraoperative mapping and monitoring of the corticospinal tracts with neurophysiological assessment and 3-dimensional ultrasonography-based navigation. Clinical article. J Neurosurg. 2011; 114(3):738–746

[11] Szelényi A, Bello L, Duffau H, et al. Workgroup for Intraoperative Management in Low-Grade Glioma Surgery within the European Low-Grade Glioma Network. Intraoperative electrical stimulation in awake craniotomy: methodological aspects of current practice. Neurosurg Focus. 2010; 28(2):E7

[12] Szelényi A, Joksimovic B, Seifert V. Intraoperative risk of seizures associated with transient direct cortical stimulation in patients with symptomatic epilepsy. J Clin Neurophysiol. 2007; 24(1):39–43

[13] Nash CL, Jr, Lorig RA, Schatzinger LA, Brown RH. Spinal cord monitoring during operative treatment of the spine. Clin Orthop Relat Res. 1977(126):100–105

[14] Marsden CD, Merton PA, Morton HB. Direct electrical stimulation of corticospinal pathways through the intact scalp in human subjects. Adv Neurol. 1983; 39:387–391
[15] Taniguchi M, Cedzich C, Schramm J. Modification of cortical stimulation for motor evoked potentials under general anesthesia: technical description. Neurosurgery. 1993; 32(2):219–226
[16] Jones SC, Fernau R, Woeltjen BL. Use of somatosensory evoked potentials to detect peripheral ischemia and potential injury resulting from positioning of the surgical patient: case reports and discussion. Spine J. 2004; 4(3):360–362
[17] Schwartz DM, Auerbach JD, Dormans JP, et al. Neurophysiological detection of impending spinal cord injury during scoliosis surgery. J Bone Joint Surg Am. 2007; 89(11):2440–2449
[18] Macdonald DB. Intraoperative motor evoked potential monitoring: overview and update. J Clin Monit Comput. 2006; 20(5):347–377
[19] Calancie B, Harris W, Broton JG, Alexeeva N, Green BA. "Threshold-level" multipulse transcranial electrical stimulation of motor cortex for intraoperative monitoring of spinal motor tracts: description of method and comparison to somatosensory evoked potential monitoring. J Neurosurg. 1998; 88(3):457–470
[20] Quiñones-Hinojosa A, Lyon R, Zada G, et al. Changes in transcranial motor evoked potentials during intramedullary spinal cord tumor resection correlate with postoperative motor function. Neurosurgery. 2005; 56(5):982–993, discussion 982–993
[21] Amassian VE, Cracco RQ. Human cerebral cortical responses to contralateral transcranial stimulation. Neurosurgery. 1987; 20(1):148–155
[22] Ulkatan S, Neuwirth M, Bitan F, Minardi C, Kokoszka A, Deletis V. Monitoring of scoliosis surgery with epidurally recorded motor evoked potentials (D wave) revealed false results. Clin Neurophysiol. 2006; 117(9):2093–2101
[23] Sloan TB. Anesthetic effects on electrophysiologic recordings. J Clin Neurophysiol. 1998; 15(3):217–226
[24] Donohue ML, Murtagh-Schaffer C, Basta J, Moquin RR, Bashir A, Calancie B. Pulse-train stimulation for detecting medial malpositioning of thoracic pedicle screws. Spine. 2008; 33(12):E378–E385
[25] Mavrogenis AF, Papagelopoulos PJ, Korres DS, Papadopoulos K, Sakas DE, Pneumaticos S. Accuracy of pedicle screw placement using intraoperative neurophysiological monitoring and computed tomography. J Long Term Eff Med Implants. 2009; 19(1):41–48
[26] Raynor BL, Lenke LG, Bridwell KH, Taylor BA, Padberg AM. Correlation between low triggered electromyographic thresholds and lumbar pedicle screw malposition: analysis of 4 857 screws. Spine. 2007; 32(24):2673–2678
[27] Shi YB, Binette M, Martin WH, Pearson JM, Hart RA. Electrical stimulation for intraoperative evaluation of thoracic pedicle screw placement. Spine. 2003; 28(6):595–601
[28] Sutter M, Eggspuehler A, Grob D, et al. The validity of multimodal intraoperative monitoring (MIOM) in surgery of 109 spine and spinal cord tumors. Eur Spine J. 2007; 16 Suppl 2:S197–S208
[29] Smith JS, Wang VY, Ames CP. Vertebral column resection for rigid spinal deformity. Neurosurgery. 2008; 63(3) Suppl:177–182

27 Neurological Complications after Surgery or Trauma to the Rigid Spine

Avi Ohry, W. S. El Masri, Stephen Eisenstein

Abstract

People who sustained spinal trauma, underwent spinal surgery, or suffer from diseases like ankylosing spondylitis, rheumatoid arthritis, and spinal disorders (stenosis, spondylolisthesis, scoliosis, kyphosis), may develop late rigid spine and neurological deterioration, which may lead to sphincter paralysis, impotence, and psychosocial-behavioral and vocational sequelae.

Keywords: ankylosing spondylitis, rheumatoid arthritis, spinal disorders, rigid spine, spinal stenosis, spondyloarthropathies, late neurological complications

27.1 Introduction

Adults who develop a rigid spine usually suffer from one or more of the following possible pathologies: ankylosing spondylitis (Bechterew disease or Marie-Strümpell disease), acquired or congenital scoliosis, Scheuermann's kyphosis, kyphoscoliosis, lumbar spinal stenosis, spondylolisthesis, rheumatoid arthritis, and more.

Patients with one problem after surgery or trauma to the spine may develop multiple additional problems, such as the following:

- New sequelae of the damaged spinal cord: motor, sensory, and autonomic nervous system, at a different level or to a different extent.
- Ongoing, unresolved original orthopaedic problem.
- Ongoing, unresolved segmental rigidity or inflexibility.
- New problems that arise (neuropathic bowel and bladder, pain, impotence, confinement to a wheelchair, immobility, weight gain, hypertension, hypercalciuria, renal problems, osteoporosis.
- New psychological, emotional, vocational, and social handicaps.

Normally, the aligned adult spine is anteroposteriorly straight and has three sagittal curves. In this manner, the body is kept erect. Spinal deformities may develop congenitally or later during growth in adolescence, due to the aging process, or due to trauma. Spinal deformities may cause hyperlordosis, kyphosis, scoliosis, rotation of vertebrae, or combinations of these deformities. These deformities, along with degeneration of disks, ligaments, and vertebrae, may cause pain, degeneration of spinal structures, breathing difficulties, as well as cosmetic and emotional problems. They require the attention of orthopaedic surgeons, experts in rehabilitation medicine, and allied health professionals. Diagnosis of adult spinal deformities is made by physical and radiological examinations and pulmonary function tests. Not all of these conditions require surgery.[1]

It is beyond the scope of this short review to define each spinal disease or deformity that can lead to a rigid spine. Generally, patients with rigid spine are prone to spinal cord or spinal nerve involvement due to falls or other trauma, vertebral spondylosis (spinal stenosis), vascular ischemia, or, rarely, spinal surgery.[2]

27.2 Spondyloarthropathies

In spondyloarthropathies, like ankylosing spondylitis (AS), psoriatic arthritis, reactive arthritis, and inflammatory bowel diseases, complications may involve spinal nerve compression, musculocutaneous lesions, aortic dysfunction, loss of spinal mobility, reduced pulmonary function, pain, and more.[3,4]

Rarely, patients with AS are referred to a department of rehabilitation medicine or to a spinal cord injury unit. Zwecker et al reported on a case of slow ascending myelopathy in a patient with AS. A 60-year-old patient suffering from AS developed, over a period of 39 years, a slow ascending myelopathy leading to tetraplegia, squamous cell carcinoma of the bladder, and amyloidosis of the small intestine secondary to neuropathic bladder and bowel. Physical examination revealed deteriorating incomplete tetraplegia with hypotonia and hyporeflexia. Neurogenic bladder and bowel developed into squamous cell carcinoma and amyloidosis. To our knowledge, flaccid tetraplegia associated with AS has never before been reported in the medical literature. The possibility of vascular compression by the ankylosed spine causing the clinical picture of flaccid tetraplegia in this patient was discussed.[5]

Recently the author AO also treated a 68-year-old man who suffered from AS and depression. During a physiotherapy session he fell down, fracturing his C2, C3, and D9 vertebrae. He was admitted to Reuth Medical Center in Tel Aviv in February 2012 on a ventilator with a tracheotomy, after surgical reduction and fixation (laminectomies at C2–C3), hemopneumothorax, paroxysmal atrial fibrillation, essential hypertension, status post–coronary bypass a year before, chronic renal failure, and tetraplegia. It was noted that after the fall he developed dorsal paraplegia, which rapidly ascended, and he became tetraplegic, with a complete lesion below C4. A few episodes of seizures were noted. Finally he was weaned from the ventilator but remained tetraplegic (American Spinal Injury Association Impairment Scale—A).

Sir Ludwig Guttmann had described thoroughly the association of Bechterew disease and tetraplegia.[6] Cervical spinal cord injury may occur during hyperextension of the neck due to an accident or careless intubation, or due to a herniated disk or vertebral cervical dislocation.[7] The management—halo vest immobilization—is usually conservative. Sometimes surgery is needed in these patients—a technique of pedicle subtraction osteotomy of the seventh cervical vertebra (C7) for correction of rigid kyphotic deformity of the cervicothoracic junction in patients with severe AS, has been described.[8] The authors reported that all patients were satisfied with the degree of correction achieved and reported alleviation of neck pain, and none suffered any neurologic deterioration.

Patients with AS may further develop osteoporosis and spinal fractures.[9] *An et al reviewed fractures in patients with ankylosing spondylitis that had been clinically diagnosed to better define the mechanism of injury, associated neurological deficit, predisposing factors, and management strategies. . . . 12 patients with 13 fractures with neurological complications were treated. . . . Management was based on the presence or absence of spinal instability. . . fractures were associated with a hyperextension mechanism. . . 10 cases resulted in a fracture by minor trauma. Posttraumatic neurological deficits were demonstrated in 11 cases and neurological improvement after surgery was observed in 5 of these cases.*

One of this chapter's authors (SE) describes two of his patients:

One patient was a middle-aged man with ankylosing spondylitis. Severe kyphosis prevented any useful forward gaze. I had done several of these operations before, with good result, via a posterior approach to L 3 usually, scooping out a good deal of vertebral cancellous bone via the pedicles, producing a posterior crush (closing wedge osteotomy), then fix and fuse in that position. He died within one hour in the recovery room because of unexplained massive intra-abdominal blood loss and despite massive blood transfusion. Postmortem examination revealed a fracture of the calcified "chalk-stick" aorta. A bitter lesson. After that, I carefully checked the preoperative X-rays of all ankylosing spondylitis patients heading for spinal osteotomy. Calcified aorta became an absolute exclusion factor for me.

The other patient was a young girl, the only case I have ever heard of, with a "one-bone" spine, a total congenital failure of segmentation from skull to sacrum. Her problem. apart from short stature, was a "chin on chest" fixed cervical kyphosis. Her life was intolerable without any forward gaze and she was not prepared to wear prism lenses. I carried out an excellent corrective osteotomy shortly before Christmas, 1987 held in a halo-vest. The problems that emerged soon after surgery [included] quadriparesis; she couldn't swallow; eventually couldn't breathe. This was the worst Christmas of my life. A brilliant young ENT surgeon managed to get a tracheostomy done. The quadriparesis slowly resolved; and a general surgeon put in a A percutaneous endoscopic gastrostomy (PEG) for feeding. The tracheostomy and the PEG remain all these years later. The fact is that this patient remains ever grateful for her improved posture even though her trachea and esophagus were destroyed by the excessive angularity of the correction. She went on to qualify for a senior clerical job, drives her own car and lives independently in her own house.

27.3 Scoliosis

Serious neurologic damage after spinal instrumentation for correction of scoliosis is relatively rare. The vascular supply to the spinal cord may be compromised after spinal distraction. Other complications are postoperative infection, rarely pneumothorax, dural tears, incorrect placement of the fusion level, late pseudarthrosis and pain.

Bar-On et al have described three patients with paraplegia following corrective surgery for idiopathic scoliosis, using Cotrel-Dubousset (CD) instrumentation, were admitted to our department over a period of 22 months. They were operated on by three different surgeons, and they were the first serious neurological complications in these surgeons' careers. The monitoring method was the "wake-up" test, applied at the end of the correction maneuver with the instrument. One patient presented paraplegia at the "wake-up" test, and the other two were paraplegic shortly after ceasing anesthesia. Electrophysiological spinal cord monitoring during surgery may reduce the risks of complications.[10] *Luckily, this complication is rare.*

Controversy remains over the role of surgical intervention in older patients with degenerative scoliosis. A few approaches have been proposed: decompression, instrumented posterior spinal fusion, anterior spinal fusion, and osteotomy.[11]

No neurologic complications were reported by Koptan et al:

The results of direct repair of spondylolysis in idiopathic scoliosis patients were very satisfactory both clinically and radiologically. Direct repair appears to be a logical alternative to spinal fusion; lumbar spine mobility was preserved, and precocious motion segments were saved with a relatively simple operation.[12]

Sixteen patients with severe and rigid idiopathic scoliosis were treated by anterior and posterior vertebral column resection (APVCR). The indication for APVCR was scoliosis of more than 90 degrees with flexibility less than 20%. Complications were encountered in four patients: one patient required ventilator support for 12 hours after anterior surgery; malposition of one pedicle screw was found in one patient; and malposition of the titanium mesh cage occurred in two patients. There were no neurologic complications, deep wound infections, or pseudarthroses.[13]

No neurologic complications, deep wound infections, or any complication of instrumentation were found at final follow-up after treatment of severe and rigid scoliosis in patients with low body weight.[14] All patients who underwent posterior spinal release, derotation, translation, segmental correction, and an in situ rod-contouring technique also seem to have avoided neurologic complications.[15]

In eight patients, the complications observed were three pseudarthroses, five hardware failures, and one transient neurologic deficit. There were no deep wound infections, deep vein thromboses, pulmonary emboli, or deaths. The average scoliosis correction was 40% (range, 5–81%), whereas the average sagittal balance was corrected 6.5 cm (range, -5–29.5 cm), on average, and coronal balance was corrected 2.5 cm (range, 1–6 cm), on average.[16] Five neurologic complications, including one late-onset paralysis and four cases of thoracic nerve root pain, were observed in the Xie et al study on posterior vertebral column resection for effective correction of severe rigid spinal deformity.[17] The authors reported that all of these neurologic complications slowly subsided.

Surgical correction or stabilization of congenital kyphoscoliosis may result in progression of kyphosis, which becomes more rigid,[18] or rarely, hemothorax, or spinal cord damage.[19,20,21,22]

Single pedicle subtraction osteotomy at the dorsolumbar level for correction of a kyphotic rigid spine seemed to be a successful operation with minimal neurologic complications.[23] Improvement of "pulmonary function and the restoration of sagittal and coronal balance are the main goals in the treatment of severe and rigid scoliosis and kyphoscoliosis."[24] These goals can be achieved by presurgical halo-gravity gradual traction. Transpedicular decancellation osteotomy may enhance neurologic recovery in patients with myelopathy due to tubercular rigid kyphosis.[25] Treatment by pedicle subtraction osteotomy of the rigid kyphotic lumbar spine can be followed by neurologic damage to the spinal cord or nerves' roots.[26,27]

Indications for correction of posttraumatic kyphotic deformity of the spine and technical aspects of the surgical procedure are reviewed. Surgical correction of posttraumatic deformity of the spine should be considered in patients presenting with a local excess of kyphosis in the fractured area superior to 20 degrees with poor functional tolerance. Severe pain, explained by objective factors such as canal or neuroforaminal compromise, with or without peripheral symptoms, angular deformity, nonunion, focal instability, and adjacent painful compensatory deformity (e.g., lumbar hyperlordosis or thoracic hypokyphosis or lordosis), is a further argument for surgery. More advanced age, litigation, and work-related trauma are negative factors. Planning of the surgical procedure includes the choice of approach(es), the corrective means (subtraction osteotomy or vertebral body reconstruction), and determining the nature and extent of osteosynthesis and fusion. Decision-making factors include level of trauma, severity of deformity, history of previous surgery in the area of deformity, bone quality, and age of the fracture. Corrective surgery of a posttraumatic deformity of the spine is a difficult procedure that should be considered only by an experienced team, after careful consideration of the indication and with the consent of a well-informed patient. Complications do occur and lead to the need for reintervention in up to 10% of our cases. However, significant complications with lasting consequences did not occur in our experience. The more severe the deformity, the better are the chances to improve the patient's condition, as long as the surgical goals are fulfilled.

27.4 Posttraumatic Kyphosis (Hermann Kummell's Disease; 1895)

Posterior osteotomy is regarded as a safe procedure for the management of rigid posttraumatic kyphosis[28] in terms of pain relief, kyphosis correction, vertebral height restoration, spinal canal integrity preservation, and reducing the risk of excessive bleeding and spinal cord injury. This condition, is actually an avascular necrosis of a damaged vertebral body.[29] The reports are scarce and the number of patients is small, so one cannot draw any conclusions.

27.5 Rehabilitation Medicine Perspective

Every patient with a rigid spine who develops spinal cord damage due to trauma or failed corrective surgery poses a challenge for the multidisciplinary rehabilitation team.[30] Even if the spinal deformity is (partially) corrected, the patient with neurologic deficits requires a comprehensive approach that will deal with the following sequelae: paralysis (motor and sensory), autonomic nervous system disorders (sphincter paralysis, impotence, autonomic dysreflexia in patients whose damage had occurred above the D7 level), sweating abnormalities, orthostatic changes, as well as basic metabolic or musculoskeletal pathologies, and more. Before trauma or surgery, a patient with a rigid spine suffers from "one problem," but whenever the spinal cord or nerve roots are involved, the situation becomes a "multiproblem" issue. Treatment and management should take into account the occupational, vocational, psychosocial, and medicolegal issues. Close cooperation between the rehabilitation team and the orthopaedic surgeon is mandatory for long-term follow-up.[30]

In our opinion, lessons learned from the complications of surgical procedures on the rigid spine are as follows: perhaps consider slow correction of the deformity, especially in ankylosing spondylitis; use somatosensory evoked potentials intraoperative monitoring; and conduct a careful, thorough discussion with patients and family members and the rehabilitation team as to whether or not to operate. A lesson from Eisenstein's case report would be to avoid corrective surgery whenever there is evidence of calcification of the aorta.

References

[1] http://www.columbianeurosurgery.org/conditions/adult-spinal-deformitiy
[2] Ohry A, Frankel HL. Rehabilitation after spinal cord injuries complicated by previous lesions. Paraplegia. 1984; 22(5):291–296
[3] Adler E, Carmon A. Ankylosing spondylitis–a review of 115 cases. Acta Rheumatol Scand. 1961; 7:219–232
[4] Hicks JE, Joe GO, Gerber LH. Rehabilitation of the patient with inflammatory arthritis and connective tissue disease. In: DeLisa JA, Gans BM, Walsh NE, eds. Physical Medicine & Rehabilitation, Principles and Practice, 4th ed. Philadelphia, PA: Lippincott Williams & Wilkins; 2005:721–763
[5] Zwecker M, Daich A, Blumen N, Zeilig G, Ohry A. Slow ascending myelopathy, tetraplegia, carcinoma of the bladder and amyloidosis in a patient with ankylosing spondylitis. Spinal Cord. 2000; 38(5):327–329
[6] Guttmann L. Tetraplegia in ankylosing spondylitis. In: Vinken PJ, Bruyn GW, eds. Handbook of Clinical Neurology. New York, NY: North Holland Publishing; 1976:175–183
[7] Rowed DW. Management of cervical spinal cord injury in ankylosing spondylitis: the intervertebral disc as a cause of cord compression. J Neurosurg. 1992; 77(2):241–246
[8] Vaněk P, Votavová M, Ostrý S, Beneš V, Pavelka K. Correction of kyphotic deformity of the cervical spine in ankylosing spondylitis using pedicle subtraction osteotomy of the seventh cervical vertebra [in Czech]. Acta Chir Orthop Traumatol Cech. 2014; 81(5):317–322
[9] An SB, Kim KN, Chin DK, Kim KS, Cho YE, Kuh SU. Surgical outcomes after traumatic vertebral fractures in patients with ankylosing spondylitis. J Korean Neurosurg Soc. 2014; 56(2):108–113
[10] Bar-On Z, Zeilig G, Blumen N, Ohry A, Azaria M. Paraplegia following surgical correction of scoliosis with Cotrel-Dubousset instrumentation. Bull Hosp Jt Dis. 1995; 54(1):32–34
[11] Silva FE, Lenke LG. Adult degenerative scoliosis: evaluation and management. Neurosurg Focus. 2010; 28(3):E1
[12] Koptan WM, ElMiligui YH, ElSharkawi MM. Direct repair of spondylolysis presenting after correction of adolescent idiopathic scoliosis. Spine J. 2011; 11 (2):133–138
[13] Zhou C, Liu L, Song Y, et al. Anterior and posterior vertebral column resection for severe and rigid idiopathic scoliosis. Eur Spine J. 2011; 20(10):1728–1734
[14] Zhou C, Liu L, Song Y, et al. Anterior release internal distraction and posterior spinal fusion for severe and rigid scoliosis. Spine. 2013; 38(22):E1411–E1417

[15] Shen F, Zhou B, Li Q, et al. Posterior-only spinal release combined with derotation, translation, segmental correction, and an in situ rod-contouring technique for treatment of severe and rigid scoliosis. J Neurosurg Spine. 2015; 22 (2):194–198

[16] Voos K, Boachie-Adjei O, Rawlins BA. Multiple vertebral osteotomies in the treatment of rigid adult spine deformities. Spine. 2001; 26(5):526–533

[17] Xie J, Wang Y, Zhao Z, et al. Posterior vertebral column resection for correction of rigid spinal deformity curves greater than 100°. J Neurosurg Spine. 2012; 17(6):540–551

[18] Reinker K, Simmons JW, Patil V, Stinson Z. Can VEPTR(®) control progression of early-onset kyphoscoliosis? A cohort study of VEPTR(®) patients with severe kyphoscoliosis. Clin Orthop Relat Res. 2011; 469(5):1342–1348

[19] Li C, Fu Q, Zhou Y, Yu H, Zhao G. Surgical treatment of severe congenital scoliosis with unilateral unsegmented bar by concave costovertebral joint release and both-ends wedge osteotomy via posterior approach. Eur Spine J. 2012; 21(3):498–505

[20] Wang S, Zhang J, Qiu G, et al. Dual growing rods technique for congenital scoliosis: more than 2 years outcomes: preliminary results of a single center. Spine. 2012; 37(26):E1639–E1644

[21] Wang Y, Zhang Y, Zhang X, et al. A single posterior approach for multilevel modified vertebral column resection in adults with severe rigid congenital kyphoscoliosis: a retrospective study of 13 cases. Eur Spine J. 2008; 17 (3):361–372

[22] Zhang JG, Wang SR, Qiu GX, et al. [The efficacy and complications of one stage posterior vertebral column resection for severe spinal deformities]. Zhonghua Wai Ke Za Zhi. 2010; 48(22):1694–1700

[23] Gavaskar AS, Naveen Chowdary T. Pedicle subtraction osteotomy for rigid kyphosis of the dorsolumbar spine. Arch Orthop Trauma Surg. 2011; 131 (6):803–808

[24] Koller H, Zenner J, Gajic V, Meier O, Ferraris L, Hitzl W. The impact of halo-gravity traction on curve rigidity and pulmonary function in the treatment of severe and rigid scoliosis and kyphoscoliosis: a clinical study and narrative review of the literature. Eur Spine J. 2012; 21(3):514–529

[25] Basu S, Rathinavelu S. Neurological recovery in patients of old healed tubercular rigid kyphosis with myelopathy treated with transpedicular decancellation osteotomy. Eur Spine J. 2012; 21(10):2011–2018

[26] Barrey C, Perrin G, Michel F, Vital JM, Obeid I. Pedicle subtraction osteotomy in the lumbar spine: indications, technical aspects, results and complications. Eur J Orthop Surg Traumatol. 2014; 24 Suppl 1:S21–S30

[27] Theologis AA, Tabaraee E, Funao H, et al. Three-column osteotomies of the lower cervical and upper thoracic spine: comparison of early outcomes, radiographic parameters, and peri-operative complications in 48 patients. Eur Spine J. 2014

[28] Wang Q, Xiu P, Zhong D, Wang G, Wang S. Simultaneous posterior and anterior approaches with posterior vertebral wall preserved for rigid post-traumatic kyphosis in thoracolumbar spine. Spine. 2012; 37(17):E1085–E1091

[29] Young WF, Brown D, Kendler A, Clements D. Delayed post-traumatic osteonecrosis of a vertebral body (Kummell's disease). Acta Orthop Belg. 2002; 68 (1):13–19

[30] Heruti RJ, Ohry A. The rehabilitation team. Am J Phys Med Rehabil. 1995; 74 (6):466–468

28 Importance of the Sagittal Balance in Correction of Rigid Spine

Pierre Roussouly, Amer Sebaaly

Abstract

Rigid spinal deformity has an increasing incidence with aging population. Correction of deformity should take into consideration the spinal sagittal balance and alignment. Sagittal balance was introduced in the late 1990s and early 2000s. Several sagittal balance parameters should be assessed. The most important parameter is the pelvic incidence (PI), which is a shape parameter and a unique anatomical feature to each individual. The PI is the sum of two positional pelvic parameters, namely, the sacral slope (SS) and the pelvic tilt (PT). These pelvic parameters affect the spinal parameters and subsequently the spinal shapes. The spinal parameters could be divided into angular parameters (lumbar lordosis, thoracic kyphosis, T1 pelvic angle, spinosacral angle [SSA], global tilt) and metric parameters (sagittal vertical axis, Barrey ratio). According to the pelvic parameters and the lumbar lordosis, Roussouly presented five types of spinal shapes. They then published a classification of the degenerative evolution of the spinal shapes according to each normal spinal shape. This chapter will review all these concepts, and will propose a treatment algorithm based on the classification of the degenerative spinal shapes.

Keywords: sagittal balance, pelvic parameters, spinal parameters, rigid spinal deformity, Roussouly classification

28.1 Introduction

Homo sapiens is the only species that uses a constantly bipedal stance for ambulation. Human bipedalism is the sole position of the species; it is stable and ergonomic. This upright position resulted in broadening of the pelvis, giving humans their characteristic sagittal spinal curves, and particularly the lordosis of the lumbar area. This change of stance resulted in a broadened pelvis by progressive sagittal positioning of the iliac wings of the pelvis in Hominidae. This results in increasing the pelvic diameter (and thus the pelvic incidence). In fact, the mean pelvic incidence of *Australopithecus afarensis* (Lucy) is thought to be around 20 degrees, whereas the mean pelvic incidence in *Homo sapiens* is around 54 degrees.

The sagittal balance concept has been one of the most discussed topics in the recent spinal, neurosurgical, and orthopaedic meetings worldwide as well as in the recent medical literature.[1] The concept and the importance of spinal balance were highlighted in France with the works of Jean Dubousset and the concepts of the "pelvic vertebra" and the "economical conus of balance,"[2] and then in Duval-Beaupère's 1998 description of pelvic incidence.[3] The overall sagittal shape and balance and their implications for spinal biomechanics were thoroughly studied by Roussouly et al.[4,5] This chapter elucidates the importance of sagittal balance in treating spinal deformity by analyzing important sagittal parameters (with a special focus on lumbar lordosis), describing the normal and degenerative spinal shapes as well as proposing surgical algorithms for treating rigid spinal deformity.

28.2 Pelvic Sagittal Parameters: The Plinth of Sagittal Balance

Initially described by During et al[6] and then defined by Legaye et al, whose work began the formal study of sagittal balance.[3] Pelvic incidence (PI) is a sagittal angle formed by the line drawn from midpoint of the upper S 1 end plate to the center of the bicoxofemoral axis, which is the center point of the overlap between the bilateral femoral heads (or hip axis) (this line is referred to as pelvic thickness) and the line perpendicular to the upper sacral end plate (▶ Fig. 28.1). Being a shape parameter, it is a unique anatomical feature in each individual and becomes set at the end of growth, regardless of the patient's position.[7] It has also been shown that there is a tendency of PI to increase linearly with age for children until the age of 10 and for adolescents to have a value similar to that in adults.[8] In asymptomatic populations, PI range varies from 33 to 85 degrees with a mean of 53 degrees in males and 56 degrees in females ($p < 0.05$).[9] Recent studies have shown differences in human races, with lower PI values in Asians (47.8 degrees) compared with Caucasian (51.9 degrees), and higher values in Hispanics (56.7 degrees) and African Americans (56 degrees).[10,11] Another study demonstrated a slight variation of PI (>3 degrees) in one person, probably due to sacroiliac joint motion.

Two sagittal "positional" pelvic parameters emerge from PI: the sacral slope (SS) and the pelvic tilt (PT) (▶ Fig. 28.1). The SS is the angle between the upper sacral end plate and the horizontal line, and PT is the angle between the pelvic thickness and the vertical axis (▶ Fig. 28.1). These parameters are governed by the mathematical relationship to the PI: $PT + SS = PI$. Because it is positional parameter, SS is often greater in the supine position (when the lower limbs are extended) than in the standing position (pelvis flexion). It diminishes when the person is sitting (pelvic extension).[7] This difference between supine and sitting angles defines the range of motion of the pelvis. To compensate the linear increase of PI with growth, PT tends to increase with age to maintain an adequate sagittal balance, whereas SS is not significantly altered by age after acquisition of walking.[12] In asymptomatic populations, PT averages 13.2 degrees and ranges between − 4.5 and 27 degrees, with a mean of 13 degrees in males and 13.6 degrees in females ($p > 0.05$), whereas SS averages 41.2 degrees, varying from 17 to 63 degrees with significant male/female difference (41 vs. 43 degrees, respectively, $p < 0.05$).[9] Some authors have proposed a way to predict the values of SS and PT. They found that SS value is two-thirds of the PI value + 7 degrees, whereas the PT value would be the remaining third of the PI value − 7 degrees.[9] Regarding the mathematical relation $PI = PT + SS$, linear relations, such as $PI = a\ PT + b$ or $PI = a\ SS + b$, are impossible, and the obtained results are wrong or at least very approximate.

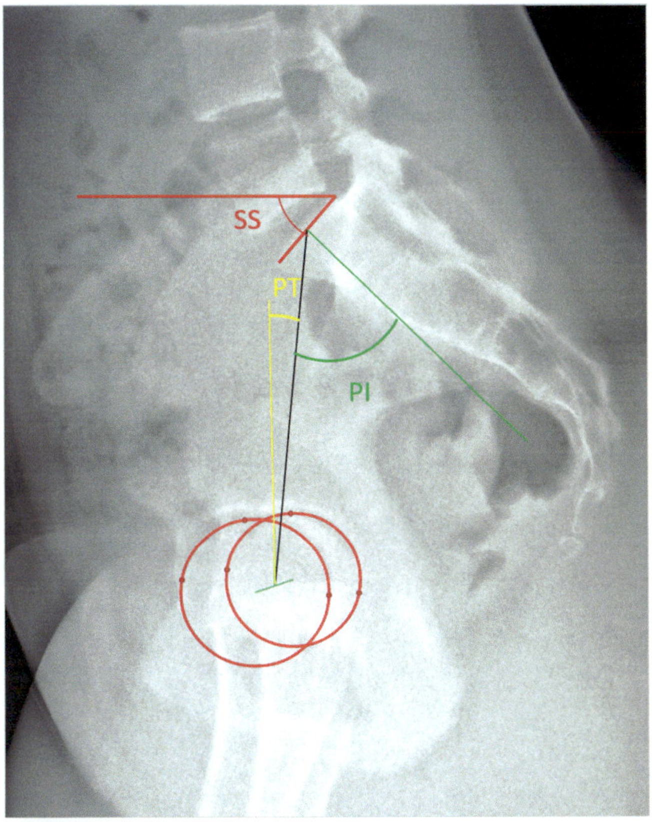

Fig. 28.1 Lateral X-rays centered over the lumbar area and showing the femoral heads. Pelvic incidence (PI) is the measured angle formed by the pelvic thickness and the perpendicular line to the upper sacral plateau. The sacral slope (SS) is the angle between the upper sacral end plate and the horizontal line, and the pelvic tilt (PT) is the angle between the pelvic thickness and the vertical axis.

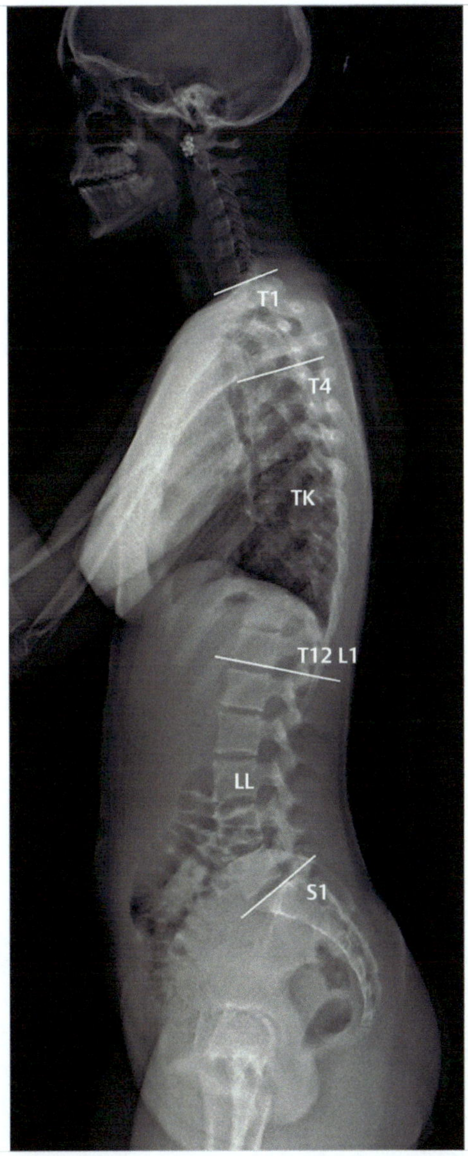

Fig. 28.2 Classical method (fixed) for measuring lumbar lordosis (LL) and thoracic kyphosis (TK). LL is measured between the upper end plates of L 1 and S 1, and TK is measured between T 1 and T 12 or T 4 and T 12.

28.3 Spinal Sagittal Parameters: Are We Speaking the Same Language?

As already mentioned, the human spine is characterized by sagittal curvatures arranged in consecutive lordosis and kyphosis curves from the cervical spine to the sacrum. This allows the body weight to be balanced above the pelvis, in turn generating an economical bipedal gait.[7] The term *lordosis* comes from the Greek word *lordos* (lórdōs, bent backward), whereas *kyphosis* originates from the Greek *kyphos* (hump). Nonetheless, there is no unanimity for the exact angular definition of lumbar lordosis. The relationship between pelvic parameters and spinal ones was initially described by Stagnara et al[13] as an array of variations of the normal spine, ranging from a "static" flat back (with low SS) to a "dynamic" curved back (with high SS).

The Scoliosis Research Society (SRS)-Schwab classification (and subsequent North American publications) defines lumbar lordosis (LL) as the angle between the upper end plate of S 1 and the upper end plate of L 1.[14] They defined the thoracic kyphosis (TK) as the angle between the lower end plate of T 12 and the upper end plate of T 1 (▶ Fig. 28.2). Since the T 1 vertebra is frequently overshadowed by the humeral head and rib cage on the lateral films, and the reliability of measuring T 1–T 5 kyphosis is low, many authors recommend measuring the of T4–T 12 angle.[15] This segmentation in the thoracic and lumbar spine is anatomical, dividing the spine into 12 thoracic and 5 lumbar vertebrae. Based on these definitions, many attempts were made to correlate pelvic and spinal parameters. Schwab et al found that restoring the LL value according to the formula LL = PI ± 9 degrees[16] was correlated to better surgical outcomes. Even though this "rule of the thumb" is helpful for novice spinal surgeons, it has several limitations. First, PI is a constitutional parameter and doesn't vary during adulthood. On the other hand, LL is a positional and very variable parameter during someone's life. Associating these two parameters with a mathematical formula seems logically unfounded. Second, albeit this formula would fit medium-range PI, with PI values in the extremes (<35 and above 70), applying this formula for correction would result in overcorrection in the low PI group and undercorrection in the high PI group. This miscorrection would thus lead to various surgical complications and undesired results. This will be further discussed in the following sections of this chapter.

The main problem with this anatomical segmentation is that, with a fixed limit (T 12 or L 1) it does consider the kyphotic and lordotic curvatures' respective lengths. Spinal parameters can also be measured using a nonfixed approach, where limits of LL and TK are based on the individual sagittal shape of the spine. In other words, the upper limit of LL would not be fixed at L 1, and LL would be measured from the upper end plate of the sacrum to the upper-limit vertebra as when measuring the coronal Cobb angle of the scoliosis.[17] Based on this concept, first described by Stagnara et al[13] and then popularized by Roussouly et al,[17] Berthonnaud et al introduced in 2005 the "inflexion point" as a limiting functional zone between LL and TK, where lordosis curvature switches to kyphosis.[18] In the sagittal plane, the pelvis and spine are considered as an open linear chain linking the head to the pelvis, in which the shape and orientation of each anatomical segment are closely related and influence the adjacent segment to maintain a stable posture with a minimum of energy expenditure.[18] Thus changes in shape or orientation at one level will have a direct influence on the adjacent segment. It is very important to realize this concept in order to understand degenerative spinal evolution discussed later in this chapter (see "Degenerative Spinal Evolution"). Roussouly et al found then that LL could be divided into two arches: the lower arch is equal to the SS and the quasi-constant upper arch of around 20 degrees.[4] The authors found LL to be highly correlated to SS and to a lesser extent to PI and PT.[4]

It is worth noting that the term *lumbar lordosis* can be confusing, and for the majority of authors may be difficult to accept that lordosis may overpass or be shorter than the lumbar area. We think it is necessary to propose a new nosology: spinal lordosis (SL) for the segment of the spine where the vertebrae are in extension (increasing angle between two successive inferior end plates), and spinal kyphosis (SK) where vertebrae are in flexion (decreasing angle between two successive inferior end plates) (▶ Fig. 28.3). The normal spine would then have three curvatures: The superior SL (SSL) in the cervical (or thoracic) area, the SK in the thoracic (with possible extension to the cervical and lumbar areas), and the lower SL (LSL) in the lumbar area (with possible extension to the thoracolumbar spine).

Few studies have compared the fixed angular approach (always L 1–S 1) and the nonfixed angle approach. In 2005, Vialle et al published a cornerstone study correlating spinal and pelvic parameters.[9] They found that "fixed LL" was correlated to SS ($R = 0.76$) and to a lesser extent to PI ($R = 0.6$) and to PT ($R = 0.24$). On the other hand, nonfixed LL (LSL; they termed it maximal LL) was better correlated to SS ($R = 0.86$) (Roussouly et al[4] found a similar result) and to a lesser extent to PI ($R = 0.6$) and to PT ($R = 0.26$). They recommended the use of maximal LL

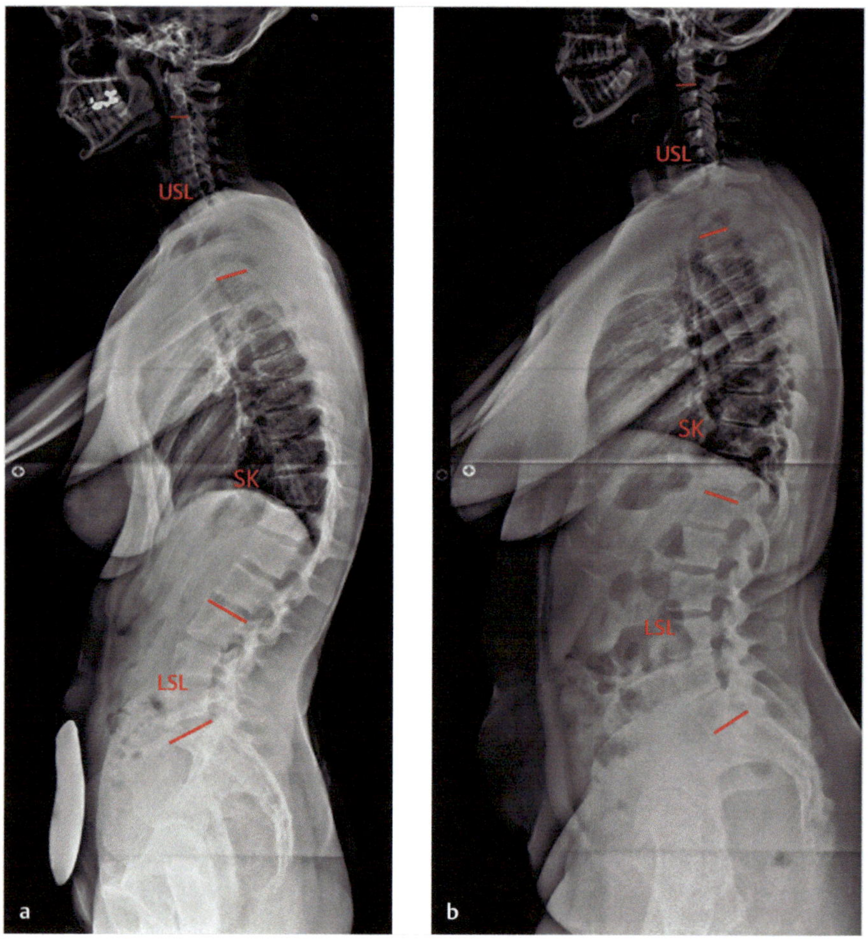

Fig. 28.3 Nonfixed method for measuring lumbar lordosis (LL) and thoracic kyphosis (TK), here referred to as spinal lordosis (SL) and spinal kyphosis (SK). **(a)** A case of an asymptomatic 30-year-old woman with a very short and steep SL (over three lumbar vertebrae) and a very long SK. **(b)** X-ray of an asymptomatic 25-year-old woman with very long lordosis (extending to T 11) and a shorter SK. LSL, lower spinal lordosis; USL, upper spinal lordosis.

as a value for LL and proposed a calculation method for all the sagittal parameters based on correlation (▶ Table 28.1). In the remaining parts of this chapter, SL (upper spinal lordosis [USL] and lower spinal lordosis [LSL]) and SK will be used.

28.4 Spinal Balance Parameters: Metric versus Angular

Why is it important to study sagittal balance? In 2001, Kumar et al found that lumbar arthrodesis with a balanced spine had the lowest incidence of adjacent segment disease (ASD) (5%) compared to that for an unbalanced spine (50%; $p = 0.02$).[19] Even when a surgeon is contemplating short-segment fixation, sagittal balance is important. The most legitimate question to follow is: What are the spinal parameters and their intended values that are required to define sagittal balance? A combination of positional pelvic parameters PT and SS, driven by the shape parameter PI, with spinal curvatures LSL and SK has to bring the global spine into a balanced situation. As for architecture, the plumb line of the top of the spine identified by the C 7 vertebral body (the first clearly visible proximal vertebra on X-rays) and its position regarding pelvic landmarks is a key factor used to evaluate the spinal global balance. Several parameters using C 7 positioning were used to identify spinal balance. With the increasing quality of recent radiographic techniques, other anatomical landmarks (e. g., the T 1 body or points on the skull) have been used.

The first and oldest parameter is the sagittal vertical axis (SVA)—the distance between the posterior superior corner of the sacrum and a plumb line from the center of the C 7 vertebra (C 7pl). Normal values in asymptomatic patients range between −3 and 3 cm[9] (▶ Fig. 28.4). Glassman et al found that coronal shift >4 cm, SVA >5 cm, and PT >25 degrees was associated with decreased quality of life scores.[20] Vital and Senegas,[21] then

Table 28.1 Calculation method

SS = 7.3 + 0.63 PI
PT = − 7 + 0.37 PI
MLL = − 16 − 1.06 SS
LL = − 2.72 − 1.1 PI + 1.1 PT − 0.31 MTK

Abbreviations: LL, lumbar lordosis; MLL, maximum lumbar lordosis; MTK, maximum thoracic kyphosis; PI, pelvic incidence; PT, pelvic tilt; SS, sacral slope.

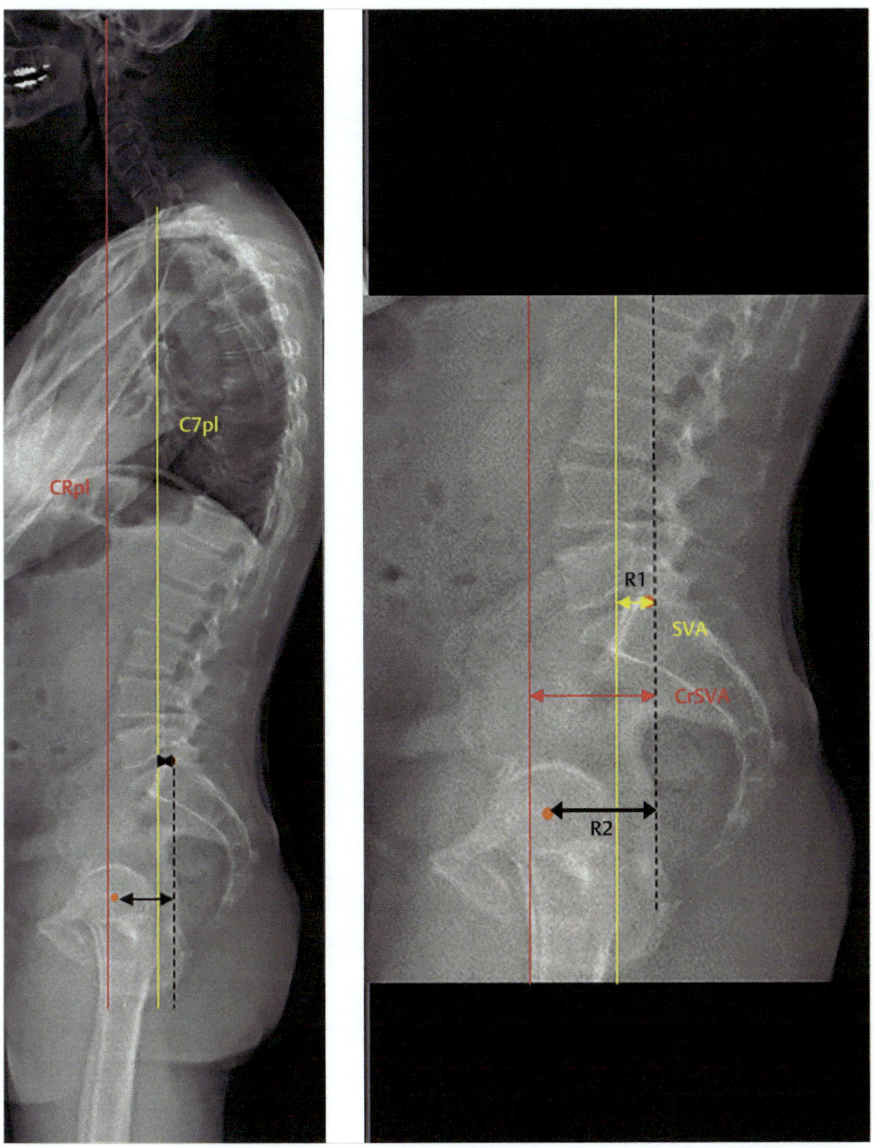

Fig. 28.4 Global metric parameters: sagittal vertical axis (SVA) is the distance between the posterior upper S 1 end plate and the C 7 plumb line (C 7pl). The cranial sagittal vertical axis (Cr SVA) is the distance between the posterior upper S 1 end plate and the cranial plumb line (CRpl). The Barrey ratio (BR) is the ratio between the SVA and the distance between the posterior upper S 1 end plate and the vertical passing through the hip axis. R1, SVA; R2, the distance between the posterior upper S1 end plate and the vertical passing through the hip axis.

more recently, Kim et al, proposed a new global metric value for sagittal balance: the cranial sagittal vertical axis (CrSVA). The CrSVA is measured using the plumb line from the external auditory meatus and the posterior border of the upper sacral end plate.[22] It was found to have a strong correlation with Oswestry disability index (ODI) and all the SRS subscores. CrSVA was also found to have a stronger predictor effect for preoperative clinical outcomes than the standard SVA.[22]

Nonetheless, there has been much criticism regarding the use of metric parameters for evaluation of global sagittal balance. First, length measurements require proper calibration of the X-rays. A known enlargement effect occurs in X-rays, depending on the position of the tube and the patient while the image is being taken; the increase in length is estimated to be around 20% of the actual size. This effect is reduced with newer acquisition techniques, such as the EOS imaging system, because of the fixed distance and the decreased cone beam artifact. Another criticism pertains to the size variation among patients, for example, when comparing the SVA in a tall man with that of a small woman. To compensate for this shortcoming, in 2007 Barrey et al suggested measuring the ratio of the SVA to the distance between the posterior corner of the sacral end plate and the vertical line passing through the hip axis.[23] This eliminates the enlarging effect of standard imaging because no calibration is needed. The Barrey ratio serves as an important parameter in studying global balance as discussed later in this chapter. It allows positioning the C 7pl regarding the anterior corner of the sacral plateau and the center of the femoral heads. The C 7pl may be behind the sacrum, between the femoral heads and the sacrum, and in front of the femoral heads.

Length measurements are dependent on the position of the patient in the X-ray machine and do not take into account the patient's effort to compensate, which is another shortcoming of SVA and CrSVA. In fact these measurements vary on the basis of the extent of pelvic retroversion or patient support in the standing position and are independent of many postural compensatory mechanisms. Angular measurements were thus introduced. Roussouly et al introduced angular parameters from C 7. The first angular measurement was positional, the C 7 vertical tilt (C 7VT), and is measured between the line joining the center of T 1 and the midpoint of the upper S 1 end plate (▶ Fig. 28.5a, b). Albeit the fact that C 7VT is simply the angular equivalent of SVA, there are few studies comparing this parameter to health-related quality of life (HRQOL) scores. The two other measurements were shape parameters: the spinosacral angle (SSA) was measured between the line joining the center of C 7 and the midpoint of the upper S 1 end plate, and the sacral plateau and the spinopelvic angle were measured with the same line (C 7–S 1) and the line of pelvic thickness between S 1 and the femoral heads. The SSA gives the value of the global spinal kyphosis. In the normal population it correlates perfectly with the SS. This demonstrates that in a balanced spine the position of C 7 over the pelvis is very stable, whatever the value of SS.

After its description SPA was carefully studied. It consists of the addition of SSA with a complementary angle of PI (SPA = SSA + 90-degree PI). Global tilt (GT) is another angular parameter recently introduced. GT is the complementary angle to the SPA, that is, the angle formed by the line joining the center of T 1 and the midpoint of the upper S 1 end plate and the pelvic thickness. GT appears to be less affected by patient positioning than the SVA and PT.[24] From a geometrical point of view, GT is the sum of PT and the C 7 vertical tilt. A GT cutoff value of 33.7 degrees was proposed by the authors for an ODI score >40.[24]

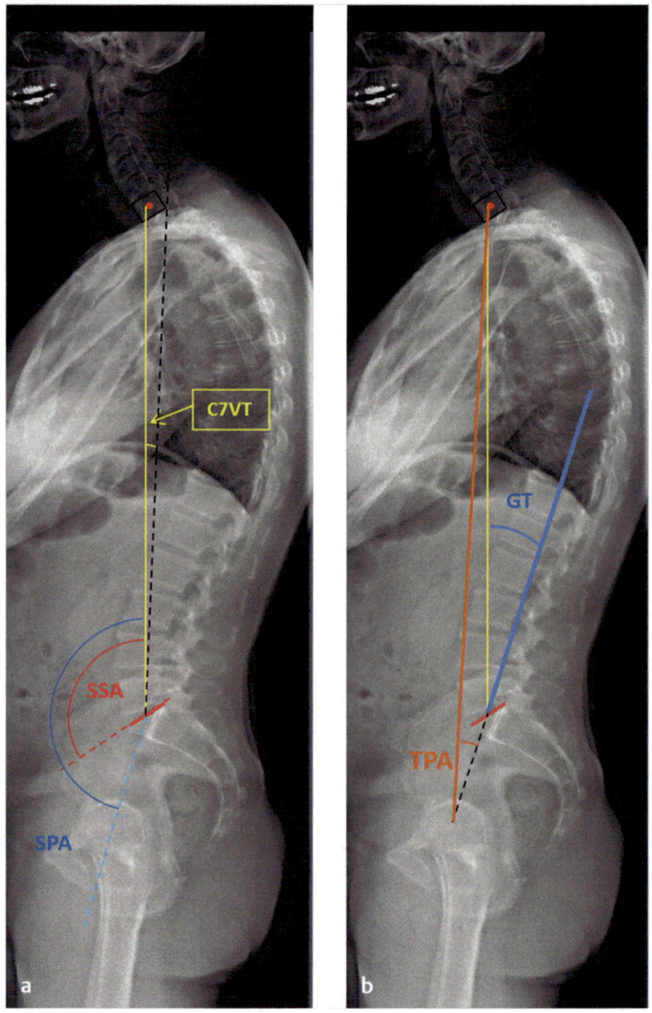

Fig. 28.5 Global angular parameters. **(a)** C 7 vertical tilt (C 7VT) is the angle between the line from the center of C 7 to the mid upper S 1 end plate and the vertical. The spinopelvic angle (SPA) is the angle between the line from the center of C 7 to the mid upper S 1 end plate and the pelvic thickness, whereas the spinosacral angle (SSA) is the angle between the line from the center of C 7 to the mid upper S 1 end plate and the upper sacral end plate. **(b)** Global tilt (GT) is none other than the supplementary angle of SPA. The T 1 pelvic angle (TPA) is the angle formed by the line from the center of T 1 to the hip axis and the pelvic thickness.

The T 1 pelvic angle (T 1PA or TPA) was first introduced by Protopsaltis et al[25] and represents the angle measured by the line from the center of T 1 to the hip axis and the pelvic thickness. TPA is related to both PT and SVA without any effect of patient compensation. It was found to correlate to HRQOL in patients with adult spinal deformity. A target TPA of <14 degrees should be the goal in preoperative planning.[25,26] Despite the absence of a comparative study between GT and TPA, the former seems more reliable because the latter relies on the femoral head axis, which may increase the error margin during the measurement given the fact that femoral heads are not always properly seen on the X-rays.[27]

All these angles are in very close proximity in geometrical construction, and it is important to recognize a truly new angle as opposed to an already described angle that is simply changed by the addition or subtraction of 90 degrees.

28.5 Spinal Shapes in the Normal Population

The classic anatomical teaching on the spinal curvatures consists of consecutive lordosis and kyphosis moving from the cervical spine to the sacrum. This succession of curvature is of primary importance for an economical bipedal gait of *homo sapiens*. As discussed earlier, Berthonnaud et al introduced in 2005 the "inflexion point."[28] Based on this theory, Roussouly et al proposed, in a study of normal volunteers, the classification of spinal shapes SK and LSL. The original study of Roussouly found near perfect correlation between LSL and SS, whereas PI and PT correlated less to the LSL.[4] Since the LSL is formed by two arches, one lower arch that equals the SS and one quasi-constant upper arch, the Roussouly classification defined four types of spinal shapes based on the SS and the extent of the LSL (▶ Fig. 28.6).[4] With lower SS values, there are two options: the lower arch of LSL tends to disappear (type 1), or the radius of the lower arch increases, close to a straight line (type 2). With higher SS values, the lower arch of LSL increases in angle and length with a higher apex of LSL (types 3 and 4).

- *Type 1:* Characterized by low SS (< 35 degrees), where the LSL is short and the SK is long, extending to the thoracolumbar area. The position of the inflexion point does not exceed the L3–L2 level, with a maximum of three vertebrae in the LSL. This is a nonharmonious back with thoracolumbar kyphosis and short hyperlordosis. The inflexion point or sagittal apex of the lordosis (SAL) is the L5 or L4–L5 disk.
- *Type 2:* Characterized by low SS (< 35 degrees) and by a longer but flat LSL (over three levels), close to a straight line. This is a harmonious flat back. The SAL is the L4 vertebra.
- *Type 3:* Characterized by medium-range SS (35-degree 35 <SS ≤45 degrees) with a well-balanced LSL between its two arches. This is a harmonious regular back. The SAL is the L3 vertebra or the L3–L4 disk.
- *Type 4:* Characterized by high SS (> 45 degrees) with increased LSL length and curvature. This is a harmonious hypercurved back. The SAL is the L3 vertebra or higher.

It was noted that types 1 and 2 had low PI values (< 50 degrees), whereas types 3 and 4 had high PI values (>50 degrees). The originality of Roussouly's classification is the introduction of a geometrical relation between SS and the lower arc of lordosis (between the S1 plateau and the horizontal line through the LSL apex), and thus with the construction of the overall spinal shape. Although several studies demonstrated a strong correlation between SS and PI,[29] the geometrical relation, PI = PT + SS, allows for the possibility of a high SS with a smaller PI if the PT is small or negative: for example, PI = 40 degrees, PT = 0 degrees, and SS = 40 degrees. Thus the original Roussouly classification could have missed a spinal shape type. A revision of the original classification was recently published and included this missed type of spinal shape.[30] The *anteverted type 3* has the same characteristics of the classical type 3 (medium SS) but with a low PT (PT ≤5 degrees). It was noted that these anteverted types had a low PI.[30] Thus there is a possibility of higher-than-expected SS with a small PI. Because LL correlates with SS, type 3 LL may be found associated with a small PI when the pelvis is anteverted (i.e., a small or negative PT). This situation is not exceptional: 16% of the recently published population could be characterized as anteverted type 3.[30]

The use of Roussouly's classification has not been popularized in North America, with detractors of this classification criticizing

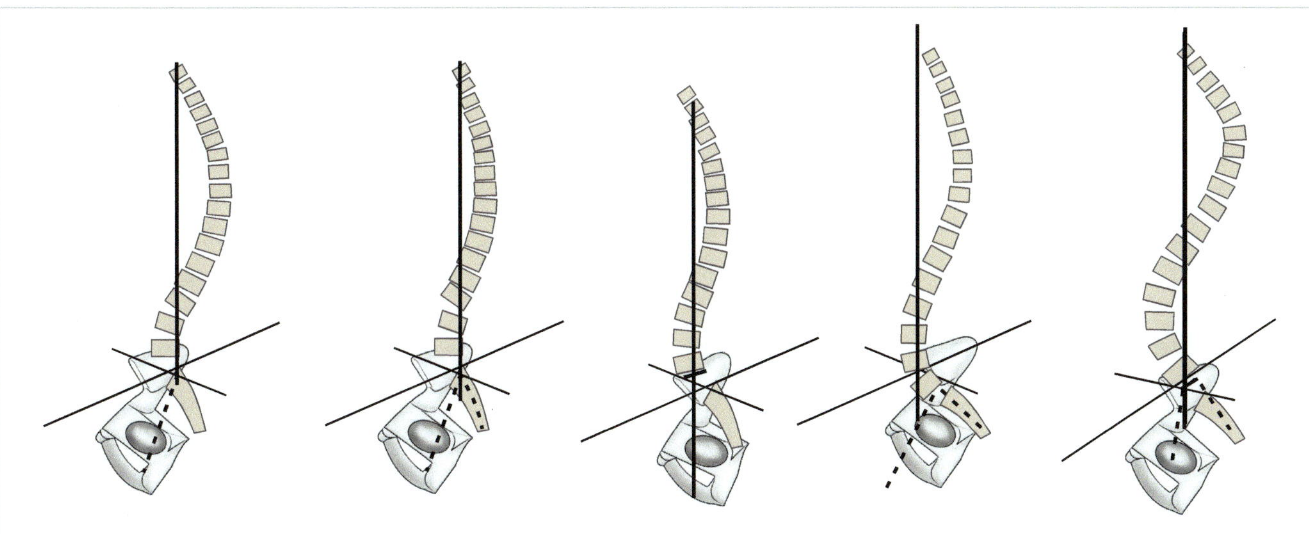

Fig. 28.6 The modified Roussouly classification.[29] Normal human spines could be divided into five different shapes according to sacral slope (SS) and pelvic incidence (PI). Types 1 and 2 have a small SS and PI, with the former having a small spinal lordosis and a long thoracic kyphosis, whereas the latter have a straight spine. Anteverted type 3 have a small PI but a high SS and a low pelvic tilt. Type 3 have a high PI and a medium-range SS, whereas type 4 have a very high PI and SS.

it for being established in the asymptomatic population and unusable in pathological conditions. Yet this classification helps in determining the high local stress zones in the spine: the greater the curvature of the lumbar spine, the greater the contact force on the posterior elements (facets in particular); the lower the curvature of the lumbar spine (i.e., flat back), the higher impact on the disks.[5] In addition, an anatomical study found that degenerative disk disease was associated with low SS, low PI patients, whereas high SS, high PI patients had a higher incidence of isthmic and degenerative spondylolisthesis.[23] This classification is important in that it will constitute the basis of the development of degenerative spine classification discussed in the next section. We may summarize this assertion as follows: a pathological spine previously had a normal shape, and the only signature of this original shape is the PI.

28.6 Degenerative Spinal Evolution

The loss of disk height is often the first phenomenon of local loss of balance inducing local kyphosis. The end point of compensation is having an upward gait and horizontal tilt of the head for a normal line of sight. If the spine is flexible, there is an increased extension of the flexible spine above and/or below this local kyphosis, with contraction of the posterior spinal muscles, which lifts the trunk vertically, requiring a painful, abnormal effort from the spinal muscles to prevent falling forward with increased pressure on the posterior facets. If the spine is rigid, with progressive kyphosis, the gravity line moves forward and the pelvis rotates backward (retroversion), inducing a decrease in the SS and an increase in PT.[31] What follows is a hyperextension of the hips, which is limited by the extension reserve (generally 10 degrees), and finally a flexion of the knees in severe forms, which is controlled by the quadriceps.[31]

It is fundamental to recognize both mechanisms. They have different clinical expressions and may be divided in local compensation and global unbalance. The first one (extension above and below the flexion accident) induces local compensations in the shape of the spine to restore a new alignment allowing slight global adaptations. The global balance is poorly disturbed and sometimes maintained. It could be, for instance, an L 3–L 4 hyperextension above an insufficient lordotic L 4–S 1 arthrodesis, or a flattening of the thoracic spine above a hypolordotic lumbar fusion. However, these local compensations are painful, either by local hyperextensive stress on the posterior facets or by muscle contracture to maintain an abnormal local positioning as thoracic hypokyphosis. These patients are difficult to diagnose because they may have pain and discomfort without global unbalance, but they do have balance problems.

The second mechanism is the well-known classical unbalance: loss of lordosis, and/or hyperkyphosis. Compensation mechanisms are unable to balance the system, either because they are surpassed or because of rigidity, leading to a retroverted pelvis and forward displacement of the C7pl. This mechanism of pelvic retroversion is linked to the PI value. The higher the PI, the greater the PT. This has a double effect: horizontal positioning of the SS and backward positioning of the whole spine regarding the femoral heads. It is limited by the hips' reserve of extension.[32] Maintaining this position is not economical and may induce muscle contractures (gluteus and hamstrings). Even if the balance seems controlled in a standing position, during walking, the forward unbalance becomes more obvious due to the hip positioning in the gait during the posterior step. When the spine is rigid, the forward unbalance causes discomfort but little pain.

Based on this, and on the Barrey ratio (BR), sagittal spinal balance can be divided into three categories (► Fig. 28.7)[33]:

1. *Type A or normal spinal balance:* This type is characterized by global balance of the trunk with a BR <100% (the C7pl is

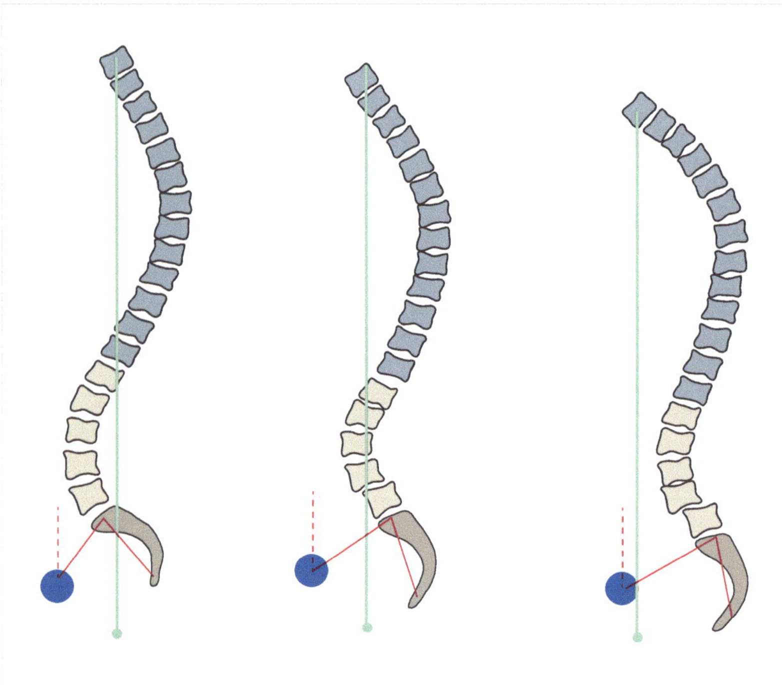

Fig. 28.7 Sagittal imbalance can be divided into three clinical scenarios. Type A is a balanced spine with a Barrey ratio (BR) < 100 % and a pelvic tilt (PT) corresponding to the pelvic incidence (PI). Type B is a spine with compensated balance in which the compensation of the sagittal imbalance begets a normal BR (< 100 %) with the caveat of a higher than normal PT. Type C is an unbalanced spine where all compensatory mechanisms have been lost.

behind the femoral heads) and normal PT (between 10 and 25 degrees). The lower limbs are completely extended in the standing position.

2. *Type B or compensated balance:* The global balance of the trunk is still normal (BR <100%) but the pelvis is retroverted (PT >25 degrees). The lower limbs show extension of the hips (the femur is straight), and the knees are in full extension.
3. *Type C or decompensated balance:* Global balance of the trunk shows a positive SVA with C7pl falling generally in front of the femoral heads, and the pelvis shows a PT in retroversion. In the lower limbs, there is extension of the hips (pelvic retroversion) and flexion of the knees. The hip extension is surpassed.

It is important to recognize the type of sagittal imbalance or compensated balance. It was found that posterior fusion in a compensated balanced position was associated with increased ASD compared to fusion patients in an unbalanced position.[19] This classification system is simplistic, and one could not develop a surgical strategy based on this classification, but there have been no attempts to classify sagittal imbalance beyond this primitive, simplistic reasoning. In fact, many attempts have been made to classify degenerative spine diseases, such as the degenerative spondylolisthesis classification[34,35] or adult deformity (Schwab-SRS classification).[14] All the parameters used in these classifications are positional parameters, without any attempt to analyze the shape of the spine and its pathological evolution. Furthermore, HRQOL scores and mechanical complications (e.g., proximal junctional kyphosis [PJK], nonunion, etc.) were correlated to some local parameters (PI, LL) or overall parameters (TPA, GT) without considering the shape of the degenerative spine.

We propose, in this chapter, a classification and degenerative evolution of the aging spine based on the initial Roussouly classification and the compensatory mechanisms for local kyphosis (▶ Fig. 28.8, ▶ Fig. 28.9, ▶ Fig. 28.10, ▶ Fig. 28.11).[36] This classification is divided into eleven types clustered into four categories:

1. *Classical types:* These are the described types 1 to 4 of the initial Roussouly classification (see earlier discussion)
2. *Anteverted types 3 and 4:* These types have respectively the same characteristics of the classical types 3 and 4 (medium and high SS) but with a low PT (PT < 5 degrees).
3. *Retroverted (or false) types:* These types arise from the four classical types with a pelvic retroversion. False types 2 and 3 have respectively the same characteristics of the classical types according to SS and LL shape, but they have a high PT (PT >25 degrees). False type 2 with TK has a low SS, a straight LL, a high PI, and high TK.
4. *Kyphotic types:* When all compensatory mechanisms are overwhelmed, kyphosis results and can be divided into two subtypes, according to the possibility of compensation in the thoracic spine:
   a) *Lumbar kyphosis shape:* Characterized by lumbar kyphosis with a hypokyphotic thoracic compensation curve.
   b) *Global kyphosis shape:* Characterized by lumbar kyphosis without a hypokyphotic thoracic compensation curve (and thus an unbalanced spine).

To simply understand this classification of spinal degenerative evolution, one must bear in mind the appropriate compensatory mechanism for local kyphosis: hyperlordosis of the adjacent mobile spine and/or retroversion of the pelvis. Considering these facts, this description of the sagittal alignment of the degenerative human spine is created by adding kyphosis to the four classical types. When a type 1 spine degenerates, compensation occurs below, in the lumbar spine, by increasing the lordosis on a short segment (thereby accentuating the type 1). On the other hand, when compensation mechanisms are inefficient, LL disappears, giving rise to the global kyphosis type, with a very small PI (▶ Fig. 28.8). Type 2 spines also have a small range of compensation. When the kyphosis occurs, either LL increases on a small arch, generating a type 1 spine (thoracolumbar kyphosis) or a global kyphosis type (with a low PI), or lumbar spine lordosis disappears, generating a lumbar kyphosis type (if the thoracic spine can compensate with a hypokyphosis) (▶ Fig. 28.9). In type 3 spines, compensation begins in the mobile spine above (loss of TK) and evolves enough to create retroversion with a straight

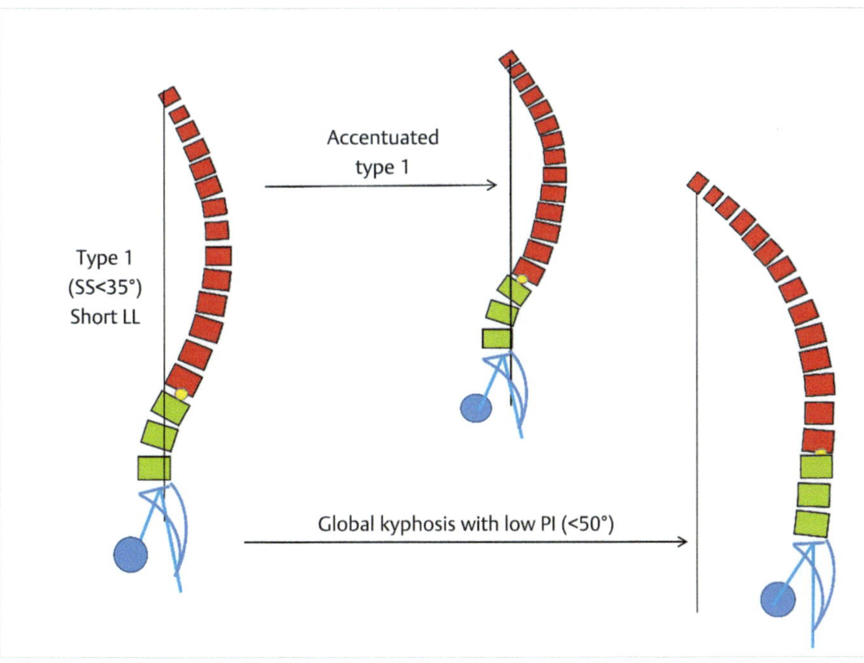

Fig. 28.8 Possible degenerative evolution of type 1 into accentuated type 1 and then global kyphosis with a low pelvic incidence.

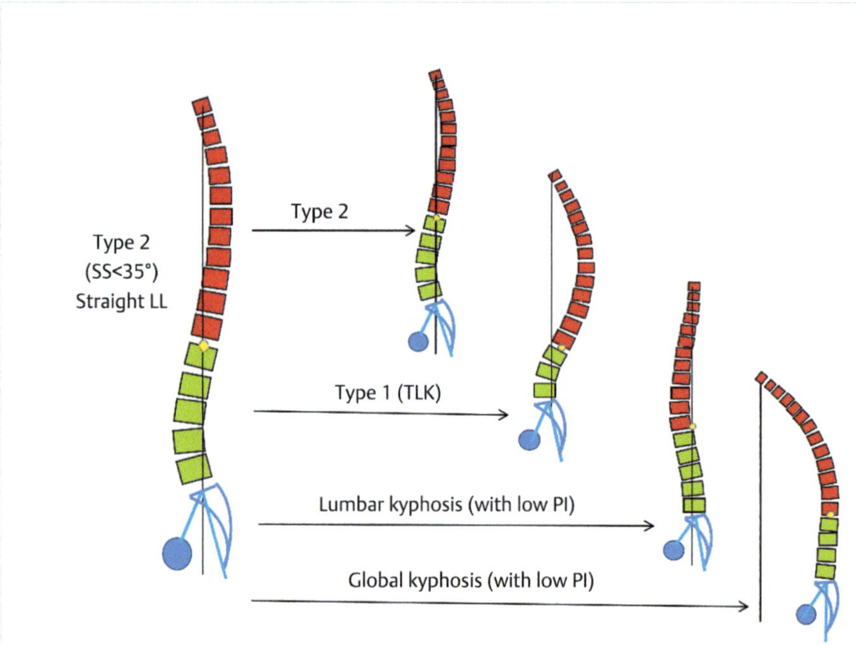

Fig. 28.9 Possible degenerative evolution of type 2 into type 1, type 2, lumbar kyphosis (with low pelvic incidence [PI]), or global kyphosis (with low PI).

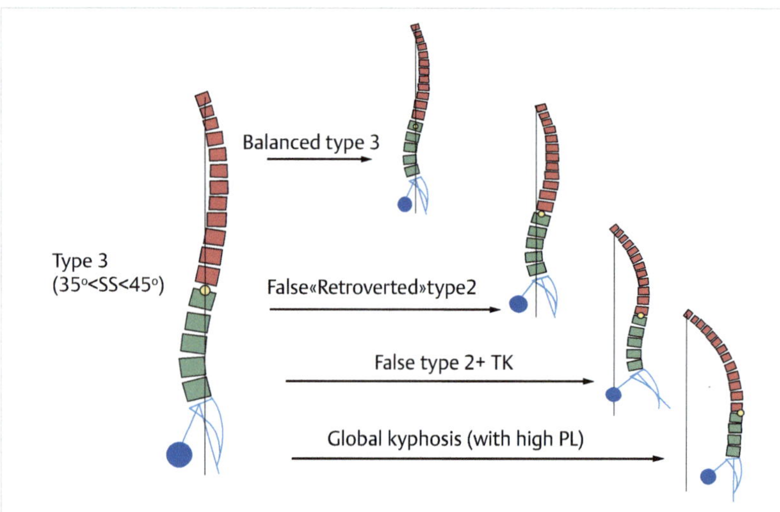

Fig. 28.10 Possible degenerative evolution of type 3 into balanced type 3, false type 2 (same as retroverted, with or without thoracic kyphosis [TK]), or global kyphosis with a high pelvic incidence (PI).

spine (false type 2) or a false type 2 with TK, when the thoracic spine is not mobile enough, with the only compensation being increased PT (retroversion of the pelvis). The ultimate evolution of type 3 is global kyphosis (with a high PI) and a maximally retroverted pelvis (▸ Fig. 28.10). Finally, a decrease of lordosis in type 4 spines induces the false type 3 spine, a type 3 shape with a retroverted pelvis. The subsequent evolution is identical to that of type 3 spines (▸ Fig. 28.11).

28.7 Surgical Strategies in Correcting Rigid Spinal Sagittal Deformity

Rigid spinal deformities require both great surgical ability and thorough preoperative preparation. Before proposing our algorithm for surgical management of adult deformity based on the foregoing proposed classification, we propose some basic rules for management. First, we believe that anterior support is of primary importance. Interbody fusion should always be done, especially if the disk opens up after posterior fixation (≥8 mm). We recommend anterior lateral interbody fusion (ALIF) for L5–S1 and oblique lateral interbody fusion (OLIF) for disks from L2 to L5 since it has shown to have a low risk of neurologic and vascular complications and low bleeding volumes.[37] Second, there is a tendency for different surgical goals between genders. In fact, males have better tolerance for undercorrection than do females, probably due to stronger posterior musculature. Finally, when the spine is not rigid, a Smith-Petersen type osteotomy or a Ponte osteotomy is preferred over a pedicle subtraction osteotomy since the former yield the same results with fewer complications.[38]

The most important aspect of the surgical strategy (▸ Fig. 28.12) in the correction of adult deformity is to avoid both under- and overcorrection, either of which could lead to several early complications (discussion follows). According to PI, the aim

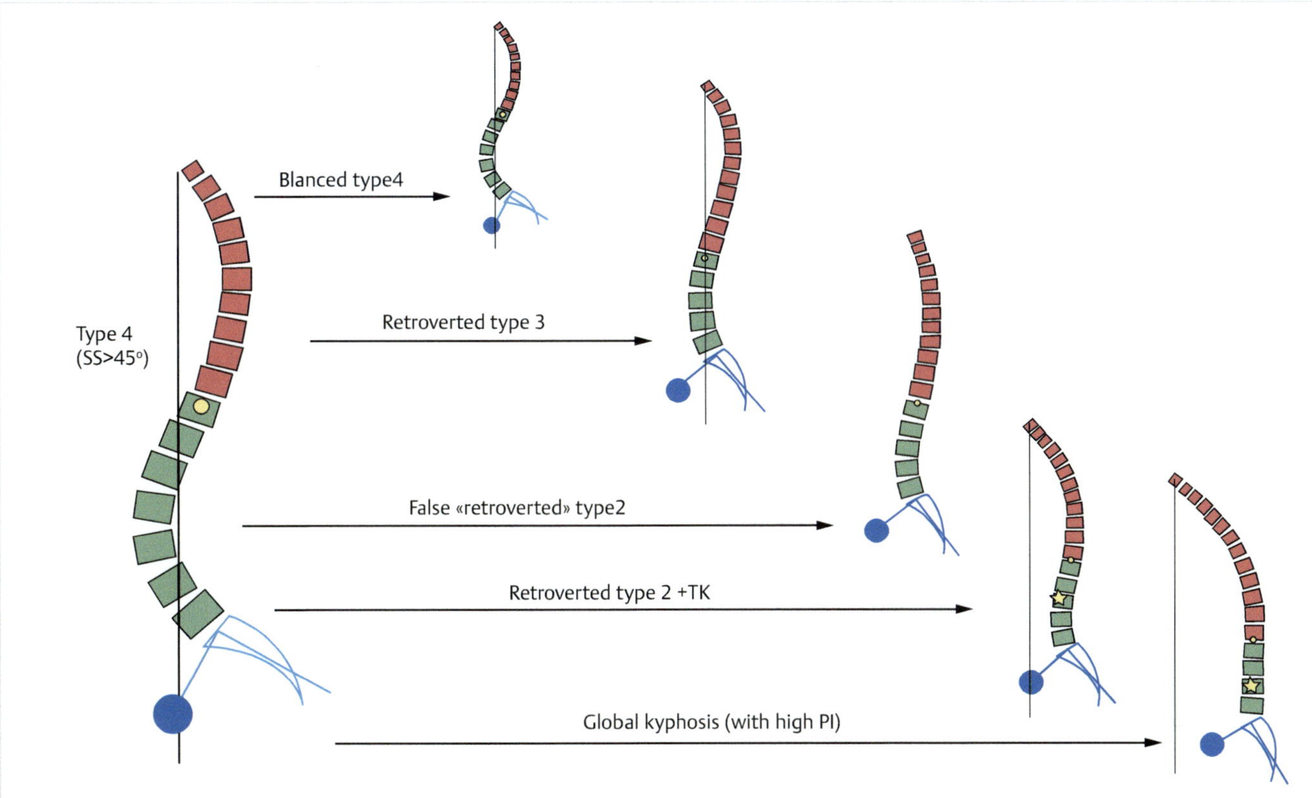

Fig. 28.11 Possible degenerative evolution of type 4. Possible degenerative evolution of type 4 into balanced type 4, retroverted or false type 3, false type 2 (with or without thoracic kyphosis [TK]), or global kyphosis with a high pelvic incidence (PI).

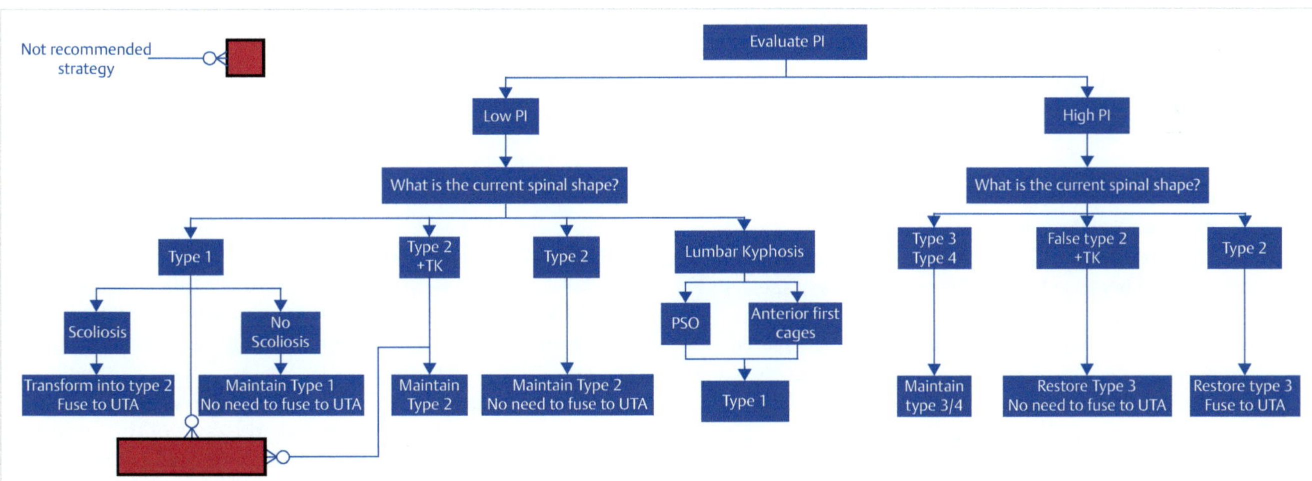

Fig. 28.12 Algorithm for treating fixed spinal deformity. PI, pelvic incidence; PSO, pedicle subtraction osteotomy; TK, thoracic kyphosis; UTA; upper thoracic area.

of the sagittal reduction is either to maintain the present shape or to restore a shape that corresponds to the pelvis shape (PI).

28.7.1 When the Pelvic Incidence Is Small (<50 degrees)

- Type 1 shapes.[39]
  - To maintain a type 1 shape in the reduction is a good option, mainly in the absence of scoliosis.
  - To turn it into a type 2 by reducing the thoracolumbar kyphosis may be a good option in cases of associated thoracolumbar scoliosis.
  - It is imperative to avoid a too long lordosis—inducing an anteverted type 3, which is always a bad option.[40]

- Type 2 shapes
  - Maintain the same type 2. It is generally not necessary to address the thoracic spine. There is a low risk of PJK if low lordosis values are maintained with an appropriate SAL.
- Type 2 with thoracic kyphosis
  - To maintain the type 2 shape, it is mandatory to reduce the thoracic kyphosis. This could be very hazardous in older patients. We recommend turning the patient's spine into a type 1 spine with a longer SK and a short distal LSL. It is always preferable to integrate the thoracic spine in the construction.
  - In any case, too much lordosis will result in an anteverted type 3 shape, which is never a good option.[40]
- Lumbar kyphosis
  - Restoration of lordosis by a posterior approach generally requires a small L 4 pedicle subtraction osteotomy (PSO) because of the rigidity of the lumbar spine.
  - Reduction of lordosis by an anterior first interbody cages (OLIF) could be a good option for opening the disk spaces and restoring the lordosis.[41]

28.7.2 When the Pelvic Incidence Is High (>50 degrees)

- Degenerative >changes with persistent type 3 or 4 spines
  - The main objective of spinal correction is to maintain the same spinal shape.
  - If the spine is well balanced with an adapted SK, it is not necessary to address the entire spine.
- Decreasing lordosis without thoracic compensation (false type 2 with TK), and retroverted pelvis (PT >25 degrees)
  - It is necessary to increase the lordosis, with either a global release (posterior column osteotomy) if the spine is still flexible, or an L 4 PSO if the spine is rigid.
  - Because there is no compensation at the thoracic level, it is not necessary to extend the fusion to the upper thoracic area.
- Decreasing lordosis with a double compensation, thoracic hypokyphosis and retroverted pelvis (false type 2)
  - When the lordosis is restored, the thoracic spine always flexes forward because the thoracic spine always seeks its original shape.
    - If the fusion stops at T 10, there is an increased risk of junctional failure. It may be necessary to extend the fusion to T 2 or T 3 depending on SK.
    - If the fusion extends to the proximal thoracic area, it is difficult to predict the precise need of kyphosis restoration. If this SK restoration is insufficient, there is an increased risk of cervicothoracic PJK, which carries a risk of proximal instrumentation loosening.
  - When restoring the lordosis, it is mandatory to respect the shape of the lordosis. The bigger angle of lordosis has to be extended distally between L 4 and S 1. If the lordosis is extended proximally, up to T 12–L 1, it reduces the space for TK and increases the risk of upper PJK. Lordosis that is too long and too strong is not a good option (see the following section).

28.8 Proximal Junctional Kyphosis: A Complication of Faulty Surgical Strategy

PJK was first described in adolescent idiopathic scoliosis[42] and Scheuermann's kyphosis.[43] The most commonly used definition for PJK is the one provided by Glattes et al: the PJK angle is determined by the angle between the lower end plate of the last instrumented vertebra and the upper end plate of the two supra-adjacent vertebrae; PJK is present when the angle is greater than 10 degrees and is at least 10 degrees greater than its preoperative value[44] (▶ Fig. 28.13). Many risk factors for PJK were described, including increased age, obesity, osteoporosis, posterior elements disruption, proximal anchor types, female sex, and others.[45] Analysis of risk factors for PJK is beyond the scope and objectives of this chapter. However, two key aspects are focused on here: the importance of accurate correction and the importance of sagittal shape.

In a recent evaluation of a large database of patients with adult deformity, accurate correction of the sagittal balance according to patient's age was evaluated.[46] Patients with accurate correction resulted in a low incidence of PJK, whereas both under- and overcorrection of the sagittal imbalance resulted in a higher incidence of this complication. One important finding is that PJK in undercorrected patients was mild (<20 degrees), whereas PJK in overcorrected patients was severe (>20 degrees) and frequently required surgical revision.

Restoring the sagittal apex of the lordosis and its effects on the incidence of PJK was recently analyzed by the authors.[47,48] When the postoperative sagittal apex of the lumbar curve was identical to the theoretical apex, PJK occurred in 13.5% of the cases, whereas it occurred in 41.4% of cases where the theoretical and actual apex were different ($p = 0.01$) with an odds ratio of 4.6. When compared to other predictive methods, restoring the sagittal apex of the lordosis was found to be the most important predictive factor (▶ Fig. 28.14). This could have several implications for degenerative spine surgery. The first implication is the choice of the level of a three-column osteotomy when treating adult deformity, which is still a debatable subject. For instance, some authors found no difference in global balance correction or complication rate with the level of PSO (comparing L 3 and L 4 osteotomy),[49] whereas others found better sagittal balance correction as well as PT correction with L 4 osteotomy compared to L 3 osteotomy.[50] We think that L 4 osteotomy is better placed to restore the apex of the lordosis at the desired theoretical value. The second implication is for the anterior correction techniques of adult scoliosis or anterior indirect decompression techniques. For instance, these techniques rely on anterior release of the diskoligament complex and to insert lordotic cages. Nonetheless, restoring the correct sagittal apex of the lordosis is important. Thus proper choice and placement of lordotic cages (very lordotic cages in L 5–S 1 and L 4–L 5 disks) helps avoid very long lumbar lordosis and decreases mechanical complications in general and PJK in particular.

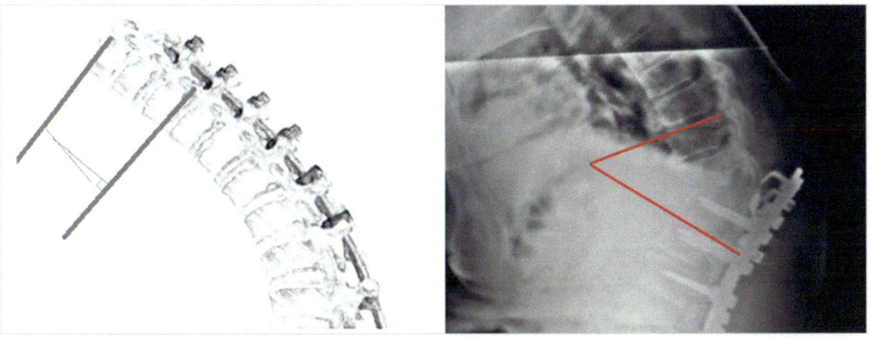

Fig. 28.13 Proximal junctional angle is defined by Glattes: angle between the lower end plate of the last instrumented vertebra and the upper end plate of two levels above.

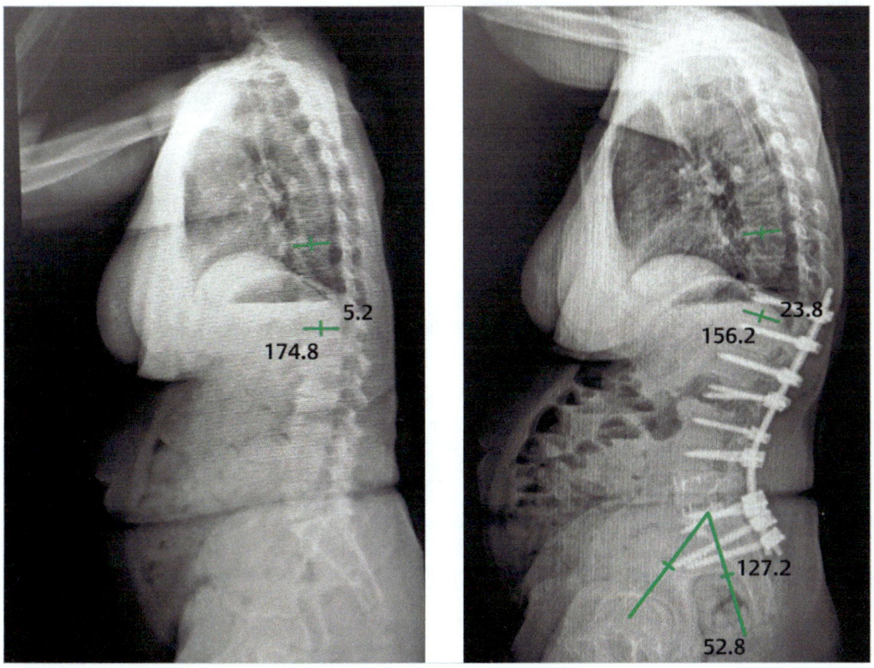

Fig. 28.14 The importance of restoring the sagittal shape of the spine. A 56-year-old woman with a type 2 spine was operated with a T 10 to iliac fusion. She was fused with a type 1 spine without extending to the upper thoracic area. Proximal junctional kyphosis developed in the early postoperative period (X-ray on day 5).

28.9 Conclusion

In conclusion, a thorough understanding of the sagittal balance is the most important factor in the treating the rigid spine deformity. PI is the single most important parameter to contemplate since it is the only stable parameter with spinal degeneration. Accurate restoring of the spinal shapes according to the pelvic incidence helps increase the surgical success rates and reduce complications rates.

References

[1] Skovrlj B, Al Maaieh M, Guzman J, Caridi J, Cho SK. The 100 classic papers in spinal deformity surgery. Spine Deform. 2014; 2(4):241–247

[2] Dubousset J. Three-dimensional analysis of the scoliotic deformity. In: Weinstein SL, ed. Pediatric Spine: principles and Practice. New York, NY: Raven Press; 1994:479–496

[3] Legaye J, Duval-Beaupère G, Hecquet J, Marty C. Pelvic incidence: a fundamental pelvic parameter for three-dimensional regulation of spinal sagittal curves. Eur Spine J. 1998; 7(2):99–103

[4] Roussouly P, Gollogly S, Berthonnaud E, Dimnet J. Classification of the normal variation in the sagittal alignment of the human lumbar spine and pelvis in the standing position. Spine. 2005; 30(3):346–353

[5] Roussouly P, Pinheiro-Franco JL. Sagittal parameters of the spine: biomechanical approach. Eur Spine J. 2011; 20 Suppl 5:578–585

[6] During J, Goudfrooij H, Keessen W, Beeker TW, Crowe A. Toward standards for posture. Postural characteristics of the lower back system in normal and pathologic conditions. Spine. 1985; 10(1):83–87

[7] Le Huec JC, Aunoble S, Philippe L, Nicolas P. Pelvic parameters: origin and significance. Eur Spine J. 2011; 20 Suppl 5:564–571

[8] Mac-Thiong J-M, Labelle H, Roussouly P. Pediatric sagittal alignment. Eur Spine J. 2011; 20 Suppl 5:586–590

[9] Vialle R, Levassor N, Rillardon L, Templier A, Skalli W, Guigui P. Radiographic analysis of the sagittal alignment and balance of the spine in asymptomatic subjects. J Bone Joint Surg Am. 2005; 87(2):260–267

[10] Zárate-Kalfópulos B, Romero-Vargas S, Otero-Cámara E, Correa VC, Reyes-Sánchez A. Differences in pelvic parameters among Mexican, Caucasian, and Asian populations. J Neurosurg Spine. 2012; 16(5):516–519

[11] Lonner BS, Auerbach JD, Sponseller P, Rajadhyaksha AD, Newton PO. Variations in pelvic and other sagittal spinal parameters as a function of race in adolescent idiopathic scoliosis. Spine. 2010; 35(10):E374–E377

[12] Mac-Thiong J-M, Berthonnaud E, Dimar JR, II, Betz RR, Labelle H. Sagittal alignment of the spine and pelvis during growth. Spine. 2004; 29(15):1642–1647

[13] Stagnara P, De Mauroy JC, Dran G, et al. Reciprocal angulation of vertebral bodies in a sagittal plane: approach to references for the evaluation of kyphosis and lordosis. Spine. 1982; 7(4):335–342

[14] Schwab F, Ungar B, Blondel B, et al. Scoliosis Research Society-Schwab adult spinal deformity classification: a validation study. Spine. 2012; 37(12):1077–1082

[15] Basques BA, Long WD, Golinvaux NS, et al. Poor visualization limits diagnosis of proximal junctional kyphosis in adolescent idiopathic scoliosis. Spine J. 2015. DOI: 10.1016/j.spinee.2015.10.040

[16] Schwab F, Patel A, Ungar B, Farcy J-P, Lafage V. Adult spinal deformity-postoperative standing imbalance: how much can you tolerate? An overview of key parameters in assessing alignment and planning corrective surgery. Spine. 2010; 35(25):2224–2231

[17] Vaz G, Roussouly P, Berthonnaud E, Dimnet J. Sagittal morphology and equilibrium of pelvis and spine. Eur Spine J. 2002; 11(1):80–87

[18] Berthonnaud E, Dimnet J, Roussouly P, Labelle H. Analysis of the sagittal balance of the spine and pelvis using shape and orientation parameters. J Spinal Disord Tech. 2005; 18(1):40–47

[19] Kumar MN, Baklanov A, Chopin D. Correlation between sagittal plane changes and adjacent segment degeneration following lumbar spine fusion. Eur Spine J. 2001; 10(4):314–319

[20] Glassman SD, Bridwell K, Dimar JR, Horton W, Berven S, Schwab F. The impact of positive sagittal balance in adult spinal deformity. Spine. 2005; 30 (18):2024–2029

[21] Vital JM, Senegas J. Anatomical bases of the study of the constraints to which the cervical spine is subject in the sagittal plane. A study of the center of gravity of the head. Surg Radiol Anat. 1986; 8(3):169–173

[22] Kim YC, Lenke LG, Lee SJ, Gum JL, Wilartratsami S, Blanke KM. The cranial sagittal vertical axis (CrSVA) is a better radiographic measure to predict clinical outcomes in adult spinal deformity surgery than the C7 SVA: a monocentric study. Eur Spine J. 2016:1–9

[23] Barrey C, Jund J, Noseda O, Roussouly P. Sagittal balance of the pelvis-spine complex and lumbar degenerative diseases. A comparative study about 85 cases. Eur Spine J. 2007; 16(9):1459–1467

[24] Obeid I, Boissière L, Yilgor C, et al. European Spine Study Group, ESSG. Global tilt: a single parameter incorporating spinal and pelvic sagittal parameters and least affected by patient positioning. Eur Spine J. 2016; 25(11):3644–3649

[25] Protopsaltis T, Schwab F, Bronsard N, et al. International Spine Study Group. TheT1 pelvic angle, a novel radiographic measure of global sagittal deformity, accounts for both spinal inclination and pelvic tilt and correlates with health-related quality of life. J Bone Joint Surg Am. 2014; 96(19):1631–1640

[26] Ryan DJ, Protopsaltis TS, Ames CP, et al. International Spine Study Group. T1 pelvic angle (TPA) effectively evaluates sagittal deformity and assesses radiographical surgical outcomes longitudinally. Spine. 2014; 39(15):1203–1210

[27] Boissière L, Takemoto M, Bourghli A, et al. Global Tilt and Lumbar Lordosis Index: Two Parameters correlating with Health related quality of life scores; but how do they truly impact disability? Spine J. 2016

[28] Berthonnaud E, Labelle H, Roussouly P, et al. A variability study of computerized sagittal spinopelvic radiologic measurements of trunk balance. J Spinal Disord Tech 2005;18:66–71.

[29] Mac-Thiong J-M, Roussouly P, Berthonnaud E, Guigui P. Sagittal parameters of global spinal balance: normative values from a prospective cohort of seven hundred nine Caucasian asymptomatic adults. Spine. 2010; 35(22):E1193–E1198

[30] Laouissat F, Sebaaly A, Gehrchen M, Roussouly P. Classification of normal sagittal spine alignment: refounding the Roussouly classification. Eur Spine J. 2017. DOI: 10.1007/s00586-017-5111-x

[31] Barrey C, Roussouly P, Perrin G, Le Huec J-C. Sagittal balance disorders in severe degenerative spine. Can we identify the compensatory mechanisms? Eur Spine J. 2011; 20 Suppl 5:626–633

[32] Hovorka I, Rousseau P, Bronsard N, et al. [Extension reserve of the hip in relation to the spine: Comparative study of two radiographic methods]. Rev Chir Orthop Repar Appar Mot. 2008; 94(8):771–776

[33] Le Huec JC, Charosky S, Barrey C, Rigal J, Aunoble S. Sagittal imbalance cascade for simple degenerative spine and consequences: algorithm of decision for appropriate treatment. Eur Spine J. 2011; 20 Suppl 5:699–703

[34] Kepler CK, Hilibrand AS, Sayadipour A, et al. Clinical and radiographic degenerative spondylolisthesis (CARDS) classification. Spine J. 2015; 15(8):1804–1811

[35] Gille O, Challier V, Parent H, et al. French Society of Spine Surgery (SFCR). Degenerative lumbar spondylolisthesis: cohort of 670 patients, and proposal of a new classification. Orthop Traumatol Surg Res. 2014; 100(6) Suppl:S311–S315

[36] Sebaaly A, Grobost P, Mallam L, Roussouly P. Description of the sagittal alignment of the degenerative human spine. Eur Spine J. 2018;27(2):489–496

[37] Silvestre C, Mac-Thiong J-M, Hilmi R, Roussouly P. Complications and Morbidities of Mini-open Anterior Retroperitoneal Lumbar Interbody Fusion: Oblique Lumbar Interbody Fusion in 179 Patients. Asian Spine J. 2012; 6(2):89–97

[38] Cho K-J, Bridwell KH, Lenke LG, Berra A, Baldus C. Comparison of Smith-Petersen versus pedicle subtraction osteotomy for the correction of fixed sagittal imbalance. Spine. 2005; 30(18):2030–2037, discussion 2038

[39] Scemama C, Laouissat F, Abelin-Genevois K, Roussouly P. Surgical treatment of thoraco-lumbar kyphosis (TLK) associated with low pelvic incidence. Eur Spine J. 2017; 26(8):2146–2152

[40] Ferrero E, Vira S, Ames CP, et al. International Spine Study Group. Analysis of an unexplored group of sagittal deformity patients: low pelvic tilt despite positive sagittal malalignment. Eur Spine J. 2016; 25(11):3568–3576

[41] Ohtori S, Mannoji C, Orita S, et al. Mini-open anterior retroperitoneal lumbar interbody fusion: Oblique lateral interbody fusion for degenerated lumbar spinal kyphoscoliosis. Asian Spine J. 2015; 9(4):565–572

[42] Lee GA, Betz RR, Clements DH, III, Huss GK. Proximal kyphosis after posterior spinal fusion in patients with idiopathic scoliosis. Spine. 1999; 24(8):795–799

[43] Lowe TG, Kasten MD. An analysis of sagittal curves and balance after Cotrel-Dubousset instrumentation for kyphosis secondary to Scheuermann's disease. A review of 32 patients. Spine. 1994; 19(15):1680–1685

[44] Glattes RC, Bridwell KH, Lenke LG, Kim YJ, Rinella A, Edwards C, II. Proximal junctional kyphosis in adult spinal deformity following long instrumented posterior spinal fusion: incidence, outcomes, and risk factor analysis. Spine. 2005; 30(14):1643–1649

[45] Liu F-Y, Wang T, Yang S-D, Wang H, Yang D-L, Ding W-Y. Incidence and risk factors for proximal junctional kyphosis: a meta-analysis. Eur Spine J. 2016; 25(8):2376–2383

[46] Sebaaly A, Sylvestre C, El Quehtani Y, et al (2018), Incidence and Risk Factors for Proximal Junctional Kyphosis: Results of a Multicentric Study of Adult Scoliosis. Clin Spine Surg 31:E178–E183

[47] Sebaaly A, Riouallon G, Obeid I, et al. Proximal junctional kyphosis in adult scoliosis: comparison of four radiological predictor models. Eur Spine J 2018;27:613–21.

[48] Sebaaly A, Gehrchen M, Silvestre C, et al. Mechanical complications in adult spinal deformity and the effect of restoring the spinal shapes according to the Roussouly classification: a multicentric study. Eur Spine J 2019;29:904–13.

[49] Lafage V, Schwab F, Vira S, et al. Does vertebral level of pedicle subtraction osteotomy correlate with degree of spinopelvic parameter correction? J Neurosurg Spine. 2011; 14(2):184–191

[50] Sebaaly A, Kharrat K, Kreichati G, Rizkallah M. Influence of the level of pedicle subtraction osteotomy on pelvic tilt change in adult spinal deformity. Global Spine J. 2016; 6(1)_suppl: s-0036-1583071-s-0036-1583071

29 Robot-Guided Surgery in Rigid Spinal Deformities

Yair Barzilay, Sajan K. Hegde, Isador H. Lieberman, Pramod K. Sudarshan, Harel Arzi, Samuel S. Bederman

Abstract

Robotic guidance is another tool at the surgeon's disposal, and like others, it does not replace the surgeon's knowledge and expertise. The first advantage of robotic guidance is preoperative planning. The fact that a surgeon must align the vertebrae, and go through each pedicle to plan implant position, thereby detecting anatomical variances of absent pedicles, upgrades the "readiness" of the surgical team. Robotic guidance allows accurate implant positioning, without the stress related to screw positioning in altered anatomy, thus removing one stressful step on the way to successful correction of the rigid deformity. It reduces radiation exposure to surgeons and operating room staff in centers that use fluoroscopic guidance for screw placement, thus reducing the risk for radiation-induced malignancy, which is a rising concern in the orthopaedic community, and it allows accurate and predictable planning and execution of osteotomies.

Surgical robots are still at their early stage of development; they can be compared to toddlers, who have just learned how to walk and are still a little unsteady. Like toddlers, surgical robots should have a bright future. The ability to perform complex tasks, without tiring and without being distracted, puts robots in an excellent position to increasingly take part in surgical procedures.

Keywords: robot guidance, rigid deformity, osteotomy, kyphoscoliosis

29.1 Introduction

Instrumentation in the setting of spinal deformity can be challenging for spinal surgeons. Pedicle screws are the preferred method of fixation, showing mechanical advantages over other methods of fixation. Deformed, hypoplastic, or absent pedicles are common, and in conjunction with unusual trajectories increase the risk of screw misplacement. Misplacement of pedicle screws, with the attendant risk of injury to the spinal cord, nerve roots, great vessels, or visceral tissue, or loss of mechanical stability, became a factor influencing surgical outcome. Revision spine surgery with altered surface anatomy increases the risk of screw misplacement as well.

In response to these issues, the use of enhanced guidance modalities seems intuitive. Moreover, navigation or other guidance systems may be used to plan and execute osteotomies, therefore potentially easing two major steps in the correction of the rigid, deformed spine.

29.2 Robotic Guidance in Spine Surgery

In recent years, a variety of robots have been introduced for different surgical applications.[1,2] Surgical robots can be divided into three broad categories: (1) Supervisory-controlled systems enable the surgeon to plan the operation offline, specifying motions that the robot must follow to perform the operation. The robot then performs the procedure autonomously with the surgeon supervising closely. (2) Telesurgical systems allow the surgeon to directly control surgical instruments held by the robot via a joystick or hand controls, with either passive or active task execution. (3) Shared-control systems allow both the surgeon and the robot simultaneous direct control of surgical instruments.[3] To date, the majority of robotically assisted spine operations have involved a shared-control system.

A recent review[4] discussed 18 robotic systems, of which 5 are clinically available. One is aimed at needle interventions, two are focused on radiosurgery, one was tested for spine surgery but is used primarily in other surgical specialties, and only one is dedicated to spine surgery. The authors concluded that the field of spine surgical robots "is still at an early stage of development but with great potential for improvement."

29.2.1 Robotic Systems in Clinical Use

To the authors' best knowledge, only one robotic system dedicated to spine surgery is available for clinical usage.[5,6,7,8,9,10,11,12,13,14] The system consists of a grid attached to a C-arm, a workstation containing a miniature robot, a computer running dedicated software that allows preoperative planning and intraoperative execution, and a screen (▶ Fig. 29.1). The bone-mounted miniature robot is a semi-active system offering surgical tool guidance while leaving performance of the actual surgical operation, such as drilling, in the surgeon's hands. The concept was first published in 2003 and 2004,[15,16] followed by lab testing,[17,18] and a clinical development phase.[19,20,21] Other systems are under different stages of development,[22,23,24,25,26] with one system at an early clinical phase[27] and others dealing with case reports or animal models of telesurgical, robot-aided surgery.[28,29,30,31,32,33,34,35]

The robotic procedure consists of five steps:

1. *Preoperative planning:* Digital Imaging and Communications in Medicine (DICOM) images of a dedicated protocol CT scan are imported by the robotic workstation software. This software can be installed on a standard laptop or desktop computer and allows for preoperative planning. The software creates two-dimensional reconstruction images of each vertebra in the region of interest with planning for virtual implant placement in the optimal position. This is a crucial step that allows for detection of abnormal anatomy, absent pedicles, and deformity, as well as determination of implant diameters and lengths.
2. *Platform attachment:* In deformity cases a clamp is connected to a spinous process after subperiosteal dissection is completed. The clamp is connected at the center of each part of the deformity, avoiding the apex region.
3. *Image acquisition and registration:* Targets for image acquisition are connected to the robotic platform, and anteroposterior and 60-degree oblique fluoroscopic images are semiautomatically registered to the preoperative CT images. The surgeon must visually verify the accuracy of the registration process before going forward.

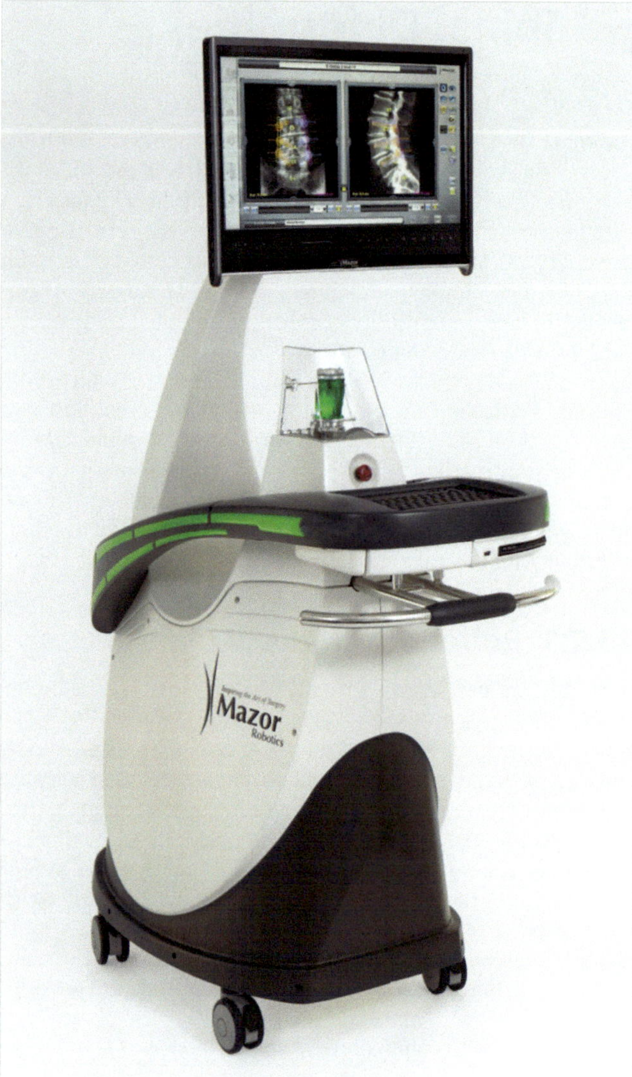

Fig. 29.1 The robotic workstation consists of a computer running software allowing preplanning, image acquisition, registration, and control of robot execution; a touch screen and a 250 g 6 degrees of freedom (DF) miniature robot.

4. *Robot assembly and motion:* The miniature robot is attached to the mounting frame, and one of three arms is connected to it, according to the software guidance. It is then instructed to move and lock into position, so that a guiding tube at the distal end of its arm is aligned with the planned screw/tool trajectory. The guiding tube, with trocar inserted, is then advanced until contact with the pedicle entry point is felt. The trocar is withdrawn and replaced with a working channel. The toothed end of the working channel is gently tapped into the bony surface anatomy of the spine to anchor the starting point and minimize skiving of the drill.
5. *Trajectory execution:* Drilling is begun through the working channel along the planned trajectory. Following drilling, a fiducial may be tapped into the pedicle, or a hollow reduction tube is placed through the working channel and advanced into the pedicle and through the posterior vertebral wall. A K-wire (KW) is then placed into the vertebral body, and the reduction tube is withdrawn. This procedure is repeated until trajectories are drilled and fiducials or KWs are placed at all levels to be treated. Instrumentation may then be placed. At this point robotic guidance is complete. The mounting system may be left attached to allow repeat robot guidance in case one of the trajectories is lost.

29.3 Robotic Surgery in Spinal Deformity

Over the past decade, we have seen major advances in our understanding and appreciation for treating patients with spinal deformities. The goals of surgical treatment of spinal deformity are to balance the spine and achieve a solid arthrodesis through the fewest levels necessary while minimizing complications.

Sagittal balance, load sharing principles, and rigid internal fixation are just a few of these breakthrough concepts that have improved our ability to balance the spine and facilitate arthrodesis. However, more work is needed to reduce perioperative complications and make surgical treatment safer and more efficient. As in degenerative nondeformity spinal conditions, robotically assisted spinal deformity surgery can help the treating surgeon with improved accuracy of screw placement and enhance surgical efficiency while reducing radiation exposure to the surgeon and patient.[5] The spinal surgeon who chooses to utilize a robot-assisted technique must be comfortable with all the components of spinal deformity surgery, including both techniques of correction and instrumentation as if there were no robotic guidance.

Techniques of robotically assisted spinal deformity surgery can be considered based on whether the patient has primarily a coronal plane or sagittal plane deformity, the region of surgery (cervical, thoracic, or lumbar), and primary deformity or revision surgery. In general, the steps of robotically assisted surgery are preoperative planning, patient positioning, platform selection with radiographic registration, and execution of robotically assisted pedicle drilling. In cases of spinal deformities or long-construct fusions there are several specific considerations that differ from the steps carried out in short-construct instrumentations.

First, preoperative planning is facilitated when the entire surgical region is captured as a single study on the preoperative CT scan. With one study, there are no disjointed segments between plans and between registration fields. If the thoracic spine and lumbar spine are separated into two distinct studies but the apex of deformity doesn't correspond to a natural regional junction (i.e., thoracolumbar junction) then some fields of registration may be too small to obtain. For example, in a case of lumbar scoliosis with the apex at L3, one registration field may be able to capture the segments at L3 and distal; however, the more proximal registration field that would typically include L3 and proximal would be artificially truncated at the thoracolumbar junction because the lumbar CT scan did not include the lower thoracic region. This would result in unnecessary radiation and inefficient use of surgical time.

In general, patient positioning is similar to what is done for the same surgery without robotic guidance. Strategic placement of neuromonitoring or electrocardiographic (ECG) leads on the patient facilitates unobstructed fluoroscopy images for successful registration. We ensure that no leads cross over the surgical field in the AP plane by placing all leads lateral to the body and distal to the field. In the case of pelvic fixation, we routinely place the leads crossing the midline distal to the pelvis. In order to avoid the leads on the oblique view, they are placed below (anterior to) the patient on the side of the C-arm. For instance, when the C-arm approaches on the right side of the patient, we place all leads on the right side lower than the patient and run the left lower ECG leads crossing the midline distal to the hips from the right to the left side. They are attached around the level of the greater trochanters. Proximal ECG leads should be above the surgical field and are typically placed over the deltoids bilaterally. The urinary catheter tube is placed with the ECG leads on the right side below the level of the abdomen. Neuromonitoring leads should also be placed appropriately to allow full image intensifier access.

Docking platforms for robotically assisted spinal surgery include the spinous process clamp (SPC), the Hover-T frame (HVT), and the table-mounted multi-directional bridge (MDB). The SPC is the most versatile because it can be mounted in any segment of the spine with a spinous process. Typically, we consider a spinal curvature as “relative” straight segments above and below apices. The SPC is placed two to three levels below or above the apex through one of the relatively straight segments. The SPC functions well in nearly all spinal deformity segments. In segments with significant rotation, the SPC can follow the rotational deformities along the line of the spinous process itself. The main disadvantage is that it requires repositioning for each distinct registration field. At the cephalad end of the curve, the SPC may be placed on the most cephalad spinous process in an effort to minimize the soft tissue exposure. With this configuration the registration typically captures only two to three levels caudal to the clamp (▶ Fig. 29.2).

The HVT frame is considered the workhorse for lumbopelvic fixation. It is relatively easy to assemble with one Schanz pin in each of the posterior superior iliac spines (PSISs) and one attachment (K-wire (KW) KW or miniclamp) at a spinous process proximal to the upper level of instrumentation. It can be used in cases of previous laminectomy and can be extended over long construct instrumentation, either in the original positioning or after flipping the two Schantz pin connectors to achieve more working length proximally (▶ Fig. 29.3). It can be maintained for multiple registration fields, all of which can be obtained at one time such that execution of pedicle drilling can continue along the entire length of the construct without repeat registration. While these features are major advantages, the system's main limitation is in cases of significant scoliosis, in which the spinal rotation and coronal shifting may limit robotic reachability (due to limitations in the working volume of the robotic arms).

Finally, the MDB (▶ Fig. 29.4) is a table-mounted platform that lies over the spine and attaches to the patient at a spinous process proximal to the operative field by a KW or clamp. While it is more cumbersome to set up intraoperatively and is not rigidly fixed to the spine distally, its major advantage is that it can accommodate for multiple drilling solutions since the bridge can be translated laterally from side to side.

Regardless of the platform used, radiographic registration can be challenging. In cases of severe deformity it is difficult to obtain fluoroscopic images that are perpendicular to the spinal segment. Severe kyphosis limits the ability to obtain an adequate AP image of each straight segment since the proximal and distal segments may overlap when one is trying to visualize each one en face. Similarly, severe scoliosis necessitates oblique imaging at very steep angles. Depending on the angular severity and the length of the C-arm, there may be limited clearance between the C-arm ends, thus either limiting the registration field or preventing an adequate image altogether. Positioning the patient's elbows may help improve the angles, but care must be taken to avoid injury to the patient's shoulders and elbows from the ends of the C-arm. Cone beam CT machines and intraoperative CT machines overcome these problems. They allow simultaneous scanning and registration and overcome the difficulties mentioned earlier. The biggest drawback of this approach is the need to perform intraoperative planning, a time-consuming step while the patient is under anesthesia. In centers where the surgical approach is done by other surgeons, the senior surgeon may plan the screws while the team is performing the surgical approach.

Once the platform has been mounted and registration is successful, we then proceed with robot-assisted pedicle drilling. The first step after registration is to ensure that the planned

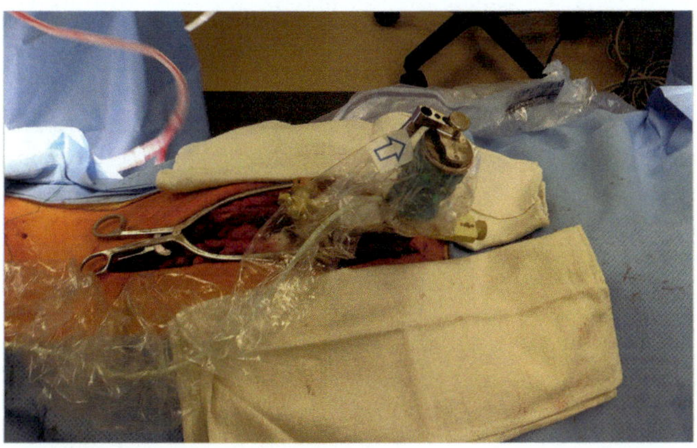

Fig. 29.2 The Spinous Process Clamp (SPC) attachment used for proximal thoracic pedicle drilling.

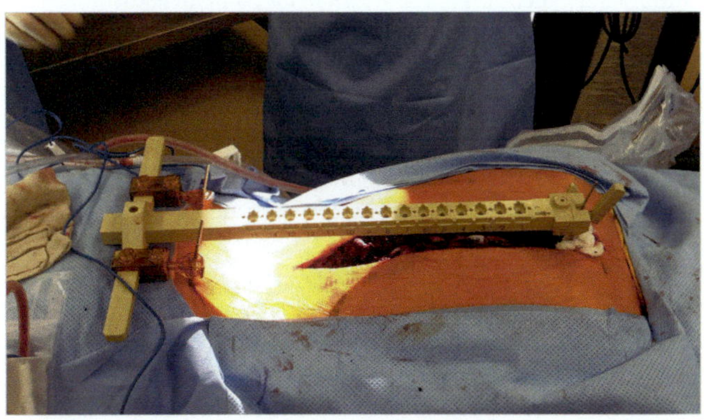

Fig. 29.3 The Hover-T frame assembled with two Schanz pins in the posterior superior iliac spines and a Kirschner wire in a superior spinous process for fixation. Flipping the position of the two Schanz pin connectors achieves more working length proximally.

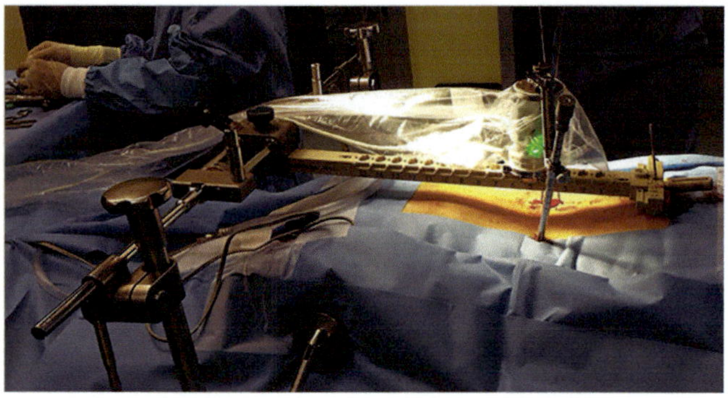

Fig. 29.4 The multidirectional bridge (MDB) is connected to the patient's anatomy through one Kirschner wire or a miniclamp proximally and to the bed bilaterally distally. It allows transverse motion of the bridge to the left and the right, thus increasing the working volume of the robot. It is an excellent platform for long instrumentation in a relatively normal appearing spine.

trajectories are reachable. Those that are not reachable may need to be adjusted on the plan to accommodate the location of the platform. Slight modifications in drilling trajectories can easily be made; however, changing them to paths that compromise fixation, hamper screw alignment, or become too dangerous should be avoided. In these situations, it may be preferable to reposition the platform once other trajectories are completed in order to reach those not achieved. Care should be taken to avoid excessive retraction of soft tissues as this may put too much pressure on the drilling tubes and thus change the desired trajectory. At the proximal or distal ends, or at the convexity of the apex of a scoliotic curve, improved exposure or percutaneous techniques for drilling may be helpful. Specifically, at the proximal end of a long construct, we routinely drill through a stab incision, either through the skin or fascia to avoid unnecessary proximal exposure that puts the adjacent interspinous ligament at risk for detachment. In cases of excessive rotation or kyphosis, rotating or tilting the table to level the robot eliminates any deforming effect of gravity during drilling. Finally, the use of intraoperative deformity reduction, such as positioning with thigh or chest extension for kyphosis or intraoperative traction for scoliosis, can improve successful registration and execution of robotically guided pedicle drilling.

29.4 Special Considerations

Some situations like spinopelvic fixation and revision spine surgery where the robot is not commonly used but can be of considerable help are mentioned in this section.

29.4.1 Pelvic Fixation

Pelvic fixation has become commonplace at the distal end of long-construct instrumented fusions. Specifically, the S2-alar-iliac trajectory (S2AI) has been shown to have significant advantages over the traditional Galveston iliac fixation technique. S2AI drilling can be achieved easily using robotic guidance. The initial CT scan should include the full pelvis in order to properly plan the drilling trajectory. Care should be taken to properly plan the drill path and ensure that there is sufficient bone on the lateral edge of the sacrum to prevent the drill from skiving off into the sacroiliac joint. Any of the mounting platforms can be used for S2AI drilling. The drilling is carried out below the mounted bridge from the contralateral side. It is imperative to drill to a depth past the sacroiliac joint (typically 50 mm or longer), rather than the standard 28 mm for pedicle drilling, in order to avoid screw malpositioning. Following the drilling, we routinely tap over a guidewire in order to ensure that the proper hole has been expanded with the tap. A standard or cannulated screw can be used once tapping has been completed.

In an early series of 14 patients (total 31 screws), there were no proximal breaches or complications related to screw placement; however, 10 screws had distal protrusions (related to short drilling and manual advancement). Overall, it was found that robotically guided S2AI drilling was accurate and feasible.[11]

29.4.2 Revision Spinal Surgery—Redrilling Pedicles, Retained Instrumentation

Proper placement of pedicle screws in revision spinal surgery can be challenging. Patients with altered normal anatomical landmarks from adjacent-level surgery, prior laminectomies, prior fusions, and malpositioned instrumentation are at higher risk for screw misplacement. While deformity correction may be the critical component of the surgery, inserting screws efficiently and safely to afford stability for correction and long-term success is of significant importance.

Robotically guided pedicle drilling in cases of altered anatomy, such as prior laminectomy or fusion without instrumentation, follows the same principles as robotic surgery in general. In the case of existing instrumentation, special considerations must be taken. While maintaining existing instrumentation can facilitate radiographic registration as the intraoperative images more closely resemble the preoperative CT scan (with instrumentation), leaving the rods may interfere with the planned drilling trajectories, and they may need to be removed after registration with the mounting platform in position. The downside here is that forcefully removing the rods may inadvertently manipulate the mounting platform and thus lead to drilling inaccuracies. Alternatively, removing the rods before registration may pose a greater challenge to successful radiographic registration. In this case, it is advisable to leave the rods in place if drilling trajectories can be planned around the rods. After robotically guided drilling, the robot and mounting platform can be removed and the rods then removed without concern

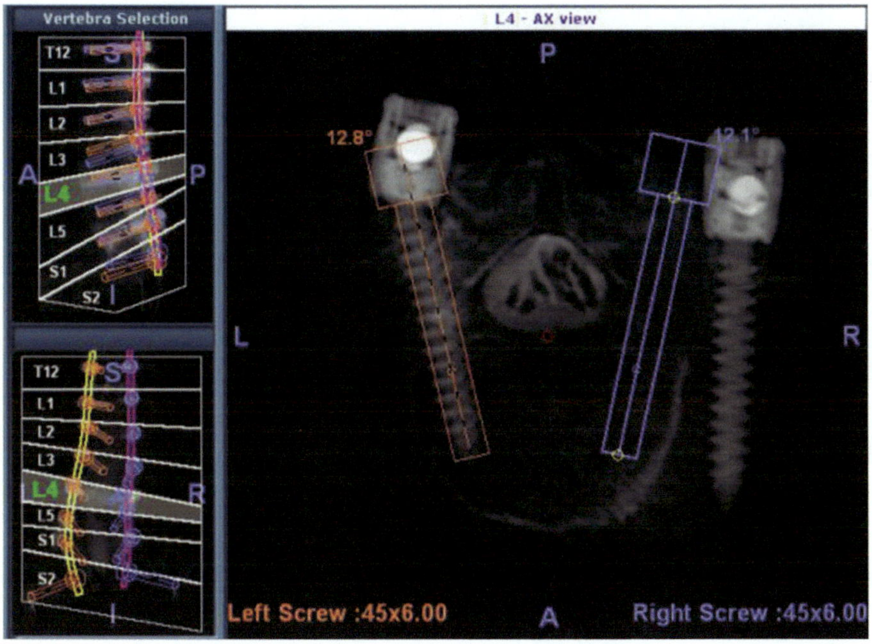

Fig. 29.5 Planning in the presence of a malpositioned screw. Since no collision is expected, the trajectory can be safely drilled with the old instrumentation left in situ, thus improving the chances of successful registration.

prior to screw insertion. If the desired trajectories cannot be drilled with the rods in place, we recommend loosening any set screws or nuts and leaving the rod loosely in place. The rods may then be easily removed after the registration but before the bridge is placed or before the robot is mounted. If the rods can be removed easily without risk of platform manipulation, then it would be best to leave the rods in for radiographic registration and then remove the rods prior to drilling.

Pedicles with malpositioned screws may be redrilled with the screws in place if the planned trajectory does not collide with the screws for the initial drilling depth (28 mm). If there will be collision, then it is preferable to leave the screws in (but not the rods) for radiographic registration and then remove them prior to robotically guided drilling (▶ Fig. 29.5).

In a series of 229 screws (26 patients) placed in revision pedicles (screw redirection, prior laminectomy, prior fusion, and adjacent-level surgery), we found 9 misplaced screws (96.1% accuracy). There were 5 lateral and 4 medial breaches, but none required revision surgery.[12]

29.5 Case Illustrations

29.5.1 Case 1

A 58-year-old woman with a history of adult degenerative scoliosis presented with progressive back pain and stooping posture over the past 5 years (▶ Fig. 29.6a, b). She underwent prolonged conservative management, including pain medication, physical therapy, and multiple facet injections. Surgery to correct the lumbar scoliosis and improve her coronal and sagittal alignment was planned using a combined anterior-posterior technique. Her preoperative CT scan identified extremely small pedicles with maximal rotation at L 1, the apex of the scoliosis (▶ Fig. 29.6c). Robotic guidance was planned with drilling of all pedicles from T 10 to S 1 with S 2AI screws. The right L 1 pedicle was avoided, but drilling of the left L 1 pedicle was successful (▶ Fig. 29.6d). The postoperative CT scan confirmed ideal screw position, and final radiographs (▶ Fig. 29.6e, f) showed improved coronal and sagittal balance with appropriate position of instrumentation.

29.5.2 Case 2

A 40-year-old woman with a history of neglected congenital scoliosis whose thoracic curve measured 130 degrees and lumbar curve measured 110 degrees (▶ Fig. 29.7a–c). She had an associated tethered cord with shortened leg and pelvic obliquity. She complained of increasing back pain, spinal imbalance, and progressive shortness of breath. She underwent T 7 vertebral column resection with T 2 to pelvis instrumented fusion. The postoperative CT scan confirmed good positioning of all pedicle screws. Her thoracic curve was reduced to 75 degrees and the lumbar curve to 60 degrees. We maintained the pelvic obliquity in order to accommodate for her leg length discrepancy (▶ Fig. 29.7d, e).

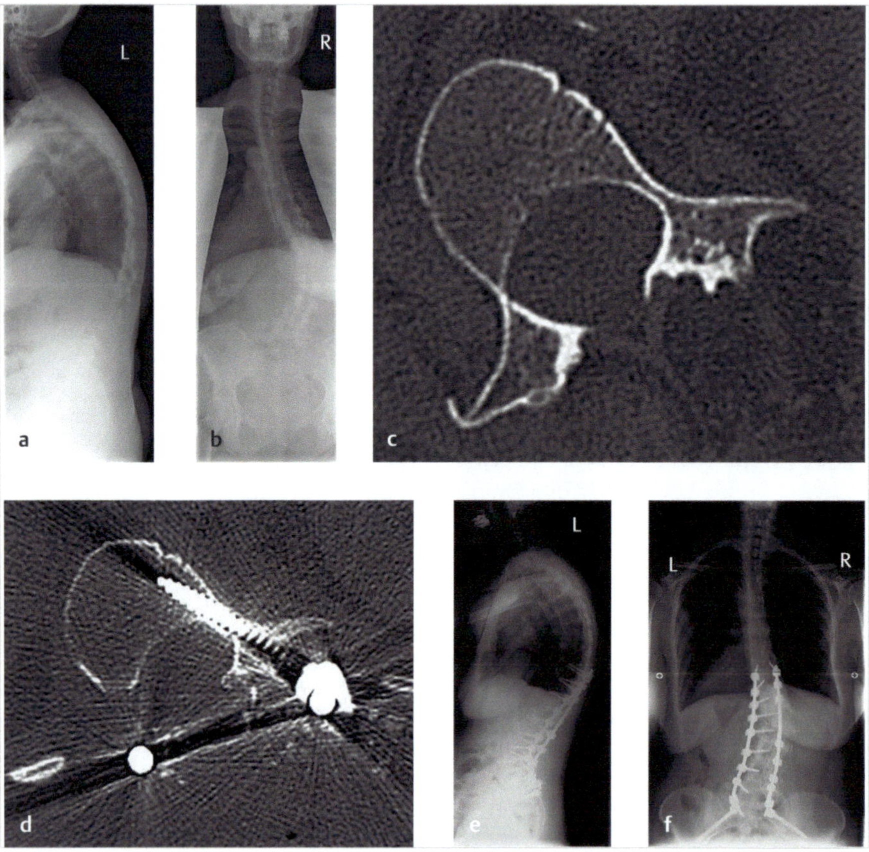

Fig. 29.6 **(a, b)** Preoperative lateral and posteroanterior radiographs and **(c)** axial CT image through L1. **(d)** Postoperative axial CT image through L1. **(e, f)** Postoperative lateral and posteroanterior radiographs showing a corrected and balanced spine.

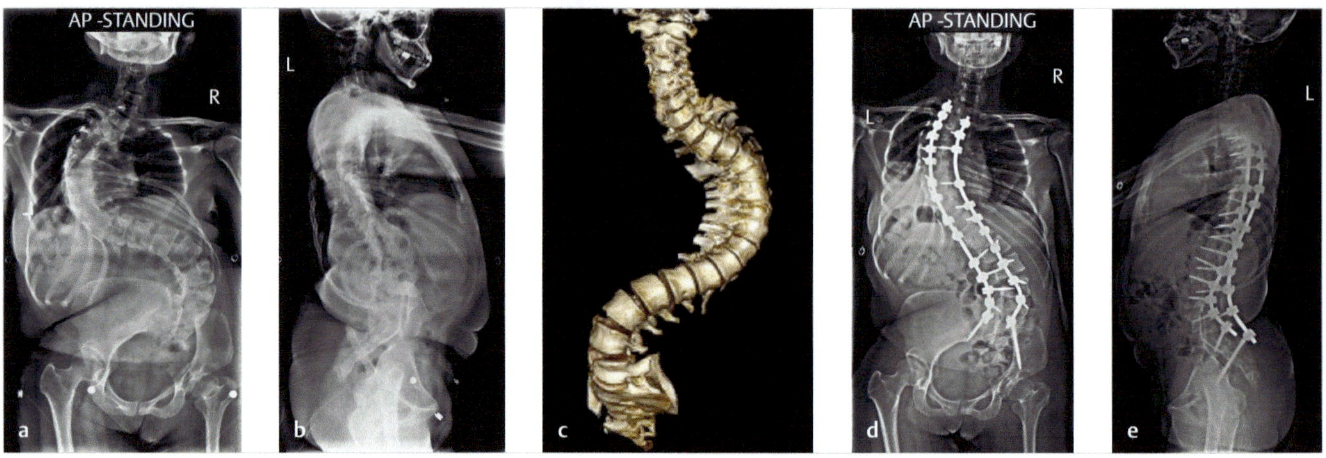

Fig. 29.7 **(a, b)** Preoperative posteroanterior and lateral radiographs and **(c)** 3-dimensional reconstruction preoperative CT image. **(d, e)** Postoperative posteroanterior and lateral radiographs showing a corrected and balanced spine.

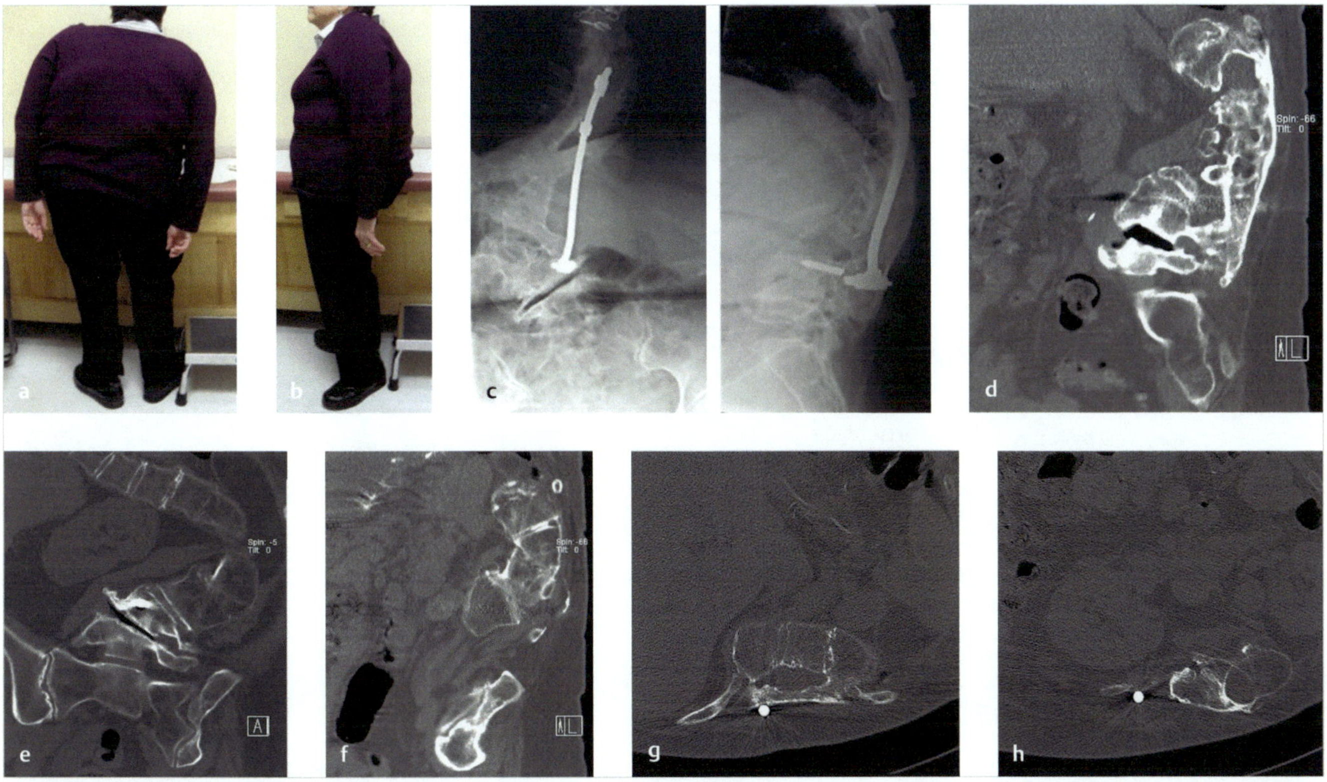

Fig. 29.8 **(a, b)** Preoperative clinical photographs and **(c)** posteroanterior and lateral radiographs. **(d–h)** Preoperative coronal, sagittal and axial T10 and L1 CT images.

(Continued)

29.5.3 Case 3

A 60-year-old woman presented after multiple spinal fusion surgeries for scoliosis, including prior anterior-posterior lumbar fusion, revisions for failure of instrumentation, prior osteotomies, and revision fusion. She complained of back pain, radiculopathy, and progressive sagittal and coronal imbalance (▶ Fig. 29.8a, b). Her radiographs demonstrated a severe spinal deformity that was fused to L4 with significant degeneration and broken posterior instrumentation (▶ Fig. 29.8c, d). The CT scan showed a solid fusion to L4 without anatomical landmarks associated with severe rotation and severe angulation (▶ Fig. 29.8e–i).

We planned a vertebral column resection of L1 with T2 to pelvis posterior instrumented fusion using robotic guidance. Robotic planning of pedicle screw instrumentation in T10 is shown in▶ Fig. 29.8i. The postoperative CT scan confirmed ideal placement of the pedicle screw despite the angulated vertebral segment (▶ Fig. 29.8j). Final radiographs and clinical photographs demonstrated good correction and placement of instrumentation (▶ Fig. 29.8k–n).

29.5.4 Case 4

A 13-year-old girl presented with a Lenke type 6C+curve. Radiographs showed a rigid lumbar curve with a Cobb angle of 60 degrees (▶ Fig. 29.9a–f). She underwent deformity correction and posterior instrumentation under robotic guidance (▶ Fig. 29.9g–j).

29.5.5 Case 5

A 14-year-old girl presented with a rapidly progressive rigid deformity in the past 12 months. Radiographs showed a rigid lumbar kyphoscoliosis with a Cobb angle of 87 degrees. A CT scan demonstrated a left-sided T10–T11 hemivertebra. She underwent excision of the hemivertebra, deformity correction, and posterior instrumentation under robotic guidance (▶ Fig. 29.10a–l).

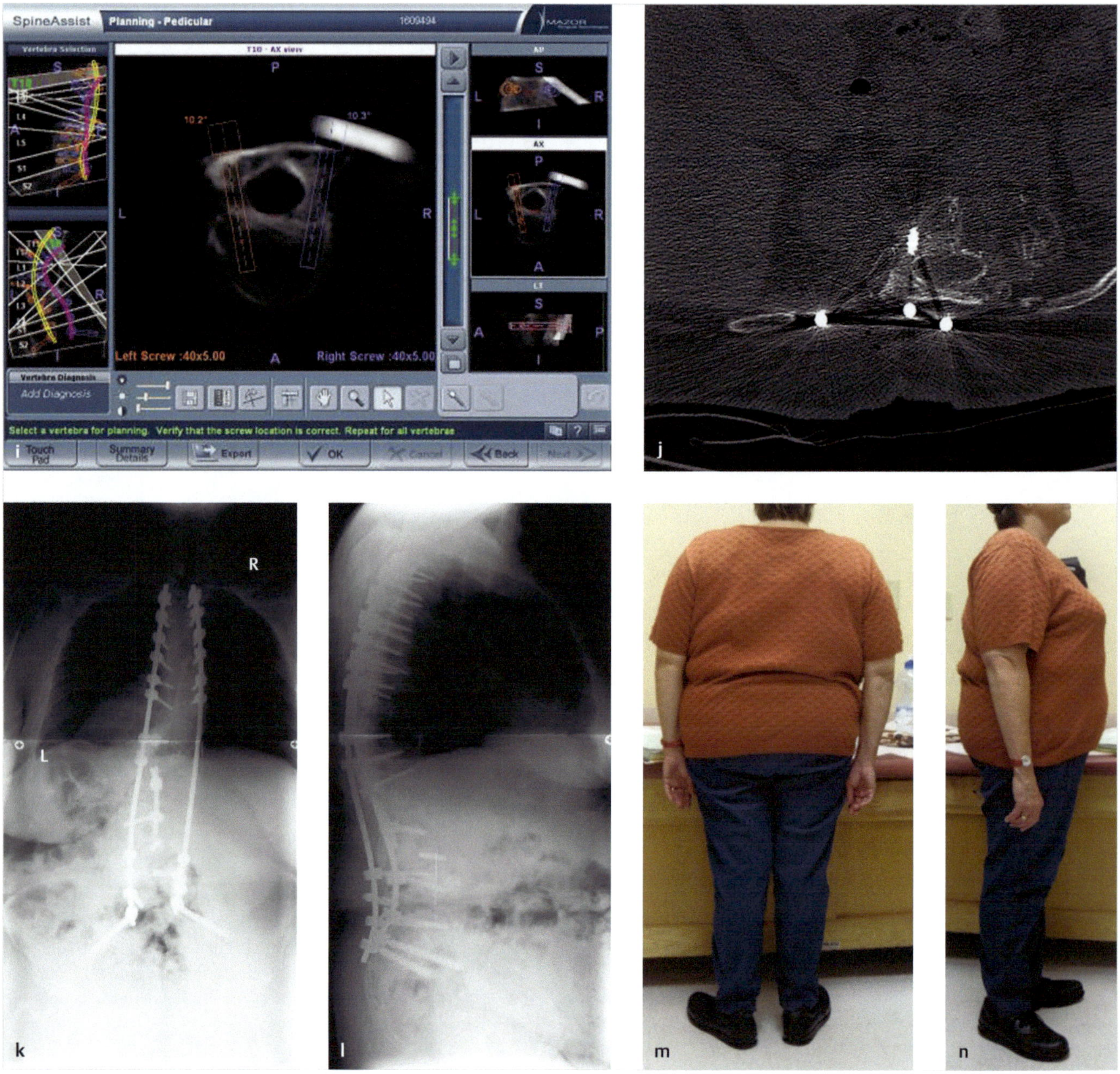

Fig. 29.8 (*Continued*) **(i)** Robot planning of T10 showing normalization of extremely titled T10 vertebral body. **(j–n)** Postoperative axial T10 CT image, posteroanterior and lateral radiographs and clinical photographs showing a corrected and balanced spine. Robot planning of T10 showing normalization of extremely titled T10 vertebral body. **(j–n)** Postoperative axial T10 CT image, posteroanterior and lateral radiographs and clinical photographs showing a corrected and balanced spine.

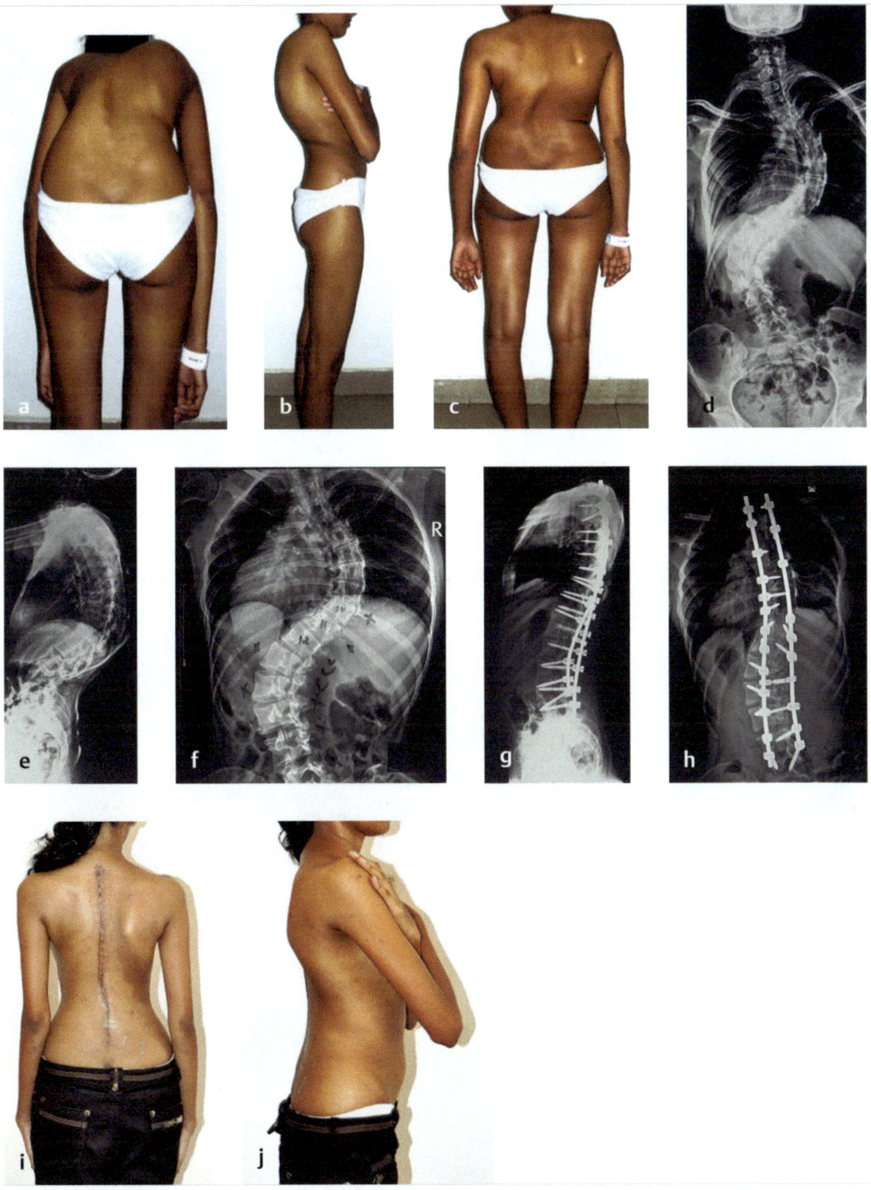

Fig. 29.9 (a–f) Preoperative radiographs and clinical photographs and traction film show the rigid nature of the curve. **(g–j)** Postoperative radiographic images and clinical photographs show a corrected and balanced spine.

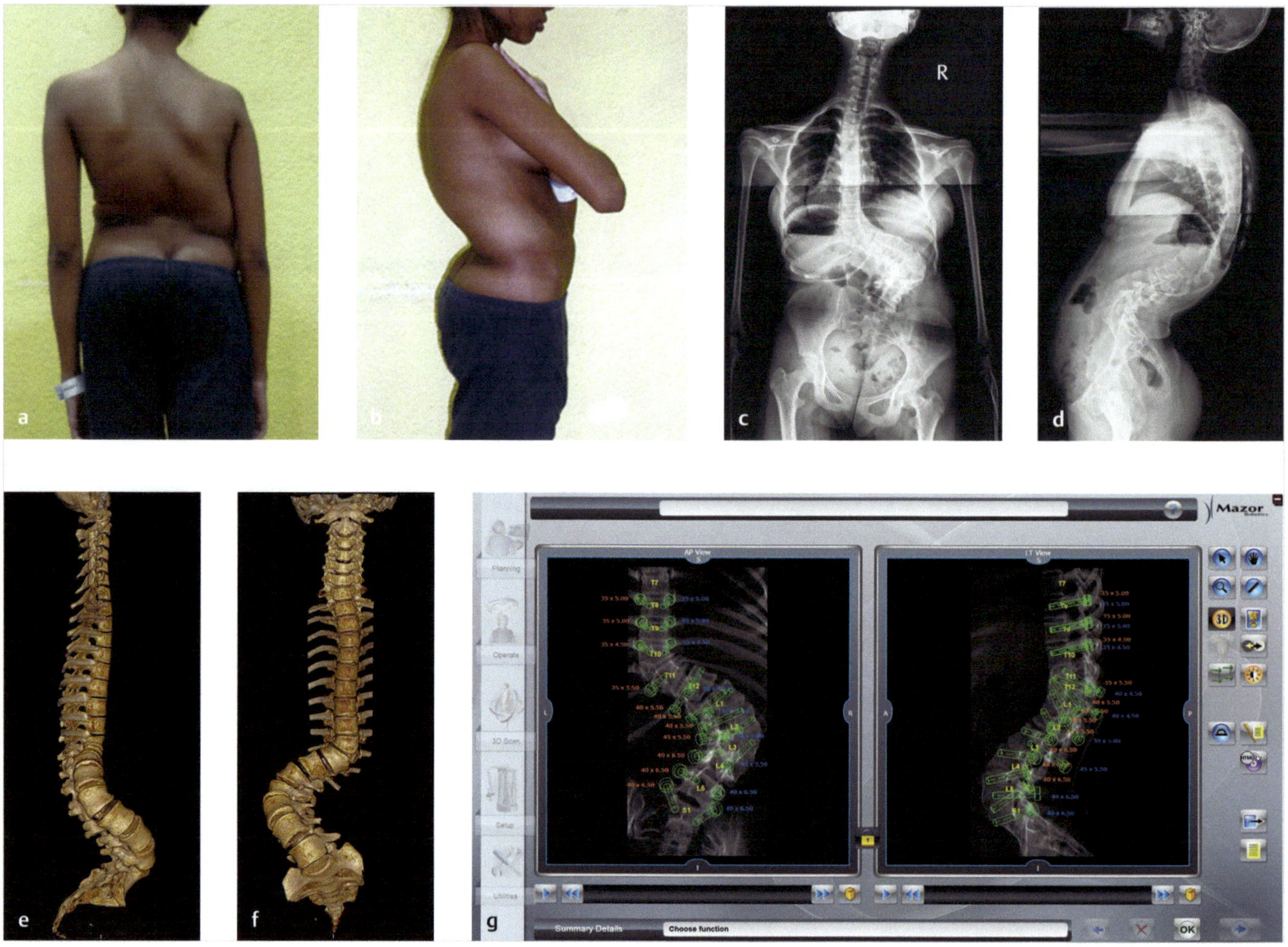

Fig. 29.10 (a–f) Preoperative clinical photos, radiographs, and three-dimensional CT. **(g)** A summary view of the preoperative plan at the robotic workstation showing screw alignment, screw diameter, and screw length at each level.

(Continued)

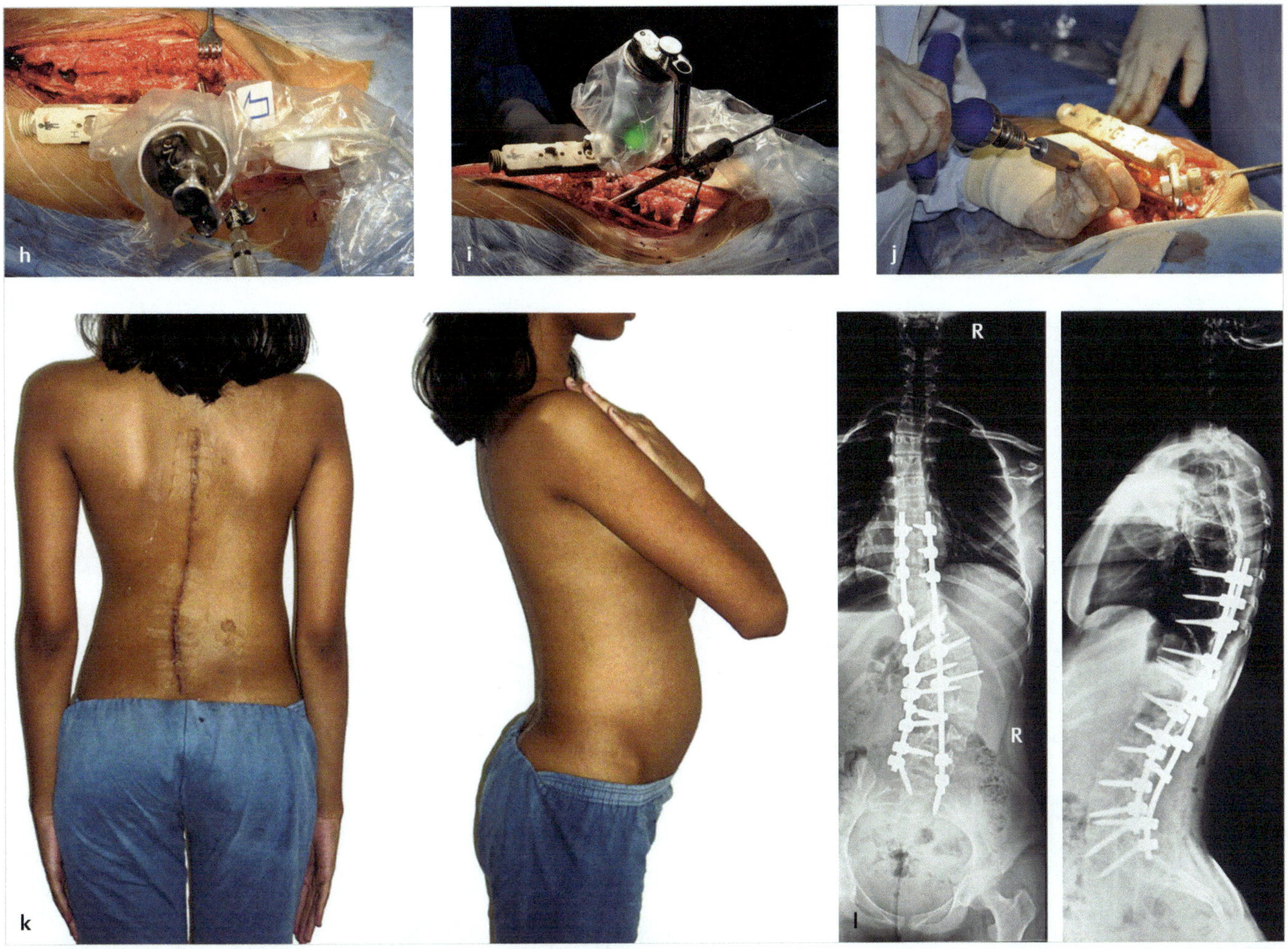

Fig. 29.10 (*Continued*) **(h–j)** Due to excessive rotation, rotating or tilting the table to level the robot, eliminates any deforming effect of gravity during drilling. Due to the exotic deformity, drilling of the right screw was done from the left side, under the bridge. **(k, l)** Postoperative clinical photographs and radiographs.

29.6 Robot-Guided Osteotomies for Rigid Deformities

In the pursuit of optimal sagittal balance, spinal surgeons are frequently resorting to multiple different osteotomies, including pedicle subtraction osteotomies. Traditionally surgeons would measure respective angles on an X-ray, estimate the amount of correction to achieve balance, and proceed to the operating room to execute the plan with crude tools and estimated landmarks. This is akin to measuring with a micrometer and cutting with a chainsaw. Currently there are preoperative planning software packages that can assist in the planning and when coupled with navigation or robotic devices can add a significant measure of efficiency and accuracy to the execution of the osteotomy.

▶ Fig. 29.11 (a-g) outlines a typical flat back syndrome revision procedure whereby the planning software was used to estimate

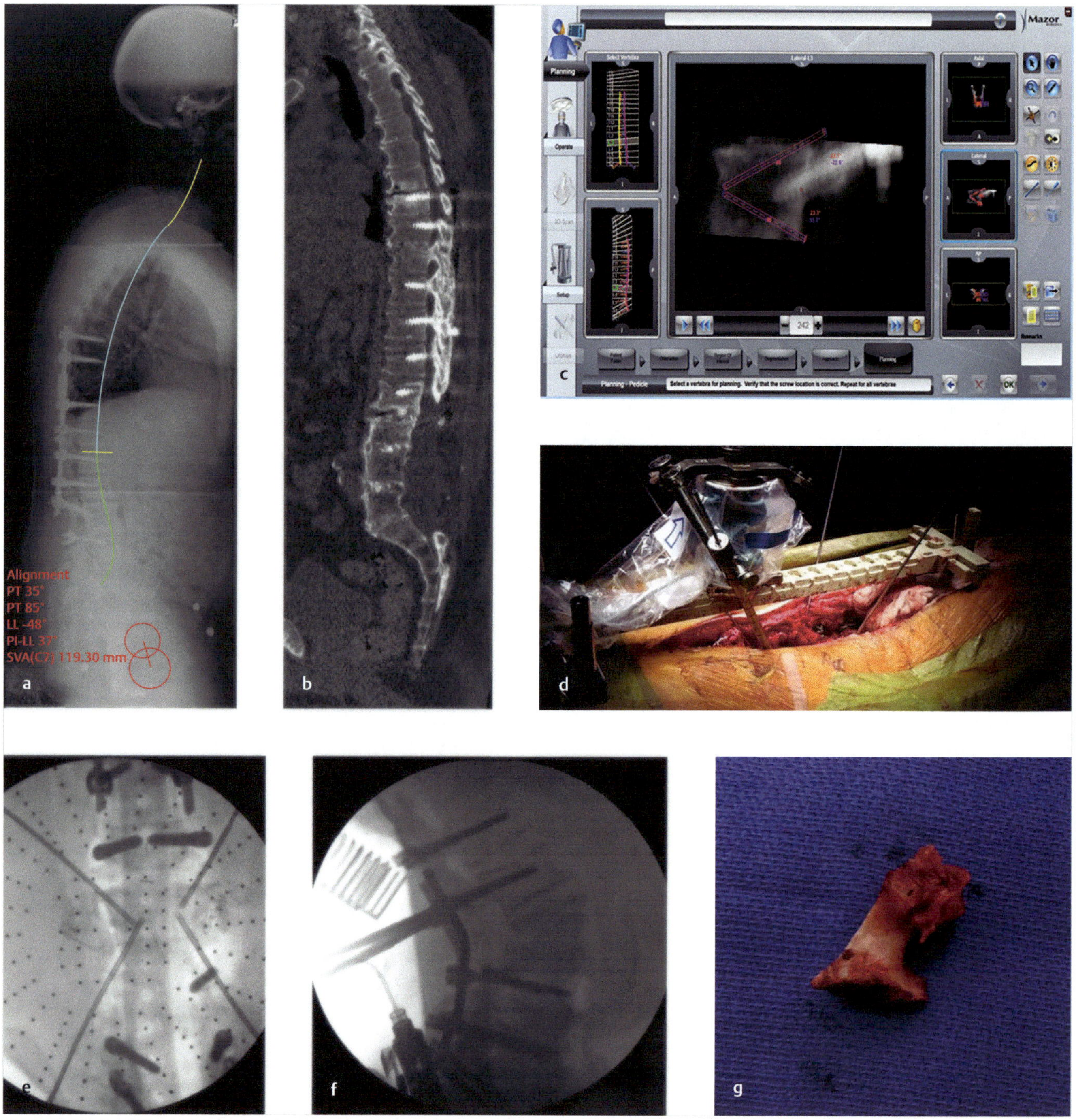

Fig. 29.11 **(a)** Preoperative standing lateral X-ray. **(b)** Preoperative supine lateral CT scan. **(c)** Preoperative plan with proposed pedicle subtraction osteotomy cuts. **(d)** Intraoperative image of robot set up and placement of K wires to guide the pedicle subtraction osteotomies. **(e, f)** Instar operative C-ram X-rays with K-wires in place and osteotomy closed. **(g)** Pedicle subtraction osteotomy removed.

the amount of correction needed, and to position the osteotomies accordingly. The osteotomies are then executed after the exposure is completed and the nerve roots are protected followed by robotically-guided placement of marker wires to outline the precise osteotomy starting point and trajectory. The path of the marker wires is then followed with the surgeon's tool of choice, be it an osteotome or ultrasonic bone scalpel, to create the osteotomy. This technique results in a precise and efficient osteotomy.

29.7 Conclusion

Robotic technologies have advanced at a gradual pace over the years since the initial robotic surgery was performed in the mid-1980s. orthopaedic robotics is both complex and challenging, being used as both a guidance tool and precision element in the execution of complicated surgeries. Advantages in the use of robotic guidance in surgery are that it is more accurate in orthopaedic implant placement; allows precise, predictable planning and execution of osteotomies; is less stressful on the surgeon and surgical team; results in less intraoperative radiation exposure for the patient, surgeons, and operating room staff; and may cause less postoperative bleeding and pain in the patient. Disadvantages to consider are the cost and the increased operative times associated with robotic systems due to set-up and learning curves.

Robotic use in orthopaedic surgeries has been widely adopted worldwide. The increase in accuracy, precision, and safety allows surgeons to perform surgeries consistently, with the least amount of damage, leading to better surgical outcomes, less pain, and quicker recovery times.

References

[1] Taylor RH, Stoianovici D. Medical robotics in computer-integrated surgery. Robotics Automation. IEEE Transactions.. 2003; 19(5):765–781

[2] Barzilay Y, Kaplan L, Liebergall M. Miniature robotic guidance for spine surgery. In: V Bozociv V, ed. Medical Robotics. Rijeka, Croatia. InTech Open 2008, accessed January 8, 2013. http://www.intechopen.com/books/medical_robotics/miniature_robotic_guidance_for_spine_surgery

[3] Nathoo N, Cavuşoğlu MC, Vogelbaum MA, Barnett GH. In touch with robotics: neurosurgery for the future. Neurosurgery. 2005; 56(3):421–433, discussion 421–433

[4] Bertelsen A, Melo J, Sánchez E, Borro D. A review of surgical robots for spinal interventions. Int J Med Robot. 2012

[5] Devito DP, Kaplan L, Dietl R, et al. Clinical acceptance and accuracy assessment of spinal implants guided with SpineAssist surgical robot: retrospective study. Spine. 2010; 35(24):2109–2115

[6] Hu X, Ohnmeiss DD, Lieberman IH. Robotic-assisted pedicle screw placement: lessons learned from the first 102 patients. Eur Spine J. 2012

[7] Kantelhardt SR, Martinez R, Baerwinkel S, Burger R, Giese A, Rohde V. Perioperative course and accuracy of screw positioning in conventional, open robotic-guided and percutaneous robotic-guided, pedicle screw placement. Eur Spine J. 2011; 20(6):860–868

[8] Pechlivanis I, Kiriyanthan G, Engelhardt M, et al. Percutaneous placement of pedicle screws in the lumbar spine using a bone mounted miniature robotic system: first experiences and accuracy of screw placement. Spine. 2009; 34(4):392–398

[9] Ringel F, Stüer C, Reinke A, et al. Accuracy of robot-assisted placement of lumbar and sacral pedicle screws: a prospective randomized comparison to conventional freehand screw implantation. Spine. 2012; 37(8):E496–E501

[10] Roser F, Tatagiba M, Maier G. Spinal robotics: current applications and future perspectives. Neurosurgery. 2013; 72 Suppl 1:12–18

[11] Bederman SS, Hahn P, Colin V, Kiester DP, Bhatia NN. Robotic guidance for S2-alar-iliac screws in spinal deformity correction. Clin Spine Surg. 2017; 30 (1):E49–E53

[12] Bederman SS, Jain N, Woolwine S, Kiester PD, Bhatia NN. Accuracy of pedicle screw placement in revision spine surgery using robotic guidance [abstract]. Global Spine J. 2015; 5:A106

[13] Schatlo B, Molliqaj G, Cuvinciuc V, Kotowski M, Schaller K, Tessitore E. Safety and accuracy of robot-assisted versus fluoroscopy-guided pedicle screw insertion for degenerative diseases of the lumbar spine: a matched cohort comparison. J Neurosurg Spine. 2014; 20(6):636–643

[14] van Dijk JD, van den Ende RP, Stramigioli S, Köchling M, Höss N. Clinical pedicle screw accuracy and deviation from planning in robot-guided spine surgery: robot-guided pedicle screw accuracy. Spine (Phila Pa 1976). 2015; 40 (17):E986–E991

[15] Shoham M, Burman M, Zehavi E, et al. Bone-mounted miniature robot for surgical procedures: Concept and clinical applications. IEEE Trans. Robotics Autom 2003;19(5):893–901

[16] Wolf A, Shoham M, Michael S, Moshe R. Feasibility study of a mini, bone-attached, robotic system for spinal operations: analysis and experiments. Spine. 2004; 29(2):220–228

[17] Lieberman IH, Togawa D, Kayanja MM, et al. Bone-mounted miniature robotic guidance for pedicle screw and translaminar facet screw placement: Part I–Technical development and a test case result. Neurosurgery. 2006; 59 (3):641–650, discussion 641–650

[18] Togawa D, Kayanja MM, Reinhardt MK, et al. Bone-mounted miniature robotic guidance for pedicle screw and translaminar facet screw placement: part 2–Evaluation of system accuracy. Neurosurgery. 2007; 60(2) Suppl 1: ONS129–ONS139, discussion ONS139

[19] Sukovich W, Brink-Danan S, Hardenbrook M. Miniature robotic guidance for pedicle screw placement in posterior spinal fusion: early clinical experience with the SpineAssist. Int J Med Robot. 2006; 2(2):114–122

[20] Barzilay Y, Liebergall M, Fridlander A, Knoller N. Miniature robotic guidance for spine surgery–introduction of a novel system and analysis of challenges encountered during the clinical development phase at two spine centres. Int J Med Robot. 2006; 2(2):146–153

[21] Shoham M, Lieberman IH, Benzel EC, et al. Robotic assisted spinal surgery–from concept to clinical practice. Comput Aided Surg. 2007; 12(2):105–115

[22] Kim S, Chung J, Yi BJ, Kim YS. An assistive image-guided surgical robot system using O-arm fluoroscopy for pedicle screw insertion: preliminary and cadaveric study. Neurosurgery. 2010; 67(6):1757–1767, discussion 1767

[23] Kostrzewski S, Duff JM, Baur C, Olszewski M. Robotic system for cervical spine surgery. Int J Med Robot. 2012; 8(2):184–190

[24] Ortmaier T, Weiss H, Döbele S, Schreiber U. Experiments on robot-assisted navigated drilling and milling of bones for pedicle screw placement. Int J Med Robot. 2006; 2(4):350–363

[25] Lee J, Hwang I, Kim K, Choi S, Chung WK, Kim YS. Cooperative robotic assistant with drill-by-wire end-effector for spinal fusion surgery. Industrial Robot: Int J.. 2009; 36(1):60–72

[26] Tian W, Han X, Liu B, et al. A robot-assisted surgical system using a force-image control method for pedicle screw insertion. PLoS One. 2014; 9(1):e86346

[27] Lonjon N, Chan-Seng E, Costalat V, Bonnafoux B, Vassal M, Boetto J. Robot-assisted spine surgery: feasibility study through a prospective case-matched analysis. Eur Spine J. 2016; ; 25(3):947–955

[28] Lee JY, Lega B, Bhowmick D, et al. Da Vinci Robot-assisted transoral odontoidectomy for basilar invagination. ORL J Otorhinolaryngol Relat Spec. 2010; 72 (2):91–95

[29] Kim MJ, Ha Y, Yang MS, et al. Robot-assisted anterior lumbar interbody fusion (ALIF) using retroperitoneal approach. Acta Neurochir (Wien). 2010; 152 (4):675–679

[30] Lee JY, O'Malley BW, Newman JG, et al. Transoral robotic surgery of craniocervical junction and atlantoaxial spine: a cadaveric study. J Neurosurg Spine. 2010; 12(1):13–18

[31] Moskowitz RM, Young JL, Box GN, Paré LS, Clayman RV. Retroperitoneal transdiaphragmatic robotic-assisted laparoscopic resection of a left thoracolumbar neurofibroma. JSLS. 2009; 13(1):64–68

[32] Ponnusamy K, Chewning S, Mohr C. Robotic approaches to the posterior spine. Spine. 2009; 34(19):2104–2109

[33] Ruurda JP, Hanlo PW, Hennipman A, Broeders IA. Robot-assisted thoracoscopic resection of a benign mediastinal neurogenic tumor: technical note. Neurosurgery. 2003; 52(2):462–464, discussion 464

[34] Yang MS, Kim KN, Yoon DH, Pennant W, Ha Y. Robot-assisted resection of paraspinal Schwannoma. J Korean Med Sci. 2011; 26(1):150–153

[35] Yang MS, Yoon DH, Kim KN, et al. Robot-assisted anterior lumbar interbody fusion in a Swine model in vivo test of the da vinci surgical-assisted spinal surgery system. Spine. 2011; 36(2):E139–E143

30 Biological Aspects of Spine Fusion—Methods to Enhance Fusion Rates

Venu M. Nemani, Matthew E. Cunningham

Abstract

Pseudarthrosis remains a significant postoperative risk after long thoracolumbar fusions to the sacropelvis for adult spinal deformity. In addition to meticulous surgical technique and rigid internal fixation, the choice and amount of graft used to promote spinal arthrodesis are critical to a successful outcome. Although iliac crest bone graft is the gold standard, there are now many different graft options available to surgeons trying to avoid the potential morbidity of harvesting autograft bone. However, a careful understanding of the biology of spinal fusion is necessary to select the proper graft for the particular clinical situation. Here we review the biology of spinal fusion, as well as discuss the characteristics of the different graft options available for use.

Keywords: spine fusion, bone graft, autograft, allograft, bone morphogenetic protein, demineralized bone matrix

30.1 Introduction

Pseudarthrosis remains a significant postoperative risk after long thoracolumbar fusions to the sacropelvis for adult spinal deformity. In addition to meticulous surgical technique and rigid internal fixation, the choice and amount of graft used to promote spinal arthrodesis is critical to a successful outcome. Although iliac crest bone graft (ICBG) is the gold standard, there are now many different graft options available to surgeons trying to avoid the potential morbidity of harvesting autograft bone. However, a careful understanding of the biology of spinal fusion is necessary to select the proper graft for the particular clinical situation. Here we review the biology of spinal fusion, as well as discuss the characteristics of the different graft options available for use.

Spinal arthrodesis is used to treat many types of spinal pathology, with etiologies including degenerative disease, trauma, congenital anomalies, tumor, as well as progressive deformity from scoliosis or kyphosis. Since the first spinal fusions were performed by Hibbs[1] and Albee[2] in 1911, numerous advances have been made in surgical techniques and spinal instrumentation; further, we now have a more detailed understanding of the biology of bone healing and fusion. However, despite these advances there is still a significant risk of pseudarthrosis estimated at 5 to 35%,[3] with the subsequent consequences of pain and poor clinical outcomes. Pseudarthrosis is an especially big problem at the thoracolumbar and lumbosacral junctions in patients undergoing long fusions to the sacrum for adult spinal deformity. Risk factors for pseudarthrosis can be categorized into patient-specific factors (smoking, diabetes, and osteoporosis) and surgeon-specific factors (surgical technique, use and type of instrumentation, choice of bone graft or graft-extender). While patient-specific factors are difficult to control, an in-depth understanding of the biology of spinal fusion can help surgeons optimize the surgeon-specific factors to decrease pseudarthrosis rates and improve outcomes. This chapter discusses the basic science behind fusion mass formation and reviews the different types of grafts available and their biological properties that enable them to act as graft-extenders.

30.2 Fusion Formation

Despite the significant advances (and increase in cost) in spinal instrumentation and grafts available, the ultimate goal of surgery remains unchanged from those performed in the early 1900s for patients with spinal deformity—to obtain a solid arthrodesis. The mechanism by which fusion occurs was first described by Boden and colleagues using a rabbit intertransverse process model in 1995.[4] Interestingly, they showed that fusion occurs via a mechanism similar to that in fracture healing, which is a combination of intramembranous and endochondral ossification. Further, they were able to define three distinct and reproducible temporal stages of healing of a spinal fusion mass: (1) the early inflammatory phase, (2) the middle reparative phase, and (3) the late remodeling phase.

The early inflammatory phase is initiated by the surgical insult to the local tissues from exposure, and further facilitated by bony decortication, which leads to the formation of a postoperative hematoma. This results in the generation and release of several proinflammatory substances, such as cytokines, tumor necrosis factor, and fibroblast growth factor. Additionally, platelet-derived growth factor, transforming growth factor-β (TGF-β), and bone morphogenetic proteins (BMPs) all can be found at the fusion site. There is also release and proliferation of polymorphonuclear leukocytes, macrophages, and lymphocytes. As the hematoma matures and transforms into a fibrovascular stroma, fibroblast-like cells are recruited to the area, and a vasculature begins to invade the fusion site. Primary membranous bone formation begins during this stage at the outer zones close to the decorticated transverse processes as defined by Boden.[4] In the central zone where bone graft has been placed, endochondral ossification is seen rather than membranous bone formation. Studies have shown a marked decrease in the rate of fusion with the use of anti-inflammatory medication,[5,6] demonstrating the importance of the inflammatory phase for bony fusion.

The middle reparative phase is characterized by increased vascularization, resorption of necrotic tissue, and differentiation of mesenchymal cells into both osteoblastic and chondroblastic cells. The fusion mass continues to evolve, with solidification of fusion in the outer zones and extension toward the less vascular central zone. Calcification of cartilaginous tissue into immature woven bone also occurs toward the end of the reparative phase.[7]

The late remodeling phase is characterized by maturation of the immature woven bone into typical lamellar bone. In the rabbit intertransverse process fusion model, this phase extends from approximately 6 to 12 weeks postoperatively. Although spinal fusion is thought to progress through these same phases in humans, this has never been shown histologically. Importantly, however, the fusion process is thought to take longer than in the described rabbit model, probably around 6 to 18 months versus 3 months in the rabbit.[7]

30.3 Properties of Bone Grafts

There are four biological properties that an ideal graft must possess to facilitate spinal fusion: (1) osteogenic—capable of directly providing cells to the newly forming bone; (2) osteoinductive—contains factors that can act in either a paracrine or endocrine fashion to recruit cells to the fusion site or promote differentiation of local cells into an osteoid-producing phenotype; (3) osteoconductive—provides a scaffold upon which new bone growth can take place and revascularization can occur; (4) mechanical strength—robust enough to provide at least partial resistance to the normal loads transmitted to the spine during routine daily activities.[8] Further, the ideal graft would not create a new clinical problem. Unfortunately, harvesting of autograft can occasionally cause symptomatic donor-site morbidity. For this reason ICBG, which is typically considered the gold standard for spinal fusion, still cannot be considered a "perfect" graft option.[9]

In addition to the foregoing biological properties, an ideal graft source needs to be easily obtainable (or manufactured), cost-effective, and plentiful. There are several situations in which the combination of iliac crest autograft and local bone may not provide sufficient graft volume to optimize the environment for spinal fusion. These situations include deformity cases, revision cases where there has been previous resection of the posterior elements and/or previous harvest of the iliac crest(s), and neuromuscular patients with a small pelvis and osteoporotic bone. These are only a few examples of the situations in which supplementation or even substitution of another type of graft would be critical to obtaining a solid arthrodesis.

30.4 Types of Grafts

In the last decade there has been an explosion in the number and types of grafts available for use. While there may never be a "perfect" graft, a surgeon can now select a graft with the desired biological properties that is tailored to the particular clinical situation (▸ Table 30.1). Here we review the general types of grafts available and their unique advantages and disadvantages.

Table 30.1 Optimal bone graft characteristics and specific products (limited list) used in spinal fusion surgery

Characteristics	Category	Examples
Osteoinductive	Bone morphogenetic protein	• InFUSE (Medtronic Sofamor Danek) • OP-1 (Stryker)
	Demineralized bone matrix	• Grafton (Osteotech) • Osteofil (Medtronic Sofamor Danek) • DBX (Synthes) • AlloMatrix (Wright Medical)
	Autograft	• Iliac crest cancellous bone
Osteoconductive	Demineralized bone matrix	• See above
	Allograft	• Cancellous chips
	Autograft	• Iliac crest cancellous bone
	Ceramics	• Calcium sulfate • β-tricalcium phosphate • Hydroxyapatite
Osteogenic	Autograft	• Iliac crest cancellous bone
	Bone marrow aspirate	• BMAC (Harvest Technologies)
Mechanical Strength	Autograft	• Fibular strut • Tricortical iliac crest
	Allograft	• Corticocancellous • Cortical strut (fibula, femoral ring)

30.4.1 Autograft

As stated earlier, autograft is still considered the gold standard for spinal fusion surgery. There are multiple potential sources of autograft depending on the procedure being performed and the clinical scenario. For one- or two-level posterior spinal fusion procedures for degenerative lumbar disease, the local bone harvested from resection of the spinous processes and laminectomy often provides sufficient bone for an intertransverse process and facet fusion. This local bone may even be sufficient if an interbody fusion (transforaminal lumbar interbody fusion or posterior lumbar interbody fusion) is also being performed concomitantly. However, in long posterior spinal fusions being performed for either adult or adolescent deformity, local bone itself typically does not provide a sufficient volume of bone for fusion. This is true even if autograft bone is harvested from bilateral iliac crests. If an anterior fusion is being performed at the thoracolumbar junction via a thoracoabdominal approach, a rib can be harvested and morselized and packed into the disk spaces. For multilevel cervical degenerative disease where a long anterior fusion is being considered, one can perform a corpectomy rather than a multilevel diskectomy and fusion to minimize the number of bony surfaces that need to heal, as well as to use the resected vertebral body for bone graft.

With regard to the biological properties of autograft bone, cancellous autograft is highly osteogenic, osteoconductive, and osteoinductive. It contains osteoblasts, a bony matrix that provides the necessary scaffolding, and growth factors such as BMPs and TGF-β. However, it lacks mechanical strength. Cortical or corticocancellous autograft has improved mechanical strength with the tradeoff of decreased osteogenic, osteoconductive, and osteoinductive properties. Important considerations when deciding to use autograft bone is the additional time and blood loss required for its harvest, and the possibility of additional complications associated with a more extensive surgical dissection. While local bone harvest does not carry the risk of donor site morbidity, there is unfortunately a significant risk of donor site morbidity with iliac crest autograft harvest, including pain, hematoma formation, wound complications, and lateral femoral cutaneous nerve injury. Although some reports state that ICBG donor site pain is as high as 60%,[10] other studies suggest that the presence of postoperative pain is multifactorial and not necessarily related to ICBG harvest.[11,12,13]

The use of autograft has generally been shown in previous studies to lead to high rates of fusion.[10,14,15,16] For single-level fusions, local bone graft has a similar rate of fusion to ICBG. Sengupta and colleagues retrospectively reviewed 76 patients treated with instrumented posterolateral fusion for spinal stenosis and reported a fusion rate of 75% with ICBG and 65% with local bone graft, determined using plain X-rays. However, when they analyzed multilevel fusions separately, the fusion rate was 66% for ICBG and only 20% for local bone.[16] Notably, there was no difference in clinical outcomes.

30.5 Osteoinductive Agents

Osteoinductive agents act by promoting the differentiation of local cells into osteoblastic and chondroblastic lineages to promote endochondral ossification. Thus they depend on the presence of pluripotent stem cells capable of differentiating into these cell types. Two osteoinductive agents commonly used today include BMP and demineralized bone matrix (DBM).

30.5.1 Bone Morphogenetic Proteins

BMPs were first discovered by Urist in 1965.[17] In this landmark study, he isolated BMPs from DBM and was the first to describe their properties, namely being able to induce bone formation in animals. BMPs are a member of the TGF-β superfamily of proteins, and act by binding to serine/threonine kinase receptors found on the surface of target cells to initiate downstream signaling. In this manner, BMPs regulate cell growth and differentiation of a wide number of cell types, with their precise function depending on the extracellular milieu.

The ability of BMPs to produce ectopic bone, induce spinal fusion, and promote fracture healing were all first shown in animal models.[18] These initial studies subsequently led to the first human trials where Boden and colleagues showed the utility of recombinant human BMP-2 (rhBMP-2) in anterior interbody fusion in the lumbar spine.[19] This and other studies ultimately led to the approval of rhBMP-2 (InFUSE, Medtronic Sofamor Danek) specifically for use in the tapered LT-Cage (Medtronic Sofamor Danek) for anterior lumbar interbody fusion by the U.S. Food and Drug Administration (FDA). Since that time, there has been an explosion of studies demonstrating the clinical utility in "off-label" uses of rhBMP-2 and BMP-7 (OP-1, Stryker) in anterior lumbar interbody fusion,[20,21] transforaminal and posterior lumbar interbody fusion,[22] anterior cervical diskectomy and fusion,[23,24] posterolateral lumbar fusion,[25,26,27,28] and spinal deformity surgery.[29,30,31] However, subsequent studies revealed a number of potential complications associated with the use of rhBMP-2, including cervical prevertebral soft tissue swelling, retrograde ejaculation, urinary retention, bony overgrowth, seroma formation, radiculitis, and increased risk of cancer.[32,33,34,35,36,37] Recently, Medtronic funded an independent assessment of the original rhBMP-2 data through the Yale University Open Data Access (YODA) project, which was published by two groups from Oregon Health and Sciences University and the University of York.[38,39] In these studies, the authors concluded that there was "little or no benefit" of rhBMP-2 compared to ICBG, and its use may be associated with increased risks not previously noted in the original industry-sponsored trials. As with any biological or pharmacological agent, the risks and benefits must be considered carefully and discussed with the patient prior to use. Despite these drawbacks and concerns, there are still particular situations, such as in patients with poor host bone and those at high risk for pseudarthrosis (i. e., long fusions to the sacrum) where BMPs may be useful and justify the associated risks and cost.

30.5.2 Demineralized Bone Matrix

DBM is created by using acid extraction to remove the mineral components of ground human corticocancellous bone. The resulting matrix contains various proteins, including collagen, as well as osteoinductive proteins, such as BMPs. This is then combined with various carrier materials to produce the final product.[7] The acid extraction process also reduces the antigenicity of DBM so immunological reactions are rare. It is well established that DBM preparations are osteoinductive[40,41,42]; however, the degree to which DBM is osteoinductive depends on how the bone was processed, the carrier, and the sterilization method. BMPs are the most well-represented osteoinductive proteins present in DBM; however, they only exist in nanogram concentrations, which is 1 million times less than the concentration of BMP that is necessary to achieve a lumbar fusion clinically.[25,43,44] Other osteoinductive proteins present in DBM include TGF-β, insulin-like growth factor, platelet-derived growth factor, and fibroblast growth factor. Together with BMPs, these proteins represent only 5% of the composition of DBM. Collagen is the largest constituent of DBM at 93%, which provides an osteoconductive surface for bone formation.[45] The other 2% is made up of residual mineral components.[46]

There have been several animal studies in rodents, rabbits, and nonhuman primates[47] showing the effectiveness of DBM products to promote spinal fusion. Martin and colleagues showed in 1999 in a rabbit posterior intertransverse process model that Grafton Flex (Osteotech) and Grafton Putty (Osteotech) were effective as graft extenders and graft enhancers when used alone or with autogenous ICBG, and in fact led to higher rates of fusion and more mature fusions when used alone than when compared to rabbits who received only ICBG.[45] A study in an intertransverse process fusion model in rats compared different preparations of DBM—Grafton Putty, DBX Putty (Synthes), and AlloMatrix injectable Putty (Wright Medical Technology)—and compared them to a control group that underwent decortication alone.[48] In this experiment, the authors found a statistically significant higher rate of fusion in animals grafted with Grafton Putty compared to the control and AlloMatrix injectable putty groups. Further, the DBX putty group only had a 50% fusion rate (3/6 animals). Another study in the same animal model examined eight different DBM formulations and found that Osteofil Paste (Medtronic Sofamor Danek) and Grafton Putty had the highest radiographic and gross evidence for fusion.[49] Given the low numbers in the majority of these studies, it is difficult to make meaningful conclusions; however, it does reinforce that different preparations of DBM have different levels of osteoinductivity.[43]

Human data are limited as to DBM's effectiveness in promoting spinal fusion. Kang and colleagues published a multicenter prospective randomized study in which they compared Grafton Matrix (Osteotech) with local bone or autogenous ICBG for single-level instrumented posterior lumbar fusion. They found equivalent rates of fusion verified by CT and equivalent clinical outcomes with no significant differences.[50]

30.6 Osteoconductive Agents

Osteoconductive agents are characterized by not having any osteogenic precursor cells capable of producing bone, as well as lacking any osteoinductive factors. Rather, they provide scaffolding on which osteoprogenitor cells can lay down mineralized bone or for formation of a cartilaginous precursor. Two types of osteoconductive agents include allograft bone and synthetic bone grafts (ceramics).

30.6.1 Allograft Bone

Allograft bone is commonly used alone, especially in anterior cervical diskectomy and fusion, and results in high rates of arthrodesis without the morbidity of autologous ICBG harvest.[53] It is also used commonly for posterior spinal fusion as a graft extender. Allografts can be used as fresh-frozen grafts, which retain their mechanical strength and some osteoinductive factors, or freeze-dried grafts, which are the least immunogenic but can lose up to 50% of their mechanical strength, and all of their osteoinductive factors are destroyed.[54] The benefit of allografts is that they are available in essentially unlimited amounts. However, the use of fresh-frozen allograft bone carries a risk of disease transmission as well as possible immunological response to the foreign tissue. Although there has never been a reported case of bacterial disease transmission due to allograft bone and only one case of viral disease transmission (HIV),[55] musculoskeletal allograft tissue accounts for the majority of recalled tissue by the FDA, with 59,476 allograft specimens recalled from 1994 to 2007.[56] The most common reasons for recall were improper donor evaluation, contamination, and recipient infections.

The differing biological and mechanical properties of cortical versus cancellous allografts make each type of graft useful for different applications. Cortical allografts can be used for anterior interbody reconstruction where mechanical support is required. Bridwell and colleagues showed in a series of patients with kyphosis or anterior column defects undergoing anterior/posterior thoracolumbar fusion that only 2 of 24 patients had collapse of their allograft at minimum 2-year follow-up.[57] At 5-year follow-up, 98.5% of the structural allografts showed incorporation.[58] Alternatively, corticocancellous or cancellous allograft can be used in isolation or as a graft extender in posterior spinal fusions where high osteoconductivity is needed.[8] Gibson and colleagues performed a prospective study of fresh-frozen allograft versus ICBG and found no difference in fusion rates after instrumented posterior spinal fusion.[59] Also, Aurori and colleagues examined the incidence of pseudarthrosis in patients undergoing spinal arthrodesis for adolescent idiopathic scoliosis (AIS) using either autograft or frozen allografts and found no difference.[60] Although allograft is a useful graft extender and even as a stand-alone graft in certain circumstances, its use may decrease in the future given the potential risks for contamination and infection, although rare, given the widespread availability of many other graft options.

30.6.2 Synthetic Bone Grafts

Synthetic bone grafts, such as ceramics, exhibit osteoconductive properties[61] and are available in a number of different formulations. Their advantages are that they are available in essentially unlimited supply, carry no potential for donor site morbidity, and are nonimmunogenic, making them a promising graft source. Only beta-tricalcium phosphate (β-TCP) and hydroxyapatite are used in spine surgery because their absorption occurs over months (β-TCP) to years (hydroxyapatite), versus calcium sulfate, which is absorbed in weeks. The disadvantages of ceramics are their brittle nature, precluding their use in load-bearing applications without rigid internal fixation.

Ceramics have been shown to be useful as bone graft extenders for posterolateral short-segment fusions.[62,63] However, their greatest utility may be combined with other graft materials (local bone, autograft) in deformity cases when large amounts of graft are needed. Ransford and colleagues performed a prospective randomized study in patients with AIS comparing autograft bone with a synthetic porous ceramic and found equivalent clinical results, although they did not formally assess fusion rates in their study.[64] Another study in patients with AIS undergoing deformity correction showed equivalent rates of fusion comparing allograft versus β-TCP as a graft extender mixed with autograft.[65] There may be increased use of these products in the future as newer ceramics are developed with even better osteoconductive properties.

30.7 Osteopromotive Agents

Osteopromotive agents do not clearly belong to one of the previously mentioned categories (osteoinductive, osteoconductive, or osteogenic) but can assist with bone formation in spinal fusion. One particular class of osteopromotive agent that has been studied previously is platelet gels. At the site of a fracture or at a bone grafting site, fibrin clot formation, platelet aggregation, and platelet degranulation initiate the healing response. Platelet granules have a variety of biologically active products within them, many of which have been shown to be beneficial for bone healing.[66] Platelet gels are formed by ultraconcentrating platelets and mixing them with thrombin to form the final product. These can then be combined with allograft, DBM, or autologous bone to assist with fusion. Although early studies in rat and sheep models suggested that platelet gels could improve fusion rates,[67,68] clinical studies have shown no benefit or even an inhibition of fusion in both the lumbar spine[69,70,71] and the cervical spine.[72] At this time, there is no evidence to support the use of platelet gels in spinal arthrodesis.

30.8 Systemic Agents

A few systemic, FDA-approved medications that are routinely used to treat osteoporosis have been recently studied as potential adjuvants to improve healing rates after spinal fusion.

Although these are not bone grafts or graft extenders per se, they can serve a complementary role in the ultimate goal of achieving a solid fusion. Given the similarities between the biological processes of fracture healing and spine fusion, these medications deserve careful study for use as adjuvants.

30.8.1 Bisphosphonates

Bisphosphonates are drugs that inhibit bone resorption and increase bone mass by three mechanisms: (1) they inhibit osteoclastogenesis in the bone marrow, (2) they reduce osteoclastic activity at bone surfaces, and (3) they promote apoptosis of osteoclasts by reducing their overall numbers.[73] All of these actions shift the balance in favor of osteoblastic activity and promote new bone formation. Several animal studies have shown mixed results with regard to their effect on fusion rates.[73,74,75] Importantly, bisphosphonate-treated animals have higher amounts of unremodeled or immature fusion mass bone, which makes sense given the important function of osteoclasts in the remodeling phase of bone healing.[76,77] There have been two human studies examining bisphosphonate therapy that have shown little to no effect on fusion rates.[78,79] Notably, there have not been any studies examining the effect of bisphosphonates on fusion in patients undergoing long fusions for spinal deformity.

30.8.2 Parathyroid Hormone

Parathyroid hormone (PTH) is an anabolic agent when administered intermittently, and acts by binding osteoblast cell surface receptors to initiate downstream signaling and increase osteoblastic activity. This leads to an overall increase in bone mass, primarily by increasing the amount of cancellous bone.[80] Animal studies have suggested a beneficial effect of PTH on fusion rates at early time points.[81] To date there has been only one study in humans, which compared PTH to bisphosphonates in patients undergoing short fusions for degenerative spondylolisthesis and found a slight decrease in rates of pedicle screw loosening at 1 year with PTH compared to bisphosphonates or controls.[82] More research is needed to determine the role for both bisphosphonates and PTH, if any, as adjuncts to improve fusion rates after surgery for spinal deformity.

30.9 Conclusions

Regardless of the type of instrumentation and graft used, the goal of surgical treatment of spinal deformity—to achieve a rigid arthrodesis—is unchanged. Proper graft selection requires a full understanding of the biology of spinal fusion, and a critical understanding of the biological and mechanical factors specific to the patient that may affect the likelihood of achieving a successful arthrodesis. For example, an adult patient with poor host physiology for bone healing will require more attention to proper graft selection compared to a patient with adolescent idiopathic scoliosis. In the coming years, we will undoubtedly see the development of newer grafts with unique properties. Understanding the principles of osteoinduction, osteoconduction, and osteogenesis with respect to spinal fusion will allow the surgeon to select the proper graft that minimizes risk to the patient, is cost-effective, and maximizes the chances of a good surgical outcome.

References

[1] Hibbs R. An operation for progressive spinal deformities. NY Med J. 1911; 93:1013

[2] Albee FH. Transplantation of a portion of the tibia into the spine for Pott's disease: a preliminary report 1911. Clin Orthop Relat Res. 2007; 460(460):14–16

[3] Ludwig SC, Kowalski JM, Boden SD. Osteoinductive bone graft substitutes. Eur Spine J. 2000; 9 Suppl 1:S119–S125

[4] Boden SD, Schimandle JH, Hutton WC, Chen MI. 1995 Volvo Award in basic sciences. The use of an osteoinductive growth factor for lumbar spinal fusion. Part I: Biology of spinal fusion. Spine. 1995; 20(24):2626–2632

[5] Dahners LE, Mullis BH. Effects of nonsteroidal anti-inflammatory drugs on bone formation and soft-tissue healing. J Am Acad Orthop Surg. 2004; 12 (3):139–143

[6] Martin GJ, Jr, Boden SD, Titus L. Recombinant human bone morphogenetic protein-2 overcomes the inhibitory effect of ketorolac, a nonsteroidal anti-inflammatory drug (NSAID), on posterolateral lumbar intertransverse process spine fusion. Spine. 1999; 24(21):2188–2193, discussion 2193–2194

[7] Grabowski G, Cornett CA. Bone graft and bone graft substitutes in spine surgery: current concepts and controversies. J Am Acad Orthop Surg. 2013; 21 (1):51–60

[8] Cheng I, Oshtory R, Wildstein MS. The role of osteobiologics in spinal deformity. Neurosurg Clin N Am. 2007; 18(2):393–401

[9] Gazdag AR, Lane JM, Glaser D, Forster RA. Alternatives to Autogenous Bone Graft: Efficacy and Indications. J Am Acad Orthop Surg. 1995; 3(1):1–8

[10] Dimar JR, II, Glassman SD, Burkus JK, Pryor PW, Hardacker JW, Carreon LY. Two-year fusion and clinical outcomes in 224 patients treated with a single-level instrumented posterolateral fusion with iliac crest bone graft. Spine J. 2009; 9(11):880–885

[11] Delawi D, Dhert WJ, Castelein RM, Verbout AJ, Oner FC. The incidence of donor site pain after bone graft harvesting from the posterior iliac crest may be overestimated: a study on spine fracture patients. Spine. 2007; 32(17):1865–1868

[12] Howard JM, Glassman SD, Carreon LY. Posterior iliac crest pain after posterolateral fusion with or without iliac crest graft harvest. Spine J. 2011; 11 (6):534–537

[13] Summers BN, Eisenstein SM. Donor site pain from the ilium. A complication of lumbar spine fusion. J Bone Joint Surg Br. 1989; 71(4):677–680

[14] Ito Z, Matsuyama Y, Sakai Y, et al. Bone union rate with autologous iliac bone versus local bone graft in posterior lumbar interbody fusion. Spine. 2010; 35 (21):E1101–E1105

[15] Rihn JA, Kirkpatrick K, Albert TJ. Graft options in posterolateral and posterior interbody lumbar fusion. Spine. 2010; 35(17):1629–1639

[16] Sengupta DK, Truumees E, Patel CK, et al. Outcome of local bone versus autogenous iliac crest bone graft in the instrumented posterolateral fusion of the lumbar spine. Spine. 2006; 31(9):985–991

[17] Urist MR. Bone: formation by autoinduction. Science. 1965; 150(3 698):893–899

[18] Lane JM. Bone morphogenic protein science and studies. J Orthop Trauma. 2005; 19(10) Suppl:S17–S22

[19] Boden SD, Zdeblick TA, Sandhu HS, Heim SE. The use of rhBMP-2 in interbody fusion cages. Definitive evidence of osteoinduction in humans: a preliminary report. Spine. 2000; 25(3):376–381

[20] Burkus JK, Gornet MF, Dickman CA, Zdeblick TA. Anterior lumbar interbody fusion using rhBMP-2 with tapered interbody cages. J Spinal Disord Tech. 2002; 15(5):337–349

[21] Burkus JK, Transfeldt EE, Kitchel SH, Watkins RG, Balderston RA. Clinical and radiographic outcomes of anterior lumbar interbody fusion using recombinant human bone morphogenetic protein-2. Spine. 2002; 27(21):2396–2408

[22] Haid RW, Jr, Branch CL, Jr, Alexander JT, Burkus JK. Posterior lumbar interbody fusion using recombinant human bone morphogenetic protein type 2 with cylindrical interbody cages. Spine J. 2004; 4(5):527–538, discussion 538–539

[23] Baskin DS, Ryan P, Sonntag V, Westmark R, Widmayer MA. A prospective, randomized, controlled cervical fusion study using recombinant human bone morphogenetic protein-2 with the CORNERSTONE-SR allograft ring and the ATLANTIS anterior cervical plate. Spine. 2003; 28(12):1219–1224, discussion 1225

[24] Boakye M, Mummaneni PV, Garrett M, Rodts G, Haid R. Anterior cervical discectomy and fusion involving a polyetheretherketone spacer and bone morphogenetic protein. J Neurosurg Spine. 2005; 2(5):521–525
[25] Boden SD, Kang J, Sandhu H, Heller JG. Use of recombinant human bone morphogenetic protein-2 to achieve posterolateral lumbar spine fusion in humans: a prospective, randomized clinical pilot trial: 2002 Volvo Award in clinical studies. Spine. 2002; 27(23):2662–2673
[26] Dimar JR, II, Glassman SD, Burkus JK, Pryor PW, Hardacker JW, Carreon LY. Clinical and radiographic analysis of an optimized rhBMP-2 formulation as an autograft replacement in posterolateral lumbar spine arthrodesis. J Bone Joint Surg Am. 2009; 91(6):1377–1386
[27] Dawson E, Bae HW, Burkus JK, Stambough JL, Glassman SD. Recombinant human bone morphogenetic protein-2 on an absorbable collagen sponge with an osteoconductive bulking agent in posterolateral arthrodesis with instrumentation. A prospective randomized trial. J Bone Joint Surg Am. 2009; 91(7):1604–1613
[28] Vaccaro AR, Whang PG, Patel T, et al. The safety and efficacy of OP-1 (rhBMP-7) as a replacement for iliac crest autograft for posterolateral lumbar arthrodesis: minimum 4-year follow-up of a pilot study. Spine J. 2008; 8(3):457–465
[29] Maeda T, Buchowski JM, Kim YJ, Mishiro T, Bridwell KH. Long adult spinal deformity fusion to the sacrum using rhBMP-2 versus autogenous iliac crest bone graft. Spine. 2009; 34(20):2205–2212
[30] Mulconrey DS, Bridwell KH, Flynn J, Cronen GA, Rose PS. Bone morphogenetic protein (RhBMP-2) as a substitute for iliac crest bone graft in multilevel adult spinal deformity surgery: minimum two-year evaluation of fusion. Spine. 2008; 33(20):2153–2159
[31] Luhmann SJ, Bridwell KH, Cheng I, Imamura T, Lenke LG, Schootman M. Use of bone morphogenetic protein-2 for adult spinal deformity. Spine. 2005; 30 (17) Suppl:S110–S117
[32] Perri B, Cooper M, Lauryssen C, Anand N. Adverse swelling associated with use of rh-BMP-2 in anterior cervical discectomy and fusion: a case study. Spine J. 2007; 7(2):235–239
[33] Carragee EJ, Mitsunaga KA, Hurwitz EL, Scuderi GJ. Retrograde ejaculation after anterior lumbar interbody fusion using rhBMP-2: a cohort controlled study. Spine J. 2011; 11(6):511–516
[34] Comer GC, Smith MW, Hurwitz EL, Mitsunaga KA, Kessler R, Carragee EJ. Retrograde ejaculation after anterior lumbar interbody fusion with and without bone morphogenetic protein-2 augmentation: a 10-year cohort controlled study. Spine J. 2012; 12(10):881–890
[35] Carragee EJ, Hurwitz EL, Weiner BK. A critical review of recombinant human bone morphogenetic protein-2 trials in spinal surgery: emerging safety concerns and lessons learned. Spine J. 2011; 11(6):471–491
[36] Glassman SD, Howard J, Dimar J, Sweet A, Wilson G, Carreon L. Complications with recombinant human bone morphogenic protein-2 in posterolateral spine fusion: a consecutive series of 1037 cases. Spine. 2011; 36(22):1849–1854
[37] Carragee EJ, Chu G, Rohatgi R, et al. Cancer risk after use of recombinant bone morphogenetic protein-2 for spinal arthrodesis. J Bone Joint Surg Am. 2013; 95(17):1537–1545
[38] Fu R, Selph S, McDonagh M, et al. Effectiveness and harms of recombinant human bone morphogenetic protein-2 in spine fusion: a systematic review and meta-analysis. Ann Intern Med. 2013; 158(12):890–902
[39] Simmonds MC, Brown JV, Heirs MK, et al. Safety and effectiveness of recombinant human bone morphogenetic protein-2 for spinal fusion: a meta-analysis of individual-participant data. Ann Intern Med. 2013; 158(12):877–889
[40] Berven S, Tay BK, Kleinstueck FS, Bradford DS. Clinical applications of bone graft substitutes in spine surgery: consideration of mineralized and demineralized preparations and growth factor supplementation. Eur Spine J. 2001; 10 Suppl 2:S169–S177
[41] Chalmers J, Gray DH, Rush J. Observations on the induction of bone in soft tissues. J Bone Joint Surg Br. 1975; 57(1):36–45
[42] Dahners LE, Jacobs RR. Long bone defects treated with demineralized bone. South Med J. 1985; 78(8):933–934
[43] Bae HW, Zhao L, Kanim LE, Wong P, Delamarter RB, Dawson EG. Intervariability and intravariability of bone morphogenetic proteins in commercially available demineralized bone matrix products. Spine. 2006; 31(12):1299–1306, discussion 1307–1308
[44] Burkus JK, Sandhu HS, Gornet MF. Influence of rhBMP-2 on the healing patterns associated with allograft interbody constructs in comparison with autograft. Spine. 2006; 31(7):775–781
[45] Martin GJ, Jr, Boden SD, Titus L, Scarborough NL. New formulations of demineralized bone matrix as a more effective graft alternative in experimental posterolateral lumbar spine arthrodesis. Spine. 1999; 24(7):637–645
[46] Lee KJ, Roper JG, Wang JC. Demineralized bone matrix and spinal arthrodesis. Spine J. 2005; 5(6) Suppl:217S–223S
[47] Louis-Ugbo J, Murakami H, Kim HS, Minamide A, Boden SD. Evidence of osteoinduction by Grafton demineralized bone matrix in nonhuman primate spinal fusion. Spine. 2004; 29(4):360–366, discussion Z1
[48] Peterson B, Whang PG, Iglesias R, Wang JC, Lieberman JR. Osteoinductivity of commercially available demineralized bone matrix. Preparations in a spine fusion model. J Bone Joint Surg Am. 2004; 86-A(10):2243–2250
[49] Lee YP, Jo M, Luna M, Chien B, Lieberman JR, Wang JC. The efficacy of different commercially available demineralized bone matrix substances in an athymic rat model. J Spinal Disord Tech. 2005; 18(5):439–444
[50] Kang J, An H, Hilibrand A, Yoon ST, Kavanagh E, Boden S. Grafton and local bone have comparable outcomes to iliac crest bone in instrumented single-level lumbar fusions. Spine. 2012; 37(12):1083–1091
[51] Jagannathan J, Shaffrey CI, Oskouian RJ, et al. Radiographic and clinical outcomes following single-level anterior cervical discectomy and allograft fusion without plate placement or cervical collar. J Neurosurg Spine. 2008; 8 (5):420–428
[52] Mummaneni PV, Burkus JK, Haid RW, Traynelis VC, Zdeblick TA. Clinical and radiographic analysis of cervical disc arthroplasty compared with allograft fusion: a randomized controlled clinical trial. J Neurosurg Spine. 2007; 6 (3):198–209
[53] Samartzis D, Shen FH, Matthews DK, Yoon ST, Goldberg EJ, An HS. Comparison of allograft to autograft in multilevel anterior cervical discectomy and fusion with rigid plate fixation. Spine J. 2003; 3(6):451–459
[54] Ehrler DM, Vaccaro AR. The use of allograft bone in lumbar spine surgery. Clin Orthop Relat Res. 2000(371):38–45
[55] Leads from the MMWR. Leads from the MMWR. Transmission of HIV through bone transplantation: case report and public health recommendations. JAMA. 1988; 260(17):2487–2488
[56] Mroz TE, Joyce MJ, Lieberman IH, Steinmetz MP, Benzel EC, Wang JC. The use of allograft bone in spine surgery: is it safe? Spine J. 2009; 9(4):303–308
[57] Bridwell KH, Lenke LG, McEnery KW, Baldus C, Blanke K. Anterior fresh frozen structural allografts in the thoracic and lumbar spine. Do they work if combined with posterior fusion and instrumentation in adult patients with kyphosis or anterior column defects? Spine. 1995; 20(12):1410–1418
[58] Molinari RW, Bridwell KH, Klepps SJ, Baldus C. Minimum 5-year follow-up of anterior column structural allografts in the thoracic and lumbar spine. Spine. 1999; 24(10):967–972
[59] Gibson S, McLeod I, Wardlaw D, Urbaniak S. Allograft versus autograft in instrumented posterolateral lumbar spinal fusion: a randomized control trial. Spine. 2002; 27(15):1599–1603
[60] Aurori BF, Weierman RJ, Lowell HA, Nadel CI, Parsons JR. Pseudarthrosis after spinal fusion for scoliosis. A comparison of autogeneic and allogeneic bone grafts. Clin Orthop Relat Res. 1985(199):153–158
[61] Baramki HG, Steffen T, Lander P, Chang M, Marchesi D. The efficacy of interconnected porous hydroxyapatite in achieving posterolateral lumbar fusion in sheep. Spine. 2000; 25(9):1053–1060
[62] Chen WJ, Tsai TT, Chen LH, et al. The fusion rate of calcium sulfate with local autograft bone compared with autologous iliac bone graft for instrumented short-segment spinal fusion. Spine. 2005; 30(20):2293–2297
[63] Epstein NE. A preliminary study of the efficacy of Beta Tricalcium Phosphate as a bone expander for instrumented posterolateral lumbar fusions. J Spinal Disord Tech. 2006; 19(6):424–429
[64] Ransford AO, Morley T, Edgar MA, et al. Synthetic porous ceramic compared with autograft in scoliosis surgery. A prospective, randomized study of 341 patients. J Bone Joint Surg Br. 1998; 80(1):13–18
[65] Muschik M, Ludwig R, Halbhübner S, Bursche K, Stoll T. Beta-tricalcium phosphate as a bone substitute for dorsal spinal fusion in adolescent idiopathic scoliosis: preliminary results of a prospective clinical study. Eur Spine J. 2001; 10 Suppl 2:S178–S184
[66] Khan SN, Fraser JF, Sandhu HS, Cammisa FP, Jr, Girardi FP, Lane JM. Use of osteopromotive growth factors, demineralized bone matrix, and ceramics to enhance spinal fusion. J Am Acad Orthop Surg. 2005; 13(2):129–137
[67] Siebrecht MA, De Rooij PP, Arm DM, Olsson ML, Aspenberg P. Platelet concentrate increases bone ingrowth into porous hydroxyapatite. Orthopedics. 2002; 25(2):169–172
[68] Walsh WR, Loefler A, Nicklin S, et al. Spinal fusion using an autologous growth factor gel and a porous resorbable ceramic. Eur Spine J. 2004; 13 (4):359–366
[69] Castro FP, Jr. Role of activated growth factors in lumbar spinal fusions. J Spinal Disord Tech. 2004; 17(5):380–384

[70] Weiner BK, Walker M. Efficacy of autologous growth factors in lumbar intertransverse fusions. Spine. 2003; 28(17):1968–1970, discussion 1971

[71] Tsai CH, Hsu HC, Chen YJ, Lin MJ, Chen HT. Using the growth factors-enriched platelet glue in spinal fusion and its efficiency. J Spinal Disord Tech. 2009; 22 (4):246–250

[72] Feiz-Erfan I, Harrigan M, Sonntag VK, Harrington TR. Effect of autologous platelet gel on early and late graft fusion in anterior cervical spine surgery. J Neurosurg Spine. 2007; 7(5):496–502

[73] Hirsch BP, Unnanuntana A, Cunningham ME, Lane JM. The effect of therapies for osteoporosis on spine fusion: a systematic review. Spine J. 2013; 13 (2):190–199

[74] Gezici AR, Ergün R, Gürel K, Yilmaz F, Okay O, Bozdoğan O. The effect of risedronate on posterior lateral spinal fusion in a rat model. J Korean Neurosurg Soc. 2009; 46(1):45–51

[75] Lehman RA, Jr, Kuklo TR, Freedman BA, Cowart JR, Mense MG, Riew KD. The effect of alendronate sodium on spinal fusion: a rabbit model. Spine J. 2004; 4(1):36–43

[76] Huang RC, Khan SN, Sandhu HS, et al. Alendronate inhibits spine fusion in a rat model. Spine. 2005; 30(22):2516–2522

[77] Sama AA, Khan SN, Myers ER, et al. High-dose alendronate uncouples osteoclast and osteoblast function: a study in a rat spine pseudarthrosis model. Clin Orthop Relat Res. 2004(425):135–142

[78] Li C, Wang HR, Li XL, Zhou XG, Dong J. The relation between zoledronic acid infusion and interbody fusion in patients undergoing transforaminal lumbar interbody fusion surgery. Acta Neurochir (Wien). 2012; 154(4):731–738

[79] Nagahama K, Kanayama M, Togawa D, Hashimoto T, Minami A. Does alendronate disturb the healing process of posterior lumbar interbody fusion? A prospective randomized trial. J Neurosurg Spine. 2011; 14(4):500–507

[80] Rosen CJ, Bilezikian JP. Clinical review 123: Anabolic therapy for osteoporosis. J Clin Endocrinol Metab. 2001; 86(3):957–964

[81] O'Loughlin PF, Cunningham ME, Bukata SV, et al. Parathyroid hormone (1–34) augments spinal fusion, fusion mass volume, and fusion mass quality in a rabbit spinal fusion model. Spine. 2009; 34(2):121–130

[82] Ohtori S, Inoue G, Orita S, et al. Comparison of teriparatide and bisphosphonate treatment to reduce pedicle screw loosening after lumbar spinal fusion surgery in postmenopausal women with osteoporosis from a bone quality perspective. Spine. 2013; 38(8):E487–E492

31 Role of Anterior Approach in the Correction of Adult Spinal Deformities

Sleiman Haddad, Ferran Pellisé

Abstract

Lumbar anterior surgery is witnessing a comeback in adult spinal deformity, mostly due to improvements in less invasive approaches and implants. It allows for direct anterior release and provides powerful correction that can restore physiological segmental alignment, increasing fusion area and avoiding posterior three-column osteotomies in well-selected patients. The authors discuss indications and potential benefits of anterior surgeries. They also review the latest literature and compare the results from combined approaches to those obtained with posterior-only approaches.

Keywords: anterior, lumbar, surgery, adult spinal deformity, scoliosis, ALIF, XLIF, OLIF

31.1 Introduction

Restoring coronal and sagittal balance with a harmonious spinopelvic alignment has been associated with significant improvement in patients' reported outcomes and fewer mechanical complications following adult spinal deformity (ASD) surgery. Deformity correction can be achieved using posterior-only surgery or with combined anterior and posterior approaches. Addition of an anterior stage allows for direct anterior release, anterior column reconstruction, better end-plate preparation, and interbody grafting. The anterior approach allows for powerful correction that can easily restore physiological segmental alignment, increasing the fusion area and avoiding posterior three-column osteotomies. The main indications for an anterior stage are deficient anterior column support over multiple segments, the need for reliable lumbosacral sagittal reconstruction when disk spaces are not already fused, and severe regular, rigid, thoracolumbar kyphoscoliosis needing multilevel circumferential release and grafting. Patients at high risk of pseudarthrosis with posterior-only surgery due to poor pedicular anchors secondary to osteoporosis or osteolysis, wide decompressions, or smoking habits, among others, may also benefit from anterior diskectomy and grafting to ensure early fusion.

After two decades of progressive decline, anterior surgery is witnessing a comeback in ASD, due mostly to improvements in less invasive approaches and implants. This chapter discusses at length the indications and potential benefits for anterior surgeries in adult deformities. It also reviews the latest literature and compares the results for combined approaches to those obtained with posterior-only approaches.

The primary goals of surgical intervention in spinal deformities are to halt curve progression, correct the deformity, and restore a balanced and stable tridimensional spinal alignment. The extent of the final correction will depend on the curve's intrinsic flexibility as much as on surgical releases and corrective maneuvers. The surgeon also aims to maintain postoperative alignment through a solid fusion that will preserve as many motion segments as possible. Fusion requires a favorable biological and mechanical environment.

Surgical goals in ASD can be obtained via anterior, posterior, or combined approaches depending, among other factors, on curve magnitude, shape, location, and flexibility. The addition of an anterior approach presents several biological and mechanical advantages as compared to posterior-only approaches. From a mechanical perspective, anterior approaches allow for direct anterior releases removing soft tissues, osteophytes, and bony bridges.[1] They also allow for the insertion of anterior, load-bearing, interbody grafts or implants providing segmental deformity correction and increasing the stability of the spinal construct. This in turn will minimize the incidence of a posterior implant loosening and failing.[2] Biologically, the disk space has a large surface area available for fusion coupled with a rich blood supply from the adjacent end plates.[3] This, combined with the placement of a bone graft in an area under compressive force, boosts the fusion potential.[4,5]

Historically, Dwyer was the first to report a scoliotic deformity correction using an anterior approach in pediatric idiopathic, neuromuscular, and congenital scoliosis.[6,7] In 1969, he performed multilevel complete diskectomies combined with vertebral screws and cable fixation on the convex side of the deformity.[6,7] Since then, anterior surgery has been widely used. In the absence of dependable posterior instrumentation with pedicle screws, early deformity surgeons relied on extensive anterior release and the powerful anterior fusion to achieve their goals in severe deformities. With advances in posterior instrumentation and surgical techniques surgeons gradually shifted to posterior-only approaches. The introduction of the pedicle screw was the main driver for this shift in practice. With the new generation of spinal implants, surgeons progressively acquired a 360-degree, circumferential control of the deformity from the back. Gradually, combined surgeries for deformity correction came to disuse over the past two decades. Vigneswaran et al reported that 38% of idiopathic deformities in the United States were treated with an anterior or a combined approach in 2000 compared to only 6% in 2012.[8] In a recent survey of spinal deformity surgeons, 97% considered posterior fusion to be the treatment of choice for adolescent idiopathic spinal deformity. A majority also supported a posterior approach to thoracolumbar Lenke 5 curves.[9]

The trend in ASD is not exactly the same. The recent rise in anterior surgeries has been driven by increasingly higher complication rates with aggressive posterior corrections (including three-column osteotomies) and the innovation in anterior approaches and implants. In addition to their high morbidity, posterior ASD corrections suffered a high rate of mechanical complications, reaching 31% in some series.[10,11,12] Pseudarthrosis and rod breakage are the most common mechanical complications associated with posterior ASD surgery, and up to 28% of patients may have a revision surgery at 2 years.[10,12,13] In parallel, less invasive anterior-access devices and implants are constantly being refined to predictably correct ASD from an anterior approach, reducing the approach-related morbidity.[14,15]

31.2 Adult Spinal Deformity

ASD comprises a heterogeneous group of patients with different deformity profiles and concerns.[16,17] There is no clear definition of ASD. On the one hand, young adult patients with neglected pediatric curves attend clinics driven mainly by deformity or cosmetic concerns. Conversely, pain and disability are the main complaints of older patients, who may have deformities with a degenerative component.[16] A third group consists of patients who have had a prior spinal surgery presenting with fixed iatrogenic deformities, mainly flatback.

Even though a proportion of ASD patients may be asymptomatic, the burden of ASD on the individual's health in patients seeking surgical attention can be very pronounced. Bodily pain, physical function, and self-image are generally the most affected domains.[18] Causes of pain in ASD include canal encroachment and neurologic compression, segmental instability, degeneration, and spinal misalignment. The goals of surgery in ASD are canal decompression, segmental stabilization, and deformity correction, restoring a biplanar trunk balance with proportionate sagittal alignment, eliminating any spinopelvic compensation.[19,20] Recent studies confirm that the lower lumbar segments play a key role in sagittal reconstruction.[19] Nearly 70% of the patient's target lordosis needs to be concentrated over the L4–S1 segments to ensure a proportionate and harmonious sagittal alignment and decrease the mechanical complication rate.[19] The lumbar distribution index becomes very relevant in ASD patients over 50 years, where sacropelvic fixation is frequently needed.[21]

Curve flexibility, apex location, and the number of segments involved in the deformity are all relevant factors to be considered when planning surgical correction and the need for anterior surgery.[22] Flexibility can be assessed clinically in the outpatient clinic. It can also be determined with bending or traction films for coronal deformities and by using bolster hyperextension and supine films for the sagittal plane. Comparing standing X-rays to supine scans can also help for assessing flexibility.[23] We recommend the routine use of two-dimensional preoperative CT scan reconstructions, which provide invaluable information related to interapophyseal joints and interbody space (vacuum sign), which can indirectly illustrate segmental flexibility and the need for anterior column support reconstruction.

We mostly use the anterior approach in ASD to restore anterior column support, to achieve reliable sagittal reconstruction of the lumbosacral area when disk spaces are not already fused, and to release and graft regular rigid thoracolumbar kyphoscoliosis. Patients at high risk of pseudarthrosis with posterior-only surgery due to poor pedicular anchors secondary to osteoporosis or osteolysis, wide decompressions, or smoking habits, among other factors, may also benefit from anterior diskectomy and grafting to ensure early fusion. This may be of great importance when fusion-enhancing proteins, such as recombinant human bone morphogenetic protein-2 (rhBMP-2) are not available or cannot be used.

In fixed angular deformities, especially angular kyphosis and flatback deformity, three-column osteotomies have a clear edge over any other technique. They allow for an all-posterior angular deformity control, which is clearly superior to combined approaches when disk spaces are already fused.

31.3 Reconstruction of the Lower Lumbar Spine and Lumbosacral Junction

There is solid evidence for the importance of the low lumbar spine in achieving a proportionate and harmonic reconstruction of sagittal spinopelvic alignment, restoring the physiological apex of lumbar lordosis.[19,24] Anterior surgery has been shown to be extremely effective for the reconstruction of the low lumbar spine in ASD, enhancing fusion, restoring sagittal alignment, and providing anterior column support.[25,26,27,28,29]

31.3.1 Access to the Lower Lumbar Spine

The anterior retroperitoneal approach (anterior lumbar interbody fusion [ALIF]) offers the most generous access to the ventral part of the disk space. It allows for complete diskectomy and insertion of a straight hyperlordotic and modular implant. The incision can be midline, paramedian, or Pfannenstiel with a retroperitoneal passage. It is generally used below the iliocaval junction, at the L5–S1 level and exceptionally at L4–L5. The main advantages of this method include an anatomical midline vision of the disk space and wide lateral exposure of the vertebral bodies, which allow effective disk space clearance and quick end plate preparation. Also, the direct anterior entry permits the use of larger and more modular implants that intimately contact the end plates. It simplifies the aggressive correction of lordosis and foraminal height restoration.[30,31] Possible complications with ALIF include retrograde ejaculation and visceral and vascular damage.

The anterior to psoas (ATP)/oblique lumbar interbody fusion (OLIF) method may involve a minimally invasive surgery (MIS) MIS entry to the disk space through a flank skin incision and retroperitoneal approach to the spine. It utilizes and develops the space between the psoas and the anterior vessels and bowels. The patient is placed in lateral or semilateral decubitus. This technique allows access to the spine from T12–S1 through one single incision without the need to dissect through the psoas muscle and risking injury to the lumbar plexus.[32,33,34] The ATP/OLIF yields to a full anterior release and disk opening, allowing the surgeon adequate anterior longitudinal ligament (ALL) release and direct posterior decompression simultaneously. The L5–S1 is easily accessible when needed.[33,35] Potential complications mainly include transient psoas weakness.[34] There is also a risk for vascular bleeding (mainly the segmental arteries), urethral and bowel injuries, and sympathetic plexus injury.[32,34,36]

The lateral lumbar interbody fusion, direct lateral interbody fusion, extreme lateral interbody fusion (LLIF, DLIF, XLIF) procedure describes the access to the disk space through a lateral retroperitoneal, transpsoas passage.[37] The patient is placed in the lateral position, and through a direct lateral incision the psoas muscle is split. Neuromonitoring guides the docking on the intervertebral disk. LLIF is appropriate for disks from L 1–L 2 to L 4–L 5. The iliac crest blocks the lateral entry to the L 5–S 1 level. Advantages of such an approach are the MIS muscle-splitting method that allows access to multiple disks.[37,38,39] Disadvantages include possible dangers of bowel or vascular injuries and, more specifically, injuries to the lumbar plexus. The plexus is at high risk of injury mainly over the lower levels, such as the L 4–L 5, as its nerve fibers cross anteriorly at the caudal levels.[39] The main disadvantage of this technique is the inability to access L 5–S 1. Vascular injury in XLIF, even if rare, can be extremely hard to manage through a lateral transpsoas approach.[39,40]

All anterior approaches rely on expert vascular mobilization and dissection. We recommend a preoperative CT-angiogram to assess the vascular anatomy prior to surgery.[41] Whenever possible, anterior approaches should be done from the left side, facing the aorta, which is more resistant to manipulation than the vena cava located on the right side of the spine.

There are very few direct studies comparing anterior techniques or comparing anterior with posterior techniques. The use of anterior stand-alone devices in ASD is not recommended, however due to the high rate of pseudarthrosis, subsidence of interbody cages, and loss of correction.[5,42,43,44,45] They are therefore used mainly as an adjunct to posterior surgery and have to be associated with posterior pedicular stabilization in a combined double-approach algorithm. Posterior osteotomies combined with compression of the vertebrae above and below can be used to increase local lordosis correction while ensuring foraminal patency.[14] Whether the anterior approach should be planned first or second is always a matter of debate. In flexible deformities where full correction can be obtained exclusively through a posterior approach, the posterior stage should be first. In rigid and partially flexible deformities with persistent disk spaces, where strict restoration of the low lumbar lordosis is needed, the anterior approach and anterior realignment with cages are usually done first unless posterior ankylosis/fusion prevents correction. In such cases three stages have been recommended by some authors (posterior + anterior + posterior).[35]

31.3.2 Restoration of Anterior Column Support

A deficient anterior column support over multiple lumbar levels in flexible deformities is one of the best indications for multilevel ALIFs (cases 1 and 2). The preoperative CT scan will typically show a vacuum phenomenon at different lumbar interbody spaces, indicating that curve correction might be easily obtained by placing the patient in hyperextension. In these cases, anterior column reconstruction is needed to ensure bony fusion and avoid posterior construct strain, collapse, and loss of correction. When lumbar deformity is flexible and correction is totally amenable through a posterior approach, restoration of anterior column support should follow posterior stabilization and is generally done from the left side. Anterior column support may also be restored from the back via transforaminal lumbar interbody fusion (TLIF) or posterior lumbar interbody fusion (PLIF). An anterior approach might be more advisable when more than two interbody spaces need reconstruction, especially if fusion-enhancing proteins such as rhBMP-2 are not available or cannot be used and the patient has a moderate to high risk of pseudarthrosis.

In a meta-analysis comparing different interbody fusion techniques, Teng et al argued that TLIF and ALIF have similar fusion rates in comparative studies ($p = 0.152$). However, ALIF had a significantly higher segmental disk and more postoperative segmental lordosis. TLIF, on the other hand, had better Oswentry disability index (ODI) scores.[46] In a matched study by Dorward et al comparing TLIF to ALIF in long constructs for spinal deformity, TLIFs had less operative time (481 vs. 595 min, $P = 0.0007$), but greater blood loss (2,011 vs. 1,281 mL, $P = 0.0002$).[47] The complication rate, including neurologic complications, was similar between both techniques. ALIFs generated more segmental lordosis than TLIFs at the L 3–S 1 segment (+ 6.9 degrees vs. − 2.6 degrees, $P < 0.0001$). Overall lumbar lordosis was nevertheless similar between both techniques (+11.5 degrees vs. +7.9 degrees, $P = 0.29$). Locally, ALIFs created significantly more lordosis at the L 4–L 5 and L 5–S 1 segments but not at the L 3–L 4 (gain of 5.3 degrees vs. 4.0 degrees, $P = 0.65$). On the other hand, TLIF patients had better coronal corrections. Bae et al studied three different techniques to treat mild to moderate sagittal deformities.[27] They compared patients having posterior-only approaches to those having posterior and anterior approaches (either with ALIF or XLIF). The authors reported similar satisfactory radiographic outcomes with these three surgical approaches. Compared with patients treated with an ALIF + PSF or a PSF-only, patients who underwent LLIF + posterior spinal fusion (PSF) had lower rates of proximal junctional kyphosis and mechanical failure at the upper-instrumented vertebra and less back pain, less disability, and better Scoliosis Research Society (SRS)-22 scores.

31.3.3 Reconstruction of Lumbosacral Segmental Sagittal Alignment

In partially flexible curves needing pelvic fixation and strict restoration of proportionate lumbosacral lordosis (70% of total lordosis over the L 4–S 1 segment), when curve rigidity prevents full posterior-only correction, if disk spaces are not already fused, the anterior approach allows for adequate release and strict deformity correction to ensure a postoperative global alignment and proportion (GAP) score <2 and avoid mechanical complications.[19] In these circumstances the anterior stage should be first, and access should be through the concavity of the lumbosacral curve. In very rare occasions, when posterior facet joints are ankylosed, a three-stage procedure (posterior release + anterior reconstruction + posterior stabilization) should be planned. The same approach can be extended cranially for release and fusion purposes (case 3).

Several reports have corroborated the utility of a combined approach. Uribe et al conducted a systematic review of minimally invasive interbody cages, including 2 ALIF, 16 XLIF, and 11 MI-TLIF studies. They described a 4-degree increase in segmental lordosis by level. They also described a significant relationship between preoperative lumbar lordosis and gains in lumbar lordosis ($r^2 = 0.413$; $P = 0.003$), wherein lower preoperative lumbarlordosis predicted a greater increase in postoperative lumbar lordosis.[48] Akbarnia et al retrospectively reviewed 17 patients treated with lateral interbody cages combined with a posterior approach from 2005 to 2011.[49] The authors achieved good deformity control with minimal blood loss (10–800 mL). Eight patients in total (47%) suffered a complication, minor or major. The most common complication was a transient quadriceps weakness (17.6%, 3/17), and only one patient had a persistent motor deficit at last follow-up (5.9%). Akbarnia et al reported a single case of vascular complication during the access surgeon approach to the spine that was repaired primarily with no further complication. Berjano et al retrospectively reviewed their 12 anterior column realignment (ACR) patients treated from 2014 to 2015.[50,51] The postoperative lordosis improved from 20 to 51 degrees (27-degree mean single-level lordosis). All patients achieved a sagittal vertical axis (SVA) less than 5 cm. Their major complication rate was 18% (2/12: one bowel perforation and one posterior wound infection). In another series by Murray et al 47 ACRs were done in a total of 31 patients from 2011 to 2014.[52] Mean lordosis improved from 32.3 to 49.9 degrees and pelvic incidence–lumbar lordosis (PI–LL) mismatch improved from 26.5 to 11 degrees. Postoperative SVA was 6.2 cm. Twenty-nine percent of their patients had a major complication: eight patients had quadriceps weakness and one retrograde ejaculation. They didn't report any vascular or bowel complications. Turner et al reported radiographic results of a retrospective multicenter study of 34 patients treated with ACR (58 ACR levels) from 2005 to 2013.[53] Again lordosis improved from 26.7 to 50.8 degrees, PI-LL from 29.4 to 6.6 degrees, and pelvic tilt (PT) from 28.3 to 22.1 degrees. A posterior osteotomy added on average 6 degrees to the 13 degrees gained by ACR without posterior osteotomy. Deukmedjian et al published a retrospective case series of seven ACR patients treated from 2010 to 2012.[54] The mean length of stay was 8.3 days. However, there have been at least 5 days of delay between the anterior and the posterior stages. They reported no blood transfusions and no vascular or visceral complications. They reported a single complication in the form of a superficial wound infection. Also Saville et al[55] reported their results with 69 hyperlordotic cages in 41 patients, the authors showed improvement in the overall mean lumbar lordosis (from 39 to 59 degrees, $p < 0.01$) and mean SVA (from 113 to 43 mm). They also reported a 20% overall complication rate, including a 4.1% transient neurologic complication rate. The mean blood loss per patient was 240 mL (range 50–900 mL). Demirkiran et al[29] reviewed their series of 8 ASD patients who underwent multilevel ACRs (≥ 2) followed by open posterior instrumentation with a minimum 1-year follow-up. They didn't report any anterior approach–related complications. Six patients had an additional posterior column osteotomy during the second stage. There was a significant increase in the lumbar lordosis and significant decreases in the sagittal vertical axis, pelvic tilt, and lumbopelvic mismatch after the first stage that was maintained with the second stage. All their patients enjoyed a significant improvement in the reported outcome measures. More recently, Hosseini et al retrospectively analyzed their results with ASD patients treated with ALIF.[26] They reviewed 39 patients, of which 33 had an additional posterior column osteotomy and instrumentation. They showed satisfactory radiographic and clinical outcomes at the 1-year follow-up. Lordosis increased from 35 to 48 degrees, and SVA was reduced from 7.8 to 3.4 cm. Fourteen patients (35.9%) experienced 26 complications (15 major and 11 minor). Eleven patients required reoperation. The most common complication was proximal junctional kyphosis (6/26 complications, 23%) followed by vertebral body/end plate fracture (3/26, 12%). Because of the hyperlordotic nature of ACR implants, it is possible to inadvertantly cause neuroforaminal stenosis. The posterior height of the cage is important to avoid such a complication.

31.4 Thoracolumbar Kyphoscoliosis and Anterior Release

In severe, regular, partially flexible or rigid thoracolumbar kyphoscoliosis, where three-column osteotomy is needed to achieve good biplanar spinal alignment and balance with posterior-only surgery, we still consider there is a place for a double approach with anterior periapical release and grafting to obtain the desired global harmonious biplanar deformity correction (scenario 3). Poor mineral bone density and high risk of pseudarthrosis are also good scenarios in which to perform anterior releases and grafting in severe adult thoracolumbar kyphoscoliosis. In most cases the goals of surgery will be wide multilevel release with complete annulotomy and interbody space grafting with morselized bone. No anterior implants or structural grafts are generally used to allow easy and gentle posterior deformity correction.

Anterior access to the thoracolumbar spine between T10–T11 and L3–L4 can be achieved retroperitoneally via a lateral thoracoabdominal route. The approach to the spine is generally done on the convex side of the deformity and can be extended caudally down to the sacrum when sacropelvic fixation with or without sagittal reconstruction is needed. It involves incision of the diaphragm and mobilization of the retroperitoneal vessels and entails a long, curvilinear incision from the lateral thorax to the medial abdomen.[56] The chest portion may be retropleural or transpleural.[57,58,59] The extent of diaphragm division depends on the exposure needed. It may be incised longitudinally at the spine or at its periphery. The lumbar portion of this exposure is always retroperitoneal. The abdominal wall musculature is divided without entering the abdomen. The peritoneal sac, aorta, kidney, ureter, and retroperitoneal fat are swept anteriorly, exposing the spine. This approach has been associated with significant morbidity. Some of the most frequent complications include lung atelectasis and pneumonia, and wound herniations.[60,61,62] In addition, this approach has been associated with other complications commonly encountered in anterior lumbar surgeries, such as damage to the major retroperitoneal vessels, ureter injury, and retrograde ejaculation caused by hypogastric sympathetic plexus injury have been reported. It should be therefore indicated with caution, balancing pros and cons of a double approach versus an aggressive posterior-only approach.

To our knowledge, no study has specifically compared posterior-only surgery to anterior release and grafting combined with a posterior approach for thoracolumbar kyphoscoliosis in ASD. The only comparative study that included these curves was the one conducted by Theologis et al.[28] In their matched cohort of thoracolumbar and lumbar curves, they found that combined approaches were used in more severe coronal and/or lumbopelvic sagittal deformities and offered better correction of major Cobb angles, lumbopelvic parameters, and SVA than posterior-only operations. Zhou et al, on the other hand, reported their results in 17 patients with anterior release and posterior fixation with a prior internal distraction for thoracolumbar severe rigid idiopathic deformities kyphoscoliosis.[63] Mean age at surgery was 22.6 years (range 15–44 years). The preoperative thoracic kyphosis was 83.5 degrees (range 60–115 degrees), and was corrected to 37.5 degrees (range 20–49 degrees) at the final follow-up. The preoperative major curve measured 110.1 degrees (range 92–145 degrees), and was reduced to 33.5 degrees (range 12–63 degrees), at the final follow-up. They reported no neurologic, wound, or mechanical complications with this sequential approach. These figures demonstrate the great potential and safety of anterior releases in rigid thoracolumbar kyphoscoliosis. The authors argued that their method is more suitable for global kyphosis, and not angular kyphosis, but it could also preclude the need for vertebral column resection (cases 4 and 5).

31.4.1 Complications of the Anterior Approaches

Complication rates with anterior surgeries range from 18 to 47%, but the rate of neurologic injuries and durotomies is extremely low.[14] Anterior approaches can have serious and life-threatening complications related to the approach and the internal adjacent structures and organs.[44] These include postoperative ileus, major vascular injury, iliac thrombosis, autonomous nerve damage, ureter injury, abdominal incision hernia, and retrograde ejaculation. In addition, there is a risk for cage subsidence, loss of correction, or even graft/implant dislocation. Despite the increased morbidity of a combined anterior-posterior approach, and increased surgical time and resources, several studies have shown a higher fusion rate, better deformity correction, and improved outcome when compared to a posterior-only approach.[25,64,65,66]

The incidence of vascular injury following anterior lumbar surgery is approximately 1% but varies according to patient demographics, number and level of lumbar spine to be fused, local vascular anatomy, and the choice of surgical approach.[67,68] The complication rate following revision lumbar surgery is three to five times higher than that for primary lumbar surgery, with vascular injury being the most common complication.[69,70] The most common type of vascular injury is venous laceration due to retraction, with the most frequently injured vessels being the left common iliac vein, the inferior vena cava, and the left iliolumbar vein.[71,72] The incidence of arterial injuries is described in 0 to 0.9%.[73] The most common artery injured is the left common iliac artery, with the highest incidence of injury occurring at the L4–L5 level. Thrombosis of the left common iliac artery is a very rare complication but can present postoperatively with pain, numbness, and decreased motor strength in the left extremity. Hypothermia and faint pulses should help the surgeon distinguish this from radicular or neurologic deficits. This emphasizes the importance of checking peripheral pulses preoperatively and in the immediate postoperative period to be alert to any changes.

Proximal deep vein thrombosis (DVT) most commonly involves the inferior vena cava and common iliac veins. Several series have documented the risk of proximal DVT during ALIF to range from 0.7 to 5%.[67] The mechanism of injury is presumed to be venous injury from retractors. Routine prophylaxis with sequential compression devices as well as intermittent release of retractors during the case is recommended to mitigate the risk.

Common visceral injuries include ureteral injury, peritoneal tears, and bowel injury. Special care must be taken to identify the ureter over the psoas and mobilize it. Ureteral stents may be helpful both for identifying the ureters in hard revision cases and for treatment of ureteral injuries. Peritoneal tears are prone to occur in patients with previous abdominal surgery or a history of intra-abdominal inflammatory processes, such as malignancy or infection. Peritoneal tears should be inspected to ensure no injury occurred to the underlying bowel and then may be repaired primarily. Bowel injury can occur during mobilization of the peritoneum and should be repaired primarily, followed by copious irrigation of the wound. The addition of antibiotics to help cover gram-negative flora should be contemplated depending on the amount of contamination that took place as well as the particular structure injured (i. e., colon vs. small bowel). Postoperative ileus ranges from 0.6 to 5.6%, with the higher incidences in transperitoneal exposures or those with multiple previous abdominal surgeries. All cases tend to resolve with medical care and/or nasogastric tube decompression.

Approach-related injury to the superior hypogastric plexus in males can result in retrograde ejaculation. The plexus sits anterior to the aorta and continues over the anterior surface of L5–S1, carrying sympathetic fibers down into the pelvis. Opening the peritoneum in the midline, aggressive traction or electrocautery use can cause injury to the plexus. The overall incidence of retrograde ejaculation has been reported to be about 4.2% in primary cases and up to 11.6% in revision cases.[69,74] In addition to injury to the superior hypogastric plexus, the lumbar sympathetic trunk is also at risk of injury as it sits on the lateral aspect of the vertebral bodies. This typically results in loss of sympathetic tone and vasodilatation on the side ipsilateral to the injury, causing patients to complain of a relative coolness in their contralateral foot. Most patients experience resolution of these symptoms after 6 months.[75]

Long-term complaints of abdominal asymmetry and pseudohernia are more commonly found in large thoracoabdominal approaches followed by thoracic approaches. Lumbar paramedian approaches had the lowest incidence of complaints related to abdominal asymmetry.[76]

Neurologic injury to the lumbar plexus is a complication that can occur during the lateral transpsoas approach. These approaches have a 10 to 19% incidence of postoperative thigh numbness, with the highest incidence occurring at L4–L5.[77] The incidence of this is not decreased by use of electromyography, which only alerts surgeons to their proximity to motor nerves.[78] The vast majority of postoperative thigh numbness tends to resolve at 3- to 6-month follow-up. Lumbar plexus-related motor deficits have an incidence of approximately 4.9%; however, these too tend to improve in incidence and severity over time.[79]

Immediate postoperative, ipsilateral iliopsoas weakness is also common and estimated between 25 and 54.9%. This is most likely due to mechanical dissection of the muscle with the retractors, and the majority of these deficits resolve by 3 months.[77]

31.4.2 Comparative Studies: Combined Approaches

Comparative studies are controversial; some studies do not show clear benefits favoring double approaches, whereas others suggest better corrections and fewer mechanical complications when approaching the spine from anterior and posterior.[65] Hsieh et al reported their results when comparing combined anterior-posterior to posterior approaches and showed a better coronal and sagittal deformity correction with combined approaches.[4]

Leveque et al compared their ACR to posterior-only approaches with PSO.[66] They excluded patients having PSO for revision surgeries with more than four levels of fusion. The mean estimated blood loss was significantly lower in the ACR group (1,466 vs. 2,910 mL, $p < 0.01$). Lumbar lordosis gain was similar in both groups (35 degrees in the PSO group, 31 degrees in the ACR group). Both groups reached similar lumbopelvic mismatch. There were three revisions in the PSO group due to pseudarthrosis versus none in the ACR group, although this did not reach significance.

Mundis et al compared 17 patients having an ACR procedure to matched patients from a retrospective database of patients having PSO for ASD.[25] Patients who underwent ACR had significantly less estimated blood loss than patients who underwent PSO (1.6 vs. 3.6 L, respectively), but no difference in the overall major complication rates was found (35.3% vs. 41.2%, respectively). There was one case of iliac vessel laceration needing vascular repair and three of quadriceps weakness. Patients achieved similar deformity corrections, and no differences were identified at 3-month or final follow-up for lumbar lordosis (51 vs. 47 degrees), pelvic tilt (25 vs. 28 degrees), and T 1 pelvic angle (23 vs. 24 degrees).

Finally, Theologis et al, on behalf of the International Spine Study Group, compared patients undergoing multiple-level lateral interbody fusions at the apex of the coronal deformity with posterior fixation to a matched cohort of adult deformity patients treated with a posterior-only approach.[28] They excluded patients receiving posterior column osteotomy or percutaneous posterior fixations. Both groups had an interbody fusion at the L 5–S 1 level. The combined-approach group had a worse coronal Cobb angle and less lordosis preoperatively. Patients in the combined group had significantly more anterior levels fused, longer operative times, and longer length of stay. They however, and contrary to the posterior-only group, could improve their spinopelvic parameters. These advantages came at the expense of having more major complications (56% vs 13%; $p = 0.02$) and postoperative leg weakness (31% vs 6%, $p = 0.07$) with no differences in clinical outcomes at 2 years. The authors of this chapter have called for clearly defined deformities that warrant the addition of multilevel anterior support to posterior fixation and L 5–S 1 interbody fusion.

The risk for a new neurological deficit following complex ASD posterior-only surgery is up to 20%, half of which do not recover at 2 years.[80,81,82] The most common major complications are still perioperative medical complications (22–27%) which could be lethal in extreme cases.[10,11] The development in anterior access techniques and instrumentation would decrease morbidity of these approaches and make them more readily available. Despite these innovations in implants and techniques, with the advances in biological engineering, ALIF may no longer be the only guarantee for interbody fusion. The spreading use of rhBMP-2 in posterior deformity correction may reduce the need for anterior cages at the L 5–S 1 disk, for example. Rahman et al proved that the utilization of 20 mg of rhBMP-2 at L 5–S 1 has the potential to be as effective and less expensive than an interbody fusion in most patients having a primary long fusion for ASD.[83]

31.5 Case Studies

We present five illustrative cases to further highlight some essential uses of anterior approaches in the correction of adult spinal deformities. Each case is presented with relevant radiological studies and parameters.

31.5.1 Case 1

A 74-year-old woman presented with rheumatoid arthritis (methotrexate), hypothyroidism, hypertension, bone mineral density T-score − 2.3 standard deviation and degenerative de novo kyphoscoliosis causing her severe axial pain and reduced walking capacity (▶ Fig. 31.1). She underwent a combined approach for periapical release, multisegmental interbody grafting, and anterior column reconstruction with lower foundation anterior structural support. The first stage consisted of a T 12–L 4 right retroperitoneal approach, anterior ligament release, and morselized bone grafting at the T 12–L 3 levels and structural lordotic cages at the L 3–L 4 and L 4–L 5 levels. The second stage consisted of a T 2 to pelvis fixation with posterior column osteotomies from T 12 to L 5 to fully mobilize the lumbar deformity.

31.5.2 Case 2

A 50-year-old woman presented with a neglected pediatric curve causing her severe axial pain (▶ Fig. 31.2). She had a rigid deformity with spontaneous periapical ankylosis and large concavity osteophytes together with segmental degeneration in the lower lumbar spine, including mild vacuum phenomenon. She underwent a combined approach for periapical release, multisegmental interbody grafting, and anterior column reconstruction with lower foundation anterior structural support. The second stage consisted of a T 9 to pelvis fixation with posterior column osteotomies from T 12 to S 1 to fully mobilize the lumbar deformity.

31.5.3 Case 3

A 47-year-old woman presented with adolescent idiopathic scoliosis fused from T 10 to L 4 as a teenager. She was referred because of severe back pain resistant to nonoperative treatment and anterior trunk shift (▶ Fig. 31.3). There was sagittal malalignment due to loss of physiological lumbosacral lordosis, which seemed to be partially flexible on CT scan. She underwent a combined approach for lumbosacral deformity correction. The second stage consisted of an L 3 to pelvis fixation with posterior column osteotomies from L 4 to S 1.

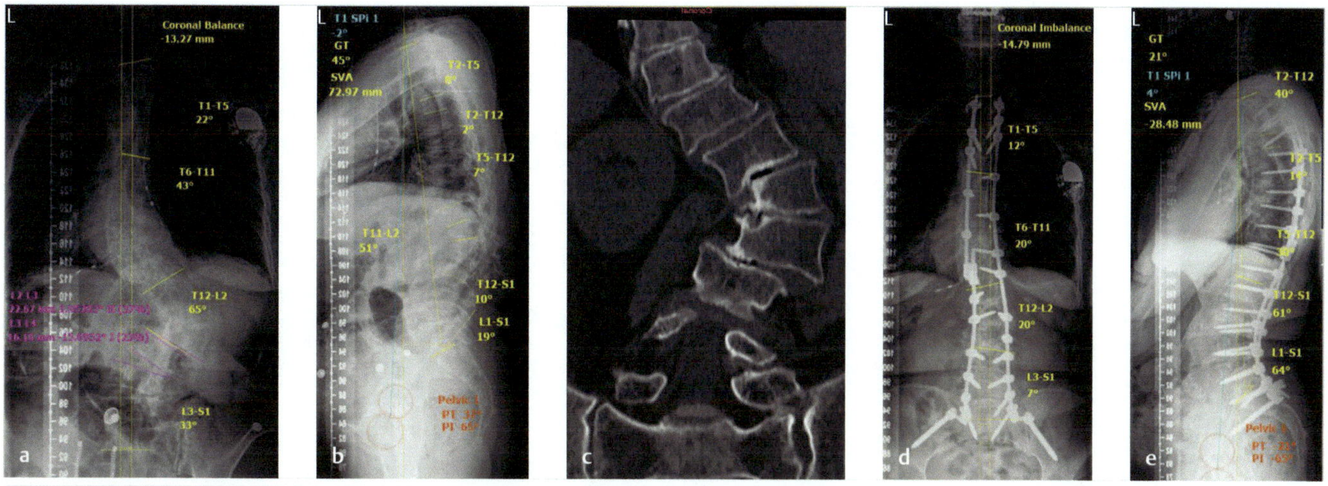

Fig. 31.1 Case 1. **(a)** Preoperative coronal and **(b)** sagittal standing X-rays and **(c)** two-dimensional CT scan reconstruction. Partially flexible deformity with mild disk vacuum, risk of pseudarthrosis and mechanical failure. **(d)** Postoperative coronal and **(e)** sagittal films showing the obtained correction 2 years after surgery.

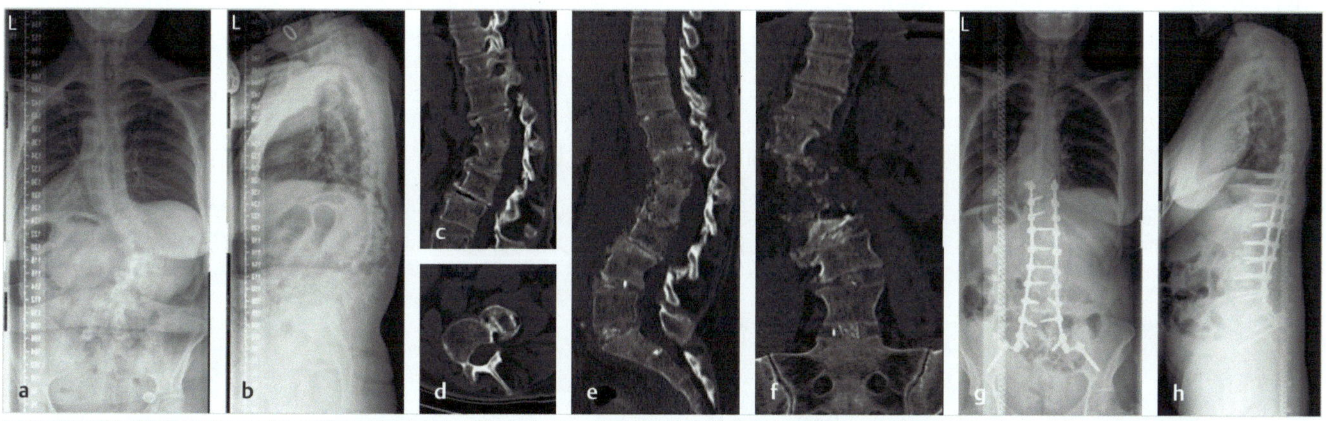

Fig. 31.2 Case 2. **(a)** Preoperative coronal and **(b)** sagittal standing X-rays and **(c, d)** two-dimensional CT scan reconstructions. The first stage consisted of a T11–S1 right transpleural retroperitoneal approach with excision of the 10th rib, osteotomy of the anterior bony bridges, anterior ligament release at the mobile segments, morselized bone grafting at T11–L4 levels, and structural anterior lumbar interbody fusion lordotic cages at the L4–L5 and L5–S1 levels and **(e, f)** structural anterior lumbar interbody fusion lordotic cages at the L4-L5 and L5-S1 levels. **(g)** Postoperative coronal and **(h)** sagittal films showing the obtained correction 2 years after surgery.

31.5.4 Case 4

An 80-year-old man with de novo degenerative scoliosis presenting with back pain, loss of trunk balance, and neurogenic claudication following multilevel decompression (▶ Fig. 31.4). He had flexible sagittal and coronal malalignment due to multilevel disk degeneration and posterior decompression, with multiple disks showing vacuum on the preoperative CT scan. He underwent a posterior-only surgery with further decompression and T12–pelvis posterior spinal fusion instrumentation associated with an L5–S1 transforaminal lumbar interbody fusion. Two weeks later he presented with construct collapse and proximal junctional failure despite having achieved adequate deformity correction. The decision was made for a combined approach revision surgery. The first stage included an extension to T10 with a prophylactic vertebroplasty at the T9 level and correction of sagittal malalignment. The anterior stage then consisted of multilevel diskectomy and bone grafting from L1 to L5. The patient didn't have any major complications.

31.5.5 Case 5

A 67-year-old woman previously decompressed and fused at L4–L5 complaining of progressive trunk deformity and back pain (▶ Fig. 31.5). She had sagittal and coronal trunk imbalance due to flexible lumbar scoliosis and a rigid lumbosacral fractional curve with a fused L4–L5 segment. She underwent a staged approach with a posterior asymmetrical pedicle subtraction osteotomy at the L4 level and posterior column osteotomies from T12 to L4 and an L5–S1 transforaminal lumbar interbody fusion cage. One week later she had anterior L1 to L4 multilevel diskectomies with anterior grafting using Moss and polyetheretherketone (PEEK) cages supplemented with autologous iliac crest bone graft.

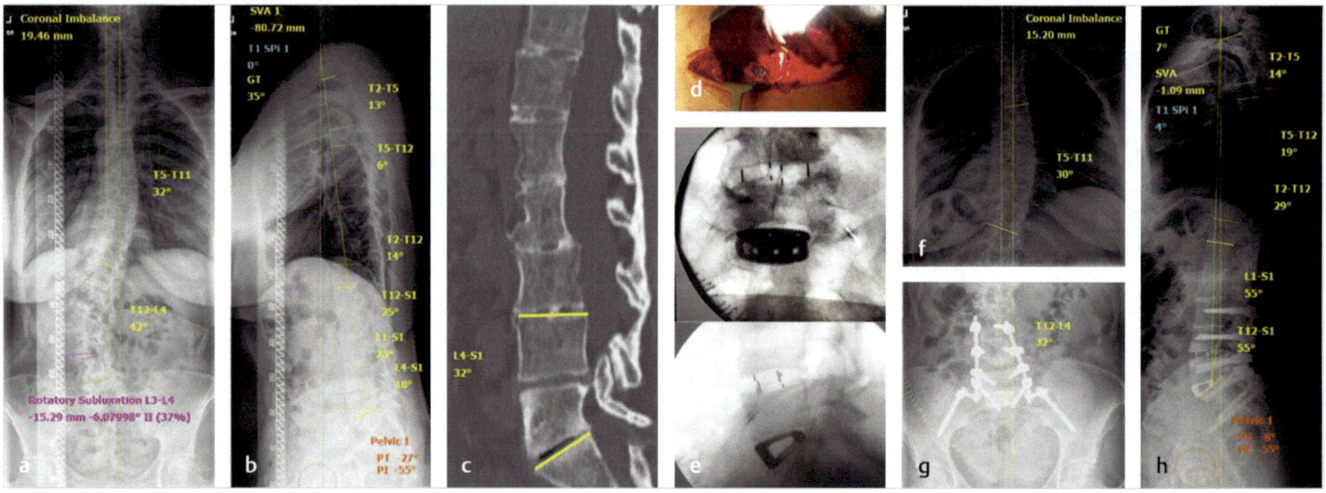

Fig. 31.3 Case 3. Strict reconstruction of lumbosacral segmental lordosis. **(a)** Preoperative whole spine coronal and **(b)** sagittal films and **(c)** lumbar two-dimensional CT scan. The first stage consisted of a left retroperitoneal approach to the lumbosacral junction, anterior ligament release, diskectomy and grafting with structural anterior lumbar interbody fusion lordotic cages at L5–S1 and L4–L5 oblique lumbar interbody fusion. The first stage **(d)** consisted of a left retroperitoneal approach to the lumbosacral junction, anterior ligament release, diskectomy and grafting with structural anterior lumbar interbody fusion lordotic cages at L5–S1 and L4–L5 oblique lumbar interbody fusion. **(e)** Intraoperative anteroposterior and **(f)** lateral fluoroscopy. **(g)** Postoperative coronal and **(h)** sagittal films showing the obtained correction 2 years after surgery.

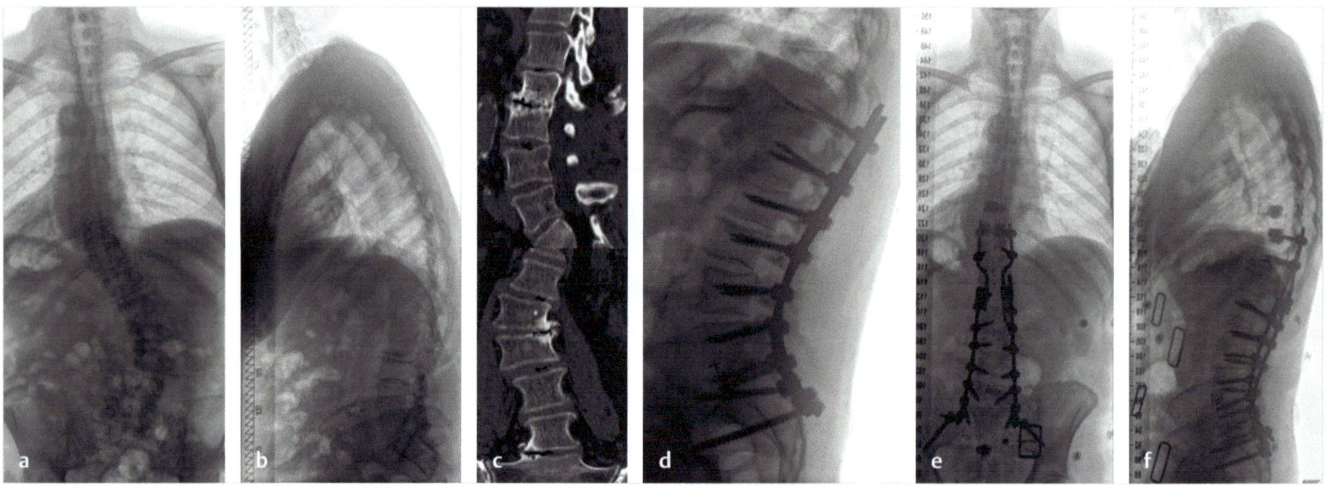

Fig. 31.4 Case 4. Failure of previous posterior-only adult spinal deformity correction due to lack of anterior column support. **(a)** Preoperative whole spine coronal and **(b, c)** sagittal films and **(d)** lumbar two-dimensional CT scan. **(e)** Postoperative coronal and **(f)** sagittal films showing the obtained correction 4 years after surgery.

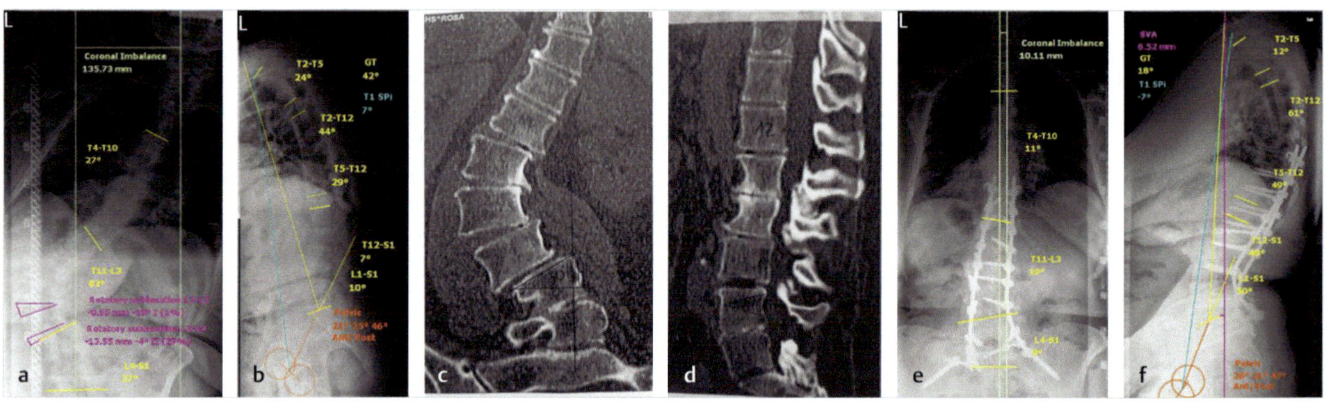

Fig. 31.5 Case 5. Posterior-only correction with multilevel anterior column support. **(a)** Preoperative whole spine coronal and **(b)** sagittal films and **(c, d)** lumbar two-dimensional CT scans. **(e)** Postoperative coronal and **(f)** sagittal films showing the obtained correction 3 years after surgery.

31.6 Conclusion

After a gradual decline, anterior approaches have reemerged as a very useful tool in the arsenal of ASD surgeons. This resurgence has been driven by the high complication rate of aggressive posterior-only procedures and improvements in anterior approaches and implants. As an adjunct to posterior surgery, anterior thoracolumbar and lumbosacral approaches offer a great deformity correction potential through wide anterior releases and interbody spacers. They also support posterior corrections by providing a solid anterior support and a favorable milieu for fusion. The main indications for anterior surgeries in ASD are severe rigid regular thoracolumbar kyphoscoliosis, the need for strict lumbosacral reconstruction in partially flexible and rigid deformities, the need for multilevel anterior column support, and a high risk of pseudarthrosis with posterior-only surgery.

References

[1] Shamji MF, Isaacs RE. Anterior-only approaches to scoliosis. Neurosurgery. 2008; 63(3) Suppl:139–148

[2] Ploumis A, Wu C, Fischer G, et al. Biomechanical comparison of anterior lumbar interbody fusion and transforaminal lumbar interbody fusion. J Spinal Disord Tech. 2008; 21(2):120–125

[3] Anderson DG, Sayadipour A, Shelby K, Albert TJ, Vaccaro AR, Weinstein MS. Anterior interbody arthrodesis with percutaneous posterior pedicle fixation for degenerative conditions of the lumbar spine. Eur Spine J. 2011; 20 (8):1323–1330

[4] Hsieh M-K, Chen L-H, Niu C-C, Fu T-S, Lai P-L, Chen W-J. Combined anterior lumbar interbody fusion and instrumented posterolateral fusion for degenerative lumbar scoliosis: indication and surgical outcomes. BMC Surg. 2015; 15(1):26

[5] Jiang S-D, Chen J-W, Jiang L-S. Which procedure is better for lumbar interbody fusion: anterior lumbar interbody fusion or transforaminal lumbar interbody fusion? Arch Orthop Trauma Surg. 2012; 132(9):1259–1266

[6] Dwyer AF. Experience of anterior correction of scoliosis. Clin Orthop Relat Res. 1973(93):191–206

[7] Dwyer AF, Newton NC, Sherwood AA. An anterior approach to scoliosis. A preliminary report. Clin Orthop Relat Res. 1969; 62(62):192–202

[8] Vigneswaran HT, Grabel ZJ, Eberson CP, Palumbo MA, Daniels AH. Surgical treatment of adolescent idiopathic scoliosis in the United States from 1997 to 2012: an analysis of 20,346 patients. J Neurosurg Pediatr. 2015; 16(3):322–328

[9] de Kleuver M, Lewis SJ, Germscheid NM, et al. Optimal surgical care for adolescent idiopathic scoliosis: an international consensus. Eur Spine J. 2014; 23 (12):2603–2618

[10] Smith JS, Klineberg E, Lafage V, et al. International Spine Study Group. Prospective multicenter assessment of perioperative and minimum 2-year postoperative complication rates associated with adult spinal deformity surgery. J Neurosurg Spine. 2016; 25(1):1–14

[11] Soroceanu A, Burton DC, Oren JH, et al. International Spine Study Group. Medical Complications After Adult Spinal Deformity Surgery: Incidence, Risk Factors, and Clinical Impact. Spine. 2016; 41(22):1718–1723

[12] Smith JS, Shaffrey E, Klineberg E, et al. International Spine Study Group. Prospective multicenter assessment of risk factors for rod fracture following surgery for adult spinal deformity. J Neurosurg Spine. 2014; 21(6):994–1003

[13] Passias PG, Soroceanu A, Yang S, et al. Predictors of Revision Surgical Procedure Excluding Wound Complications in Adult Spinal Deformity and Impact on Patient-Reported Outcomes and Satisfaction: A Two-Year Follow-up. J Bone Joint Surg Am. 2016; 98(7):536–543

[14] Saigal R, Mundis GM, Jr, Eastlack R, Uribe JS, Phillips FM, Akbarnia BA. Anterior Column Realignment (ACR) in Adult Sagittal Deformity Correction: Technique and Review of the Literature. Spine. 2016; 41 Suppl 8:S66–S73

[15] Phan K, Mobbs RJ. Evolution of Design of Interbody Cages for Anterior Lumbar Interbody Fusion. Orthop Surg. 2016; 8(3):270–277

[16] Bess S, Boachie-Adjei O, Burton D, et al. International Spine Study Group. Pain and disability determine treatment modality for older patients with adult scoliosis, while deformity guides treatment for younger patients. Spine. 2009; 34(20):2186–2190

[17] Acaroğlu RE, Dede Ö, Pellisé F, et al. European Spine Study Group. Adult spinal deformity: a very heterogeneous population of patients with different needs. Acta Orthop Traumatol Turc. 2016; 50(1):57–62

[18] Pellisé F, Vila-Casademunt A, Ferrer M, et al. European Spine Study Group, ESSG. Impact on health related quality of life of adult spinal deformity (ASD) compared with other chronic conditions. Eur Spine J. 2015; 24(1):3–11

[19] Yilgor C, Sogunmez N, Boissiere L, et al. European Spine Study Group (ESSG). Global Alignment and Proportion (GAP) Score: Development and Validation of a New Method of Analyzing Spinopelvic Alignment to Predict Mechanical Complications After Adult Spinal Deformity Surgery. J Bone Joint Surg Am. 2017; 99(19):1661–1672

[20] Boissière L, Takemoto M, Bourghli A, et al. European Spine Study Group (ESSG). Global tilt and lumbar lordosis index: two parameters correlating with health-related quality of life scores-but how do they truly impact disability? Spine J. 2017; 17(4):480–488

[21] Yilgor C, Sogunmez N, Yavuz Y, et al. European Spine Study Group. Relative lumbar lordosis and lordosis distribution index: individualized pelvic incidence-based proportional parameters that quantify lumbar lordosis more precisely than the concept of pelvic incidence minus lumbar lordosis. Neurosurg Focus. 2017; 43(6):E5

[22] Bridwell KH. Decision making regarding Smith-Petersen vs. pedicle subtraction osteotomy vs. vertebral column resection for spinal deformity. Spine. 2006; 31(19) Suppl:S171–S178

[23] Sharma A, Pourtaheri S, Savage J, et al. The Utility of Preoperative Magnetic Resonance Imaging for Determining the Flexibility of Sagittal Imbalance. Neurosurgery. 2018; 83(3):465–470

[24] Laouissat F, Sebaaly A, Gehrchen M, Roussouly P. Classification of normal sagittal spine alignment: refounding the Roussouly classification. Eur Spine J. 2018; 27(8):2002–2011

[25] Mundis GM, Jr, Turner JD, Kabirian N, et al. International Spine Study Group. Anterior Column Realignment has Similar Results to Pedicle Subtraction Osteotomy in Treating Adults with Sagittal Plane Deformity. World Neurosurg. 2017; 105:249–256

[26] Hosseini P, Mundis GM, Jr, Eastlack RK, et al. Preliminary results of anterior lumbar interbody fusion, anterior column realignment for the treatment of sagittal malalignment. Neurosurg Focus. 2017; 43(6):E6

[27] Bae J, Theologis AA, Strom R, et al. Comparative analysis of 3 surgical strategies for adult spinal deformity with mild to moderate sagittal imbalance. J Neurosurg Spine. 2018; 28(1):40–49

[28] Theologis AA, Mundis GM, Jr, Nguyen S, et al. for the International Spine Study Group. Utility of multilevel lateral interbody fusion of the thoracolumbar coronal curve apex in adult deformity surgery in combination with open posterior instrumentation and L5-S1 interbody fusion: a case-matched evaluation of 32 patients. J Neurosurg Spine. 2017; 26(2):208–219

[29] Demirkiran G, Theologis AA, Pekmezci M, Ames C, Deviren V. Adult Spinal Deformity Correction with Multi-level Anterior Column Releases: Description of a New Surgical Technique and Literature Review. Clin Spine Surg. 2016; 29 (4):141–149

[30] Rao PJ, Loganathan A, Yeung V, Mobbs RJ. Outcomes of anterior lumbar interbody fusion surgery based on indication: a prospective study. Neurosurgery. 2015; 76(1):7–23, discussion 23–24

[31] Rao PJ, Ghent F, Phan K, Lee K, Reddy R, Mobbs RJ. Stand-alone anterior lumbar interbody fusion for treatment of degenerative spondylolisthesis. J Clin Neurosci. 2015; 22(10):1619–1624

[32] Silvestre C, Mac-Thiong JM, Hilmi R, Roussouly P. Complications and Morbidities of Mini-open Anterior Retroperitoneal Lumbar Interbody Fusion: Oblique Lumbar Interbody Fusion in 179 Patients. Asian Spine J. 2012; 6(2):89–97

[33] Sato J, Ohtori S, Orita S, et al. Radiographic evaluation of indirect decompression of mini-open anterior retroperitoneal lumbar interbody fusion: oblique lateral interbody fusion for degenerated lumbar spondylolisthesis. Eur Spine J. 2017; 26(3):671–678

[34] Abe K, Orita S, Mannoji C, et al. Perioperative Complications in 155 Patients Who Underwent Oblique Lateral Interbody Fusion Surgery: Perspectives and Indications From a Retrospective, Multicenter Survey. Spine. 2017; 42(1):55–62

[35] Molloy S, Butler JS, Benton A, Malhotra K, Selvadurai S, Agu O. A new extensile anterolateral retroperitoneal approach for lumbar interbody fusion from L1 to S1: a prospective series with clinical outcomes. Spine J. 2016; 16 (6):786–791

[36] Orita S, Inage K, Sainoh T, et al. Lower Lumbar Segmental Arteries Can Intersect Over the Intervertebral Disc in the Oblique Lateral Interbody Fusion

Approach With a Risk for Arterial Injury: Radiological Analysis of Lumbar Segmental Arteries by Using Magnetic Resonance Imaging. Spine. 2017; 42 (3):135–142

[37] Ozgur BM, Aryan HE, Pimenta L, Taylor WR. Extreme Lateral Interbody Fusion (XLIF): a novel surgical technique for anterior lumbar interbody fusion. Spine J. 2006; 6(4):435–443

[38] Arnold PM, Anderson KK, McGuire RA, Jr. The lateral transpsoas approach to the lumbar and thoracic spine: A review. Surg Neurol Int. 2012; 3(4) Suppl 3: S198–S215

[39] Malham GM, Parker RM, Goss B, Blecher CM. Clinical results and limitations of indirect decompression in spinal stenosis with laterally implanted interbody cages: results from a prospective cohort study. Eur Spine J. 2015; 24 Suppl 3:339–345

[40] Barbagallo GM, Albanese V, Raich AL, Dettori JR, Sherry N, Balsano M. Lumbar Lateral Interbody Fusion (LLIF): Comparative Effectiveness and Safety versus PLIF/TLIF and Predictive Factors Affecting LLIF Outcome. Evid Based Spine Care J. 2014; 5(1):28–37

[41] Capellades J, Pellisé F, Rovira A, Grivé E, Pedraza S, Villanueva C. Magnetic resonance anatomic study of iliocava junction and left iliac vein positions related to L5-S1 disc. Spine. 2000; 25(13):1695–1700

[42] Mummaneni PV, Dhall SS, Eck JC, et al. Guideline update for the performance of fusion procedures for degenerative disease of the lumbar spine. Part 11: interbody techniques for lumbar fusion. J Neurosurg Spine. 2014; 21(1):67–74

[43] Rao PJ, Phan K, Giang G, Maharaj MM, Phan S, Mobbs RJ. Subsidence following anterior lumbar interbody fusion (ALIF): a prospective study. J Spine Surg. 2017; 3(2):168–175

[44] Than KD, Wang AC, Rahman SU, et al. Complication avoidance and management in anterior lumbar interbody fusion. Neurosurg Focus. 2011; 31(4):E6

[45] Pellisé F, Puig O, Rivas A, Bagó J, Villanueva C. Low fusion rate after L5-S1 laparoscopic anterior lumbar interbody fusion using twin stand-alone carbon fiber cages. Spine. 2002; 27(15):1665–1669

[46] Teng I, Han J, Phan K, Mobbs R. A meta-analysis comparing ALIF, PLIF, TLIF and LLIF. J Clin Neurosci. 2017; 44:11–17

[47] Dorward IG, Lenke LG, Bridwell KH, et al. Transforaminal versus anterior lumbar interbody fusion in long deformity constructs: a matched cohort analysis. Spine. 2013; 38(12):E755–E762

[48] Uribe JS, Myhre SL, Youssef JA. Preservation or Restoration of Segmental and Regional Spinal Lordosis Using Minimally Invasive Interbody Fusion Techniques in Degenerative Lumbar Conditions: A Literature Review. Spine (Phila Pa 1976). 2016;41 Suppl 8:S50–S58

[49] Akbarnia BA, Mundis GM, Jr, Moazzaz P, et al. Anterior column realignment (ACR) for focal kyphotic spinal deformity using a lateral transpsoas approach and ALL release. J Spinal Disord Tech. 2014; 27(1):29–39

[50] Berjano P, Damilano M, Ismael M, Longo A, Bruno A, Lamartina C. Anterior column realignment (ACR) technique for correction of sagittal imbalance. Eur Spine J. 2015; 24 Suppl 3:451–453

[51] Berjano P, Cecchinato R, Sinigaglia A, et al. Anterior column realignment from a lateral approach for the treatment of severe sagittal imbalance: a retrospective radiographic study. Eur Spine J. 2015; 24 Suppl 3:433–438

[52] Murray G, Beckman J, Bach K, Smith DA, Dakwar E, Uribe JS. Complications and neurological deficits following minimally invasive anterior column release for adult spinal deformity: a retrospective study. Eur Spine J. 2015; 24 Suppl 3:397–404

[53] Turner JD, Akbarnia BA, Eastlack RK, et al. Radiographic outcomes of anterior column realignment for adult sagittal plane deformity: a multicenter analysis. Eur Spine J. 2015;24 Suppl 3:427–432

[54] Deukmedjian AR, Dakwar E, Ahmadian A, Smith DA, Uribe JS. Early outcomes of minimally invasive anterior longitudinal ligament release for correction of sagittal imbalance in patients with adult spinal deformity. ScientificWorldJournal. 2012; 2012:789698

[55] Saville PA, Kadam AB, Smith HE, Arlet V. Anterior hyperlordotic cages: early experience and radiographic results. J Neurosurg Spine. 2016; 25(6):713–719

[56] Heitmiller RF. The left thoracoabdominal incision. Ann Thorac Surg. 1988; 46 (2):250–253

[57] McCormick PC. Retropleural approach to the thoracic and thoracolumbar spine. Neurosurgery. 1995; 37(5):908–914

[58] Mirbaha MM. Anterior approach to the thoraco-lumbar junction of the spine by a retroperitoneal-extrapleural technic. Clin Orthop Relat Res. 1973 (91):41–47

[59] Barone GW, Eidt JF, Webb JW, Hudec WA, Pait TG. The anterior extrapleural approach to the thoracolumbar junction revisited. Am Surg. 1998; 64 (4):372–375

[60] Ikard RW. Methods and complications of anterior exposure of the thoracic and lumbar spine. Arch Surg. 2006; 141(10):1025–1034

[61] Hodgson AR, Stock FE. The Classic: Anterior spinal fusion: a preliminary communication on the radical treatment of Pott's disease and Pott's paraplegia. 1956. Clin Orthop Relat Res. 2006; 444(444):10–15

[62] Nakai S, Zielke K. Chylothorax–a rare complication after anterior and posterior spinal correction. Report on six cases. Spine. 1986; 11(8):830–833

[63] Zhou C, Liu L, Song Y, Liu H, Zeng J, Yang X. Anterior release posterior internal distraction and subsequent posterior spinal fusion for the treatment of severe kyphoscoliosis. Eur Spine J. 2015; 24(7):1560–1567

[64] Mundis GM, Akbarnia BA, Phillips FM. Adult deformity correction through minimally invasive lateral approach techniques. Spine. 2010; 35(26) Suppl: S312–S321

[65] Good CR, Lenke LG, Bridwell KH, et al. Can posterior-only surgery provide similar radiographic and clinical results as combined anterior (thoracotomy/thoracoabdominal)/posterior approaches for adult scoliosis? Spine. 2010; 35 (2):210–218

[66] Leveque JC, Yanamadala V, Buchlak QD, Sethi RK. Correction of severe spinopelvic mismatch: decreased blood loss with lateral hyperlordotic interbody grafts as compared with pedicle subtraction osteotomy. Neurosurg Focus. 2017; 43(2):E15

[67] Brau SA. Mini-open approach to the spine for anterior lumbar interbody fusion: description of the procedure, results and complications. Spine J. 2002; 2(3):216–223

[68] Inamasu J, Guiot BH. Vascular injury and complication in neurosurgical spine surgery. Acta Neurochir (Wien). 2006; 148(4):375–387

[69] Schwender JD, Casnellie MT, Perra JH, et al. Perioperative complications in revision anterior lumbar spine surgery: incidence and risk factors. Spine. 2009; 34(1):87–90

[70] Wagner WH, Regan JJ, Leary SP, et al. Access strategies for revision or explantation of the Charité lumbar artificial disc replacement. J Vasc Surg. 2006; 44 (6):1266–1272

[71] Baker JK, Reardon PR, Reardon MJ, Heggeness MH. Vascular injury in anterior lumbar surgery. Spine. 1993; 18(15):2227–2230

[72] Faciszewski T, Winter RB, Lonstein JE, Denis F, Johnson L. The surgical and medical perioperative complications of anterior spinal fusion surgery in the thoracic and lumbar spine in adults. A review of 1223 procedures. Spine. 1995; 20(14):1592–1599

[73] Brau S, Delamarter R, Schiffman M, Williams L, Watkins RG. 56. Vascular injury during anterior lumbar surgery. Spine J. 2003; 3(5):93

[74] Sasso RC, Kenneth Burkus J, LeHuec J-C. Retrograde ejaculation after anterior lumbar interbody fusion: transperitoneal versus retroperitoneal exposure. Spine. 2003; 28(10):1023–1026

[75] Hamdan AD, Malek JY, Schermerhorn ML, Aulivola B, Blattman SB, Pomposelli FB, Jr. Vascular injury during anterior exposure of the spine. J Vasc Surg. 2008; 48(3):650–654

[76] Kang B-U, Choi W-C, Lee S-H, et al. An analysis of general surgery-related complications in a series of 412 minilaparotomic anterior lumbosacral procedures. J Neurosurg Spine. 2009; 10(1):60–65

[77] Le TV, Burkett CJ, Deukmedjian AR, Uribe JS. Postoperative lumbar plexus injury after lumbar retroperitoneal transpsoas minimally invasive lateral interbody fusion. Spine. 2013; 38(1):E13–E20

[78] Dakwar E, Cardona RF, Smith DA, Uribe JS. Early outcomes and safety of the minimally invasive, lateral retroperitoneal transpsoas approach for adult degenerative scoliosis. Neurosurg Focus. 2010; 28(3):E8

[79] Pumberger M, Hughes AP, Huang RR, Sama AA, Cammisa FP, Girardi FP. Neurologic deficit following lateral lumbar interbody fusion. Eur Spine J. 2012; 21 (6):1192–1199

[80] Street JT, Lenehan BJ, DiPaola CP, et al. Morbidity and mortality of major adult spinal surgery. A prospective cohort analysis of 942 consecutive patients. Spine J. 2012; 12(1):22–34

[81] Fehlings MG, Kato S, Lenke LG, et al. Incidence and risk factors of postoperative neurological decline after complex adult spinal deformity surgery: results of the scoli-risk-1 study. Spine J. 2018

[82] Kelly MP, Lenke LG, Shaffrey CI, et al. Evaluation of complications and neurological deficits with three-column spine reconstructions for complex spinal deformity: a retrospective Scoli-RISK-1 study. Neurosurg Focus. 2014; 36(5): E17

[83] Rahman RK, Buchowski JM, Stephens B, Dorward IG, Koester LA, Bridwell KH. Comparison of TLIF with rhBMP-2 versus no TLIF and higher posterolateral rhBMP-2 dose at L5-S1 for long fusions to the sacrum with sacropelvic fixation in patients with primary adult deformity. Spine. 2013; 38(26):2264–2271

32 Osteotomies in Spinal Tuberculosis—Adult Care

S. Rajasekaran, Rishi Mugesh Kanna, Ajoy Prasad Shetty

Abstract

Kyphosis is one of the major adverse sequelae of spinal tuberculosis. Since the disease is predominantly destroying the vertebral body and is chronic and progressive, most patients have kyphosis of varying degrees, even at first presentation. Patients younger than 10 years with severe disease, contiguous multilevel destruction, and thoracolumbar disease are more prone to severe kyphosis. Post-tubercular kyphosis can result in cosmetic disfigurement, painful costopelvic impingement, respiratory complications, and neurologic deficit due to chronic cord compression. Corrective surgery in the form of osteotomy is often required in both the active and healed stages. In patients with kyphosis and active disease, the aims of surgery are debridement, stabilization, and anterior reconstruction so that the spine heals in appropriate sagittal alignment. This can be performed through direct anterior corpectomy and stabilization, a posterior-only approach for anterior decompression/reconstruction and posterior stabilization, and combined anterior and posterior reconstruction performed through two separate approaches. In the healed stages, patients present with either severe kyphosis alone or with neurologic deficit. Corrective osteotomy is performed to correct the kyphosis within safe limits for normal functioning of the spinal cord. This can be performed through posterior vertebral column resection, pedicle subtraction osteotomy, and closing-opening wedge osteotomy.

Keywords: spinal tuberculosis, kyphosis, deformity, osteotomy

32.1 Introduction

Kyphosis, apart from neurologic deficit, is the most feared complication of spinal tuberculosis. Kyphosis is a pathognomonic feature of the disease as most patients with spinal tuberculosis will have some degree of kyphosis. Modern antitubercular chemotherapy is very effective in achieving a disease cure, but up to 60% of patients can develop significant kyphosis. Kyphotic deformity affects the biomechanics of the spine, resulting in pain, respiratory insufficiency, neurologic deficit, and poor cosmesis and often requires surgical correction (▸ Fig. 32.1).

32.2 Pathophysiology of Kyphosis in Spinal Tuberculosis

The etiology and progression of kyphosis are different in the active and healed phase of the disease. Tuberculosis preferably affects anterior structures in more than 95% of the patients, leading to kyphosis. The partially destroyed vertebrae have to collapse until there is contact with healthy vertebrae, resulting in kyphosis. In the healed stages of the disease, adults do not show any progression of deformity after healing and consolidation of the vertebra occur. Children, however, show a tendency toward increased kyphosis, even after healing, due to the disproportionate growth between the anterior and posterior structures.

32.2.1 Kyphosis during the Acute Phase of Tuberculosis

The vertebral body (paradiskal region) is the most common site of involvement for spinal tuberculosis. Gradually as the disease progresses, the vertebral body and the disk become structurally weak, resulting in progressive collapse of the disk and the adjoining vertebral body. The intact posterior bony elements, ligaments, and facet joint capsule act as a restraint initially. Adequate antitubercular chemotherapy and bracing at this stage prevent further vertebral destruction, and the kyphosis progresses only until the adjacent intact vertebral bodies meet each other anteriorly (▸ Fig. 32.2). In untreated patients, however, the kyphosis gradually worsens due to further destruction, insufficiency of the posterior restraints, and facetal subluxation resulting in severe kyphosis. The severity of collapse during the active phase is mainly influenced by the *severity of vertebral destruction, the level of the lesion, and the age of the patient*, with children showing more collapse for the same degree of vertebral destruction.[1]

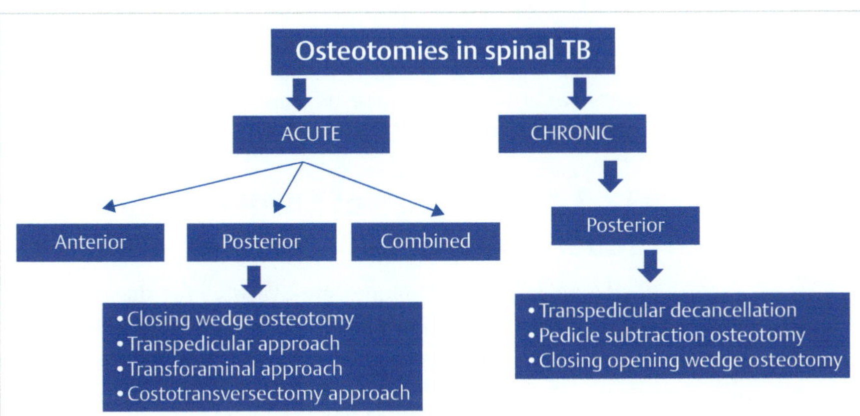

Fig. 32.1 Osteotomies performed for kyphosis correction in active and healed stages of spinal tuberculosis.

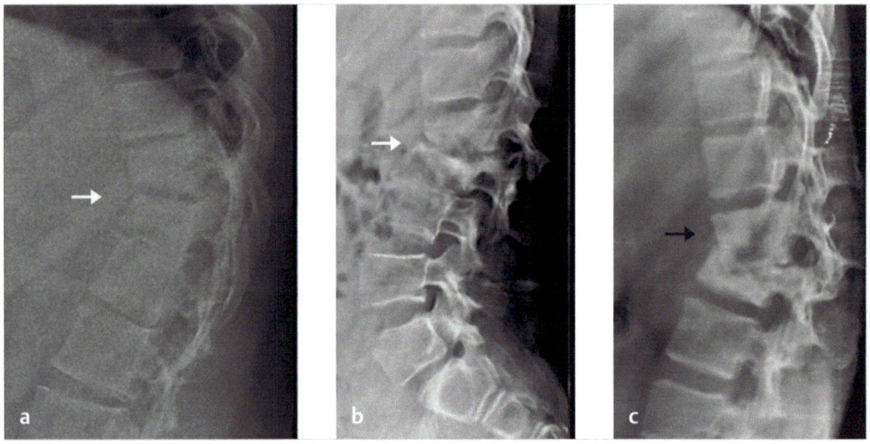

Fig. 32.2 Varying degrees of kyphosis observed in patients with active spinal tuberculosis. **(a)** Mild, **(b)** moderate, and **(c)** severe, angular. The *arrows* (white and black) indicate the vertebral level of spinal tuberculosis and the severity of kyphosis is appreciated.

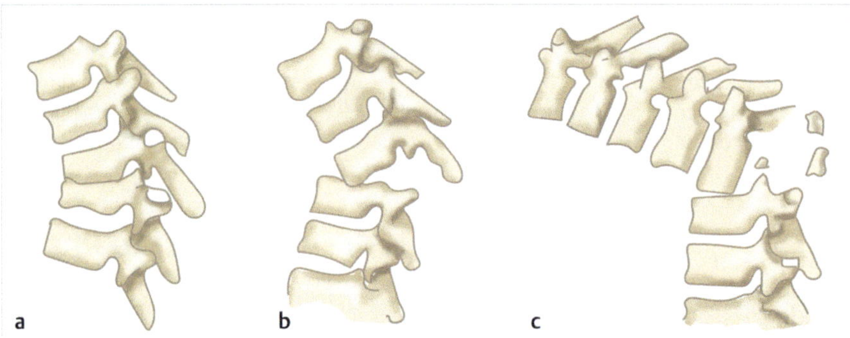

Fig. 32.3 During the healing phase of tuberculosis, restabilization occurs by one of three methods. **(a)** In patients with minimally destroyed vertebrae with intact facet joints, restabilization occurs with a wide contact area. **(b)** In patients with dislocation of a single facet joint, restabilization occurs by point of contact. **(c)** In patients with loss of two or three vertebrae, the facets dislocate at multiple levels, and the superior segment rotates by 90 degrees so that its anterior surface can rest on the superior surface of inferior vertebra.

32.2.2 Healing Patterns in Spinal Tuberculosis

Without surgical intervention, healing in tuberculosis occurs by approximation of intact vertebral bodies anteriorly (▶ Fig. 32.3). Three different types of healing of the vertebra have been identified during the healing phases of tuberculosis, depending on the initial severity of vertebral body damage.[2]

Type A healing is seen in patients where the destruction is minimal and the partially destroyed vertebral bodies come into contact over a large contact area. This pattern is commonly seen in adults and in the early paradiskal type, and in the lumbar region.

Type B healing is seen in patients with a vertebral body loss of more than one and there is subluxation or dislocation of the facet joint. The superior vertebra rotates where its anteroinferior margin comes into point of contact with the superior surface of the inferior normal vertebra.

Type C healing occurs when the vertebral body loss involves more than two vertebrae. The superior normal vertebra rotates more than 90 degrees so that the anterior surface of the superior vertebra comes into contact with the superior surface of the inferior vertebra.

32.2.3 Kyphosis Progression in the "Healed" Phase

In adults, the deformity acquired at the end of disease healing remains static and does not worsen further. In contrast, the posttuberculous kyphosis in children is a dynamic deformity with variable progression during growth (▶ Fig. 32.4). Three different patterns of kyphosis progression have been observed in a study of 63 children with spinal tuberculosis followed over 15 years. In type 1 progression, the deformity worsens during growth; in type II progression there is spontaneous correction of the deformity; and in type III progression, there is no major change during growth. To identify children who could develop worsening kyphosis during the growth period, four radiological "spine-at-risk" signs have been identified by Rajasekaran: (1) dislocation of one or more facet joints in the lateral view, (2) retropulsion of the diseased vertebra, (3) lateral translation seen in the anteroposterior view, and (4) the "toppling sign."[3]

32.3 Surgical Treatment of Kyphosis in Spinal Tuberculosis

During the active phase of the disease, patients with severe lesions of the thoracic spine, with the loss of more than one vertebral body, the involvement of more than three contiguous vertebral bodies, a kyphosis of>30 degrees, and, in children, with two or more spine-at-risk signs are at risk for a kyphosis and may require surgical stabilization.

32.3.1 Principles of Surgery in Active Tuberculosis

Different surgical techniques are available for the prevention and management of kyphosis during active spinal tuberculosis. In the active phase, in addition to kyphosis correction, essential steps include debridement of paravertebral and epidural abscess, circumferential decompression of the spinal cord, and spinal stabilization. Treatment planning requires consideration of the following: the extent of vertebral body involvement, the number of vertebrae involved and the presence of cord compression with pus and granulation tissue, neurologic status of the patient, and severity of kyphosis.

Many different techniques are available for kyphosis correction in active spinal TB:

- Single-stage kyphosis correction by anterior approach and stabilization.
- Single-stage transpedicular approach and posterior stabilization (posterior closing wedge osteotomy).
- Single-stage kyphosis correction by posterior-only transforaminal approach and interbody fusion.
- Single-stage kyphosis correction by posterior costotransversectomy or anterolateral approach and posterior stabilization.
- Single- or two-staged anterior decompression, kyphosis correction, and reconstruction followed by posterior instrumentation (two separate approaches: Kyphosis correction by combined anterior and posterior approach).

32.3.2 Single-Stage Kyphosis Correction by Anterior Approach and Stabilization

In this technique, the diseased vertebra is accessed through a direct anterior approach. The type of approach varies depending on the primary region of spine that has been affected by the disease. The routinely used approaches are a Smith–Robinson approach for subaxial cervical spine lesions (▶ Fig. 32.5), a sternotomy approach for lesions from T 2–T 4, a lateral thoracotomy approach for lesions from T 5 to T 11, a thoracoabdominal approach for T 12–L 1 lesions, and a retroperitoneal approach for L 2–L 4 lesions. Once the affected vertebral region is reached, the prevertebral fascia is incised to let out the tuberculous abscess. The disks above and below the infected body and the necrotic bone tissue are removed until a bleeding bone surface is reached. After adequate debridement, kyphosis is corrected by reconstructing the anterior defect with a cage or a structural allograft. A single screw rod suffices in most patients, but a double screw construct may need to be used if the kyphosis correction has been significant or the vertebral dimensions are wide. The limitations of the anterior approach include poor access to the upper thoracic, lower lumbar, and lumbosacral regions, difficulties of working around a diseased lung, risks of injury to viscera and the vascular structures, and inadequate deformity correction.

32.3.3 Single-Stage Transpedicular Approach and Posterior Correction (Posterior Closing Wedge Osteotomy)

In patients with early disease and with a deformity of less than 40 degrees, a posterior transpedicular decompression, wedge resection of posterior elements with posterior stabilization (posterior closing wedge osteotomy) enables kyphosis correction and ensures disease healing (▶ Fig. 32.6). The transpedicular

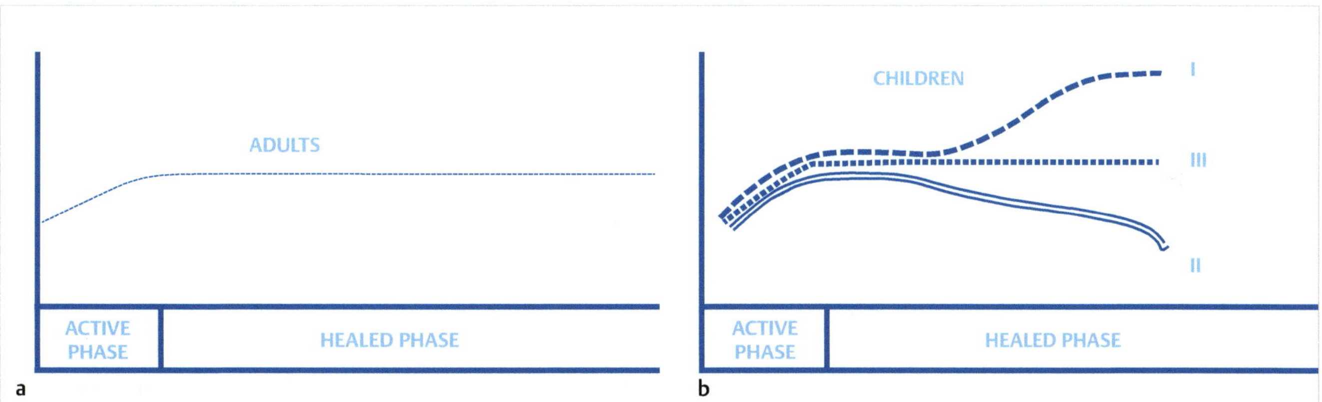

Fig. 32.4 Deformity progression in healed tuberculosis in adults and children. **(a)** In adults, the deformity remains the same during the healed phase. **(b)** In children, the deformity can either worsen (type I), remain static (type III), or improve (type II) during the healed phase.

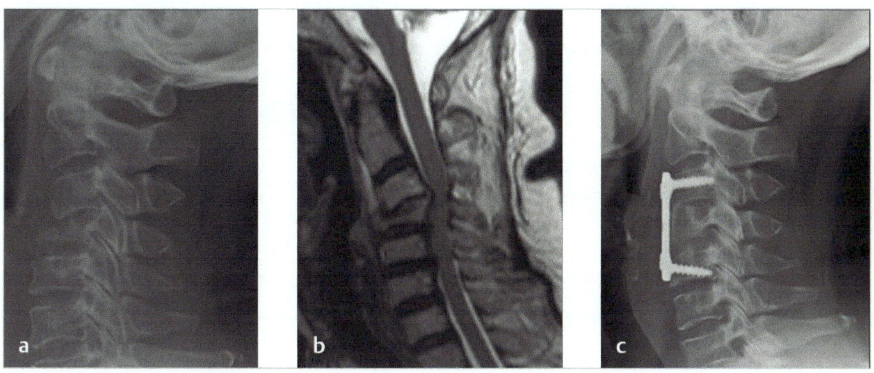

Fig. 32.5 **(a)** Lateral radiograph of the cervical spine showing pathological collapse of the C 4 vertebra resulting in local kyphosis. **(b)** Sagittal MRI shows C 4 collapse causing cord compression with epidural abscess. **(c)** The lesion has been treated by anterior corpectomy, reconstruction with iliac crest graft, and fixation with a plate.

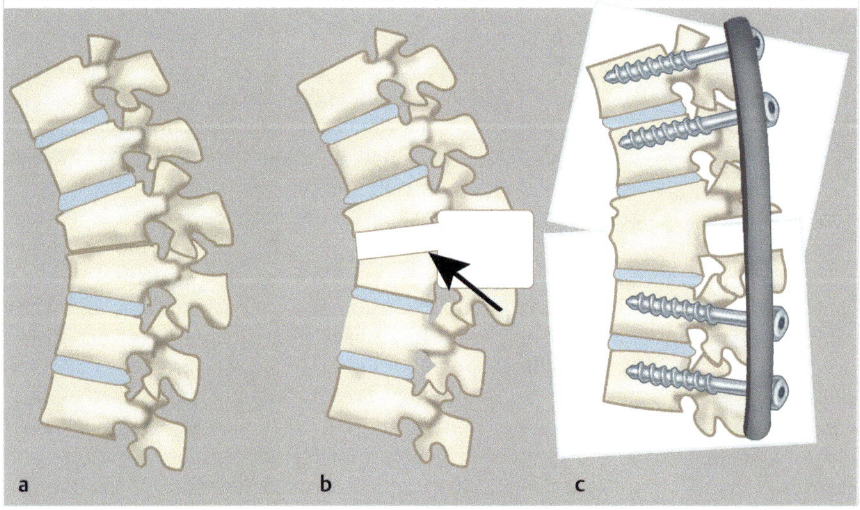

Fig. 32.6 Diagrammatic representation of a posterior closing wedge osteotomy in spinal tuberculosis. **(a)** Vertebrae in brown color represent the infected and collapsed vertebrae. **(b)** Disk space debridement is done (*black arrow*) through a posterior approach. **(c)** Posterior lamina and facets are resected to close the posterior osteotomy and fixed with pedicle screws and rod.

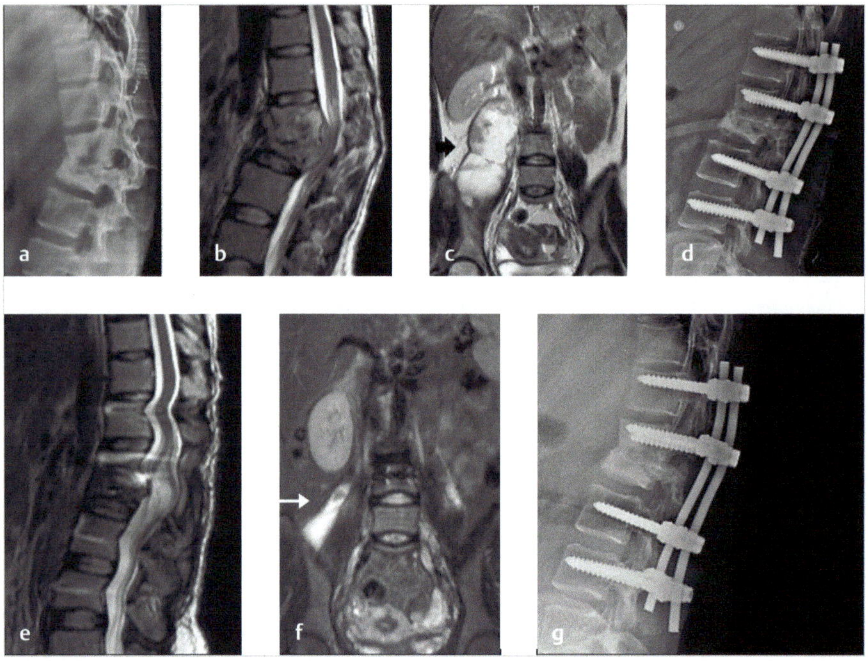

Fig. 32.7 **(a)**Lateral radiograph and **(b)** sagittal MRI show collapse of T 12–L 1 vertebra causing kyphosis and epidural abscess. **(c)** The coronal MRI shows a huge abscess (*black arrow*) in the paraspinal region. **(d)** Patient has been treated by debridement and posterior closing wedge osteotomy with kyphosis correction. **(e, f)** Follow-up MRI scans at 9 months show good resolution of the abscess (*white arrow*) and **(g)** the radiograph shows a healed lesion.

approach serves as a good portal for debridement of the vertebral body and decompression of the spinal cord. Gokce et al reported correction of sagittal balance in 12 patients with kyphosis through transpedicular decompression and posterior column shortening osteotomy.[4] The authors reported correction of kyphosis from 51.1 to 23 degrees in the lower dorsal and dorsolumbar spine. Lee et al compared single-stage transpedicular decompression and posterior instrumentation with anterior decompression fusion and anterior instrumentation ($n = 7$) in an active TB spinal lesion and reported equal kyphosis correction in both groups.[5]

Technique

The technique can be used for spinal tuberculosis anywhere from T 1 to the lumbosacral junction. A standard posterior midline approach is performed. Pedicle screws are inserted cephalad and caudad to the diseased level, and a rod is inserted on the side contralateral to the planned transpedicular approach. At the diseased level, a laminectomy is performed to relieve cord compression. The transpedicular approach is then started by using a pedicle probe and creating a tract across the pedicle into the diseased vertebral body. A screw-tap or a high-speed bur or a curet is now used to widen the pedicle canal. The track is used to remove the perivertebral abscess and necrotic bone tissue. When more anterior bone tissue needs to be removed, the transverse process is resected at its base to allow more medial angulation to enter the disk and infected body. Once the desired amount of debridement is achieved, the anterior bone gap is assessed. If the anterior defect is wide, a cage of the appropriate size, filled with bone grafts, is packed into the intervertebral space, which enables good correction of the kyphosis. If the defect is less than 10 mm, the facet joints are excised bilaterally, and posterior elements are compressed across the screws to correct the deformity (▶ Fig. 32.7).

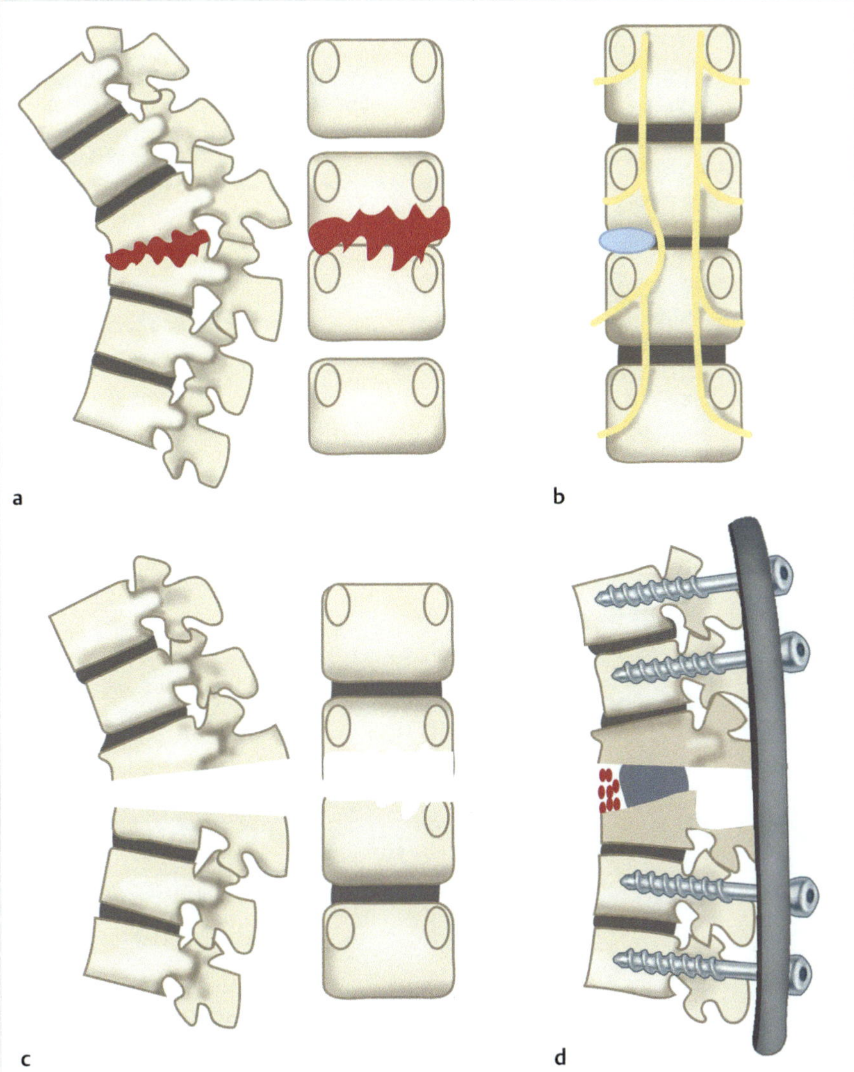

Fig. 32.8 Diagrammatic representation of posterior transforaminal debridement and fusion in active spinal tuberculosis. **(a)** The affected vertebrae (tan) have collapsed in kyphosis with abscess formation (maroon). **(b)** After posterior decompression, the disk and infected vertebra are accessed through the transforaminal route (*blue oval*). **(c)** The gap between the vertebrae shows the area of debridement. **(d)** The deformity has been corrected through pedicle screws and rods, and the interbody debrided disk space is filled with bone graft and cage.

32.3.4 Single-Stage Kyphosis Correction by Posterior-Only Transforaminal Approach and Interbody Fusion

The transforaminal approach is a variant of the transpedicular approach where anterior decompression and reconstruction are performed through the transforaminal space (▸ Fig. 32.8). In the lumbar spine, it is preferred because the lumbar roots and thecal sac can be retracted without risking neurologic injury. Even cages of size >20 mm can be safely inserted transforaminally. Zaveri et al studied 15 patients treated by transforaminal debridement and fusion for TB. The mean preoperative local lordosis of −3.7 degrees was corrected surgically to a mean of 5 degrees.[6]

Technique

A posterior midline approach is performed with the patient in the prone position. Pedicle screws are inserted at one or two levels adjacent to the involved region. The screws are fixed to a contoured rod on one side with distraction at the involved segment. Decompression of the neural elements is performed through a laminectomy along with removal of the facet joints. The proximal part of the superior facet of the distal vertebra is removed to allow access to the transforaminal region. The disk and the infected vertebral bone can be accessed through this space. Epidural granulation and diseased tissue within the disk space are thoroughly excised. The anterior third of the disk space is packed with morselized bone graft, and an adequately sized interbody cage packed with bone is introduced. Pedicle screws on both sides are then fixed to precontoured rods under compression, aiding in kyphosis correction (▸ Fig. 32.9).

32.3.5 Single-Stage Kyphosis Correction by Posterior Costotransversectomy or Anterolateral Approach and Posterior Stabilization

The costotransversectomy approach involves excision of the medial 4 cm of the rib along with the rib head to gain a more oblique access anteriorly into the vertebral body. It is performed in the thoracic spine, and when the amount of vertebral destruction requires a larger anterior reconstruction.

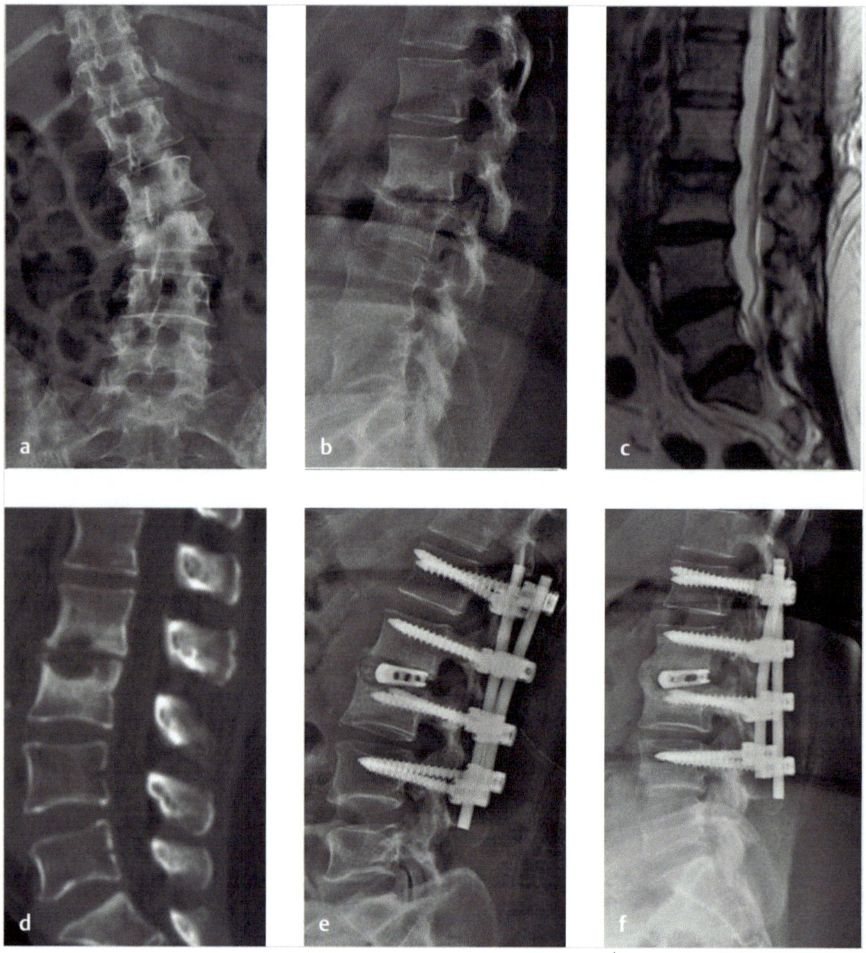

Fig. 32.9 **(a)** Anteroposterior and **(b)** lateral radiographs show asymmetric collapse of the L2–L3 disk space and adjoining vertebrae. **(c)** Sagittal MRI and **(d)** CT scans show the eroded disk space with paravertebral collection. **(e)** Posterior kyphosis correction with transforaminal reconstruction, which **(f)** has healed nicely at 9 months.

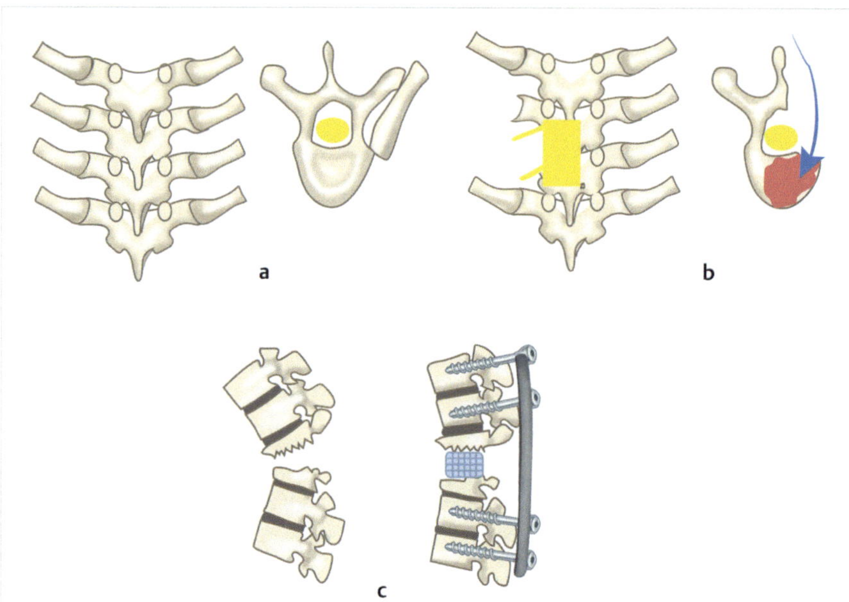

Fig. 32.10 Diagrammatic representation of a costotransversectomy approach and anterior reconstruction through a posterior approach. **(a)** Adequately wide posterior approach to at least two vertebrae above and below the lesion and laterally up to 4 cm of the ribs is necessary. **(b)** Lamina, facet joints, transverse process, and the medial 5 cm of the ribs are removed to reach the vertebra and paravertebral region. **(c)** After thorough debridement, the anterior defect is filled with a cage and stabilized posteriorly with screws and rods.

Technique

The authors prefer a midline longitudinal incision over the affected segment in the prone position. The technique can also be performed in the lateral decubitus position, where longitudinal paramedian, semicircular, or T-shaped incisions are used to access the spine circumferentially. The paraspinal muscles are dissected from the midline subperiosteally and retracted beyond the tip of the transverse process. Posterior instrumentation is placed at two to three levels cephalad and caudad to the pathology, and a temporary rod is assembled on the contralateral side (▶ Fig. 32.10).

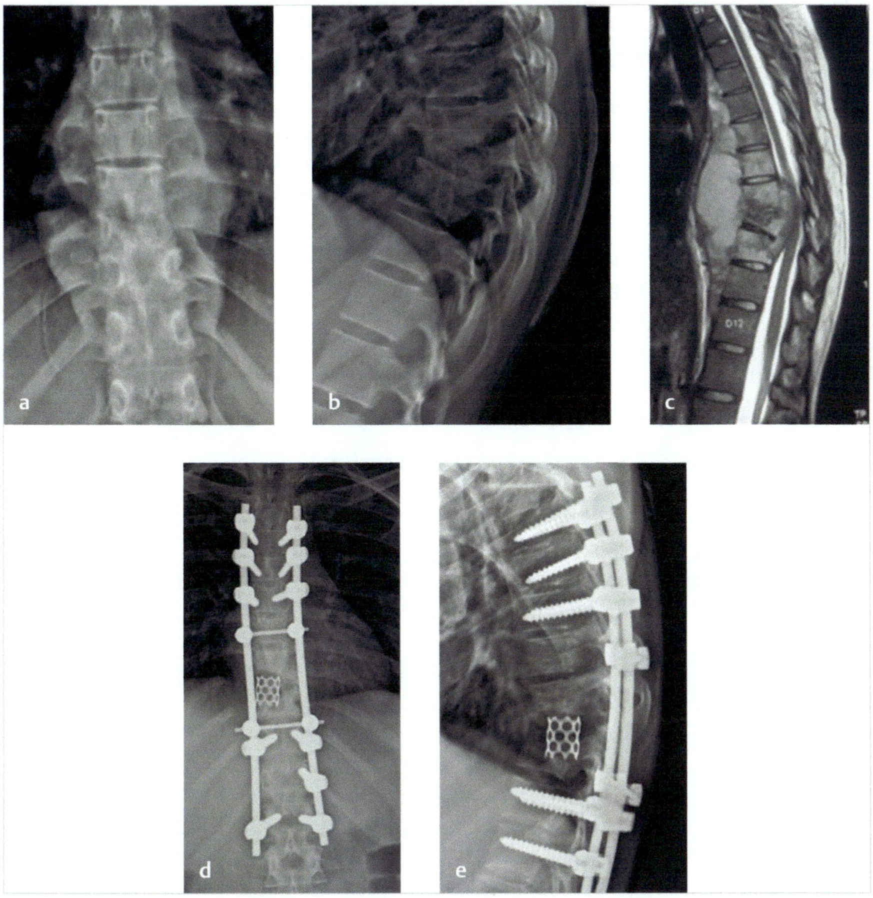

Fig. 32.11 An 18-year-old woman with acute tubercular kyphosis and paravertebral abscess formation. **(a)** Anteroposterior radiograph of the thoracic spine shows paravertebral shadows suggestive of abscess formation. **(b)** Lateral view of the thoracic spine shows T8 and T9 vertebral collapse. **(c)** Sagittal T2-MRI image shows prevertebral abscess, T7-T10 spondylodiscitis and epidural abscess formation causing cord compression, postoperative AP **(d)** and lateral views **(e)** indicate that she has been treated by posterior pedicle screw stabilization and anterior reconstruction through a costotransversectomy approach.

On one side, the medial 5 cm of the ribs to be resected are exposed subperiosteally while preserving the intercostal neurovascular bundle. The costotransverse ligaments are cut, and the rib is divided laterally at its posterior angle. The transverse process is also cut at its base, exposing the lateral surface of the pedicle. The rib is then followed up to its articulation with the vertebral body and disarticulated from the vertebral body. Excision of the rib opens up the prevertebral abscess. More than one rib can be excised to offer a wider longitudinal exposure. The parietal pleura is dissected off the vertebral body and pushed anteriorly, exposing the lateral part of the vertebral body. The intercostal vessels can be ligated, and the intercostal nerve is traced back to the neural foramina. The ipsilateral lamina, facet joint, and pedicle are removed to decompress the spinal cord. The anterior vertebral body is debrided. Anterior struts graft or cage is placed into the anterior defect, correcting the deformity. Rods are placed into the posterior pedicle screws and compressed to load the graft and hold it firmly in position (▸ Fig. 32.11).

32.3.6 Kyphosis Correction by Combined Anterior and Posterior Approach

Here the correction of kyphosis is achieved in two stages, where anterior decompression and reconstruction are performed initially, followed by posterior instrumentation. After anterior decompression by a transthoracic retropleural or retroperitoneal approach, the gap is filled by the bone graft or a cage. Two to three weeks later, supplemental posterior pedicle screw stabilization surgery is performed. The techniques are similar to those already described. With the advent of modern spinal instrumentation, kyphotic deformity can be corrected adequately from a posterior-only approach. Since the two procedures can be performed through either a costotransversectomy or a transforaminal approach, the combined approach is not popular now.

32.4 Surgery for Kyphosis Correction in Healed Tuberculosis

Intervention to prevent deformity must be done early because surgery in the early stages is relatively simple, enables deformity correction, and prevents future kyphosis. In contrast, surgery for an established kyphotic deformity, especially in the presence of neurologic deficit, is difficult, with significant complication rates. Various surgical treatment methods have been described in the literature involving either a single-stage anterior or posterior corrective surgery and combined anterior and posterior techniques. Each technique has its own advantages and disadvantages, and adopting a particular technique would depend on the patient's deformity, neurologic status, and general condition, as well as the severity and flexibility of the deformity and the surgeon's experience and expertise with the procedure.

Single-stage anterior procedures have not been advocated for posttubercular kyphosis correction because of difficulties in approaching the concavity of the angular kyphosis, possibilities of lung adhesions, and inadequate deformity correction risks of neurologic deficits. Similarly, combined anterior and posterior procedures are a major surgical undertaking and have the associated problems of an anterior approach. Posterior procedures are preferred at this time. The advantages of the posterior approach include familiarity of the approach, direct access to the apex of the deformity from behind, and the ability to achieve circumferential decompression of the cord, lengthen the anterior column, and shorten the posterior column, which helps in achieving kyphosis correction without altering the length of the cord and provides strong posterior instrumentation. Posterior-only procedures for the correction of postinfection kyphotic deformities include the transpedicular decancellation osteotomy, pedicle substraction osteotomy, single-stage global reconstruction by an extrapleural approach, and closing opening wedge osteotomy (posterior vertebral column resection). Unlike other sagittal plane deformities, posttubercular kyphosis provides less anterior vertebral bone for performing a transpedicular resection or pedicle subtraction osteotomy (PSO). These are indicated in mild to moderate deformities. Complex procedures such as the closing opening wedge osteotomy are useful in gross kyphosis but can be associated with significant complications and protracted recovery.

32.4.1 Transpedicular Decancellation Osteotomy

In this technique, after an extended laminectomy, the apical vertebral body is decancellated through the pedicles, and the posterior column is shortened by pedicle screw instrumentation. Bezer et al studied sixteen patients with angular kyphotic deformity who underwent transpedicular decancellation osteotomy with at least 5 years of follow-up.[7] There were 6 male and 10 female patients with a mean age of 51.0. The mean preoperative angle of kyphosis was 29.9 degrees (range, 9–97 degrees), which was corrected to 12.2 degrees (range, 0–43 degrees) postoperatively. The mean localized angle of kyphosis at the last follow-up was 13.9 degrees (range, 2–43 degrees).

32.4.2 Pedicle Subtraction Osteotomy

A PSO involves a V-shaped resection of the vertebral column through the posterior elements, pedicles, and vertebral body. The hinge is anterior near the anterior longitudinal ligament. All three columns are shortened, the maximum being at the posterior column. The osteotomy is then closed in such a way as to accomplish bone-on-bone in the posterior, middle, and anterior columns. Kalra et al studied 15 patients with kyphosis and healed spinal tuberculosis and performed a wedge resection of the vertebra using a transpedicular approach.[8] The wedge was removed from the apex of the deformity. The mean preoperative kyphosis was 58.8 degrees (34 –100 degrees). The mean immediate postoperative kyphosis was 13.7 degrees. A mean correction of 44.2 degrees (18–70 degrees) was obtained. At a mean follow-up of 26.8 months, the mean loss of correction was 4.2 degrees.

32.4.3 Single-Stage Kyphosis Correction through Extrapleural Approach

Anil Jain et al corrected posttubercular kyphosis through an extrapleural anterolateral (costotransversectomy) approach, as described earlier. Instead of a posterior midline approach, the authors used a T-shaped incision, with the vertical part over the midline, and the transverse part over the affected region of kyphosis.[9] The mean kyphosis was 58.5 degrees (range, 35–76 degrees), which was corrected to a mean 27.3 degrees. All but one patient with neural deficit showed complete neural recovery, and no neurologically intact patient had neural deterioration.

32.4.4 Closing Opening Wedge Osteotomy (Vertebral Column Resection)

This technique ensures complete resection of the internal kyphosis (retropulsed posterior vertebral border that causes cord compression), anterior column lengthening, posterior column shortening, and correction of the deformity through a single-stage posterior approach (▶ Fig. 32.12). The disadvantages are that the procedure is risky, requires expertise, and requires intensive care backup and perioperative neural monitoring. For posttubercular kyphosis of more than 60 degrees with or without neurologic deficit, this technique is preferred.

Technique

The procedure is a modification of the procedure described by Kawahara et al.[10] The surgery is performed under general anesthesia. The patient is placed prone over two bolsters with adequate padding of the bony prominences. In patients with severe kyphosis, particular care should be taken to prevent hyperextension of the neck, and pressure on the eyes and abdomen. When necessary, the table may be appropriately "broken" to accommodate the deformity.

Through a midline incision extending three or four vertebrae above and below the involved segment, the paraspinal muscles are dissected subperiosteally until reaching the tips of the transverse processes. This enables dissection under the surface of the transverse processes at the sides of the target vertebra so that circumferential decompression can be performed. Pedicle screws are inserted into two or three vertebrae above and below the lesion. The apex of the kyphosis is identified, and a wide laminectomy is performed at the involved levels, including the facet joints. A temporary rod is placed to maintain spinal stability while the surgeon proceeds to perform resection of the anterior kyphosis. The pedicles and intercostal nerve roots are identified at the level of kyphosis. In the thoracic region, one or two nerve roots can be safely sacrificed by ligating about 3 to 4 cm away from the intervertebral foramen. The spinal branch of the segmental artery, which runs along with the nerve root, should also be ligated and divided. The ligatures should be left long and maintained till the end of the procedure because they can be used as landmarks and also to gently lift the dura during the terminal stages of resecting the internal gibbus. The utmost care is taken while retracting the nerve roots to avoid traction on the cord (▶ Fig. 32.13).

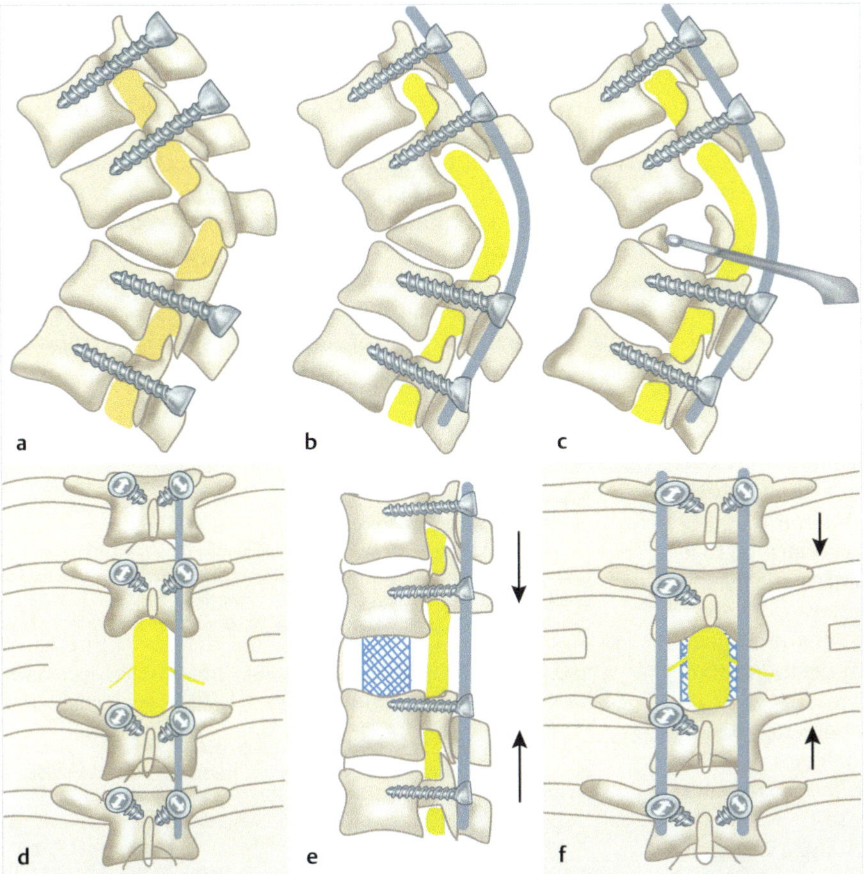

Fig. 32.12 Diagrammatic representation of posterior closing opening wedge osteotomy. **(a)** Pedicle screws are inserted at least two levels above and below the lesion. **(b)** Laminectomy is performed at the apex, and the vertebrae are stabilized with a temporary rod. **(c)** After ligating the nerve roots on either side, **(d)** the anterior kyphotic mass is excised. **(e)** The anterior void is reconstructed with a cage and **(f)** closed posteriorly with definitive rods placed over the pedicle screws.

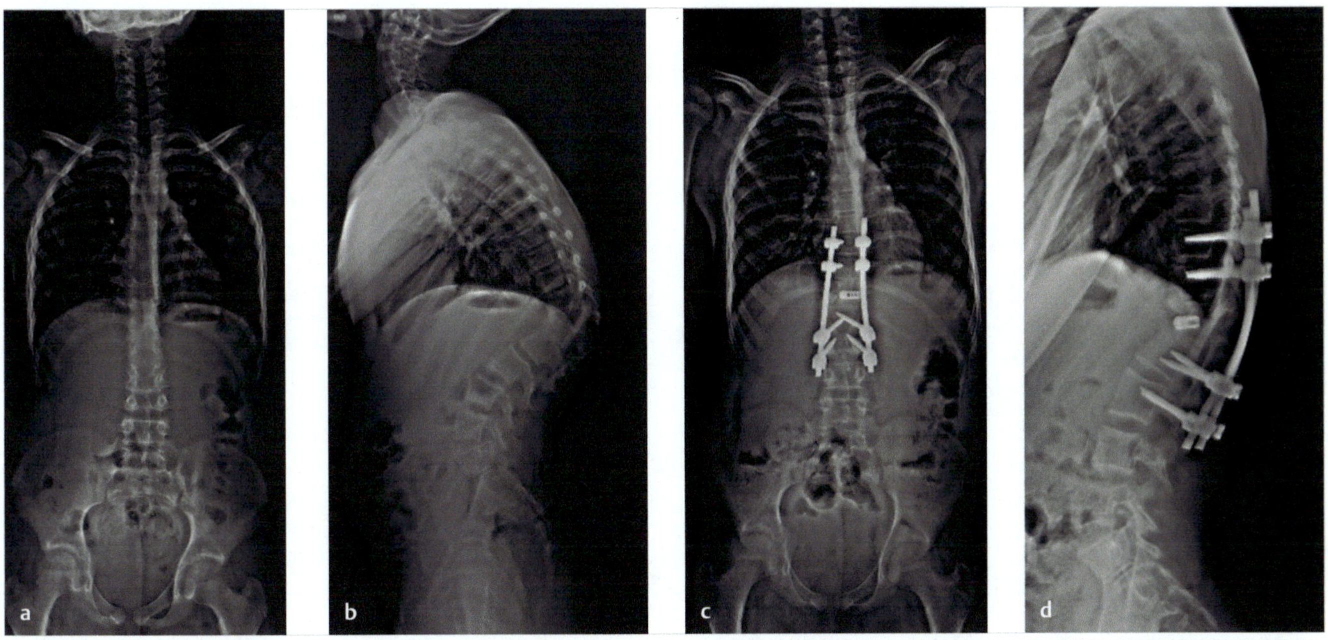

Fig. 32.13 This 24-year-old man presented with a healed post-tubercular kyphosis. In the AP **(a)** and lateral **(b)** whole spine radiographs, the angle of thoracolumbar kyphosis measured 92 degrees. The deformity was corrected through a posterior closing-opening wedge osteotomy. Postoperative AP **(c)** and lateral **(d)** radiographs show good correction of kyphosis. The final kyphosis achieved was 29 degrees.

The ribs at the affected level are transected 3 to 4 cm lateral to the costotransverse joint, and the pleura is bluntly separated from the ribs. The rib heads at the corresponding level, as well as the transverse process, are then carefully excised, remaining extrapleural. Blunt dissection is performed anteriorly on both sides through the plane between the pleura and the vertebral body. The viscera and vessels are carefully dissected anteriorly away from the anterior aspect of the vertebral body with a spatula and blunt finger dissection. While the integrity of the end plates of adjacent vertebrae is maintained, the vertebral body is carefully removed using a curet, rongeur, or high-speed bur in a wedge shape approximating the angular deformity. The posterior vertebral cortex is kept intact, and its early removal will lead to troublesome bleeding from the epidural veins and will also increase the chance of neurologic deficits as the cord then continuously descends down into the working area of the bur and other sharp instruments. A second temporary rod is then attached to the screws on the opposite side. The initial rod is removed, and the decompression procedure is repeated on that side. At the end of the decompression, a circumferential exposure of the spinal cord is obtained. Then the posterior vertebral cortex at the apex of the deformity is finally removed under direct vision using a diamond burr and a 1 mm Kerrison's rongeur from the lateral direction.

Using contoured rods, shortening is carefully done to produce a concertina collapse of the wedge and correction of the deformity. The entire procedure should be performed slowly and gradually with frequent pauses so that the cord is not shortened suddenly. The anterior defect is measured, and a vertebral spacer, such as the Harms titanium mesh cage with autograft inside, is carefully inserted into the intervertebral gap. A wake-up test is performed to ensure neurologic stability. The rods are firmly secured, and further packing of the chip grafts is performed along the posterolateral gutter.

32.5 Conclusion

Uncomplicated spinal tuberculosis is now mainly a medical disease, but many patients end up with considerable kyphosis. The severity of deformity in spinal tuberculosis depends on the extent of vertebral destruction, level of the lesion, and age of the patient, with more severe deformities seen in children and in lesions involving the thoracolumbar spine. In children, the kyphosis may continue to progress during growth, even after the disease is cured, and they should be followed up till completion of growth. The presence of two or more "spine-at-risk" radiologic signs indicates the possibility of severe late collapse in children. Surgical procedures performed in the active stage to prevent deformity are simple and have lower morbidity compared to surgical correction of established deformities. There are numerous surgical procedures available for prevention and correction of deformities from which the surgeon may choose depending on his preference and expertise. With the refinement of surgical technique and rigid spinal instrumentation providing three-column support, a posterior-only approach for prevention and correction of deformity in spinal tuberculosis is now preferred.

References

[1] Rajasekaran S. The problem of deformity in spinal tuberculosis. Clin Orthop Relat Res 2002; (398):85–92

[2] Rajasekaran S, Prasad Shetty A, Dheenadhayalan J, Shashidhar Reddy J, Naresh-Babu J, Kishen T. Morphological changes during growth in healed childhood spinal tuberculosis: a 15-year prospective study of 61 children treated with ambulatory chemotherapy. J Pediatr Orthop 2006;26(6):716–724

[3] Rajasekaran S. The natural history of post-tubercular kyphosis in children. Radiological signs which predict late increase in deformity. J Bone Joint Surg Br 2001;83(7):954–962

[4] Gokce A, Ozturkmen Y, Mutlu S, Caniklioğlu M. Spinal osteotomy: correcting sagittal balance in tuberculous spondylitis. J Spinal Disord Tech 2008;21 (7):484–488

[5] Lee SH, Sung JK, Park YM. Single-stage transpedicular decompression and posterior instrumentation in treatment of thoracic and thoracolumbar spinal tuberculosis: a retrospective case series. J Spinal Disord Tech 2006;19 (8):595–602

[6] Zaveri GR, Mehta SS. Surgical treatment of lumbar tuberculous spondylodiscitis by transforaminal lumbar interbody fusion (TLIF) and posterior instrumentation. J Spinal Disord Tech 2009;22(4):257–262

[7] Bezer M, Kucukdurmaz F, Guven O. Transpedicular decancellation osteotomy in the treatment of posttuberculous kyphosis. J Spinal Disord Tech 2007;20 (3):209–215

[8] Kalra KP, Dhar SB, Shetty G, Dhariwal Q. Pedicle subtraction osteotomy for rigid post-tuberculous kyphosis. J Bone Joint Surg Br 2006;88(7):925–927

[9] Jain AK, Dhammi IK, Prashad B, Sinha S, Mishra P. Simultaneous anterior decompression and posterior instrumentation of the tuberculous spine using an anterolateral extrapleural approach. J Bone Joint Surg Br 2008;90 (11):1477–1481

[10] Kawahara N, Tomita K, Baba H, Kobayashi T, Fujita T, Murakami H. Closing-opening wedge osteotomy to correct angular kyphotic deformity by a single posterior approach. Spine 2001;26(4):391–402

33 Osteotomies in Tuberculosis—Pediatric Care

Alexander Mushkin

Abstract

Spinal tuberculosis in pediatric patients is frequently associated with multiple vertebral lesions and could be complicated by kyphosis. The diagnosis should be confirmed by culturing or molecular-genetic study of the pathological tissues that are harvested from the zone of bone lesions or from the paravertebral abscesses.

Long-term chemotherapy is the basis for treatment of tuberculosis. Operative treatment in the form of angular kyphosis or compression of the spinal cord is absolutely indicated in cases of orthopaedic or neurological complications of spinal tuberculosis. Simultaneous debridement, kyphosis correction by posterior instrumentation, and anterior fusion by bone transplant alone or with titanium mesh cage are the best options for complete recovery and restoration of spinal balance.

Keywords: spinal tuberculosis, children, kyphosis, abscesses, surgery

33.1 Introduction

Tuberculosis (TB) spondylitis is infectious damage to the spine caused by *Mycobacterium tuberculosis* complex. The majority of cases of TB spondylitis develop as a result of *M. tuberculosis humanus* generalization from the infected lung or lymph nodes; in the endemic areas the disease might appear due to other strains.[1,2,3,4] Extremely rare spondylitis in children could be caused by dissemination of vaccine steam*M. tuberculosis bovis* BCG (bacille Calmette-Guerin) as a result of the pathological process of anti-TB vaccination.[5]

The morphological basis of TB spondylitis is a necrotic granulomatous inflammation that relates it to primary chronic osteomyelitis of the spine. In patients with a primary and secondary immune insufficiency, the morphological pattern could be unusual due to the incomplete phagocytosis and the inability to form a typical cellular and tissue composition in TB granulomas.[6,7]

There are fundamental differences between TB in pediatric and adult spines[4,8]:

- The tendency for multilevel damage with total or subtotal lesions of several vertebral bodies leads to spinal collapse and early kyphosis. The deformity in particular is the first clinical symptom that parents can distinguish.
- TB spondylitis frequently occurs at an early age. Due to the continuing growth of the posterior spinal column and dislocation of facets, the natural history of kyphosis is associated with a deformity progression. In children younger than 10 years, kyphosis greater than 30 degrees and involvement of the cervicothoracic or thoracolumbar junction are the factors leading to inevitable deformity progression.[1,8,9]
- Back pain and neurologic disorders are less severe in children than in adults. Nonreversible ischemic changes in the spinal cord with gross neurologic compromise (e.g., complete paraplegia, pelvic disorders) rarely develop in children despite the severe deformity of the spinal canal and spinal cord compression by bone sequesters and abscesses. Due to the high compensatory potential the clinical signs of myelopathy in children are more prone to neurologic improvement after the elimination of pathological substrates.[3,8]
- Tuberculosis spondylitis may develop in children with a normal immune reaction or in those who are immunocompromised as a result of a primary disease (e.g., chronic granulomatous disease, interferon gamma interleukin-12–linked immune deficit, etc.)[6] or an acquired one (e.g., human immunodeficiency virus infection).[7]

33.2 Diagnosis of Spinal Tuberculosis in Children

World Health Organization (WHO) guidelines (2011)[10] suggest two levels of diagnosis of extrapulmonary TB (including the TB spondylitis):

1. *The determined but unproven diagnosis* is stated when it is based on the clinical, anamnesis, instrumental, radial, and other data but does not require microbiological or histological confirmation.
2. *The proven or confirmed* cases can be established if *M. tuberculosis* is verified in the material from the damaged vertebrae or the paravertebral tissues.

Tissue samples for proven or confirmed cases are most quickly obtained by CT-navigated, fine-needle aspiration biopsy (for abscesses) or trepan-biopsy followed by examination, including bacterioscopy, culture incubation, as well as detection of fragments of mycobacteria by DNA amplification techniques (polymerase chain reaction) or mutations in the genes responding for drug resistance (X-pert MTB/RIF Assay), thereby reducing the verification period to several hours or a few days.[2,11] Spinal TB can be considered proven on the basis of clinical and radial data without bacteriological confirmation in the world's regions where such investigations cannot be done. The immune and blood-based serologic tests, as interferon-gamma release assays and tuberculin skin tests should not be used for confirmation of TB spondylitis because they reflect only the TB infection, not the appropriate method for its activity verification and specificity for the local spinal damage.[11]

33.3 Principles of Treatment

The current treatment of TB in children is based on the combination of anti-TB chemotherapy and surgery.

The chemotherapy regimens (the combination of drugs and the treatment duration) is established according to WHO recommendations and based on the data of drug sensitivity (or resistance) of *M. tuberculosis*, which must be established as early as possible. Treatment effectiveness is determined by the disappearance of abscesses and radiologic signs of bone healing after the initial phase of chemotherapy, which continues for a minimum of 2 months in cases caused by drug-sensitive *M. tuberculosis*, and 6 months in cases of multidrug-resistant *M. tuberculosis*. The total duration of TB treatment regimens can range from 6 to 24 months and includes initial and continuation phases depending on the disease category.[10,11]

Indications and methods for the surgical treatment of spinal TB in children significantly differ in active cases and their consequences. The correction of spinal deformity provides not only cosmetic benefits but also creates the balance required for spinal growth that is essential for preventing secondary post-TB kyphosis (PTK). All operations include correction of severe deformity, especially in PTK, and carry a risk of neurologic complications. Thus, in these cases, it is preferable to monitor evoked potentials and, if possible, check motor control with a wakeup test.

The absolute indications for surgical treatment in *active* TB spondylitis in children include the following complications of spinal lesions:

- *Neurologic disorders:* These can include complete or incomplete paraplegia, bladder and bowel dysfunction caused by spinal cord compression or spinal cord tension within the spinal canal due to its deformity or an epidural abscess.
- *Spinal deformity:* Widespread vertebral damage with active growth of the posterior column and the tendency for fibrous changes of the soft tissues during the healing process lead to the development of severe rigid angular kyphosis that cannot be corrected by external fixation, neither during an active process nor during remission or full healing with the formation of the solid bone block. The most severe deformities develop in the damaged cervicothoracic (▶ Fig. 33.1) and thoracolumbar spine, and in the thoracic level.[12,13,14,15]
- *Ineffective initial course of chemotherapy:* In patients who have not had neurologic or orthopaedic complications this can be confirmed by persistence of abscesses and vertebrae lesions that are detected on the control CT or MRI scan.
- *Chronic back pain caused by spinal instability:* When chronic pain cannot be resolved by a brace and medications (note: this pain is rare in young children and is more typical for adolescents and adults).

The aims for surgery in *active* TB spondylitis in children include the following:

- Remove the pathological tissues—abscesses, necrosis, sequesters.
- Release the spinal cord.
- Restore the anterior spinal support.
- Correct the deformity.
- Create balanced growth of the anterior and posterior spinal columns.

The principal stages of surgery correspond to the following goals:

1. *Removal of pathological tissues and spinal cord decompression:* The out-cavity approaches are used for the anterior spine: extrapleural (thoracic spine, Th2–Th11–T 11), thoracophrenic (thoracolumbar spine, Th12–L 1), retroperitoneal (lumbar spine, L2–L4), ilioinguinal (lumbosacral level, L5–S2). The cervical and cervicothoracic spine (C3–Th1) are the most accessible for an anterior approach. Lateral submandibular or direct transoral approaches could both be useful for suboccipital spondylitis (Oc–C1–C2), but the last one is preferable. After opening the abscesses, their contents must be removed as completely as possible; vertebral bodies are opened up until the healthy surfaces are reached. The pathological contents of the spinal canal (sequesters, necrosis, and granulomatous tissues) must be removed with the dural sac release.
2. *Anterior fusion*: After debridement a trial correction is held by hand pressure on the top of the kyphosis (in young children) or by a temporary interbody spreader (in adolescents) to assess spinal mobility. If the trial maneuver successfully leads to complete correction of the deformity, anterior fusion can be performed by autologous bone (rib, iliac crest, fibular

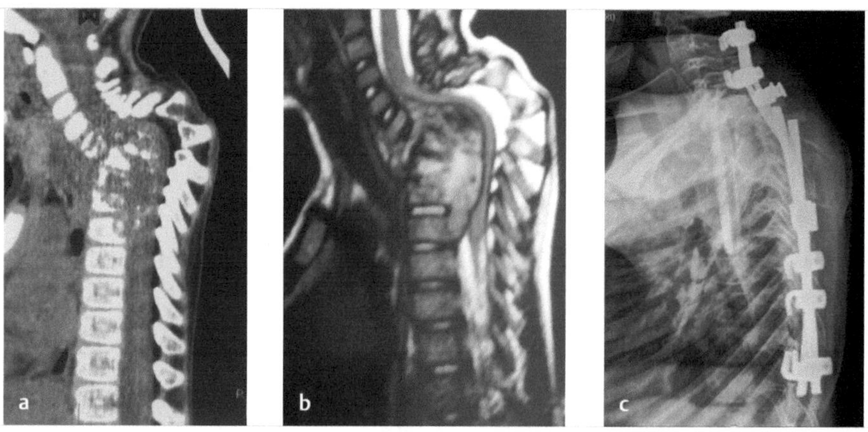

Fig. 33.1 An active tuberculosis spondylitis C 5–Th8 in a 4-year-old boy. **(a)** Preoperative CT and **(b)** MRI show the extensive lesion of the spine, including the total damage of C6–Th4, subtotal Th5, large focuses in Th6–Th8 with large epidural and prevertebral abscesses. Despite the rough deformity and compression of the spinal cord over a large area, neurologic disorders correspond to Frankel grade D. The operation (two-stage, one-narcosis surgery) was performed from two approaches: abscesses, C5–Th6 vertebral body sequestered fragments and focuses inside Th7 and Th8 were removed through the posterolateral thoracic access; Th1 and Th2 neural arcs were removed via a posterior approach along with instrumentation C2–Th9 and kyphosis correction. **(c)** The operation was finished by anterior fusion with cortical allograft (postoperative lateral X-ray). In the early postoperative period, neurologic disorders increased to Frankel grade C, followed by complete recovery to Frankel grade E during the 2 months postsurgery.

graft), cortical allograft, or a combination of bone and a titanium cage.[1]

3. *Posterior instrumentation:* This is the main method currently used for deformity correction, along with software for the spinal stability in reconstruction. In order to ensure the stability of instrumentation and to prevent the growth of deformity, the length of instrumentation should exceed by one or two segments cranial and/or caudal to the length of the anterior fusion. The implant has to have a low profile, especially in young children. The hooks can be used inside the instrumented zone, but hooks or pedicle screws may be used at the end fixed vertebrae. Before the rods are inserted they are modeled regarding the restored lateral contour of the spine, and they are established at a moderate tension, accompanied by visual correction of the deformity;
4. *Deformities exceeding 50 degrees that cannot be effectively corrected without additional posterior spinal osteotomy:* In such cases, the posterior osteotomy and instrumentation have to be completed before the final anterior fusion. One or two neural arcs with facets are removed at the apex of the kyphosis, and instrumentation is performed under compression (the "shortening of the spine"). The bone-inducted transplants are placed inside the instrumented zone. After this procedure, the anterior support is restored by bone grafts or bone grafts in combination with a titanium mesh. The posterior wound is closed completely, and access to the vertebral bodies is drained by a device for active aspiration, usually for 1 to 2 days.
5. *Cervicothoracic spondylitis, complicated by severe kyphosis in children:* In these cases the instrumentation uses connecting constructions (▶ Fig. 33.2). After the separate fixation of the cervical and thoracic spine and the resection of the neural arc (or arcs) on the top of the kyphosis (usually Th1 and/or Th2), the cervical and thoracic rods on each side are connected with the simultaneous extension of the head and cervical spine. This operation and corrective manipulations are best performed with the head previously fixed in a halo ring or a Mayfield bracket.

In most cases, all surgical goals can be met in a single surgical session ("one narcosis surgery") performed using combined approaches or a posterior approach only. An obstacle to completing the surgery using only a posterior approach is the necessity to ensure an adequate view for the debridement and extended anterior fusion. This could require sacrifice of the spinal root (roots), which can be performed relatively safely only on the thoracic level, with local abscesses and insignificant kyphosis.

Correction of kyphosis in active spondylitis using only a posterior approach followed by a closed wedge osteotomy to shorten the posterior spinal column in cases of multilevel lesions and severe deformity (>50 degrees) can give rise to shirring of the dura mater, which leads to increased risk for postoperative neurologic disorders. Thus, the majority of specialists prefer to use a combination of approaches and methods of stabilization, which allow them to shorten the posterior column and lengthen the anterior column (so-called closing-opening osteotomy).[13] Despite these limitations, studies show that the complete surgery can be performed using a posterior approach only in the different levels, including cervicothoracic and thoracolumbar levels.[14,15]

The removal of the posterior spinal implants in young children is performed no sooner than 1.5 to 2 years after reconstructive surgery. The indication for this is the solid anterior and posterior bone fusion proven by CT. The resorption of bone graft in the area of anterior fusion can be an evidence of spondylitis progression or pseudarthrosis. This requires a repeat operation, which can be carried out without posterior reinstrumentation if the instrumentation is stable. The appearance of seromas above the posterior elements usually depends on destabilization, and requires the surgeon to repeat the instrumentation.

33.3.1 Surgical Treatment of the Consequences of Tuberculosis Spondylitis in Children

Depending on the complete or incomplete healing of TB spondylitis in early childhood, especially if it was surgically treated,

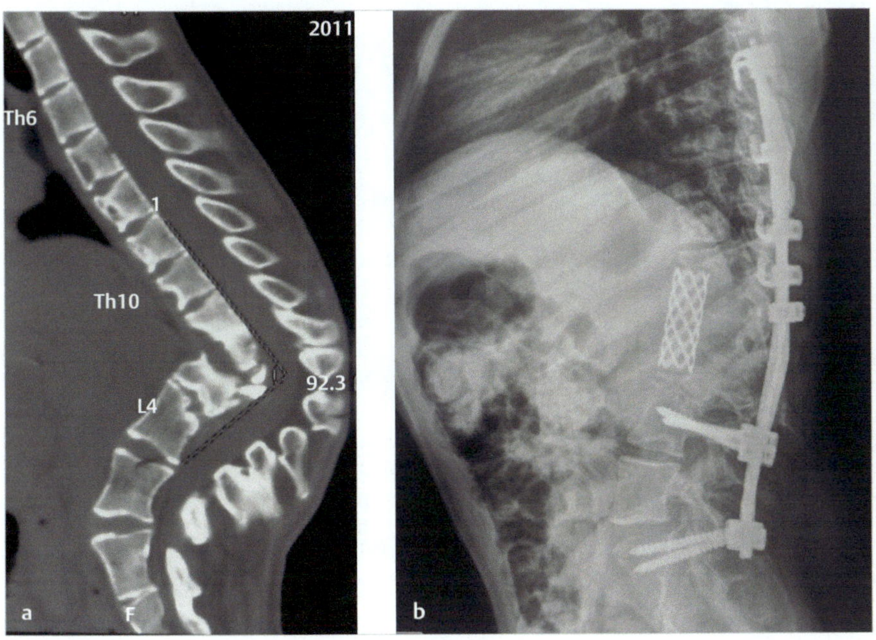

Fig. 33.2 **(a)** Inactive, but not completely healed ("hushed") tuberculosis spondylitis Th7, Th8, Th11–L3 in a 16-year-old girl. The diagnosis was established at 6 years of age when debridement was done without fusion (the data about cultural identification of the isolate are absent). The 18-month anti-TB treatment led to the remission of spondylitis, and there were no neurologic, bladder, or bowel disorders. However, a rough kyphosis complicated by pain was formed. **(b)** The spinal reconstruction was provided from two approaches accompanied by anterior titanium mesh with autologous-bone stabilization. The hybrid instrumentation (hooks and pedicle screws) was used due to residual cavities in the thoracic vertebrae. The postoperative period was without complications. *Note:* During the operation in the fragments of the bodies the necrotic masses were found. The isolates were verified as a *Mycobacterium tuberculosis bovis*, nonvaccine steam.

the consequences can give rise to a unique pathology.[16] As a rule, the deformities increase gradually throughout the period of childhood; however, during puberty and the skeletal growth spurt they progress rapidly. By the end of the growth period (16–18 years) the previously affected spine becomes a conglomerate of bone. Deformities that develop during the processes involved in the healing of TB and the active growth of the child can include both typical single-plane kyphosis and combined kyphoscoliosis. A compensatory hyperlordosis can be observed in the adjacent levels but usually below the kyphosis. The deformity progression, as well as complaints of back pain during this period, can also be signs of the absence of true bone block or of instability in the contacts between the adjustment segments and the area of the previous fusion. Increased post-TB deformity in the adolescent and adult as a rule is accompanied by a typical deformity of the spinal canal with the narrowing or complete disappearance of the anterior epidural space. The local blood flow also changes: as a result of fibrosis and prior surgical procedures, segmental vessels may be reduced, which increases the risk of myeloischemia as in the natural post-TB course and also after surgery.

Correction of severe spinal deformities at the period of the remission (▶ Fig. 33.2a, b) or complete healing (▶ Fig. 33.3) of local TB spondylitis is possible only through the circular spine osteotomy. The operation can be performed in one stage from the posterior approach and includes the successive stages of release, temporary instrumental fixation, vertebral osteotomy, instrumental correction, and final instrumentation with a fusion.[12,13] Preplanning of the size of resection and extension of instrumentation is carried out on the basis of X-ray and CT studies: the spinal cord is visualized by MRI and controlled by neural monitoring during the procedure.

Due to spontaneous facet's ankylosis or the previous fusion, the spine from the back usually represent as a single bone bar. According to the preoperative planning the posterior column osteotomy, using an osteotome, a high-speed bur, and bone rongeurs, continues until the complete release of the spinal canal; in the thoracic region costotransversectomy is done without damaging the pleura. If vascularized rib or periosteum was used for anterior fusion during primary reconstruction (this type of fusion was popular in the 1980s), the bone-bridge extending from the ribs to the vertebrae has to be removed. Thereafter, the anterior longitudinal ligament is separated from the side to the front and the defenders are inserted. According to the preplanned extension of instrumentation, pedicle screws are inserted into supporting vertebrae, and the temporary rod is fixed on the one side to prevent spontaneous displacement of the spine at the moment of complete vertebrotomy.

The upper level of instrumental fixation should not finish on the apical vertebra of kyphosis. The posterior wall of the spinal canal is then removed, a wedge vertebrotomy is done with a circular release of the dural sac. Upon reaching the visually defined mobility of the spine, the second rod is inserted on the contralateral side, and due to the stage by stage alternating tensions and rods modeling on both sides, the deformity is corrected, accompanied by convergence or complete contact of the vertebral bodies. The residual postlaminectomy defect is covered by bone grafts.

In cases of operative neurologic disorders, recorded by the neural monitoring, the correction has to be stopped, the tension should be reduced until the restoration of evoked potentials, and a wakeup test can be used as an additional control. Instrumentation is carried out under continued motor control followed by at least 24 hours of medications.

If the patient with PTK has a long-term (more than 2 years) severe neurologic disorder estimated as complete paraplegia (Frankel types B and A), the target and principles of planned surgery differ from the ones described here. In these cases, the irreversible changes in spinal cord are usually revealed on MRI (atrophy, myelomalacia), and the possibility for neurologic recovery is extremely low. The indication for treatment in these situations is to improve the patient's quality of life. The clinical evidence of spinal instability (back pain or deterioration of kyphosis) could be a reaction to continuous instrumentation,

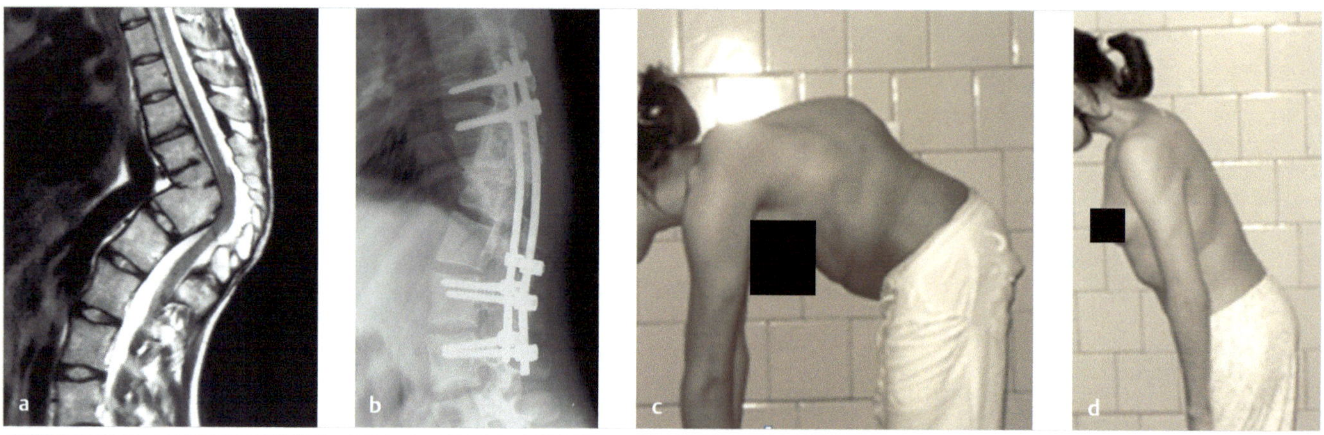

Fig. 33.3 Consequences of tuberculosis spondylitis Th9–L1: post-TB kyphosis in a 15-year-old girl. Radical surgery consisting of debridement and anterior fusion (i.e., "Hong Kong surgery," developed by AR Hodgson and FE Stock, who employed the technique in Hong Kong in the 1940s and 1950s) had been performed at 3 years of age, and solid fusion had been achieved. The complaints at examination included increasing spinal deformity during the last 3 years with pain in the lower thoracic and upper lumbar spine. **(a)** The preoperative sagittal MRI scan revealed a solid bone block with a degenerated disk above it and multilevel edema of the spaces between the spinous processes. **(b)** Closed-wedge osteotomy (Schwab 4 vertebrotomy) was done through a posterior approach with instrumentation and **(c, d)** achieved a good cosmetic effect and complete pain relief.

while vertebral column resection is provided to improve the patient's position for social adaptation, especially for sitting and wheelchair mobility.

References

[1] Tuli SM. Tuberculosis of the spine: a historical review. Clin Orthop Relat Res. 2007; 460(460):29–38

[2] Marquez L, Starke JR. Diagnosis and management of TB in children: an update. Expert Rev Anti Infect Ther. 2011; 9(12):1157–1168

[3] Luk KDK, Leong JCY, Ho EKW. Tuberculosis of the spine. In: Weinstein SL, ed. The Pediatric Spine: Principles and Practice. 2nd ed. Philadelphia, PA: Lippincott Williams & Wilkins; 2001:635–648

[4] Eisen S, Honywood L, Shingadia D, Novelli V. Spinal tuberculosis in children. Arch Dis Child. 2012; 97(8):724–729

[5] Marík I, Kubát R, Filipský J, Galliová J. Osteitis caused by BCG vaccination. J Pediatr Orthop. 1988; 8(3):333–337

[6] Mushkin AY, Galkina EV, Malyarova EY, Kondratenko IV, Kovalenko KN, Vatutina VV. Mycobacterial bone lesions in children with primary immune insufficiency (clinical, diagnostic and tactic peculiarities). Curr Paediatr. 2011; 10:60–64

[7] Walters E, Duvenhage J, Draper HR, et al. Severe manifestations of extrapulmonary tuberculosis in HIV-infected children initiating antiretroviral therapy before 2 years of age. Arch Dis Child. 2014; 99(11):998–1003

[8] Kumar R. Spinal tuberculosis: with reference to the children of northern India. Childs Nerv Syst. 2005; 21(1):19–26

[9] Rajasekaran S. Natural history of Pott's kyphosis. Eur Spine J. 2013; 22 Suppl 4:634–640

[10] World Health Organization. Guidelines for the Programmatic Management of Drug-Resistant Tuberculosis, 2011 Update. Geneva: World Health Organization; 2011

[11] TB CARE I. International Standards for Tuberculosis Care. 3rd ed. TB CARE I, The Hague, 2014

[12] Pang X, Li D, Wang X, et al. Thoracolumbar spinal tuberculosis in children with severe post-tubercular kyphotic deformities treated by single-stage closing-opening wedge osteotomy: preliminary report a 4-year follow-up of 12 patients. Childs Nerv Syst. 2014; 30(5):903–909

[13] Rajasekaran S, Vijay K, Shetty AP. Single-stage closing-opening wedge osteotomy of spine to correct severe post-tubercular kyphotic deformities of the spine: a 3-year follow-up of 17 patients. Eur Spine J. 2010; 19(4):583–592

[14] Zhang HQ, Wang YX, Guo CF, et al. One-stage posterior focus debridement, fusion, and instrumentation in the surgical treatment of cervicothoracic spinal tuberculosis with kyphosis in children: a preliminary report. Childs Nerv Syst. 2011; 27(5):735–742

[15] Zhang HQ, Wang YX, Guo CF, et al. One-stage posterior approach and combined interbody and posterior fusion for thoracolumbar spinal tuberculosis with kyphosis in children. Orthopedics. 2010; 33(11):808

[16] Schulitz KP, Kothe R, Leong JC, Wehling P. Growth changes of solidly fused kyphotic bloc after surgery for tuberculosis. Comparison of four procedures. Spine. 1997; 22(10):1150–1155

34 Osteotomies for Adult Degenerative Scoliosis

Yigal Mirovsky, Yossi Smorgick

Abstract

A balanced spine is a significant predictor of the clinical outcome for patients with adult spinal deformity. To achieve a balanced spine, osteotomies often need to be performed. In this chapter we will review the different osteotomies in the spine with mobile disks and in the rigid spine.

In the spine with mobile disks, correction can be performed with the Smith-Petersen osteotomy (SPO) and the Ponte osteotomy. With these osteotomies, one can achieve a sagittal correction across the apex of the curve of 5 to 15 degrees per level with a low risk for complications. In the rigid spine, we can achieve correction with the pedicle subtraction osteotomy (PSO), bone–disk–bone osteotomy (BDBO), and vertebral column resection (VCR). With these osteotomies up to 30 to 60 degrees of correction can be achieved, but with a higher rate of complications.

Early complications include major blood loss and neurologic complication, while late complications include adjacent segment disease, instrumentation failure, and pseudarthrosis. It appears that the risk factors for adjacent segment disease are sagittal imbalance and facet joint injury during surgery.

Restoration of sagittal balance decreases the rate of subsequent pseudarthrosis, and is associated with better clinical results. The goal of surgery is not only to relieve pain and correct deformity, but also to minimize complications related to surgery. According to the amount of correction needed, the extent of surgery may range from posterior osteotomies to PSO and up to complete resection of a vertebral body.

Keywords: Smith-Petersen osteotomy, Ponte osteotomy, pedicle subtraction osteotomy, bone–disk–bone osteotomy, vertebral column resection

34.1 Introduction

Global sagittal balance is a significant predictor of the clinical status of patients with adult deformity. Positive sagittal balance, defined as an anterior deviation of the C7 plumb line from the S1 sagittal vertical axis (SVA), was found in a survey of patients to be more significantly associated with pain than curve location, magnitude, and coronal balance.[1] Restoration of the sagittal balance was found to decrease the rate of subsequent pseudarthrosis. The preoperative plan should aim to obtain a pelvic tilt of less than 25 degrees and to restore the lumbar lordosis so that it matches and exceeds the pelvic incidence angle.[2]

To achieve these goals of adequate balance restoration of the rigid spine in the coronal and sagittal planes, the spine should be released. This can be done through an anterior approach followed by posterior stabilization, but these combined surgeries have an increased complication rate. The "all posterior" approach has gained popularity in recent years. The amount of correction should be calculated according to the preoperative standing X-rays. Bending films are necessary to evaluate the flexibility of the curves and whether or not a balanced spine might be achieved only by positioning the patient on the operating table, or if further correction is needed with osteotomy.

34.2 Selection of Fusion Levels

One of the issues under constant debate is the preoperative decision about the extent of fusion, the amount of correction necessary to achieve coronal and sagittal balance, and the method of fixation. The following are some of the more accepted criteria for fusion[3,4,5]:

- Fusion should not stop at the apex of the curve where the stress on the adjacent level is increased.
- When compensatory hypokyphosis of the thoracic spine is present, fusion should not stop between T 5 and T 9 because this region will become the new apex of the thoracic curve.
- Junctional kyphosis should be included in the fused area to decrease the likelihood of adjacent-level failure.
- Any lateral subluxation should be included in the fused curve.
- Segments with degenerative disks, spondylolisthesis, and retrolisthesis adjacent to an instrumented segment should not be left unfused.
- A horizontal upper instrumented vertebra is preferred to an oblique one.
- Stopping fusion in mobile segments of lumbar curves may lead to disk degeneration, segmental collapse, and translational instability in the segment above the fusion. This will lead to decompensation and secondary kyphosis.
- Selecting T 10 as the upper instrumented vertebra in lumbar curves might be a good decision. Through its attachment to the rib cage, the T 10 vertebra is more stable, and some surgeons believe that fusing to T 10 will decrease the risk of adjacent-level disease compared to fusion that stops below.[6] On the other hand, it has been reported that fusion to T 11 or T 12 is acceptable when the upper instrumented vertebra is above the upper end of the curve.
- Fusion to the sacrum is indicated when there is preexisting pathology at the L 5–S 1 disk, such as spinal stenosis, spondylolisthesis, prior decompression, marked degenerative changes, and lumbosacral obliquity. The disadvantage of fusion to S 1 is the highly reported nonunion rate of up to 42% compared to only 4% following fusion to L 5.[7] To reduce the rate of pseudarthrosis at the lumbosacral junction, rigid anchorage to the sacrum and pelvis has been suggested. This includes wider and bicortical screws at S 1, the addition of sacral and alar screws, iliac screws, and S 2-alar-iliac screws. Anterior support either through an anterior approach or as posterior lumbar interbody fusion or transforaminal lumbar interbody fusion with a cage and bone graft will further increase the rigidity of the construct.
- Fusion to L 5 should be considered if the L 5–S 1 disk is healthy. It preserves a motion segment, the surgery is less demanding, and the likelihood of nonunion is decreased. On the other hand, excessive stresses are located at L 5–S 1 because it is a junction between two major rigid lever arms,

the pelvis and the instrumented spine.[8] Indeed, radiologic signs of L5–S1 disk degeneration have been reported in 58 to 61% of cases following fusion to the L5. Many of the patients were found symptomatic but L5–S1 disk degeneration was associated with less lordosis correction and increased risks of sagittal imbalance and reoperation.[8] The L5 is the natural lower fused vertebra in degenerative scoliosis since the apex of the curve is usually at L2–L4, and the L4–L5 disk is frequently degenerated. On the other hand, extension to the sacrum removes the last motion segment of the spine so there is less ability to compensate for improper realignment, the surgery is longer, and more extensive with greater blood loss and a higher pseudarthrosis rate, and there may be subsequent degeneration of the sacroiliac joints.

34.3 Spine with Mobile Disks

When the deformed spine segments include mobile disks, correction of the deformity might be achieved by positioning the patient in extension on the operating table and by adding posterior osteotomies to release the posterior elements. The osteotomies should be located at the most deformed segments, but if anterior ossification is present a more mobile cranial segment might be preferable.[9,10]

34.3.1 Two Main Surgical Techniques Described in This Category

Deformity correction of the spine with mobile disks is usually done with posterior osteotomies. The two main types of posterior osterotomies are the Smith-Petersen osteotomy and the Ponte osteotomy.

Smith-Petersen Osteotomy

In 1945, Smith-Petersen described a one- or two-level posterior column osteotomy for the goal of coronal and sagittal deformity correction through a posterior-only approach.[9] Its goal was to release a rigid kyphotic spine in patients with rheumatoid arthritis and ankylosing spondylitis. This is an extension osteotomy involving removal of the posterior ligaments, including the supraspinous, intraspinous, and ligamentum flavum, and removal of the facets. Correction of the sagittal curve through a single level is somewhat better compared with the later-described Ponte osteotomy. It includes shortening of the posterior column by closing the posterior gap through compression and lengthening the anterior column with a controlled release, or opening of the anterior structures using a cantilever technique. A symmetrical closure of the posterior gaps can correct some coronal imbalance as well. Smith-Petersen and some later surgeons performed this surgery in patients with ankylosing spondylitis.

Ponte Osteotomy

In 1984, Ponte described a posterior closing wedge osteotomy for the treatment of flexible Scheuermann's kyphosis.[11] The procedure includes removal of the ligamentum flavum, the inferior articular processes of the cephalad vertebra, and the superior articular processes of the caudal vertebra. Correction over multiple levels is achieved by sequential closure with gradual compression. As with the Smith-Petersen osteotomy (SPO), asymmetrical closure can also correct some coronal imbalance. The nerve roots should be checked after correction to exclude any impingement of the nerves in the intervertebral foramen. There are some basic points that should be considered when planning correction with posterior osteotomy. It has been found that about 1 mm of bone removal posteriorly correlates with about 1 degree of correction, and that the maximum correction possible following closure of the gap in both the SPO and Ponte osteotomies is approximately 5 to 15 degrees per level.[12]

The ideal patients for Ponte osteotomy are those with a type 1 sagittal deformity. These patients have a long, gradual, rounded kyphosis at multiple levels with a positive C7 plumb line in the range of 6 to 8 cm, such as in Scheuermann's kyphosis. Both SPO and Ponte osteotomies might also be suitable at the apex of rigid scoliosis, but greater global correction is expected with a more caudal osteotomy due to the longer lever arm.

Compared to pedicle subtraction osteotomy (PSO), which will be described later, SPO and the Ponte osteotomy are less demanding surgeries; they offer reduced operative time, less blood loss, and decreased rates of neurologic deficit. The osteotomy performed in SPO and Ponte osteotomies does not violate the anterior column, and the posterior gap created along several segments is small so that good bone apposition is achieved following closure of the gap. Thus anterior column support is not mandatory in these cases, and the rate of fusion following these procedures is very high.[13] SPO has a greater tendency toward coronal decompensation, especially if there is residual lumbar scoliosis with substantial rotation. Coronal imbalance is caused by the difference in radius of curvature between the convexity and the concavity. Asymmetric wedge resection—slightly bigger on the convexity—might prevent this coronal decompensation. Performing SPOs at neutral and stable vertebral segments has been suggested to prevent decompensation.

34.4 Spine with Decreased Disk Mobility

When the disks are fused or when a more aggressive approach is needed to correct the sagittal and coronal balance, the osteotomy should include not only the posterior column but also the vertebral bodies and the disks since posterior column release would be insufficient, and procedures aimed at gaining motion in the anterior column are needed.

The two main procedures described in this category are the PSO and vertebral column resection (VCR). Both are indicated in patients with an ankylosed spine either following surgery or due to ankylosing spondylitis and diffuse idiopathic skeletal hyperostosis. They are also indicated in patients with a type 2 sagittal deformity when the imbalance is greater than 12 cm.

34.4.1 Pedicle Subtraction Osteotomy

In 1985, Thomasen[14] described a three-column osteotomy pedicle subtraction osteotomy (PSO). The PSO was first described in correction of kyphotic deformity in patients with ankylosing spondylitis. This is a posteriorly based V-shaped resection that removes the posterior elements, including the lamina, ligaments, and pedicles, and it continues to the anterior column with removal of the central and lateral part of the vertebral body. It is an entirely bony resection, but for more aggressive correction the cephalad disk may be included with the resected bone. In the same year, Heinning[15] described a similar procedure in which intravertebral decancellation is performed, leaving the vertebral cortex as an eggshell instead of wedge resection of the entire width of the vertebral body. In both procedures, correction is achieved by closing the osteotomy. In cases of rigid and significant coronal deformity, both the coronal and sagittal curves can be addressed by asymmetric PSO with its base pointed more to the convex part of the curve. Another possibility for correcting the coronal component of the curve is compressing the convex side following PSO more than the concave side. Less sagittal correction is achieved following both the posterolateral-based PSO and asymmetric closure of the gap. In the latter, there is also less bone to bone contact. Unlike the Ponte osteotomy, where correction is hinged on the posterior column, or the SPO where the pivot is on the middle column, PSO obtains correction through an anterior cortical hinge with bone to bone contact. Hinging on the anterior cortex prevents lengthening the anterior column while correction is achieved through shortening of the posterior and middle columns. With this maneuver, the fusion potential is maximized while avoiding stretch on the major vessels and viscera anterior to the spine. PSO is a more powerful tool for correction of sagittal imbalance. It allows 30 to 40 degrees of segmental and 10 to 15 cm of global sagittal correction. It can be performed for thoracic deformity, but as with SPO and Ponte osteotomies the more distally it is performed the more correction is gained. Ideally the L3 or L4 should be the osteotomy site where the vertebral bodies are higher and the lever arm from C7 is longer.

The surgical technique includes exposure of the posterior elements up to the tip of the transverse processes. Pedicle screws are then inserted in at least two vertebrae above and two below the planed osteotomy level. Wide laminectomies at the level of the osteotomy and the vertebra above are performed. The nerve roots at the level of the osteotomy and the level above should be exposed bilaterally all the way lateral to the pedicles. The transverse process at the level of the osteotomy is resected, and the lateral border of the vertebral body from the disk above and the one below is released from the soft tissue. The segmental vessels are coagulated, and the pedicles of the osteotomized vertebra are resected down to the vertebral body. At this stage, we usually insert a temporary rod on one side while working on the contralateral side to prevent translation of the spine. A wedge osteotomy is then performed with the wide base posteriorly. The osteotomy lines should meet at a short distance from the anterior vertebral wall. At this stage of the surgery, we use fluoroscopy to ensure that the osteotomy line starts a short distance from the disks above and below and that the anterior cortex of the vertebral body is preserved. This is a crucial step since the anterior vertebral wall acts as a hinge through which the osteotomy is closed. An intact anterior wall will prevent translation during closure of the osteotomy. The dura is next released anteriorly from any adhesions. The posterior longitudinal ligament is incised, and the posterior wall of the vertebral body is pushed into the cavity with reverse curettes or similar instruments. The osteotomy site is then closed over the rods by compressing the screws above and below the osteotomy and by bending the rods in situ. Some companies have developed special instruments to achieve safe closure of the wedge while maintaining the integrity of the anterior vertebral wall. Prior to closure of the osteotomy site, the gap created should be checked for any bone fragments in the cavity that might prevent closure of the cavity. After closure of the gap, the dural sac and nerve roots should be checked to exclude dural buckling or nerve impingement.

At the end of surgery, the cancellous bone obtained from the osteotomy is used for posterolateral fusion, but the main concern is with the gap created at the osteotomy site. Many solutions have been suggested to bridge this gap, such as cortical allografts with the shape of the letter H, a rib graft, or three cortical grafts, but the rate of failure with readmitted patients due to breakage of the rods secondary to nonunion at the osteotomy level is high. To solve this problem we now include several steps:

- We exchange the rods used while performing in situ bending with a new one that is shaped according to the new curve of the spine in order to prevent sharp angles that weaken the rods.
- We use at least one rigid rod.
- We add two additional small rods connected to each long rod at the osteotomy level (▶ Fig. 34.1d).
- We aim for interbody fusion above and below the osteotomy. This can be done with an anterior cage, but we have found it is safe to perform it with a transforaminal lumbar interbody fusion.

PSO is technically challenging and is prone to complications, but the long-term follow-up shows satisfactory clinical and radiologic outcomes. In Kim et al's study,[16] 35 patients were followed for more than 5 years. Some worsening of the SVA was noted with time, and 29% had pseudarthrosis that was revised after 2 to 5 years. At follow-up, 87% reported their satisfaction level as being very good, 76% reported a good self-image, 69% reported good function, and 66% had fair pain subscales. Radiographically no significant regional radiologic changes were found between the postoperative second year and final follow-up. Better results were associated with SVA that was less than 8 cm at final follow-up.

Bone–Disk–Bone Osteotomy

In a bond–disk–bone osteotomy (BDBO), the area of bone resection during the osteotomy is extended to include the disk with its adjacent end plates. For even more extensive correction, both disks and the adjacent end plates are resected. Depending on the extent of resection, up to 47 to 60 degrees of correction can be achieved following these procedures compared to 35 degrees on average with PSO. These extensive osteotomies are indicated in severe sagittal curves where correction following PSO is not enough to balance the spine and when the disk above or below the osteotomized vertebra is the apex of the curve. The amount of correction achieved approaches the rates of VCR without the need to sacrifice nerve roots.[17]

With BDBO, the potential risk of nonunion with rod breakage and loss of correction is decreased compared to that with PSO. In PSO, the movable disks above and below the osteotomy are left intact. This increases the stress along the rods. BDBO is a bone to bone contact procedure with the upper and lower screws closer to the osteotomized area, thereby increasing the stability of the construct and reducing the risk for pseudarthrosis.

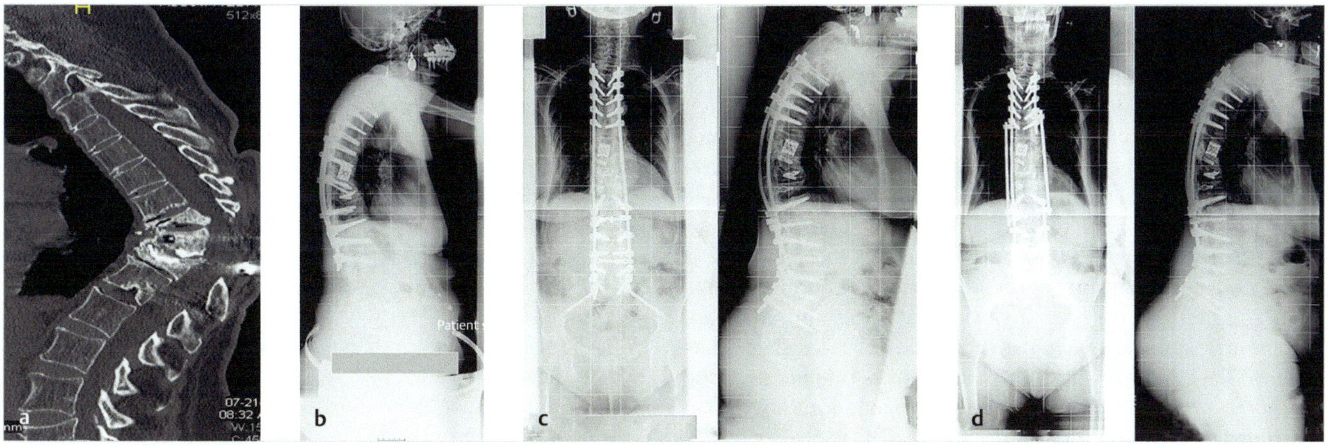

Fig. 34.1 (a) A-68-year-old woman with severe painful upper back pain as a result of a T9 fracture with sagittal imbalance following cementation and T10–T12 posterior spine fusion for T11 osteoporotic fracture. (b) Painful fracture of the lower instrumented vertebra 7 months following vertebral column resection of T9 with T3–L3 fusion and anterior cage replacing the resected T9 vertebra. (c) Long fusion down to the sacrum with S2-alar-iliac screws was performed with good clinical and radiologic results. (d) One year later, painful loss of correction occurred following pseudarthrosis associated with rod breakage and loss of correction. Two additional rods were used to bridge the broken rods. The fusion mass was reinforced with iliac autograft, demineralized bone, and bone morphogenetic protein with good clinical and radiologic results.

The surgical technique is similar to PSO. Since more bone is resected, the stability of the construct should be increased by adding more instrumented pedicles with at least three vertebra below and above the osteotomy site. The wide laminectomies should include the vertebrae above and below the disk space in the area planned for resection. In BDBO, the anterior column is significantly shortened so an anterior cage can be placed anteriorly through the same approach or through an anterior approach before compression in order to preserve the length of the anterior column.

Vertebral Column Resection

Compared to the previously described procedures VCR provides the greatest degree of correction, with more than 60% correction at the coronal plane and 45 to 72% in the sagittal plane.[13,18] It enables manipulation of the spine in every direction, controlling both the anterior and posterior columns of the deformed spine, all through one approach. It is a highly demanding procedure with a high potential for neurologic complications and is reserved for severe rigid multiplanar deformities, sharp congenital deformities, and posttraumatic angulated deformities and when resection of the whole vertebral body is indicated as with spondyloptosis, hemivertebra, and spinal tumors (▶ Fig. 34.1a, b). The procedure involves complete resection of the posterior elements posteriorly and the vertebral body with its adjacent disks anteriorly. It can be performed as a combined anterior and posterior procedure or through an all-posterior approach.[13,19] The all-posterior approach has gained popularity since it enables translational and rotational correction of the spinal column with controlled manipulation of both the anterior and posterior columns simultaneously through a single approach.

The first surgical steps are identical to those described with PSO and BDBO. Following pedicle screw insertion, usually three above and below the vertebra to be removed, a wide laminectomy and complete exposure and release of the nerve roots is performed. In the thoracic spine, the nerve roots are ligated and incised at the level of vertebral resection. This enables access to the lateral walls of the vertebral body. The rib heads and about 5 cm of the ribs are resected bilaterally. Careful subperiosteal dissection is performed along the lateral and down to the anterior wall of the vertebra. At this stage, a temporary rod is connected to the screws on one side to prevent vertebral translation. On the opposite side (usually the convex side), the disks above and below the planned resection level are removed, followed by piecemeal removal of the pedicle and vertebral body. The same surgical steps are carried out on the other side following replacement of the temporary rod to the contralateral side. The anterior longitudinal ligament with a slice of bone connected to it is preserved as a barrier from the great vessels anteriorly and as a safety measure to prevent vertebral translation. As with PSO, a reverse curette or similar curved instrument is used to push the remaining posterior vertebral wall into the gap. A cage filled with autologous bone from the resected vertebra is placed anteriorly to provide an anterior support. The cage should be similar in length to the gap created following the vertebrectomy in order to prevent neurologic deficit due to excessive shortening of the vertebral column. In the thoracic spine, the cage can be inserted posterolaterally since there is enough room following resection of the nerve roots. In the lumbar spine, ligation of the nerve roots has serious neurologic consequences so the cage should be placed through a second anterior approach, or posteriorly with an elongated cage. The spinal canal is checked to ensure that there is no residual bone or disk tissue anterior to the dura, and a second rod is then placed. Deformity correction is performed gradually by compression and in situ contouring over the anteriorly placed cage. The correction should be done under neurologic monitoring. As with PSO we usually replace these rods with new countered rods and connect them to two shorter rods that bridge the osteotomy site.

34.5 Complications

Spinal osteotomies are extensive and complex procedures. Most patients are in the more advanced age group, many of them with serious comorbidities and poor bone quality so it is not surprising that these long surgeries are associated with a high rate of complications. An increase of 10% in the mortality rate has been reported among individuals 80 years of age and older who had extensive thoracolumbar spinal fusion.[20]

The postoperative complications can be divided into major and minor complications. The major complications primarily include pulmonary complications (pneumonia, pulmonary embolism, and respiratory failure), then renal, cardiac, gastrointestinal problems; neurologic deficits; dural tears; and superficial and deep wound infection. Minor complications include ileus, transient delirium, and urinary tract infection. Risk factors for developing major complications have been identified as advanced age, sagittal deformity, preoperative kyphosis, long fusion constructs, three or more medical comorbidities, excessive blood loss, and revision surgery. Cho et al reported that the overall complication rate was 68% in 47 patients with degenerative lumbar scoliosis and an average age of 66.6 years following decompression and fusion with pedicular screws. This was composed of 30% early perioperative complications and 38% late complications. By excluding minor complications, the complication rate decreased to 55%.[21] The overall incidence of major complications following VCR was 42%, similar to those who underwent posterior spinal fusion.[22]

Analysis of the Scoliosis Research Society morbidity and mortality database focused on 578 patients with rigid sagittal deformity undergoing surgery found a 29% complication rate. They had a higher complication rate than those who had undergone other surgical procedures. As the level of complexity increases, so does the complication risk. There was an increase in complication rates from no osteotomy (17.0%), to SPO (28.1%), to PSO (39.1%), to VCR (61.1%).[23]

Several studies have shown a direct relation between the length of fusion and the risk of major complications, but Daubs et al found that once a procedure extends to at least a five-level fusion, the addition of more fusion levels did not significantly increase the complication rate or hospital stay and had no effect on the outcomes.[24]

Infection is another major risk in all spine surgeries. Intravenous prophylactic antibiotics should be used. We routinely use normal saline irrigation mixed with first-generation cephalosporin. It seems that this practice has lowered our infection rate.

Superior mesenteric artery syndrome is a rare condition of gastric outlet obstruction that results from extrinsic compression of the third portion of the duodenum between the superior mesenteric artery anteriorly and the aorta and spine posteriorly. It is a rare condition with a reported incidence of less than 1% following spinal deformity correction surgery.

34.5.1 Early Complications

As in any spinal procedure, major neurologic problems can occur, especially when there is manipulation of the foraminal space, retraction of the thecal sac or nerve roots, and elongation or shortening of the spinal column. Neurologic complications generally result from either contusion or an ischemic insult and sometimes from both. Ischemic insult can be the result of stretching of an important spinal cord blood vessel during correction, prolonged hypotension, and ligation of the anterior segmental arteries.

Besides contusion or ischemia, there may be unrecognized intraspinal pathology within the deformity, such as an unrecognized Chiari malformation with secondary hydromyelia, or tethered cord, both of which add unanticipated risk to the surgical correction. To exclude such anomalies, we routinely perform preoperative “all spine MRI” for every patient.

In the SPO, closure of the wedge posteriorly opens the disk space anteriorly. There is a concern that this could result in injury of the major vessels, particularly the abdominal aorta. Mainly at risk are patients with ankylosing spondylitis. Specific to the SPO are complications such as intraspinal hematoma, intestinal obstruction, and superior mesenteric artery syndrome.

The reported incidence of neurologic deficits following PSO is in the range of 3.6 to 15% and is higher, with 2 to 27% of patients following VCR.[25,26,27,28] It is most likely caused by either direct insult during decompression and bone resection, nerve distraction following curve correction, or from subluxation, residual dorsal impingement of bone fragments or the posterior longitudinal ligament, dural buckling, or a combination of these. In most of the cases, some if not complete recovery is expected. The deficits are usually unilateral and never proximal to the osteotomy; they often do not correspond to the level of osteotomy and are not detected by neuromonitoring.[27] Therefore, it is important to perform proper inspection of the spinal cord and nerve roots prior to and during closure of the osteotomy to detect any subluxation or bone spikes that might impinge on neural structures and if necessary enlarge the central canal and intervertebral foramen. A wake-up test following closure of the osteotomy should be considered, and prompt motor function evaluation should be performed following surgery.

Major blood loss defined as blood loss over 4 L was reported in 24% (range 0–66%) of 423 patients in eight centers following VCR. It was more common in patients 60 years or older, in those who had revision surgery, or when more than one osteotomy was performed. In these patients, major blood loss was associated with longer operative times and a higher risk of developing intra- and postoperative complications.[22] In PSO, there is substantial mobilization of the dura, and the blood loss is greater than that associated with the SPO.

Preoperative autologous blood donation, antifibrinolytic administration, and blood salvage with cell saver can be used to minimize the blood loss.

34.5.2 Late Complications

Late complications include adjacent segment disease, instrumentation failure, and pseudarthrosis. Adjacent segment disease might present as facet or disk degeneration leading to degenerative listhesis and spinal stenosis. In osteoporotic patients, fracture of the lower instrumented vertebra or the upper adjacent vertebra with proximal junctional kyphosis is the typical mode of failure (▶ Fig. 34.1b). It appears that the risks for adjacent segment disease are sagittal imbalance and facet joint injury during surgery.

Instrumentation failure results from screw loosening, pullout, or fatigue fractures of the screws or rods at the most distal and proximal part of the fixation. According to our experience there is a different mode of failure in the normal and osteoporotic spine. In the osteoporotic bone, the screw usually comes out, whereas in the normal bone, fatigue fractures of the construct are more frequently seen. For the proximal screws, cement augmentation may reduce the risk of screw loosening, whereas cementation of the adjacent vertebra might prevent fracture of the vertebra in the osteoporotic spine. Caustal screw loosening is common in patients with sagittal imbalance, mainly at the L5 vertebra. To prevent failure of fixation in the distal part of the instrumentation, we usually extend the fixation in long constructs to the sacrum and ileum, usually with S2 alar screws, and add anterior L5–S1 support with a cage (▶ Fig. 34.1c, d).

Pseudarthrosis most commonly occurs at L5–S1 when fused to the sacrum, but it also occurs at the thoracolumbar or cervicothoracic junctions. Risk factors for pseudarthrosis include older age, thoracolumbar kyphosis of more than 20 degrees, decreased lumbar lordosis, and sagittal imbalance. A prospective multicenter study with a minimum of 1-year follow-up assessed the rates and risk factors of rod fracture following surgery for adult spinal deformity. It was found in 18 of 200 patients (9%) at a mean of 14.7 months (range 3–27 months).[29] Twelve of the 18 patients with rod fracture had undergone revision surgery in which pseudarthrosis was confirmed intraoperatively. PSO is associated with a significantly higher rate of rod fracture compared with cases in which a PSO is not performed. The rate of rod fracture following PSO was 22%. In 10 of the 11 cases of rod fractures the fractures occurred at or adjacent to the level of the osteotomy.

Placement of interbody spacers adjacent to the osteotomized level and use of either unilateral or bilateral satellite rods did not demonstrate a significant reduction in the rate of rod fracture.

Restoration of sagittal imbalance is critical in order to improve clinical outcome. A higher pelvic incidence angle and larger pelvic tilt are associated with sagittal decompensation due to insufficient correction, since in these patients a higher degree of correction of lumbar lordosis is needed. The degree of lumbar lordosis correction should exceed the measured pelvic incidence by 7 to 10 degrees. To reduce the risk of mechanical complications related to the instrumentation, we now use a multirod construct, usually bilateral satellite rods. We try to get closure of the osteotomy with bone-to-bone contact, sometimes with an **H**-shaped autograft.

34.6 Conclusion

Global sagittal balance is a significant predictor of the clinical status of patients with adult deformity. Restoration of the sagittal balance was found to decrease the rate of subsequent pseudarthrosis and is associated with better clinical results. To achieve good sagittal balance it is necessary in rigid curves with a severe Cobb angle, coronal imbalance, and sagittal imbalance to perform osteotomy of the vertebral column. The surgical planning should aim to restore the lumbar lordosis to match and exceed the pelvic incidence angle with a pelvic tilt of less than 25 degrees.

The goal of surgery is not only to relieve pain and correct deformity but also to minimize complications related to surgery, as the incidence of complications is relatively high. According to the amount of correction needed the extent of surgery may range from posterior osteotomies to PSO and up to complete resection of a vertebral body. Longer fusions with extensive osteotomies are prone to general complications including significant blood loss, neurologic complications and higher rate of reoperations. The more extensive the osteotomy is and the longer the fusion is the higher is the likelihood of blood loss and neurologic and general complication and the higher is the rate of reoperations. Accordingly, surgeons should attempt to seek a trade-off between the benefits of surgery and the risks of complications. One should consider the patient's general condition, not just that of the spine, when choosing surgical options.

Despite the extensive surgery and the high rate of complications most of these patients are satisfied with the results. We often tell patients that they should expect a long path to recovery, but when they ultimately overcome all the complications they will most likely be satisfied with the results.

References

[1] Glassman SD, Bridwell K, Dimar JR, Horton W, Berven S, Schwab F. The impact of positive sagittal balance in adult spinal deformity. Spine. 2005; 30 (18):2024–2029

[2] Lafage V, Bharucha NJ, Schwab F, et al. Multicenter validation of a formula predicting postoperative spinopelvic alignment. J Neurosurg Spine. 2012; 16 (1):15–21

[3] Aebi M. The adult scoliosis. Eur Spine J. 2005; 14(10):925–948

[4] Bridwell KH. Selection of instrumentation and fusion levels for scoliosis: where to start and where to stop. Invited submission from the Joint Section Meeting on Disorders of the Spine and Peripheral Nerves, March 2004. J Neurosurg Spine. 2004; 1(1):1–8

[5] Diebo BG, Henry J, Lafage V, Berjano P. Sagittal deformities of the spine: factors influencing the outcomes and complications. Eur Spine J. 2015; 24 Suppl 1:S3–S15

[6] Shufflebarger H, Suk SI, Mardjetko S. Debate: determining the upper instrumented vertebra in the management of adult degenerative scoliosis: stopping at T10 versus L1. Spine. 2006; 31(19) Suppl:S185–S194

[7] Edwards CC, II, Bridwell KH, Patel A, et al. Thoracolumbar deformity arthrodesis to L5 in adults: the fate of the L5-S1 disc. Spine. 2003; 28(18):2122–2131

[8] Boachie-Adjei O, Gupta MC. Adult scoliosis + deformity. AAOS Instructional Course Lectures. 1999; 48:377–391

[9] Smith-Petersen MN, Larson CB, Aufranc OE. Osteotomy of the spine for correction of flexion deformity in rheumatoid arthritis. Clin Orthop Relat Res. 1969; 66(66):6–9

[10] La Marca F, Brumblay H. Smith-Petersen osteotomy in thoracolumbar deformity surgery. Neurosurgery. 2008; 63(3) Suppl:163–170

[11] Ponte A, Vero B, Siccardi GL. Surgical treatment of Scheuermann's hyperkyphosis. In: Winter R, ed. Progress in Spinal Pathology: Kyphosis. Bologna, Italy: Aulo Gaggi; 1984:75–81

[12] Geck MJ, Macagno A, Ponte A, Shufflebarger HL. The Ponte procedure: posterior only treatment of Scheuermann's kyphosis using segmental posterior shortening and pedicle screw instrumentation. J Spinal Disord Tech. 2007; 20 (8):586–593

[13] Suk SI, Chung ER, Kim JH, Kim SS, Lee JS, Choi WK. Posterior vertebral column resection for severe rigid scoliosis. Spine. 2005; 30(14):1682–1687

[14] Thomasen E. Vertebral osteotomy for correction of kyphosis in ankylosing spondylitis. Clin Orthop Relat Res. 1985; 194(194):142–152

[15] Heinning CA. Eggshell procedure. In: Luque ER, ed. Segmental Spinal Instrumentation. Thorofare, NJ: Slack; 1984:221–230

[16] Kim YJ, Bridwell KH, Lenke LG, Cheh G, Baldus C. Results of lumbar pedicle subtraction osteotomies for fixed sagittal imbalance: a minimum 5-year follow-up study. Spine. 2007; 32(20):2189–2197

[17] Domanic U, Talu U, Dikici F, Hamzaoglu A. Surgical correction of kyphosis: posterior total wedge resection osteotomy in 32 patients. Acta Orthop Scand. 2004; 75(4):449–455

[18] Hamzaoglu A, Alanay A, Ozturk C, Sarier M, Karadereler S, Ganiyusufoglu K. Posterior vertebral column resection in severe spinal deformities: a total of 102 cases. Spine. 2011; 36(5):E340–E344

[19] Lenke LG, O'Leary PT, Bridwell KH, Sides BA, Koester LA, Blanke KM. Posterior vertebral column resection for severe pediatric deformity: minimum two-year follow-up of thirty-five consecutive patients. Spine. 2009; 34(20):2213–2221

[20] Cloyd JM, Acosta FL, Jr, Cloyd C, Ames CP. Effects of age on perioperative complications of extensive multilevel thoracolumbar spinal fusion surgery. J Neurosurg Spine. 2010; 12(4):402–408

[21] Cho KJ, Suk SI, Park SR, et al. Complications in posterior fusion and instrumentation for degenerative lumbar scoliosis. Spine. 2007; 32(20):2232–2237

[22] Bianco K, Norton R, Schwab F, et al. International Spine Study Group. Complications and intercenter variability of three-column osteotomies for spinal deformity surgery: a retrospective review of 423 patients. Neurosurg Focus. 2014; 36(5):E18

[23] Smith JS, Sansur CA, Donaldson WF, III, et al. Short-term morbidity and mortality associated with correction of thoracolumbar fixed sagittal plane deformity: a report from the Scoliosis Research Society Morbidity and Mortality Committee. Spine. 2011; 36(12):958–964

[24] Daubs MD, Lenke LG, Cheh G, Stobbs G, Bridwell KH. Adult spinal deformity surgery: complications and outcomes in patients over age 60. Spine. 2007; 32 (20):2238–2244

[25] Yang BP, Ondra SL, Chen LA, Jung HS, Koski TR, Salehi SA. Clinical and radiographic outcomes of thoracic and lumbar pedicle subtraction osteotomy for fixed sagittal imbalance. J Neurosurg Spine. 2006; 5(1):9–17

[26] Ahn UM, Ahn NU, Buchowski JM, et al. Functional outcome and radiographic correction after spinal osteotomy. Spine. 2002; 27(12):1303–1311

[27] Buchowski JM, Bridwell KH, Lenke LG, et al. Neurologic complications of lumbar pedicle subtraction osteotomy: a 10-year assessment. Spine. 2007; 32 (20):2245–2252

[28] Lenke LG, Newton PO, Sucato DJ, et al. Complications after 147 consecutive vertebral column resections for severe pediatric spinal deformity: a multicenter analysis. Spine. 2013; 38(2):119–132

[29] Smith JS, Shaffrey E, Klineberg E, et al. International Spine Study Group. Prospective multicenter assessment of risk factors for rod fracture following surgery for adult spinal deformity. J Neurosurg Spine. 2014; 21(6):994–1003

Index

Note: Page numbers set **bold** or *italic* indicate headings or figures, respectively.

2

22q11 deletion syndrome 77

A

Achondroplasia 78
Active bending, in rigid spinal deformities 34
Active forces 33
Adams technique, for posterior column osteotomy 22
Adjacent segment disease 280
Adolescent idiopathic scoliosis (AIS) 190
- anterior approach for adult deformity in **256**, *258*
- early-onset scoliosis versus 84
- nonidiopathic scoliosis versus 108
- proximal junctional kyphosis in 228
- severe
-- anterior release with open thoracotomy for 110
-- combined anterior posterior release for 110
-- computed tomography of 108
-- definition of **108**
-- definitive instrumentation in **117**
-- derotation in **116**
-- distraction timing in 116
-- first posterior surgery for **114**
-- halo traction for *109*, *110*, 111, *113*
-- intraoperative spinal cord monitoring in **114**, 116
-- magnetically controlled growing rods for 111, **113**, **116**, *117*
-- mini-laminotomy technique for **114**
-- pedicle entry point in **114**
-- pedicle screws for **111**, *112*, **114**
-- physical examination in 108
-- pitfalls and difficulties in surgical management of **108**
-- posterior release in *115*
-- posterior staged technique for **111**
-- posterior-only approaches for **110**, 111, *113*
-- preferred operative technique for **111**
-- preoperative study of **108**
-- radiologic study of 108
-- screw placement in **114**
-- second stage of posterior surgery in **116**, *117*
-- surgical treatment of **110**
-- thoracoplasty in **117**
-- vertebral column resection for 110
- spinal osteotomies for **22**
-- complications of **26–27**
-- PCO versus PSO **26**
-- pedicle subtraction **23**, *115*
-- posterior column **22**
-- preoperative considerations in **26**
- spinal rigidity in 84
Adult degenerative scoliosis
- decreased disk mobility with **277**
- fusion levels in, selection of **276**
- mobile disks with **277**
- osteotomies for **276**
-- bone-disk-bone **278**
-- complications of **279**
-- pedicle subtraction 277, *279*
-- Ponte **277**
-- Smith-Petersen **277**
- vertebral column resection for 277, **279**
Adult spinal deformity **190**, **252**
- *See also* specific types
- anterior approach for **251**
-- access to lower lumbar spine in **252**
-- case studies of **256**, *257–258*
-- classification of **191**
-- comparative studies of **256**
-- complications of **255**
-- in tuberculosis 261
-- neurologic injury in 255
-- pain in 252
-- reconstruction of lower lumbar spine and lumbosacral junction in **252**
-- release in thoracolumbar kyphoscoliosis **254**, 256, *257*
-- restoration of anterior column support in **253**, **256**, *258*
-- restoration of lumbosacral segmental sagittal alignment in **253**, **256**, *258*
-- surgical goals in 251
-- vascular anatomy in 253
-- vascular injury in 255
-- visceral injury in 255
Aebi classification **191**
Airway assessment **204**
AIS, *see* Adolescent idiopathic scoliosis
Allograft bone **247**
Anesthesia **203**
- airway assessment for **204**
- bispectral index monitoring with **205**
- blood pressure monitoring with 206
- induction and maintenance of **205**
- neurophysiologic monitoring with 203, **205**
- postoperative management of **207**
- preexisting conditions and **203**
- preoperative assessment for **203**
- wake-up test and **207**
Angular balance parameters **221**, *222*
Ankylosing spinal disorders **176**
- *See also* specific disorders
Ankylosing spondylitis (AS) 176
- clinical presentation of 176
- etiology of 176
- pathogenesis of 176
- pedicle subtraction osteotomy for 23
- posterior column osteotomy for 22
- three-dimensional CT reconstruction of *176*
- with fracture **176**
-- cervical 177
-- posterior surgical approach for 178
-- thoracolumbar 177, *178*
-- treatment of 177
- with kyphotic deformity 176, *177*, **178**
-- cervical osteotomy for 180, *181*
-- loss of horizontal gaze in 178–179
-- lumbar osteotomy for 178
-- opening-wedge osteotomy for 178
-- pedicle subtraction osteotomy for 178, *179–180*
-- preoperative imaging/planning for 178, *179*
-- Smith-Petersen osteotomy for 178
-- surgical goals in 178
Anterior approach, for adult spinal deformities **251**
- access to lower lumbar spine in **252**
- case studies of **256**, *257–258*
- comparative studies of **256**
- complications of **255**
- in tuberculosis 261, 263
- neurologic injury in 255
- reconstruction of lower lumbar spine and lumbosacral junction in **252**
- release in thoracolumbar kyphoscoliosis **254**, 256, *257*
- restoration of anterior column support in **253**, **256**, *258*
- restoration of lumbosacral segmental sagittal alignment in **253**, **256**, *258*
- surgical goals in 251
- vascular anatomy in 253
- vascular injury in 255
- visceral injury in 255
Anterior column support, restoration of **253**, **256**, *258*
Anterior lateral interbody fusion 226
Anterior lumbar interbody fusion 252–253
Anterior retroperitoneal approach 252
Anterior superior iliac spine compression test 171
Anterior to psoas (ATP)/oblique lumbar interbody fusion 252
Anteroposterior discordance 2, *3*
Anteversion 225
Antifibrinolytics 207, 280
Apical vertebrectomy
- for neuromuscular spinal deformity 20
- for rigid spinal deformities **55**
Arthrogryposis 78
AS, *see* Ankylosing spondylitis
Autograft **245**
- cortical 245
- corticocancellous 245
- fusion rates with 246
Autologous blood donation 206–207, 280
Avascular necrosis, posttraumatic vertebral **122**
Axial loading, and spinal injury 121

B

Bamboo spine 176
Barrey ratio *221*, 222, 224
BDBO, *see* Bone-disk-bone osteotomy
Bending
- in rigid spinal deformities 34
- in thoracic insufficiency syndrome 58
Bilateral modified Salter osteotomy 172, *173*
Billot test 33–34
Bipedalism 223
Bispectral index (BIS) monitoring **205**
Bisphosphonates, for spinal fusion **248**
Block vertebrae 190
Blood conservation techniques **206**, 280
Blood pressure monitoring, in spinal surgery 206
Blood supply, spinal **203**
Bone grafts
- for pedicle subtraction osteotomy 278
- for spinal fusion
-- allograft **247**
-- autograft **245**
-- iliac crest, as gold standard 244–245
-- mechanical strength of 245
-- osteoconductive characteristics of 245
-- osteogenic characteristics of 245
-- osteoinductive characteristics of 245
-- properties of 245
-- selection of 244
-- synthetic **247**
-- types of **245**
Bone morphogenetic proteins **246**
Bone-disk-bone osteotomy (BDBO) 93, 185–186, **278**
Bone-Disk-Bone Osteotomy (BDBO) **81**
Boston-type thoracolumbosacral orthosis 16
Bracing
- for early-onset scoliosis **86**
- for idiopathic scoliosis 49
- for neuromuscular spinal deformities 16
- for Parkinson disease-related spinal deformities 135
Butterfly hemivertebra 2

C

C7 vertical tilt 222
Camptocormia 135, *136*
Cancellous autograft 245
Cardiovascular system, spinal surgery and **204**
Casting
- for early-onset scoliosis **86**
- for thoracic insufficiency syndrome **59**
CBVA, *see* Chin-brow vertical angle
Cell salvage 206–207, 280
Central venous pressure 206
Ceramic (synthetic) bone grafts **247**

Cerebral palsy, rigid spinal deformity in 77
Cervical deformities
- assessment and preoperative planning in **154**
- chin-brow vertical angle in 151, *152*
- clinical symptoms and natural history of **151**
- Cobb method in 152, 153
- computed tomography of 154
- corrective osteotomies for **151**
- curve rigidity and degree of deformity **155**
- functional disability and pain with 151
- Harrison posterior tangent method in 153
- Jackson physiological stress line method in 152
- location of *154*
- MRI of 153, *154*
- neck tilt in 153
- neurologic exam with 152
- neurologic status with **155**
- occiput-to-wall measure in 152
- osteotomy for
-- anterior **155**
-- closing-wedge 156
-- combined **157**
-- opening-wedge 156
-- pedicle subtraction 156
-- posterior **156**, *157*
-- types of **155**
- physical examination of **151**
- previous surgery and **155**
- radiographic evaluation of *152*, *153*
- sagittal vertical axis in 153
- T1 slope in 153
- thoracic inlet angle in 153
Cervical fractures, with ankylosing spondylitis 177
Cervicothoracic kyphotic deformity **160**
- anterior support in 161
- causes of 159–160
- corrective osteotomies for **159–160**
-- anterior opening/posterior closing 161
-- opening wedge 161
-- patient positioning for 160
-- patient preparation for **160**
-- pedicle subtraction 161, *162*
-- posterior closing-wedge 161
-- technical considerations in **160**
- preoperative evaluation of **159**
- rods for 161
- sublaminar wire fixation for 161
- vertebral column resection for 161
Cervicothoracic spondylitis, in pediatric tuberculosis 273
Charcot arthropathy of spine **121**
Chevron osteotomy 185
Children, *see* specific deformities and procedures
- congenital upper thoracic deformities and vertebral malformations in **39**
- early-onset scoliosis in **84**
- halo traction in **50**
- osteotomies in, in children under age 10 **49**
- rigid spinal deformities in **189**
-- classification of **191**
-- surgery for, in older children and adolescents **37**
-- surgery for, in young children **36**
- spinal tuberculosis in **271**
Chin-brow vertical angle (CBVA) 151, *152*
Circumferential vertebral column resection 63
Closing-opening-wedge osteotomy, for spinal tuberculosis **268**, *269*
Closing-wedge osteotomy 156
- *See also* specific types
- for cervicothoracic kyphotic deformity 161
- for congenital spinal deformities 63
- for posttraumatic spinel deformities 126
- for spinal tuberculosis, adult 263, *264*
- for spinal tuberculosis, pediatric *274*
Coffin-Lowry syndrome 78
Compensated balance *224*, 225
Complete facet joint resection **50**, *52*
Computed tomography 94
- *See also* specific disorders
Computed tomography myelography 94
Computer-assisted surgery, for sacropelvic pathologies **173**, *174*
Congenital spinal deformities **1**, **190**
- *See also* Congenital vertebral malformations, specific types
- classification of **191**
- definition of 1
Congenital vertebral malformations (CVMs) 1, 190
- *See also* specific types
- age of patient at diagnosis 3–4
- classification of 1
- epiphysiodesis for *6*, *7*
- hemivertebra resection for **6**, *8*
- imaging modalities for 1
- observation of **6**
- pedicle subtraction osteotomy for *8*, *9–10*
- perioperative considerations **4**
- prognosis of **3**
- rotation and rib distortion with 4
- site of anomaly in 3–4
- surgery for
-- decisions on **1**
-- image guidance for 4
-- patient positioning for 4
-- revision 5
- syndromes of 1
- tolerance for blood loss in 1
- treatment options and principles in **6**
- type of anomaly in 3
- upper thoracic deformities with, surgical management of children with **39**
- vascular anomalies with 4
- vertebral column decancellation for **11**
- vertebral column resection for **9**
Cord tethering, posttraumatic **122**
Coronal balance, *see* specific disorders
- radiologic assessment of 94
Coronal decompression 28
Coronal plane deformity, pure, type III osteotomy for **52**
Cortical autograft 245
Corticocancellous autograft 245
Cranial sagittal vertical axis (CrSVA) 221
Crankshaft phenomenon 33–34, 37, 87, 93, 184
CrSVA, *see* Cranial sagittal vertical axis
CVMs, *see* Congenital vertebral malformations

D

Decompensated balance *224*, 225
Degenerative scoliosis, adult
- decreased disk mobility with **277**
- fusion levels in, selection of **276**
- mobile disks with **277**
- osteotomies for **276**
-- bone-disk-bone **278**
-- complications of **279**
-- pedicle subtraction 277, *279*
-- Ponte **277**
-- Smith-Petersen **277**
- vertebral column resection for 277, **279**
Degenerative spine evolution **224**
- anteverted types 3 and 4 225
- classical types 225
- kyphotic types 225
- retroverted (or false) types 225
- type 1 225
- type 2 *226*
- type 3 *226*
- type 4 *227*
Demineralized bone matrix **246**
Derotation, in severe idiopathic scoliosis **116**
Diffuse idiopathic skeletal hyperostosis (DISH) 176
- clinical presentation of 180
- monastic way of life and 180, *182*
- morphological changes in *177*
- physical findings in 180
- with fracture **180**, *182*
DiGeorge syndrome 77
Direct lateral interbody fusion 252
DISH, *see* Diffuse idiopathic skeletal hyperostosis
Diskectomy, in vertebral column resection 9
Disks
- decreased mobility in **277**
- mobile **277**
Docking platforms, for robot-guided surgery 233
Donaldson-Stagnara distraction 34
Duchenne muscular dystrophy
- bone density in 80
- preoperative workup in 79
- rigid spinal deformity in 75
Dystrophic scoliosis 15

E

Early-onset scoliosis (EOS)
- casting and bracing for **86**
- classification of 84
- clinical and radiographic evaluation of **84**
- compression-based techniques for 86–87
- CT scan of *87*
- distraction techniques for 86–87
- extra measures for **90**, 91
- flexibility/rigidity criteria in 84
- growing rods for 86, **88**, *89*
-- magnetically controlled 86, **88**
- growth-friendly techniques for 85–87
- growth-guided systems for 86–87
- halo traction in 85, **90**
- hemiepiphysiodesis for 86, **88**
- history and physical examination in **84**
- idiopathic, treatment algorithm for 85, *86*
- imaging system/three-dimensional modeling techniques for **85**
- Luque trolley for 86, **88**
- MRI of **85**, *87*
- nonoperative management of 85
- operative management of **86**
- osteotomies for 85, **91**
- plain radiographs of **85**, *87*
- possibility or proof of progression in 85
- posterior instrumentation without fusion for **88**, *89*
- resolution versus progression of 84
- rigid spine deformities in **84**
- Shilla system for 86, **89**
- spinal fusion and posterior instrumentation with and without anterior release for **88**
- spinal fusion for 86, *87*, *90*
- temporary internal distraction rods for 85, 88, **91**
- treatment goals in 84
- treatment of **85**
- vertical expandable prosthetic titanium rib for 86, **88**
Eggshell procedure 11, 23, **54**
- *See also* Pedicle subtraction osteotomy
Electromyography, intraoperative 67, **212**
Elementectomy, posterior **50**, *52*
Enlargement effect, in X-rays 222
Enneking classification, of spinal tumors 138–139, 148
EOS, *see* Early-onset scoliosis
Epiphysiodesis *6*, *7*
Evoked potentials 203, 205
- in posterior vertebral column resection 67
- in revision surgery 184
- in severe idiopathic scoliosis procedures **114**
- in syndromic rigid spine surgery 80, 82
Expandable pedicle screws 131
External passive forces 33
Extreme lateral interbody fusion 252

F

Facet joint resection
- complete **50**, *52*
- partial **50**
Factor VII, recombinant 207
Failed instrumentation, secondary correction after **93**
- *See also* Revision surgery
Flatback syndrome 123, 159, 242
Flexion injuries 121
Flexion-extension radiography 94

Fractures
- ankylosing spondylitis with **176**, *177–178*
- DISH with **180**
- osteoporotic 130
-- *See also* Osteoporotic rigid spine deformities
- pelvic 170
- traumatic 120
-- *See also* Posttraumatic spine deformity

Fulcrum, in rigid spinal deformities 34

G

Galveston technique 18, 104
GAP score 253
Gastrointestinal problems, with neuromuscular spinal deformity 13, 17
Global alignment and proportion score (GAP) 253
Global kyphosis shape 225
Global tilt (GT) 222
Grade 1 osteotomies 123, 185
Grade 2 osteotomies 123, 185
Grade 3 osteotomies 123, 185, *186*
Grade 4 osteotomies 52, 123, 185, **186**
Grade 5 osteotomies 123, 185, **186**, *187*
Grade 6 osteotomies 123, 185, **186**
Growing rods
- for early-onset scoliosis 86, **88**, *89*
- for idiopathic scoliosis
-- in children under age 10 49
-- severe adolescent 111, **113**, **116**, *117*
- for neuromuscular scoliosis 20
- for thoracic insufficiency syndrome 59
- magnetically controlled 86, **88**, **113**, **116**, *117*

Growth inhibition 2
Growth-sparing techniques
- for early-onset scoliosis 85–87
- for idiopathic scoliosis, in children under age 10 49
- for neuromuscular spinal deformity **20**
- for thoracic insufficiency syndrome 59

GT, *see* Global tilt

H

Halo traction
- complications with **50**
- contraindications to **91**
- in children under age 10 **50**
- in congenital spinal deformities 5
- in early-onset scoliosis 85, **90**
- in patients with neurologic deficits 63, **64**, *67*, 69, *71*
- in rigid spinal deformities 34, **50**
- in severe idiopathic scoliosis *109*, *110*, 111, *113*
- indications for **90**
- long-term 50
- management of 50, *51*
- placement technique for **50**

Halo-femoral traction 91
Halo-tibial traction 91
Hand-dependent sitters 13
Hanging radiographs, in thoracic insufficiency syndrome 58
Harrington instrumentation, for neuromuscular scoliosis 18
Hemiepiphysiodesis 86, **88**
Hemilamina 2
Hemivertebra (HV) 2, 190
- anterior 1
- anteroposterior discordance or dissociated 2, *3*
- butterfly 2
- double, with unilateral bar 3
- epiphysiodesis for **6**
- fully segmented 2–3
- kyphosis and kyphoscoliosis with 4
- lateral-sided 1
- nonsegmented or incarcerated 2, 4
- observation of **6**
- posterior 1
- semisegmented 2, 4
- unilateral unsegmented 3
- upper thoracic 39–40, 43–44

Hemivertebra resection **6**
- advantages and indications for 6
- fluoroscopy in 7
- posterior approach in *8*
- thoracic 7

Hemodilution 206
Hibbs-Ferguson technique, for posterior osteotomy 50
Hip joint, preoperative examination of 94
Hongkong surgery *274*
Hook fixation
- in osteoporotic rigid spinal deformities 132
- in upper thoracic congenital deformities 41, 44–45

Horizontal gaze, loss of 178–179
Hover-T Frame (HVT) 233
Howarth technique, for posterior osteotomy 50
Hurler's disease 77
HV, *see* Hemivertebra
HVT, *see* Hover-T Frame
Hydroxyapatite-coated titanium pedicle screws 131
Hyperkyphosis
- neuromuscular disorders and 13–14
- pure, type I osteotomy for **51**

Hyperlordosis
- neuromuscular disorders and 13–14, 18
- type II osteotomy for **52**

I

ICBG, *see* Iliac crest bone graft
Idiopathic spinal deformities **190**
- *See also* Adolescent idiopathic scoliosis
- classification of **191**
- spinal osteotomies for **22**
-- complications of **26–27**
-- in children under age 10 **49**
-- PCO versus PSO **26**
-- pedicle subtraction **23**, *115*
-- posterior column **22**
-- preoperative considerations in **26**

Iliac crest bone graft (ICBG) 244–245
Iliac osteotomy 172, *173*
Iliac wing compression test 171
Inflammatory phase, in spinal fusion 244
Inflexion point 223
Instrumentation failure 280
Interbody fusion 226, 252

J

Junctional deformities
- causes of 159
- corrective osteotomies for **159**
- preoperative evaluation of **159**

K

King classification **191**
Knee joint, preoperative examination of 94
Kümmell disease **122**, **216**
Kyphectomy, in spina bifida (myelomeningocele) 15, **102**
- outcome of *105*, *106*
- patient positioning for 103
- preoperative checklist for 103
- preoperative imaging for *104*
- prerequisites for 102
- surgical technique of **103**, *104–105*

Kyphoscoliosis
- congenital 1, **4**
- multiplanar, type IV osteotomy for *53*
- neurofibromatosis and 15
- neuromuscular 14
- rigid 33
- secondary correction of **95**, *97*
- thoracolumbar, anterior release for **254**, 256, *257*

Kyphosis
- ankylosing spondylitis with **178**
- cervical 151
-- *See also* Cervical deformities
- congenital 1, **4**
-- blood supply compromise with 4
-- type 1 (anterior failure of formation) 4
-- type 2 (anterior or anterolateral failure of segmentation) 4
-- type 3 (mixed anomalies) 4
- in normal populations 223
- in spinal tuberculosis 261
-- during acute phase **261**, *262*
-- pathophysiology of **261**
-- surgical techniques for 263
-- surgical treatment of **262**
- junctional 159
- local, degenerative spine evolution and 224
- neurofibromatosis and 15
- neuromuscular 13–14
- posttraumatic (Kümmell disease) **122**, **216**
- proximal junctional **228**
- pure, type I osteotomy for **51**
- rigid 33
- secondary correction of **96**, *97–98*
- spina bifida and 15
- thoracic, definition of 219
- with myelomeningocele 102

L

La Chapelle technique, for posterior column osteotomy 22
Laminectomy defect, reconstruction of **98**, *100*
Late remodeling phase, of spinal fusion 244
Lateral lumbar interbody fusion 252
Lenke classification 22, 108, **191**
Lordoscoliosis, secondary correction of **97**, *98–99*
Lordosis 219
- in normal populations 223
- lumbar 221
-- definition of 219
-- measurement of *219–220*
- secondary correction of **97**, *98–99*
- spinal 220
-- lower 220
-- superior 220

Lower lumbar spine
- access to **252**
- reconstruction **252**

Lower motor neuron 13
Lower spinal lordosis (LSL) 220
LSL, *see* Lower spinal lordosis
Lumbar kyphosis shape 225
Lumbar lordosis 221
- definition of 219
- measurement of 219–*220*

Lumbar osteotomy 178
Lumbar spine, lower
- access to **252**
- reconstruction of **252**

Lumbosacral junction reconstruction **252**
Lumbosacral kyphotic deformity
- causes of 159
- corrective osteotomies for **159**, **165**
-- patient positioning for 166
-- patient preparation for **166**
-- pedicle subtraction 166, *168*
-- revision rates in 167
-- Smith-Petersen 166
-- technical considerations in **166**
-- transdiskal wedge 167
- preoperative evaluation of **159**
- vertebral column resection for 166–167

Lumbosacral segmental sagittal alignment, restoration of **253**, **256**, *258*
Luque principle 18
Luque trolley 49, 86, **88**

M

Magnetic resonance imaging 94
- *See also* specific disorders

Magnetically controlled growing rods
- for early-onset scoliosis 86, **88**
- for severe idiopathic scoliosis **113**, **116**, *117*

Marfan syndrome 76
Margerl/AO thoracolumbar classification 121
McMaster-Bradford technique, for posterior column osteotomy 22
MDB, *see* Multidirectional Bridge
Meiss technique, for posterior column osteotomy 22
Meningocele 102
Metric balance parameters *221*

Middle reparative phase, of spinal fusion 244
Mini-laminotomy technique **114**
Mobile disks **277**
Modulation techniques, for neuromuscular spinal deformity **20**
Motor evoked potentials, *see* Transcranial motor evoked potentials
Mucopolysaccharidoses 77, 79–80
Multidirectional Bridge (MDB) 233, *234*
Myelomeningocele
- kyphectomy in patients with 15, **102**
-- outcome of *105*, *106*
-- patient positioning for 103
-- preoperative checklist for 103
-- preoperative imaging for *104*
-- prerequisites for 102
-- surgical technique of **103**, *104–105*
- spinal deformity with *15*
Myelopathy, deformities in patients with
- cervical 151
- osteotomies for **63**
- progressive, vertebral column resection for **68**
Myopathic conditions 13

N

Neck tilt 153
Neglected spinal deformities
- anterior approach in **256**, *257*
- pelvic obliquity correction in **98**, *99–100*
Neurofibromatosis 78
- spinal deformity with **15**
Neurologic complications **214**
- *See also* specific complications and procedures
- in anterior approaches 255
- in pedicle subtraction osteotomy 215, 280
- in scoliosis **215**
- in spondyloarthropathies **214**
- rehabilitation medicine viewpoint of **216**
Neurologic deficit, deformities in patients with
- 3D models of 64, 66, 69
- halo traction for 63, **64**, *67*, 69, *71*
- history and physical examination of **63**
- multidisciplinary approach for 63
- osteotomies in **63**
-- minimizing blood loss in 66
-- patient positioning for 65
-- spinal cord monitoring in **67**
-- surgical outcomes in 69, *72–73*
-- surgical technique for **65**
- preoperative evaluation of **63**
- preoperative imaging of 63, *64*, *65*, 69–72
Neurologic examination
- in cervical deformities 152
- preoperative, in revision surgery 93
Neurologic system, spinal surgery and **204**
Neuromuscular spinal deformities **13**, **190**
- clinical problems associated with **13**
- etiology and natural history of **13**
- gastrointestinal problems with 13, 17
- growth-related development of 14
- neurofibromatosis and **15**
- nonoperative treatment of **16**
- observation and monitoring of 16
- patterns of **14**
- respiratory compromise with 13, 17
- seating adaptations for 16
- spina bifida and *15*
- surgical treatment of **16**
-- anterior correction in **19**
-- combined two-stage anterior and posterior approach in 19
-- correction techniques in **18**
-- excessive blood loss in 17
-- first- and second-generation instrumentation techniques in **18**
-- fusion levels in **19**
-- growth preservation/modulation techniques in **20**
-- intraoperative and postoperative complications of **17**
-- intraoperative management in **19**
-- life-threatening complications of 17
-- medical considerations—preoperative assessment in **17**
-- noninvasive ventilation in 17, 20
-- patient impairment and cooperation in 18
-- posterior apical vertebrectomy in 20
-- quality of life/life expectancy after **20**
-- superior mesenteric artery syndrome in 18
-- third-generation instrumentation for **18**
-- thoracotomy or thoracoabdominal approach in 19
- treatment principles for **16**
- types of **15**
Neurophysiologic intraoperative monitoring (NIOM) **209**
- anesthesia considerations in 203, **205**
- clinical applications of **212**
- in posterior vertebral column resection **67**
- in revision surgery 184
- in rigid spine deformity correction **209**
- in severe idiopathic scoliosis procedures **114**, 116
- in syndromic rigid spine surgery 80, 82
- multimodality approach in **212**
- tools for **209**
NIOM, *see* Neurophysiologic intraoperative monitoring
Nondystrophic scoliosis 15
Noninvasive ventilation 17, 20
Normal balance 224

O

Oblique lateral interbody fusion 226
Oblique lumbar interbody fusion 252
Occiput-to-wall measure 152
Oncological staging 138, **139**, 148
Opening-wedge osteotomy, *see* specific types
- for ankylosing spondylitis 178
- for cervical deformities 156
- for cervicothoracic kyphotic deformity 161
- for posttraumatic spinel deformities 126
OPLL, *see* Ossification of the posterior longitudinal ligament
Ossification centers 1, *2*
Ossification of the posterior longitudinal ligament (OPLL) 176
Osteochondrodystrophies 78
Osteoconductive agents **247**
Osteoinductive agents **246**
Osteoporosis 130
Osteoporotic rigid spine deformities **130**
- epidemiology of **130**
- etiology of **130**
- MRI of 130, *131*
- pedicle screws in
-- cement leakage from 132
-- expandable 131
-- hydroxyapatite-coated titanium 131
-- improving stability of **131**
-- PMMA augmentation of 131, 132
- progression of 132
- prophylactic vertebroplasty for 132, *133*
- proximal junctional kyphosis and adjacent segment disease with 132
- radiographic evaluation of 132
- surgical correction of **132**
-- complications of **132**
-- fixation options for 132
-- osteotomies in 132
-- strategy for 132
- treatment philosophy for **130**
Osteoporotic vertebral compression fractures 130
Osteopromotive agents **247**
Osteotomies, *see* specific types and procedures
- grade 1 123, 185
- grade 2 123, 185
- grade 3 123, 185, *186*
- grade 4 52, 123, 185, **186**
- grade 5 123, 185, **186**, *187*
- grade 6 123, 185, **186**
- in adult degenerative scoliosis **276**
- in cervical deformities **151**
- in children under age 10 **49**
- in congenital upper thoracic deformities 41, 44
- in early-onset scoliosis **91**
- in idiopathic spinal deformities **22**, *115*
- in junctional correction **159**
- in osteoporotic rigid spinal deformities 132
- in patients with neurologic deficit **63**
-- minimizing blood loss in 66
-- patient positioning for 65
-- spinal cord monitoring in **67**
-- surgical outcomes in 69, *72–73*
-- surgical technique for **65**
- in posttraumatic spine deformity 120, 123, *124–125*
- in revision surgery 93, **184**
-- *See also* specific procedures
- in rigid sacropelvic pathologies 171
- in rigid spinal deformities **49**, 194, 226
-- robot-guided **242**
- in rigid spinal deformities, syndromic **75**
- in spinal tuberculosis, adult **261**
- in spinal tuberculosis, pediatric **271**
- in spinal tumor en bloc resection **138**, *147*, 149
- neurologic complications of 215
- Schwab classification of 8, 50, 52, 78, 123, 185
- type II—hyperlordotic deformity **52**
- type III—pure coronal plane deformity **52**
- type I—pure hyperkyphotic deformity **51**
- type IV—multiplanar kyphoscoliotic deformity *53*
- type V—eggshell 11, 23, **54**
- type VI—vertebral column resection or apical vertebral resection **55**
Overcorrection 226

P

Pain assessment 94
Paralytic scoliosis **190**
Parathyroid hormone, for spinal fusion **248**
Parkinson's disease, spinal deformities in patients with **135**
- bracing for 135
- camptocormia in 135, *136*
- long fusions for, poor results of 135, *137*
- medical management of 135
- progression/worsening of 135
- sacral and iliac screws for 136
- surgical management of 135
- variability of trunk position in 135
Partial facet joint resection **50**
Passive bending, in rigid spinal deformities 34
Patient positioning **206**
- *See also* specific procedures
PCO, *see* Posterior column osteotomy
Pedicle redrilling, robot-guided **234**, *235*
Pedicle screws, *see* specific procedures using
- expandable 131
- hydroxyapatite-coated titanium 131
- in adult degenerative scoliosis 278
- in congenital vertebral malformations 4, 6
- in hemivertebra resection 7
- in idiopathic spinal deformity correction 22, 49, **111**, *112*, **114**
-- in pedicle subtraction osteotomy 25
-- in posterior column osteotomy 22
- in neuromuscular scoliosis correction 18
- in osteoporotic rigid spine deformities **131**, 132
- in posttraumatic spine deformity 120, 126
- in revision surgery 187
- PMMA augmentation of 131, 132
- redrilling for **234**
- robot-guided placement of 231, **234**, *235*

Pedicle subtraction osteotomy (PSO)
– asymmetric (convex-based) 52
– blood loss in 280
– development of 23
– extended 23, 52
– for adult degenerative scoliosis 277, *279*
– for ankylosing spondylitis with kyphotic deformity 178, *179–180*
– for cervical deformities 156
– for cervicothoracic kyphotic deformity 161, *162*
– for congenital spinal deformity *8*, *9*
–– adjacent osteotomies in 8
–– two-level 8, *10*
– for idiopathic spinal deformity **23**, *115*
–– case illustration of **26**, *27–31*
–– complications of **26–27**
–– indications for **25**
–– limiting factor in 23
–– patient positioning for 25
–– PCO versus **26**
–– preoperative considerations for **26**
–– technique of **25**
– for kyphosis in tuberculosis **268**
– for lumbosacral kyphotic deformity 166, *168*
– for osteoporotic rigid spinal deformities 132
– for posttraumatic spine deformity 123, 126–127
– for revision surgery 93, 185
– for rigid spinal deformities 194
– for syndromic rigid spine 75, **81**
– for thoracolumbar kyphotic deformity 164
– neurologic complications of 215, 280
– pseudoarthrosis in 281
Pelvic deformity 170
– *See also* Sacropelvic pathologies, rigid
Pelvic fixation, robot-guided **234**
Pelvic girdle reconstruction 171
Pelvic incidence (PI) 218, *219*, 221, 223
– too high (50 degrees) **228**
– too small (50 degrees) **227**
Pelvic obliquity correction, in neglected congenital scoliosis **98**, *99–100*
Pelvic osteotomies **172**
– bilateral modified Salter 172, *173*
– posterior iliac 172, *173*
Pelvic tilt (PT) 218, *219*, 221, 223, 276
Pelvis plain radiography 94
Peripheral vascular examination 94
PI, *see* Pelvic incidence
Platelet gels 247
PMMA, *see* Polymethylmethacrylate
Polymethylmethacrylate (PMMA) augmentation, of pedicle screws 131, 132
Ponte osteotomy
– for adult degenerative scoliosis **277**
– for cervical deformities 156
– for congenital spinal deformities 9
– for osteoporotic rigid spinal deformities 132
– for revision surgery 93, 185
– for rigid spinal deformities 37, 226
– for syndromic rigid spine **80**
– for thoracolumbar kyphotic deformity 164
Posterior apical vertebrectomy, for neuromuscular spinal deformity 20
Posterior column osteotomy (PCO) **22**
– anterior approaches versus 256
– case illustration of **23**, *24*
– Cobb angle improvements with 22
– complications of **26–27**
– development of 22
– for adult degenerative scoliosis 277
– for cervical deformities **156**, *157*
– for lumbosacral kyphotic deformity 166
– for osteoporotic rigid spinal deformities 132
– for posttraumatic spine deformity 120, 123, 127
– for thoracolumbar kyphotic deformity 164
– indications in idiopathic deformity **22**
– patient positioning for 23
– preoperative considerations for **26**
– PSO versus **26**
– technique of **23**
Posterior elementectomy **50**, *52*
Posterior iliac osteotomy 172, *173*
Posterior longitudinal ligament, ossification of 176
Posterior vertebral column resection (PVCR)
– for deformities in patients with neurologic deficit 63
– for lumbosacral kyphotic deformity 167
– for progressive myelopathy **68**
– for revision surgery 93, 187
–– complications of **99**
–– correction of kyphoscoliosis deformity in **95**, *97*
–– correction of kyphosis deformity in **96**, *97–98*
–– correction of lordosis/lordoscoliosis deformity in **97**, *98–99*
–– correction of scoliosis deformity in *95*, *96*
– for severe rigid pelvic obliquity, in neglected congenital scoliosis **98**, *99–100*
– indications for 93
– reconstruction of laminectomy defect after **98**, *100*
– spinal cord monitoring in **67**
Postoperative care and complications **207**
Posttraumatic kyphosis (Kümmell disease) **122**, **216**
Posttraumatic spine deformity (PTSD) **120**, **204**
– anterior surgical approaches for **126–127**
– biomechanics and pathology of **121**
– Charcot arthropathy in **121**
– classification of **121**
– combined anterior–posterior surgical approaches for **126**
– complications of **128**
– deforming forces and **121**
– epidemiology of **120**
– evaluation of **121**
– neurologic complications with 124, **214**
– nonoperative management of **123**
– normal thoracolumbar alignment versus **121**
– operative management of **123**
– osteotomies for 123, *124–125*
–– closing-wedge 126
–– opening-wedge 126
–– pedicle subtraction 123, 126–127
–– posterior column 123, 127
–– technical considerations in **127**
– pedicle screw fixation for 120, 126
– posterior column osteotomy for 120
– posterior surgical approaches for **126–127**
– presentation and physical exam of **122**
– radiographic evaluation of **122**
– restoring stability and alignment in 120
– sacropelvic 170
– spectrum of injury in 120
– surgical indications and planning in **123**
– transforaminal lumbar interbody fusion for 127
– type I 123
– type II 123
– vertebral column resection for 123
– vicious cycle of progression in 120
Posttraumatic syringomyelia **122**
Posttraumatic tethering **122**
Posttraumatic vertebral avascular necrosis **122**
Preexisting conditions **203**
Preoperative assessment **203**
– *See also* specific disorders and procedures
Pressure sores 13
Proximal junctional kyphosis **228**
– correction of sagittal balance in 228, *229*
– definition of 228, *229*
– risk factors for 228
Pseudoarthrosis 244, 280–281
– biology of fusion and 244
– risk factors for 244
PSO, *see* Pedicle subtraction osteotomy
PT, *see* Pelvic tilt
PTSD, *see* Posttraumatic spine deformity
PVCR, *see* Posterior vertebral column resection

R

Recombinant factor VII 207
Rehabilitation medicine **216**
Respiratory compromise 204
– with deformities in patients with neurologic deficit 63
– with idiopathic scoliosis 49
– with neuromuscular spinal deformity 13, 17
– with thoracic insufficiency syndrome 58
Respiratory failure, in thoracic insufficiency syndrome 58
Respiratory system, spinal surgery and **204**
Retained instrumentation, in robot-guided revision surgery **234**
Retrograde ejaculation, anterior approach and 255
Retroversion 225
Rett syndrome 76
Revision surgery
– challenges and risks of 93
– complications of **99**
– correction of kyphoscoliosis deformity in **95**, *97*
– correction of kyphosis deformity in **96**, *97–98*
– correction of lordosis/lordoscoliosis deformity in **97**, *98–99*
– correction of scoliosis deformity in *95*, *96*
– for congenital vertebral malformations 5
– for rigid spinal deformities **93**
– goals of 93
– osteotomies in 93, **184**
–– *See also* specific procedures
–– approaches for 184
–– general indications for **184**
–– grade 1 185
–– grade 2 185
–– grade 3 185, *186*
–– grade 4 185, **186**
–– grade 5 185, **186**, *187*
–– grade 6 185, **186**
–– spinal cord monitoring in 184
– patient history in **93**
– physical examination for **93**
– preoperative evaluation for **93**
– preoperative imaging studies for **94**
– robot-guided **234**
– surgical technique in **94**
Rib vertebral angle difference (RVAD) 85
Rib(s)
– CVMs and distortion of 4
– fused 4
– hypoplastic 4
– supplementary 4
Rigid spinal deformities **35**, **189**
– aging spine and etiologies in **35**
– algorithm for treating *227*
– anatomopathology of 33
– assessment of flexibility/rigidity in **34**, 49, *197*, *198–201*
– Billot test in 34
– classification of **191**
– definition of **33**, **189**
– Donaldson-Stagnara distraction in 34
– facet joint resection for
–– complete **50**, *52*
–– partial **50**
– fulcrum in 34
– growing spine and etiologies in **34**, 189
– halo traction in 34, **50**
– historical perspective on 189
– in early-onset scoliosis **84**
– location of **194**
– mature spine and etiologies in **34**
– measurement of **33**
– MRI monitoring of 33
– natural history of **33**
– osteoporotic **130**
–– *See also* Osteoporotic rigid spine deformities
– osteotomies for 226
–– *See also* specific conditions and procedures
–– in children under age 10 **49**
–– outcome and complications of **56**

-- pedicle subtraction 194
-- posterior 50
-- robot-guided **242**
-- three-column 50, **51**
-- type II–hyperlordotic deformity **52**
-- type III–pure coronal plane deformity **52**
-- type I–pure hyperkyphotic deformity **51**
-- type IV-multiplanar kyphoscoliotic deformity *53*
-- type V-eggshell **54**
-- type VI-vertebral column resection or apical vertebral resection **55**
- passive and active bending in 34
- pediatric **189**
-- classification of **191**
-- surgery for, in older children and adolescents **37**
-- surgery for, in young children **36**
- physiopathology of **33**
- preoperative evaluation in 35
- reduction, local and global **34**
- sacropelvic **170**
-- *See also* Sacropelvic pathologies, rigid
- sagittal balance correction in **218**
- secondary correction, after failed instrumentation **93**
- shape and severity of *195, 196*
- structural, involving entire spine 33
- structural, involving significant part of spine 33
- structural, localized on a few spinal units 33
- structural, referred to as iatrogenic 33
- supine traction in 34
- surgical complications in, neurologic **214**
- surgical indications in **35**
- surgical strategies for correcting **226**
- surgical techniques and approaches in **36**, **194**
-- combined anterior–posterior 194
-- for aging spine **37**
-- for anterior rigidity 36
-- for craniocervical junction 36
-- for lesions extending to multiple levels **36**
-- for localized pathology **36**
-- for older children and adolescents **37**
-- for posterior or posterolateral rigidity 36
-- for young children **36**
-- neuromonitoring **209**
-- patient assessment and strategy for **194**
-- posterior-only 194
-- robot guidance in **231**
- suspension in 34
- syndromic **75**, 189
-- *See also* Syndromic rigid spine
- treatment principles for 38
- with thoracic insufficiency syndrome **58**
Robot-guided osteotomies **242**
- for flatback syndrome 242
Robot-guided surgery **234**
- case illustrations of **235**, *236–241*
- categories of robots for 231
- docking platforms for 233
- for rigid spinal deformities **231**
- for sacropelvic pathologies 173, *174*
- image acquisition and registration in 231, 233
- patient positioning for 232
- pelvic fixation in **234**
- platform attachment in 231, 233
- preoperative planning in 231–232
- procedures for 231
- redrilling pedicles in **234**
- retained instrumentation in *235*
- revision **234**
- robot assembly and motion in 232
- robot systems in clinical use **231**
- special considerations in **234**
- trajectory execution in 232–233
- workstation for 231, *232*
Rods
- for cervicothoracic kyphotic deformity 161
- for kyphectomy, in spina bifida 104–*105*
- for neuromuscular scoliosis 18
- for osteoporotic rigid spinal deformities 132
- for upper thoracic congenital deformities 41
- growing
-- for early-onset scoliosis 86, **88**, *89*
-- for idiopathic scoliosis, in children under age 10 49
-- for neuromuscular scoliosis 20
-- for severe idiopathic scoliosis 111, **113**, **116**
-- for thoracic insufficiency syndrome 59
-- magnetically controlled 86, **88**, **113**, **116**
- temporary internal distraction
-- for early-onset scoliosis 85, 88, **91**
-- for severe idiopathic scoliosis 111
Roussouly classification 223, 225
RVAD, *see* Rib vertebral angle difference

S

Sacral alar-iliac screws, for neuromuscular scoliosis 18
Sacral deformity 170
- *See also* Sacropelvic pathologies, rigid
Sacral osteotomies **172**
Sacral slope (SS) 218, *219*, 221, 223
Sacropelvic pathologies, rigid
- computer-assisted surgery for **173**, *174*
- corrective strategies and management of **170**
- gait abnormalities with 170
- genitourinary malfunction with 170
- nonsurgical care in 171
- osteotomies for 171
-- bilateral modified Salter 172, *173*
-- pelvic **172**
-- posterior iliac 172, *173*
-- sacral **172**
- pain with 170
- pelvic girdle reconstruction for 171
- presenting symptoms of **170**
- radiographic evaluation of **171**
- salvage procedures for 171, **172**
- surgical indications in 171
- x, y, and z axes in 171
Sagittal balance **218**
- *See also* specific disorders and procedures
- bipedalism and 223
- categories of 224
- degenerative spine evolution and **224**
- importance of studying 221
- in adult degenerative scoliosis 276, 281
- in normal populations *223*
- lumbosacral segmental, restoration of **253**
- metric versus angular parameters of *221, 222*
- positive, definition of 276
- preoperative evaluation of 94
- proximal junctional kyphosis and **228**, *229*
- radiologic assessment of 94
- spinal parameters of **219**
- surgical strategies for correcting **226**
-- when pelvic incidence is too high (50 degrees) **228**
-- when pelvic incidence is too small (50 degrees) **227**
- type A (normal) 224
- type B (compensated) *224*, 225
- type C (decompensated) *224*, 225
Sagittal index 122
Sagittal vertical axis (SVA) 153, 159, 221, 276
Salter pelvic osteotomy, bilateral modified 172, *173*
Scheuermann's kyphosis **190**
- Ponte osteotomy for 277
- proximal junctional kyphosis in 228
Schwab classification, of osteotomies 8, 50, 52, 78, 123, 185
Schwab-Scoliosis Research Society classification **192**, 219
Scoliosis
- adult degenerative **276**
-- *See also* Adult degenerative scoliosis
- cervical 151
-- *See also* Cervical deformities
- congenital 1
-- *See also* Congenital vertebral malformations
-- classification of **191**
-- neglected, correction of severe rigid obliquity in **98**, *99–100*
- early-onset, *see* Early-onset scoliosis
- neurofibromatosis and 15
- neurologic complications in **215**
- neuromuscular 13, **190**
-- *See also* Neuromuscular spinal deformities
- paralytic **190**
- rigid 33
-- *See also* Rigid spinal deformities
-- osteotomies for **49**
- secondary correction of *95, 96*
- spina bifida and 15
Scoliosis, idiopathic **190**
- *See also* Adolescent idiopathic scoliosis (AIS)
- classification of **191**
- spinal osteotomies for **22**
-- complications of **26–27**
-- in children under age 10 **49**
-- PCO versus PSO **26**
-- pedicle subtraction **23**
-- posterior column **22**
-- preoperative considerations in **26**
Seating adaptations 16
Secondary correction, *see* Revision surgery
Segmental spine stabilization, for neuromuscular scoliosis 18
Shared-control robot systems 231
Shilla technique 36, 49, 59, 86, **89**
Shprintzen–Goldberg syndrome 78
Sitting balance 79
SL, *see* Spinal lordosis
Smith-Petersen osteotomy (SPO)
- complications of 280
- for adult degenerative scoliosis **277**
- for ankylosing spondylitis with kyphotic deformity 178
- for cervical deformities 156, *157*
- for idiopathic spinal deformities 22
- for lumbosacral kyphotic deformity 166
- for osteoporotic rigid spinal deformities 132
- for revision surgery 185
- for rigid spinal deformities 50, 226
- for syndromic rigid spine 75, **80**
- for thoracolumbar kyphotic deformity 164
Somatosensory evoked potentials (SSEPs) 205, 209, *210–211*
- in posterior vertebral column resection 67
- in revision surgery 184
- in severe idiopathic scoliosis surgery 114, 116
- in syndromic rigid spine surgery 80
SPA, *see* Spinopelvic angle
SPC, *see* Spinous Process Clamp
Spina bifida
- kyphectomy in 15, **102**
-- outcome of *105, 106*
-- patient positioning for 103
-- preoperative checklist for 103
-- preoperative imaging for *104*
-- prerequisites for 102
-- surgical technique of **103**, *104–105*
- spinal deformity with *15*
Spina bifida occulta 102
Spinal angiography 94
Spinal cord
- anatomy and physiology of **203**
- blood supply to **203**
Spinal fusion, *see* specific disorders and procedures
- biological aspects of **244**
- bisphosphonates in **248**
- bone grafts for
-- allograft **247**
-- autograft **245**
-- iliac crest, as gold standard 244–245
-- mechanical strength of 245
-- osteoconductive characteristics of 245
-- osteogenic characteristics of 245
-- osteoinductive characteristics of 245
-- properties of 245
-- selection of 244
-- synthetic **247**
-- types of **245**

- for adult degenerative scoliosis **276**
- for early-onset scoliosis 86, *87*, *90*
-- with posterior instrumentation **88**
- for thoracic insufficiency syndrome **59**
- fusion formation in **244**
-- inflammatory phase of 244
-- late remodeling phase of 244
-- middle reparative phase of 244
- indications for 244
- methods to enhance fusion rates in **244**
- osteoconductive agents in **247**
- osteoinductive agents in **246**
- osteopromotive agents in **247**
- parathyroid hormone in **248**
- pseudoarthrosis with 244
- systemic agents in **247**
Spinal lordosis (SL) 220
Spinal muscular atrophy
- bone density in 80
- rigid spinal deformity in 75–76
Spinal osteotomies, *see* Osteotomies
Spinal sagittal parameters **219**
Spinal shapes
- in normal population *223*
- in rigid spinal deformities *195*, *196*
Spinal tuberculosis, adult, kyphosis in 261
- combined anterior and posterior approach for 263, **267**
- during acute phase **261**, *262*
- healing patterns in *262*
- osteotomies for **261**
- pathophysiology of **261**
- pedicle subtraction osteotomy for **268**
- single-stage correction by anterior approach and stabilization 263
- single-stage correction by posterior costotransversectomy or anterolateral approach and posterior stabilization 263, **265**, *266–267*
- single-stage correction by posterior-only transforaminal approach and interbody fusion 263, *265*, *266*
- single-stage correction through extrapleural approach **268**
- single-stage transpedicular approach and posterior correction of 263, *264*
- surgical correction in healed phase **267**
- surgical goals in 261
- surgical principles in active phase **262**
- surgical treatment of **262**
- transpedicular decancellation osteotomy for **268**
- vertebral column resection for **268**, *269*
Spinal tuberculosis, pediatric, *see* Tuberculosis spondylitis
- adult spinal tuberculosis versus 271
- diagnosis of **271**
- osteotomies in **271**
- surgical indications and methods in 272
- treatment principles for **271**
Spinal tumors
- en bloc resection of
-- anatomical features in **139**
-- case report of **147**, *148*
-- definition of 138
-- essential surgical criteria in **140**
-- indications for 138
-- osteotomy to finalize *147*, 149
-- surgical approach for **140**
-- surgical planning for **138**
-- surgical tips and techniques for **140**
-- type 1 (single anterior approach) 140, *141*
-- type 2A (single posterior approach) 140, *141*
-- type 2B (single posterior approach with surgical sequence) 140, **141**, *142*
-- type 2C (single posterior approach with sagittal osteotomy) 140, **142**, *143*
-- type 3A (sequential anterior and posterior approaches) 140, **142**, *143*
-- type 3B (sequential anterior and posterior approaches) 140, **143**, *144*
-- type 3C (sequential anterior and posterior approaches for eccentric tumors) 140, **144**, *145*
-- type 4 (posterior, anterior contralateral, and anterior ipsilateral approaches) 140, **144**, *145*
-- type 5 (posterior followed by simultaneous anterior/posterior approaches) 140, **145**, *146*
-- type 6 (anterior contralateral, posterior, and simultaneous anterior/posterior approaches) 140, *146*
- Enneking classification of 138–139, 148
- extension of 138, **140**, 148
- margin of 138
-- functional relevance of **139**
-- planning and approach for 139
- metastatic 138
- palliative treatment of 138
- primary 138
- Weinstein-Boriani-Biagini staging system for 138–139, 148
Spinopelvic angle (SPA) 222
Spinosacral angle (SSA) 222
Spinous Process Clamp (SPC) 233
SPO, *see* Smith-Petersen osteotomy
Spondyloarthropathies, *see* specific types
- neurologic complications in **214**
SS, *see* Sacral slope
SSA, *see* Spinosacral angle
SSEPs, *see* Somatosensory evoked potentials
SSL, *see* Superior spinal lordosis
Superior mesenteric artery syndrome 18, 128, 280
Superior spinal lordosis (SSL) 220
Supervisory-controlled robot systems 231
Supine traction, in rigid spinal deformities 34
Suspension, in rigid spinal deformities 34
SVA, *see* Sagittal vertical axis
Syndromic rigid spine **75**, 189
- bone density in 80
- coronal and sagittal imbalance in 75, 81
- definition and classification of **75**
- imaging studies of **79**
- multidisciplinary approach to 78
- osteotomies in **75**
-- blood loss in 82
-- bone–disk–bone **81**
-- complications of **82**
-- goals of 75, **78**
-- indications for **75**
-- outcome of **83**
-- pedicle subtraction 75, **81**
-- Ponte **80**
-- positioning and perioperative measures in **80**
-- postoperative care in **82**
-- Smith-Petersen 75, **80**
-- spinal cord monitoring in 80, 82
-- surgical aspects and technique in **80**
-- types of **78**
- patient history and physical findings in **78**
- preoperative workup of **78**
- prevalence of 75
- sagittal imbalance in 75, 81
- syndromes associated with 76
- type I deformity 75, 81
- type II deformity 75, 81
- vertebral column resection for 75, **81**
Synthetic bone grafts **247**
Syringomyelia, posttraumatic **122**

T

T1 pelvic angle (TPA) 222
T1 slope 153
TcMEPs, *see* Transcranial motor evoked potentials
Telesurgical systems 231
Temperature, during spinal surgery 206
Temporary internal distraction rods (TIDRs)
- contraindications to 91
- for early-onset scoliosis 85, 88, **91**
- for severe idiopathic scoliosis 111
Tethering, posttraumatic **122**
Thoracic inlet angle 153
Thoracic insufficiency syndrome (TIS) **58**
- care in **58**
- casting for **59**
- causes of 58
- definition of 58
- flexibility, bending, and traction in 58
- hanging radiographs of 58
- multidisciplinary team for 58
- respiratory failure in 58
- severely collapsing chest cavity deformity in 58
- surgical treatment of spinal deformities in **58**
-- discussion with patients, parents, and caregivers 58
-- fusion in **59**
-- mortality risk without 59
-- nonfusion devices and thoracospinal elongation in **59**, *60–61*
-- risks and ability to perform procedure 58
- treatment options for **59**
- vertical expandable prosthetic titanium rib for 59
Thoracic kyphosis
- definition of 219
- measurement of *219–220*
Thoracic spine, upper, congenital deformities with vertebral malformations in **39**
Thoracolumbar alignment, normal **121**
Thoracolumbar fractures, with ankylosing spondylitis 177, *178*
Thoracolumbar kyphoscoliosis, anterior release for **254**, 256, *257*
Thoracolumbar kyphotic deformity
- anterior column corpectomy and cage implant for 164, *165*
- causes of 159, 162
- corrective osteotomies for **159**, **162**
-- anterior lengthening procedures in 164
-- patient positioning for 163
-- patient preparation for **163**
-- pedicle subtraction 164
-- Ponte 164
-- posterior 164
-- Smith-Petersen osteotomy 164
-- technical considerations in **164**
- preoperative evaluation of **159**
Thoracolumbar trauma 120
- *See also* Posttraumatic spine deformity
Thoracolumbosacral orthosis 16
Thoracoplasty, in severe idiopathic scoliosis **117**
Three-column osteotomy 6, 8–*9*, 50, **51**, 93
TIDRs, *see* Temporary internal distraction rods
TIS, *see* Thoracic insufficiency syndrome
TPA, *see* T1 pelvic angle
Tranexamic acid 207
Transcranial motor evoked potentials (TcMEPs) 205, 209, *210*
- in posterior vertebral column resection 67
- in revision surgery 184
- in severe idiopathic scoliosis surgery 114, 116
- in syndromic rigid spine surgery 80
Transdiskal osteotomy 8, 167
Transforaminal lumbar interbody fusion 127, 253
Transpedicular decancellation osteotomy **268**
Transpedicular screws, in upper thoracic congenital deformities 45
Triggered EMG (TrgEMG) 67
Tuberculosis, *see* Spinal tuberculosis
Tuberculosis spondylitis 271
- anterior fusion in 272
- cervicothoracic 273
- consequences of, surgical treatment of **273**, *274*
- diagnosis of 271
- Hongkong surgery for *274*
- morphological basis of 271
- posterior instrumentation in 273
- removal of pathological tissues and spinal cord decompression in 272
- spinal deformity in 272
-- exceeding 50 degrees in 273
- surgical goals in 272
- surgical indications in 272
Tumors, *see* Spinal tumors

Type I osteotomy—pure hyperkyphotic deformity **51**
Type II osteotomy—hyperlordotic deformity, osteotomies **52**
Type III osteotomy—pure coronal plane deformity, osteotomies **52**
Type IV osteotomy—multiplanar kyphoscoliotic deformity, osteotomies *53*
Type V osteotomy—eggshell, osteotomies 11, 23, **54**
Type VI osteotomy—vertebral column resection or apical vertebral resection **55**

U

Undercorrection 226
Upper motor neuron 13
Upper thoracic spine
- anatomy and biomechanics of 39
- congenital deformities of, with vertebral malformations
-- age distribution of 40, 44
-- course and progression of 39
-- gender distribution of 39–40, 43–44
-- instrumentation for 45
-- localization of hemivertebrae 40, 43–44
-- preoperative imaging of 40
-- surgical approach and technique in 40–*41*, 44
-- surgical indications in 40
-- surgical management of **39**
-- surgical outcomes in 42, **43**, *45–46*, 47
-- treatment principles for 42

V

VACTERL association 78
VEPTR, *see* Vertical expandable prosthetic titanium rib
Vertebra(e)
- growth of 1
- ossification centers of 1, *2*
Vertebral avascular necrosis, posttraumatic **122**
Vertebral column decancellation **11**, 23, **54**, **268**
Vertebral column resection
- blood loss in 280
- circumferential 63
- combined anterior—posterior approach for 9
- complications of 280
- for adult degenerative scoliosis 277, **279**
- for cervicothoracic kyphotic deformity 161
- for congenital vertebral malformations **9**
- for deformity in patients with neurologic deficit 63
- for kyphosis in tuberculosis **268**, *269*
- for lumbosacral kyphotic deformity 166–167
- for neuromuscular spinal deformity 20
- for posttraumatic spine deformity 123
- for progressive myelopathy **68**
- for revision surgery 93, 185–186, *187*
-- complications of **99**
-- correction of kyphoscoliosis deformity in **95**, *97*
-- correction of kyphosis deformity in **96**, *97–98*
-- correction of lordosis/lordoscoliosis deformity in **97**, *98–99*
-- correction of scoliosis deformity in *95*, *96*
- for rigid spinal deformities **55**, 194
- for severe idiopathic scoliosis 110
- for severe rigid pelvic obliquity, in neglected congenital scoliosis **98**, *99–100*
- for syndromic rigid spine 75, **81**
- neurologic complications of 215
- posterior approach for 9, *11*, **55**
- spinal cord monitoring in **67**
- surgical challenges and procedures in 9
Vertebral fractures
- osteoporotic 130
-- *See also* Osteoporotic rigid spine deformities
- traumatic 120
-- *See also* Posttraumatic spine deformity
Vertebral malformations, congenital, *see* Congenital vertebral malformations
Vertebrectomy, *see* Vertebral column resection
Vertical expandable prosthetic titanium rib (VEPTR)
- for early-onset scoliosis 86, **88**
- for idiopathic scoliosis, in children under age 10 49
- for neuromuscular scoliosis 20
- for thoracic insufficiency syndrome 59

W

Wake-up test 215
- in AIS surgery 114, 116
- in cervicothoracic surgery 160
- in patients with neurologic deficit 67–68
- in patients with syndromic rigid spine 82
- in pedicle subtraction osteotomy 280
- in revision surgery 184
- in spinal tuberculosis surgery 270
WBB, *see* Weinstein-Boriani-Biagini (WBB) staging system
Wedge osteotomy 156
- *See also* specific types
- for ankylosing spondylitis 178
- for cervical deformities 156
- for cervicothoracic kyphotic deformity 161
- for congenital spinal deformities 63
- for posttraumatic spinel deformities 126
- for spinal tuberculosis **268**, *269*
- for spinal tuberculosis, adult 263, *264*
- for spinal tuberculosis, pediatric *274*
Wedge vertebra 2, 4, 190
Weinstein-Boriani-Biagini (WBB) staging system 138–139, 148
Wheelchair-bound children
- neuromuscular spinal deformity in 13, 16
- seating adaptations for 16
- sitting balance in 79
Windswept/windblown posture 14
Wire fixation
- for cervicothoracic kyphotic deformity 161
- for neuromuscular scoliosis 18